First Aid: Taking Action

NATIONAL SAFETY COUNCIL

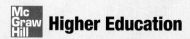

Mc Graw Hill **Higher Education**

Boston   Burr Ridge, IL   Dubuque, IA   New York   San Francisco   St. Louis
Bangkok   Bogotá   Caracas   Kuala Lumpur   Lisbon   London   Madrid   Mexico City
Milan   Montreal   New Delhi   Santiago   Seoul   Singapore   Sydney   Taipei   Toronto

Other titles available from the National Safety Council

National Safety Council: *Standard First Aid, CPR, and AED*, 2e
National Safety Council: *First Aid*, 2e
National Safety Council: *CPR and AED*, 2e
National Safety Council: *Bloodborne and Airborne Pathogens*
National Safety Council: *Pediatric First Aid, CPR, and AED*, 2e
National Safety Council: *Basic Life Support: Healthcare and Professional Rescuers*

About the National Safety Council

Founded in 1913, the National Safety Council (NSC) is a nonprofit membership organization devoted to making our world a safer place. Its mission is to educate and influence people to prevent accidental injury and death. For more than 90 years, the National Safety Council has been the leader in protecting life and promoting health in the workplace. The Council has helped make great improvements in safety with an expanded focus on safety on the roads and in the home and community. Working through its 48,000 members, and in partnership with public agencies, private groups, and other associations, the Council serves as an impartial information gathering and distribution organization. The NSC disseminates safety, health, and environmental materials through a network of regional offices, chapters, and training centers.

The NSC's First Aid and CPR/AED courses have grown to meet the changing needs of emergency responders at all levels of expertise. Upon completing this course, you will join millions of first aiders and emergency responders trained to protect life and promote health.

Author Acknowledgements

Many National Safety Council staff and affiliates have contributed to the production of this book and we would like to acknowledge the following people for their assistance:

Paul Satterlee MD, Medical Director, for reviewing and providing oversight of the content;

Tom Lochhaas, Editorial Services, for providing technical writing services;

Donna M. Siegfried, Executive Director, Emergency Care, for providing vision and support;

Barbara Caracci, Director of Emergency Care Programs and Training, for providing oversight of content and interfacing with McGraw-Hill staff on all areas of production;

Donna Fredenhagen, Product Manager, for providing marketing support;

Kathy Safranek, Project Administrator, for providing day-to-day assistance.

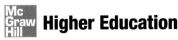

The McGraw·Hill Companies

Higher Education

FIRST AID: TAKING ACTION

Published by McGraw-Hill, a business unit of The McGraw-Hill Companies, Inc., 1221 Avenue of the Americas, New York, NY 10020. Copyright © 2007 by The National Safety Council. All rights reserved. No part of this publication may be reproduced or distributed in any form or by any means, or stored in a database or retrieval system, without the prior written consent of The McGraw-Hill Companies, Inc., including, but not limited to, in any network or other electronic storage or transmission, or broadcast for distance learning.

Some ancillaries, including electronic and print components, may not be available to customers outside the United States.

♲ This book is printed on recycled, acid-free paper containing 10% postconsumer waste.

1 2 3 4 5 6 7 8 9 0 QPD / QPD 0 9 8 7 6

ISBN-13 978–0–07–352200–5
ISBN-10 0–07–352200–7

Publisher, Career Education: *David T. Culverwell*
Senior Sponsoring Editor: *Claire Merrick*
Editorial Coordinator: *Michelle L. Zeal*
Outside Managing Editor: *Kelly Trakalo*
Senior Marketing Manager: *Lisa Nicks*
Senior Project Manager: *Sheila M. Frank*
Senior Production Supervisor: *Laura Fuller*
Lead Media Project Manager: *Audrey A. Reiter*
Senior Media Producer: *Renee Russian*

Senior Coordinator of Freelance Design: *Michelle D. Whitaker*
Cover/Interior Designer: *Studio Montage*
(USE) Cover Images: © *National Safety Council/Rick Brady, photographer*
Lead Photo Research Coordinator: *Carrie K. Burger*
Photo Research: *Pam Carley/Sound Reach*
Compositor: *Electronic Publishing Services Inc., NYC*
Typeface: *11.5/13 Minion*
Printer: *Quebecor World Dubuque, IA*

Photo Credits: Figure 11.1: © Tierbild Okapia/Photo Researchers, Inc.; Figures 11.2, 11.3: © Dr. P. Marazzi/Photo Researchers, Inc.; Figure 11.4: © Custom Medical Stock Photo; Figure 11.6: © Dr. P. Marazzi/Photo Researchers, Inc.; Pages 164, 165: © Dr. P. Marazzi/Photo Researchers, Inc.; Page 166: © Image courtesy Bradley R. Davis; Figure 12.5: © Dr. P. Marazzi/Photo Researchers, Inc.; Figure 12.7: © Mediscan; Page 217: © Mediscan; Figure 15.8: © Custom Medical Stock Photo; Figure 18.3 A: www.poison-ivy.org; Figure 18.3 B: Courtesy M. D. Vaden, Certified Arborist, Oregon; Figure 18.3 C: © Gilbert Grant/Photo Researchers, Inc., Figure 18.4: © Bill Beatty/Visuals Unlimited; Figure 20.2 A: © Tom McHugh/Photo Researchers, Inc.; Figure 20.2 B: © Educational Images Ltd./Custom Medical Stock Photo; Figure 20.2 C: © Jim Merli/Visuals Unlimited; Figure 20.2 D: © Suzanne L. Collins/Photo Researchers, Inc.; Figure 20.3 B: © Robert Noonan/Photo Researchers, Inc.; Figure 20.5 A: © Brad Mogen/Visuals Unlimited; Figure 20.5 B: Photo by Scott Bauer, Agricultural Research Service, USDA; Figure 20.6: © Caliendo/Custom Medical Stock Photo; Figure 20.9: © A.N.T./Photo Researchers, Inc.; Page 320 (top): © Mediscan; Page 320 (bottom): © SIU/Visuals Unlimited; Page 361: Courtesy Kelly Trakalo; Figure 24.5: © Custom Medical Stock Photo; Page 401: Courtesy NOAA Photo Library, OAR/ERL/National Severe Storms Lab (NSSL). All other photographs © National Safety Council/Rick Brady, photographer.

NATIONAL SAFETY COUNCIL MISSION STATEMENT
The mission of the National Safety Council is to educate and influence people to prevent accidental injury and death.

Library of Congress Cataloging-in-Publication Data

First aid : taking action / National Safety Council. — 1st ed.
    p.   cm.
Includes index.
ISBN 978–0–07–352200–5 — ISBN 0–07–352200–7
1. First aid in illness and injury. 2. Medical emergencies. I. National Safety Council.

RC86.7.F57   2007
616.02'52—dc22   2006042563
                                                CIP

www.mhhe.com

Table of Contents

Index of Skills

Welcome to your first aid course with *First Aid: Taking Action,* developed by the National Safety Council. *First Aid: Taking Action* is a comprehensive and reader-friendly first aid textbook designed both for lay people and more highly trained healthcare personnel and professional rescuers. You will learn everything you need to know to provide basic life support and first aid in an emergency.

Unlike smaller texts and other training materials designed for a short course, *First Aid: Taking Action* has been developed for a comprehensive course covering all emergency and other first aid situations that may be encountered. Some topics, such as first aid in remote locations or emergency childbirth, may not be covered in all first aid courses using this text, but the majority of the text focuses on care for injuries and sudden illness that almost anyone may encounter at almost any time.

First Aid: Taking Action is unique as a textbook in maintaining a dual focus throughout. The primary goal is to teach people *what to do* in different emergencies, and many of the text's features are designed to present this practical information concisely and visually in a manner that aids retention. At the same time, since people remember key information longer and can better apply it in real-life situations when they understand the underlying principles, the text also discusses what is happening within the body in emergencies and how and why first aid actions are effective.

Primary Themes

To promote more effective learning and retention, *First Aid: Taking Action* applies certain themes consistently in all chapters where appropriate.

- **Injury and illness prevention.** It is much better to take actions to stay safe and healthy by preventing injury and illness than merely to know how to respond to emergencies after they occur. Learners are given useful, specific information as well as general principles they can apply in their own lives.

- **Current statistics** show how common various injuries and illnesses are, helping motivate learners to be prepared for encountering them. Statistics related to age and other groups also help learners to understand who is most likely to be involved in certain kinds of emergencies. NSC has collected data on accidents/injuries for over 80 years, and the NSC's annual publication *Injury Facts* is the most convenient, easy-to-use, and authoritative source of accident/injury data.

- **When to call 9-1-1 (or local emergency number) or see a healthcare provider.** Although the need to call for help in a life-threatening emergency is usually obvious, many instances of injury or sudden illness may seem less serious. Those giving first aid are often unsure whether to call 9-1-1, transport a victim oneself to a hospital emergency department, or perhaps just call a healthcare provider. This issue is considered throughout the text. While key principles are emphasized that are easily remembered and can be applied in different situations, specific guidelines are also provided for special circumstances.

- **Emphasis on the key principles of first aid.** Learners are sometimes intimidated by what seems a large number of specific injuries or illnesses all with their own particular first aid steps. Although this text does describe the specific first aid for specific injuries and illnesses, the recurring emphasis on basic principles helps learners to organize and remember this information and promotes self-confidence even in situations when a lesser action might be forgotten. Some of these key principles are:
  - Stay calm.
  - Call 9-1-1 (or local emergency number) for all serious emergencies and whenever in doubt.
  - Remember your own safety.
  - Act quickly.
  - Check the victim.
  - Do no harm.
  - Ask others for help.
- **Variations on key principles** are also often important, such as when first aid is given in a different way for infants or children or when a problem is more severe in an elderly victim. Such variations are discussed, when appropriate, in a way that promotes a fuller understanding rather than simply stating the differences. These variations also help learners to see the immediate relevance of first aid in their own lives: being prepared to help family members young or old, co-workers, and one's peers.
- **Current events** related to first aid are reported in boxes whenever they will help to enrich learners' understanding of first aid or the prevention of injury and illness. Including information on current and changing technology, for example, helps learners to understand the larger context of first aid in an evolving world, as well as the need to stay current in one's skills and knowledge after completing the course.

Key Features

First Aid: Taking Action has been designed for use in a range of different settings, from the college classroom to training courses in healthcare or industry. Key features help learners focus on essential information and promote retention, while allowing course instructors to vary their teaching approach to best meet the needs of their particular students.

- **Chapter Preview.** This listing of topics at the opening of the chapter provides learners with a brief overview of chapter core content. ▶
- **Opening Scenario.** Each chapter opens with a visual scene and a typical first aid situation. The scenario pertains to information discussed in the chapter and helps learners apply their knowledge. ▶

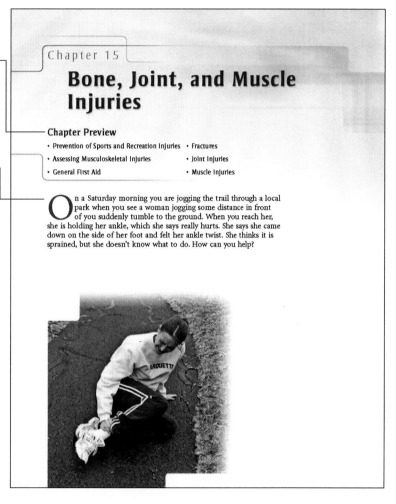

Chapter 15

Bone, Joint, and Muscle Injuries

Chapter Preview
- Prevention of Sports and Recreation Injuries
- Assessing Musculoskeletal Injuries
- General First Aid
- Fractures
- Joint Injuries
- Muscle Injuries

On a Saturday morning you are jogging the trail through a local park when you see a woman jogging some distance in front of you suddenly tumble to the ground. When you reach her, she is holding her ankle, which she says really hurts. She says she came down on the side of her foot and felt her ankle twist. She thinks it is sprained, but she doesn't know what to do. How can you help?

- **First aid steps** are highlighted for all significant injuries and sudden illnesses in a concise, visual format. These steps are structured to make it easy to see what actions to take immediately, what things *not* to do (*Alerts*), and what additional actions to take while waiting for help to arrive. ▶
- **Skills** are presented visually as an easy-to-follow step-by-step procedure. ▼

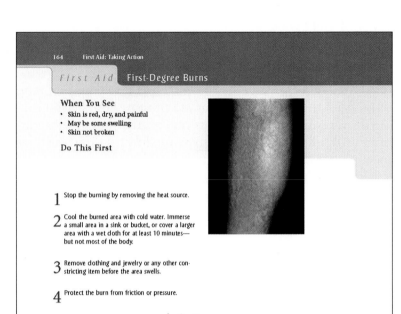

First Aid **First-Degree Burns**

When You See
- Skin is red, dry, and painful
- May be some swelling
- Skin not broken

Do This First

1 Stop the burning by removing the heat source.

2 Cool the burned area with cold water. Immerse a small area in a sink or bucket, or cover a larger area with a wet cloth for at least 10 minutes— but not most of the body.

3 Remove clothing and jewelry or any other constricting item before the area swells.

4 Protect the burn from friction or pressure.

ALERT
- Do not put butter on a burn.
- Do not use ice on a burn because even though it may relieve pain, the cold may cause additional damage to the skin. Ice-cold water should not be used longer than 10 minutes.

Additional Care
- Aloe vera gel can be used on the skin for comfort.

y and cool the area. continually adding d constricting cloth- rn with a dry, loose, urns, do not apply o the burn. While

waiting for emergency personnel, treat the victim for shock by having the victim lie down, elevating the legs, and maintaining normal body temperature. Monitor the victim's breathing and give basic life support (BLS) if needed (see First Aid: "Third-Degree Burns").

Controlling Bleeding   119

Skill **Controlling Bleeding**

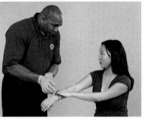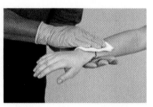

1 Put on gloves.

2 Place a sterile dressing on the wound and apply direct pressure with your hand.

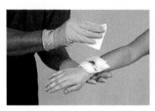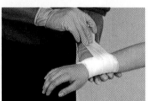

3 If needed, put another dressing or cloth pad on top of the first and keep applying pressure.

4 Apply a roller bandage to keep pressure on the wound.
5 If appropriate, treat the victim for shock (see Chapter 10), and call 9-1-1.

ALERT
- Use your bare hands only if no barrier is available, and then wash immediately.
- Do not put pressure on an object in a wound.
- Do not put pressure on the scalp if the skull may be injured.
- Do not use a tourniquet to stop bleeding except as an extreme last resort because the limb will likely be lost (see Chapter 24).

- **Learning Checkpoints** appear in key places within chapters to help learners confirm their understanding of preceding topics. Correct answers and explanations are located in **Appendix G.**

62 First Aid: Taking Action

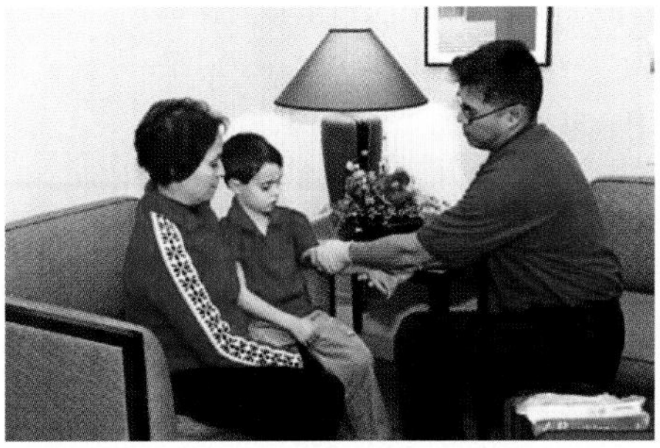

Figure 4-6 Involve the child's parent or guardian in the history and physical examination.

Learning Checkpoint 2

1. When is the secondary assessment performed?
   - **a.** Immediately before giving CPR when needed
   - **b.** In all victims, right after the initial assessment
   - **c.** After checking for responsiveness
   - **d.** After determining that there are no life-threatening conditions
2. Write what each letter in the SAMPLE history stands for

   S = ________________ **P** = ________________

   A = ________________ **L** = ________________

   M = ________________ **E** = ________________
3. Describe what signs and symptoms of injury you are looking for as you examine each part of a victim's body.

   ____

   ____

   ____

- **Learning Outcomes** are listed at the end of each chapter to help learners confirm their expectation of learning chapter topics and skills. ▶
- **Review Questions** in multiple choice format are included at the end of each chapter. These questions help learners review chapter content and continue to reinforce knowledge and skills. Answers are provided in **Appendix G**. ▶
- **References and Resources** are provided at the end of each chapter for further information. ▶

Concluding Thoughts

Remember to check for normal breathing in any unresponsive victim. If an unresponsive victim is gasping or is not breathing, give two rescue breaths to move oxygen into the victims lungs, and then start chest compressions as you will learn in Chapter 6.

Learning Outcomes

You should now be able to do the following:

1. List ways to prevent drowning and SIDS.

2. Describe the age categories for adults, children, and infants related to differences in basic life support skills.

3. Explain how to give rescue breaths via a barrier device, the mouth, the nose, or a stoma, and to an infant.

Review Questions

1. For the purposes of BLS, when does an infant become a child?
   a. At six months
   b. At one year
   c. At 15 pounds
   d. At 25 pounds

2. Rescue breaths are given with the victim in what position?
   a. On the back
   b. On the side
   c. On the back or the side
   d. In the position in which the victim is found

3. How long should it take to deliver one rescue breath?
   a. ½ second
   b. 1 second
   c. 1½ seconds
   d. 2 seconds

4. Why should a barrier device be used with rescue breaths?
   a. To help get more air into the victim
   b. To prevent vomiting
   c. To protect against infectious disease
   d. To prevent air from entering the esophagus

5. Vomiting during rescue breaths may result from
   a. blowing in too forcefully.
   b. blowing in for too long.
   c. blowing in too fast.
   d. All of the above

References and Resources

American Heart Association. www.americanheart.org

First Candle/SIDS Alliance, SIDS Q & A. Available from: www.firstcandle.org

American Heart Association. 2005 International consensus on cardiopulmonary resuscitation (CPR) and emergency cardiovascular care (ECC) science with treatment recommendations. *Circulation*, 112(22). November 29, 2005.

National Center for Injury Prevention and Control. Water-related injuries: fact sheet. Available from: www.cdc.gov/ncipc/factsheets/drown.htm

National Safe Kids Campaign. www.safekids.org

National Safety Council. www.nsc.org

- **Appendix of Advanced Skills.** **Appendix A** describes and discusses a wide range of additional basic life support skills. Such skills are often included in the training of healthcare personnel or professional rescuers. Instructors and participants have a choice of completing either the layperson or professional level of basic life support. ▶

- **Appendix of Skill Performance Checklists. Appendix B** includes key skill performance checklists to monitor the learner's proficiency during practice. ▼

Appendix
A Advanced Resuscitation Techniques

The skills included in this appendix are typically not taught to lay rescuers. Healthcare providers and rescuers at higher levels of training may be trained in some or all of these skills. As always, never attempt a skill in which you have not been appropriately trained. This appendix discusses the following topics:

- Definition of pediatric victims
- Assessment skills
  - Call first vs. call fast
  - Jaw thrust
  - Assessing breathing
  - Pulse check for circulation
- Ventilation skills
  - Rescue breathing without chest compressions
  - Resuscitation masks
  - Cricoid pressure
  - Airway suctioning
  - Bag-valve masks
  - Supplemental oxygen
  - Oral and nasal airways
- CPR skills
  - Hand position for chest compressions
  - Compressions for bradycardia in child
  - CPR
  - Two-rescuer CPR
- AED skills
- Special resuscitation situations
  - Trauma
  - Hypothermia
  - Near-drowning

PEDIATRIC VICTIMS
...ild as 1 to 8 years of age (to about 55 lbs and ...ches) for all BLS skills including AED use. For ...ED, healthcare providers also consider a child to ...r rescue breathing and CPR, however, healthcare ...der a victim a child from age 1 up to the onset of

Appendix
B Performance Checklists for Key Skills

- **Disaster Preparation Appendices.** Four appendices cover preparedness for types of natural disasters that may occur in your geographic area: earthquakes, floods, hurricanes, and tornadoes. ▶

Preventing Emergencies

First aid skills are important for helping victims of medical emergencies, but obviously it is better to avoid such emergencies altogether. You may have heard people refer to someone as "accident-prone," but have you ever considered what that really means? Accidents almost always occur when people do not use common sense or follow appropriate safety guidelines for the activity. Being "accident-prone" is not a genetic flaw—it is usually a simple lack of safety awareness that results in not making the effort to act safely. Everyone knows, for example, that driving under the influence of alcohol results in tens of thousands of deaths every year as well as countless injuries and disabilities. All of these could be prevented if everyone followed one simple guideline. This is more a matter of attitude than a need to learn something new.

Other injuries result, however, from a lack of information about the risks of certain activities or guidelines for doing them safely. These guidelines *can* be learned. Being aware of risks, and acting in ways to stay safe from them, begins with being motivated—when one deliberately chooses to avoid injury rather than run the risk. This text includes statistics throughout, such as the fact that every year in the United States almost five million victims of motor vehicle crashes are seen in emergency departments with serious injuries, along with 35 million people with other kinds of injuries. In other words, injuries are so common that unless you choose to try to prevent them, you yourself are likely to become such a statistic. The point of such statistics is not to scare you but to highlight the fact that injuries, illness, and deaths do not happen only to *other people.* They can happen to anyone who does not act to avoid them. It is not just accident-prone people who are hurt; it is all of us who are not safety conscious.

Some people argue there are actually no "accidents" at all—in the sense of something that "just happens." Injuries do not just happen. **Since they can be prevented, they occur only when someone fails to prevent them.** When you start thinking of your health and well-being in that way, you understand you do have the power to stay well—it is simply up to you to decide to do so. This book describes many of the common causes of injuries and illnesses that can be prevented, although it is beyond the scope of this book to cover prevention in detail for every activity.

Following are general guidelines for injury prevention:

- In your home, take steps to prevent fires, accidental poisonings, and other injuries. Look for hazards and correct them.
- In the workplace, always follow safety procedures required by the Occupational Safety and Health Administration (OSHA). If you have received safety training, use it. It takes only one lapse from a safety procedure to lose a life.
- Use common sense when driving or engaging in activities that involve injury risks. As you will learn in **Chapter 1**, the huge majority of injuries seen in hospital emergency departments result from motor vehicle crashes, falls, or being struck by or against an object or cut or pierced by an object.

These are just general principles for preventing common injuries. Chapters throughout this text contain additional, specific injury-prevention information for particular types of injuries. Remember: it is always better to take a minute to consider safety issues before starting an activity than to have to cope later with an injury. This is true in all settings: at school, at work, in your home, when driving, when engaged in sports or recreational activities, and so on. Emergencies can occur anywhere, at any time, and the great majority of those that do occur could have been prevented.

Preventing Illness: A Healthy Lifestyle

Literally millions of people die every year of illnesses that could largely have been prevented by living healthier lifestyles. Following are some of the most common diseases and conditions leading to death, a high percentage of which could be prevented:

- Heart disease (causing heart attacks)
- Stroke
- High blood pressure (contributes to both heart attacks and strokes)
- Diabetes
- Cancer (some, like lung cancer caused by smoking, can be prevented)

Virtually all adults know the importance of healthful living, yet many still are overweight, get too little exercise, eat poorly, smoke, drink too much, and so on. In most cases lifestyle habits are formed in childhood and adolescence when the individual is not thinking about distant health concerns. Entrenched habits can then be very hard to break. Fortunately, the media and programs in schools and communities are increasingly focusing on the importance of forming healthful habits from an early age, with the hope that more youth will grow into adulthood with healthier lifestyles and a lower risk of developing a preventable illness. The most serious preventable risk factors for the common diseases just listed are:

- Smoking
- High cholesterol levels (preventable with diet, exercise, and medication if needed)
- High blood pressure (preventable with diet, exercise, and medication if needed)
- Physical inactivity
- Obesity and overweight
- Stress

A healthy lifestyle, therefore, begins with avoiding these risk factors: stop smoking, eat a diet low in fats and sugars, exercise regularly, manage your weight, and learn to cope with stress. **Chapter 6** describes these strategies for healthful living in more detail.

A longer life is not the only result of a healthy lifestyle. Quality of life is also improved: you have more energy, generally feel healthier, and feel better about yourself. As someone trained in first aid, the stronger and healthier you are, the more fit you are to be able to help others in times of need.

Complete the "Healthy Lifestyle Self-Assessment" to see what you already know—or do not know—about specific ways you can improve your health. But do not be concerned if you are unsure of some of the answers, as you will be learning more about these topics as you read later chapters. The correct answers are provided in **Appendix G.**

Healthy Lifestyle Self-Assessment

> *Circle True or False for each of the following statements:*
>
> True   False   1. Smokers have a risk two to four times higher for cardiovascular disease than nonsmokers.
>
> True   False   2. For a 2000-calorie intake, people should eat about 4 cups of fruit and 8 cups of vegetables daily.
>
> True   False   3. At least half the grain products you eat should come from whole grains.
>
> True   False   4. Natural saturated fats and trans fats are generally healthier than unsaturated fats.
>
> True   False   5. Limit your salt intake to approximately 3 tsp per day.
>
> True   False   6. Pregnant women can have up to two glasses of wine a day but should not exceed that limit.
>
> True   False   7. Your cholesterol level is higher if you are relatively sedentary.
>
> True   False   8. To reduce the risk of chronic disease in adulthood, engage in at least 30 minutes of moderate-intensity physical activity on most days of the week.
>
> True   False   9. Body weight affects one's health only after approximately age 30.
>
> True   False   10. Hypertension increases your risk for both heart attack and stroke.

Concluding Thoughts

Although most injuries and many illnesses can be prevented, some emergencies will still inevitably occur, and people like you trained in first aid and basic life support skills will always be needed. The skills you will learn in the following chapters may help save a life—perhaps a loved one or family member. Remember: injuries and sudden illness don't only happen to "other people."

Publisher's Acknowledgements

Trent Applegate HSD, MPH, ATC
Applied Health Science Department
Indiana University-Bloomington
Bloomington, IN

David Beymer
Physical Education Department
Hartnell College
Salinas, CA

Jay Bradley MED, LAT, ATC
HPER Department
IUPUI
Indianapolis, IN

Susan Brown
Physical Education/Athletics Department
Johnson City Community College
Overland Park, KS

Rod Compton
Assistant Professor, First Aid and Safety
Program Director
Department of Health, Education and Promotion
East Carolina University
Greenville, NC

Chris Coughlin
Emergency Medical Technology
Glendale Community College
Glendale, AZ

Dean C. Dieter, RN, ND, CS, CEN
Assistant Professor of Nursing
Pennsylvania State University-School of Nursing
University Park, PA

Debra DiMatteo
Physical Education Department
College of Dupage
Glen Ellyn, IL

Christopher L. Fink
School of Physical Activity and Educational Services
The Ohio State University
Columbus, OH

Pat Graman, MA, ATC
Health Promotion and Education
University of Cincinnati
Cincinnati, OH

Alisa Grimes
Department of Public Health
Western Kentucky University
Bowling Green, KY

Dana Hale, MS, ATC
Health and Physical Education Department
Itawamba Community College
Fulton, MS

Carrie Hammond, CMA, LPRI
Medical Assistant Department
Utah Career College
West Jordan, UT

Elisa Elizabeth Hutson McNeill
Health and Kinesiology Department
Texas A&M University
College Station, TX

Deb Kaye, EMT-B
Health Department
Dakota County Technical College
Minnesota Safety Council
Rosemount, MN

Patrick Kincaid
Division of Kinesiology
University of Michigan
Physical Education Department
Ann Arbor, MI

Harriette Lavenue
Health and Sport Sciences Department
The University of Memphis
Memphis, TN

Marguerite Moore, MS, ATC
Kinesiology Department
Michigan State University
East Lansing, MI

Toni Morris, RN, MS, MFA
Community Medicine Department
West Virginia University
Morgantown, WV

Peggy Oberstaller
Health, PE and Athletics Department
Lane Community College
Eugene, OR

Tona Palmer
Health and Human Performance Department
Oklahoma State University
Stillwater, OK

Sandra L. Raborn
Health-Wellness Department
Daytona Beach Community College
Daytona Beach, FL

Carol M. Reed
School of Physical Education, Sport
and Exercise Science
Ball State University
Muncie, IN

Robb S. Rehberg, PhD, ATC, NREMT
Coordinator of Clinical Education,
Athletic Training Education Program
Department of Exercise and Movement Sciences
William Paterson University of New Jersey
Wayne, NJ

Vicki H. Sageser
Kinesiology and Health Promotion
University of Kentucky
Lexington, KY

Danielle Schortzmann Wilken
Department Head
Allied Health Department
Goodwin College
East Hartford, CT

Mary Segle
Physical Education Department
Shoreline Community College
Seattle, WA

Karen Skrbich
HPER Department
University of Minnesota-Duluth
Duluth, MN

Steve Underwood
HHP Department
University of Tennessee at Chattanooga
Chattanooga, TN

Green T. Waggener, PhD, MPH
Kinesiology and Physical Education Department
Valdosta State University
Valdosta, GA

First Aid: Taking Action

NATIONAL SAFETY COUNCIL

Chapter 1

Preparing to Act

Chapter Preview

- What Is First Aid?
- The Need for First Aid
- Deciding to Help

- Staying Prepared
- The Emergency Medical Services System
- Legal Concepts in First Aid

You are staying late at work to catch up on a project, when a co-worker returns to the office to pick up something she forgot. While she is in her office, her young son, whom she left in the reception area, is running around. He falls and hurts his arm, and you hear him crying and come out to see if you can help. His mother calms him while you get a first aid kit.

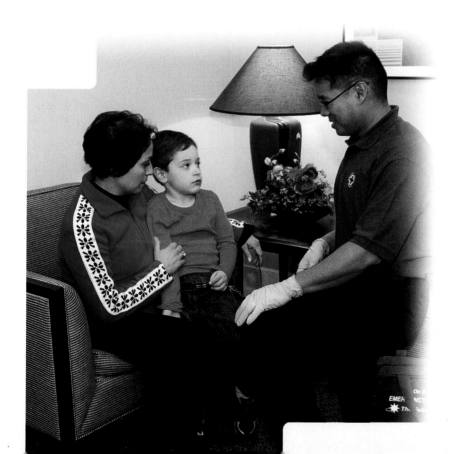

First aid training is important because injuries and sudden illness occur frequently. People of all ages, in all places, may experience an injury or sudden illness requiring immediate attention when a doctor or medical professional is not present. Often the person needing first aid is a family member or loved one. In many cases the victim's life or well-being depends on actions that first aiders take during the first few minutes before emergency healthcare workers take over.

This chapter will help you become prepared to act in an emergency. It explains the need for first aid and how to decide to help when you recognize an emergency. You will also learn what it means to be prepared, your role in the Emergency Medical Services (EMS) system, and relevant legal issues in first aid.

WHAT IS FIRST AID?

First aid is the immediate help given to a victim of injury or sudden illness until appropriate medical help arrives or the victim is seen by a healthcare provider. First aid is typically given by a friend or family member, a co-worker, or a bystander at the scene with minimal or no medical equipment. First aid is generally not all the treatment the person needs, but it helps the victim for the usually short time until advanced care begins. First aid can also be simple care given when medical attention is not needed, such as caring for a small wound.

The primary goals of first aid are to:

- Keep the victim alive until he or she receives medical care
- Prevent the victim's condition from getting worse
- Help promote early recovery from the injury or illness
- Ensure the victim receives appropriate medical care

Other goals include reassuring the victim and providing comfort until medical care is provided.

Most first aid does not require extensive training or equipment. With the first aid training in this course and a basic first aid kit, you can perform first aid in most situations.

THE NEED FOR FIRST AID

In the United States every year:

- Almost 40 million visits are made to emergency departments because of injuries.
- Two million people are hospitalized because of injuries.
- 140,000 die from injuries.
- Over 800,000 heart attacks occur, resulting in 180,000 deaths.
- 162,000 die from strokes.

Tables 1-1 and 1-2 list the most common causes of injuries for which the victim goes to a hospital emergency department, and the annual deaths resulting from the most common types of injuries. Figures 1-1 and 1-2 show the most common types of injuries occurring in the workplace.

In many cases these deaths could have been prevented. In other cases the victim might have lived if a trained first aider had been present to

Table 1-1

Injuries Annually Treated in Hospital Emergency Departments

Falls	7,989,000
Motor vehicle crashes	4,582,000
Struck by or against object	4,209,000
Cut or pierced by object	2,544,000
Overexertion and strenuous movements	1,686,000
Assault	1,608,000
Bites and stings (other than dog bites)	998,000
Poisoning (includes drug overdose)	750,000
Burns	516,000
Attempted suicide	438,000

Source: National Safety Council, Injury Facts 2005.

Table 1-2

Annual Deaths Due to Selected Accidental Injuries

Motor vehicle crashes	45,549	Assault by sharp objects	2,074
Suicide	31,655	Bicycle crashes	767
Poisoning (includes drug overdose)	17,550	Cold exposure	646
Falls	16,257	Water transport/boating accidents	617
Assault by firearm	11,829	Other breathing threats	583
Choking	4,934	Electrocution	454
Drowning	3,447	Heat exposure	350
Smoke, fire, flames	3,159	Burns	102
Mechanical forces	2,871	Venomous animals and plants	76

Source: National Safety Council, Injury Facts 2005.

give help until medical help arrived. This text therefore describes both injury and illness prevention and the care to give until help arrives. With what you learn in this first aid course, you can help make a difference and maybe save a life.

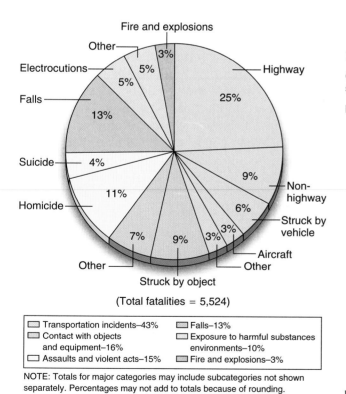

Figure 1-1 The manner in which workplace fatalities occurred. (Source: U.S. Department of Labor, Bureau of Labor Statistics. Census of Fatal Occupational Injuries, 2002.)

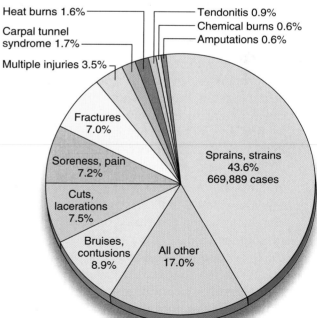

Figure 1-2 Occupational injuries and illnesses involving days away from work. (Source: Bureau of Labor Statistics, U.S. Department of Labor. Survey of Occupational Injuries and Illnesses, 2001.)

Learning
Checkpoint ①

1. True or False: When first aid is given, the victim does not need further medical attention.

2. True or False: First aid given promptly can save lives and reduce the severity of injuries.

DECIDING TO HELP

Recognizing the need for first aid and knowing what first aid to give are the first steps in preparedness, but you also need to make the conscious decision to help in an emergency. This is not always an easy decision. You may hesitate to act because of any of the following common concerns:

- *You may be worried about not doing the right thing.* Remember that you have first aid training. This course will teach you all you need to know to be able to help. Once you call for help, professionals will arrive very soon. Usually you are needed to help only for a few minutes.

- *You may think someone else would provide better care.* Do not delay giving first aid because you hope someone else will do it. Many people are naturally shy about stepping forward in an emergency, but unless someone else has already begun to help the victim and is obviously trained in what to do, it is up to you to help the victim. People without first aid training can assist you, such as by calling 9-1-1, going to get first aid supplies, or helping calm a victim they know. But do not let precious minutes pass while waiting to see if someone else will help.

- *You may not be sure it is an emergency.* This first aid course will teach you the signs of an emergency when an injured or suddenly ill person needs help right away. When in doubt, call 9-1-1 and tell the dispatcher what you see. It is better to make the call and find out later the victim's condition was not so serious after all, than to not call and allow a victim's condition to deteriorate before seeking care.

- *You may be upset by the sight of blood or the injury.* Some injuries can be very upsetting, especially those involving blood, badly burned skin, vomiting, and other factors. You may have to muster your self-control. Try to focus on the immediate tasks at hand to prevent the experience from overwhelming you. You may

need to look away and take a deep breath. You may need to ask others to help. Those who are easily upset may gain from learning stress reduction techniques along with first aid in order to stay in control in an emergency. If you react strongly to photographs of severe injuries such as those in this text, and if you feel you might have difficulty acting in an emergency because of such factors, talk with your instructor about relaxation techniques that may be appropriate for you.

- *You may be worried about catching a disease from the victim.* Most of us would not worry about helping a family member or friend because of a fear of disease, but we may be reluctant to touch a stranger. Because some diseases can be transmitted through contact with another person's blood or other body fluids, this is—and should be—a concern. As discussed in **Chapter 2**, you should take steps in any emergency to prevent disease transmission. When you give first aid using the precautions you will learn in this course, you will not face a higher risk of contracting a disease.

STAYING PREPARED

An emergency can occur at any time in any place, and most emergencies occur without warning. One moment you are enjoying dinner with friends, and the next moment someone at the table is choking on food and unable to breathe. A child running through a meadow trips and falls on broken glass and suddenly is bleeding severely. A co-worker abruptly clutches his chest and collapses. In each of these cases you need to act immediately, for the victim may have only minutes to live unless you give first aid. Therefore it is essential to always be prepared to act as needed.

Being prepared means knowing what to do—but it also means *feeling* ready and taking steps to ensure you do not lose precious time when responding to an emergency:

- *Know the appropriate first aid techniques.* This first aid course will teach you what to do in all emergencies involving injury or sudden illness.
- *Be confident in your skills.* Sometimes people at the scene of an emergency hesitate to help. Remember that *you* have first aid training, however, and you should feel confident that you can help the victim. Never hesitate or wait for others to act—remember that the victim's life may depend on acting quickly.
- *Have a personal first aid kit at home and in your car.* Be sure first aid kits are well stocked with the right supplies. Keep emergency phone numbers, such as EMS, the Poison Control Center, and other emergency agencies, in a handy place.
- *Know whether your community uses 9-1-1 or a different emergency telephone number.* Note that this text says "Call 9-1-1" throughout. If your community does not use the 9-1-1 system, call your local emergency number instead. Some companies have an internal emergency number employees are expected to call, and that department will then call EMS.
- *When teaching children to call 9-1-1, say "nine-one-one" and never "nine-eleven."* Young children are known to lose valuable time searching for an "eleven" button on the telephone keypad.
- *If you or your significant others have a medical condition, be sure that information is available to others in an emergency.* Information should include the telephone numbers of healthcare providers, allergies, and any prescription medications. People with certain medical conditions such as diabetes, epilepsy, and severe allergies are advised to wear a medical alert bracelet or necklace to alert others in an emergency (**Figure 1-3**).

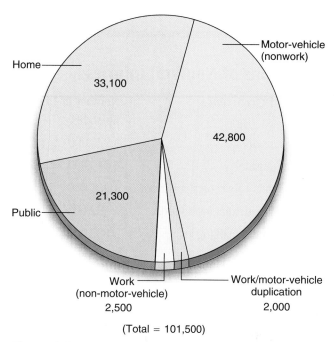

Figure 1-4 Unintentional injury deaths by class, United States, 2003. (National Safety Council, Injury Facts 2004.)

People with certain illnesses or conditions may also carry medications for emergency use. For example, people with severe allergies may carry an emergency kit such as an EpiPen,® or some people with heart conditions may carry nitroglycerine tablets.

Most accidental injury deaths occur as a result of motor vehicle crashes, followed by injuries in the home, public places, and work (**Figure 1-4**). First aiders therefore need to be prepared to give first aid in any place at any time. As **Figure 1-5** shows, home and community unintentional injury deaths have continued to rise in the last decade. **Table 1-3** shows the locations of nonfatal injuries that typically require first aid.

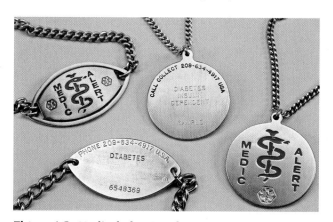

Figure 1-3 Medical alert jewelry.

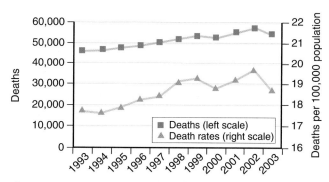

Figure 1-5 Home and community deaths and death rates, United States 1993–2003. (National Safety Council, Injury Facts 2004.)

Table 1-3

Locations of Nonfatal Injuries

Place of Occurrence	Number of Injury Episodes	Place of Occurrence	Number of Injury Episodes
Home (inside)	5,926,000	Sport facility/recreation area/lake/river/pool	3,039,000
Home (outside)	4,949,000	Industrial/construction/farm	1,089,000
School/child care center/preschool	1,261,000	Trade/service area	1,082,000
Hospital/residential institution	392,000	Other public building	661,000
Street/highway/parking lot	3,832,000	Other (unspecified)	1,482,000

Source: Schiller JS, Adams PF, Coriaty Nelson Z. Summary health statistics for the U.S. population: National Health Interview Survey, 2003. *National Center for Health Statistics. Vital Health Stat 10(224). 2005.*

Your First Aid Kit

Keep a well-stocked first aid kit in your home and vehicle, and know where one is kept at work or at school. Take one with you on recreational activities. A cell phone is also helpful in most emergencies.

Make sure your first aid kit includes the items shown in **Figure 1-6**. Note that you may not necessarily use all items in a kit just because they are there. For example, first aiders do not give medications such as aspirin or acetaminophen. However, some adult victims may choose to take such medications themselves.

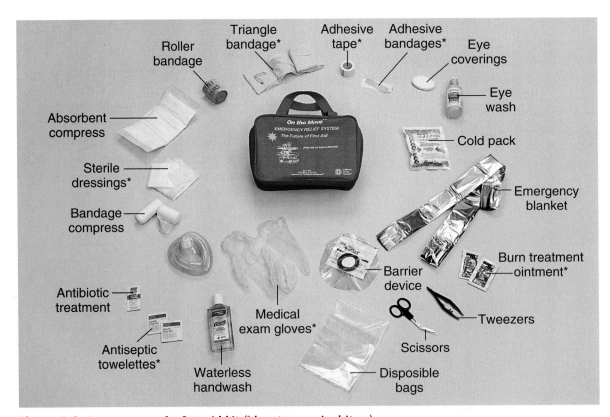

Figure 1-6 Components of a first aid kit (*denotes required item).

Learning
Checkpoint ②

1. Being prepared for an emergency means

   a. knowing what to do.

   b. being ready to act anytime, anywhere.

   c. knowing how to get medical care for a victim.

   d. All of the above

2. It is a good idea to have a first aid kit

   a. in your home.

   b. in your car.

   c. on recreational outings.

   d. All of the above

THE EMERGENCY MEDICAL SERVICES SYSTEM

People trained in first aid are the first link in the **Emergency Medical Services (EMS)** system. The EMS system in the United States is a comprehensive network of professionals linked together to provide appropriate levels of medical care for victims of injury or sudden illness.* As a first aider, your role in the system, in addition to giving the victim first aid until he or she is seen by advanced caregivers, is to make sure the EMS system responds as quickly as possible to help the victim, by calling 9-1-1. In most communities help will arrive within minutes.

The Emergency Medical Services system includes a number of different professionals with different levels of training and responsibilities (**Box 1-1**).

When to Call EMS

Call 9-1-1 immediately if you recognize a life-threatening injury or illness. A life-threatening emergency is one in which a problem threatens the victim's breathing or circulation of blood (i.e., cardiac arrest or severe bleeding), as described in later chapters. If you are alone with the victim and not near a telephone, shout

for help and ask someone to call 9-1-1. Do not try to transport a victim to the emergency department yourself. Movement may worsen his or her condition, or the victim may suddenly need additional care on the way. An ambulance also can usually reach the emergency room faster than you can, and the EMTs can provide care as needed on the way. If you are not sure whether a situation is serious enough to call, do not hesitate—call 9-1-1. It is better to be safe than sorry.

If the victim is responsive and may not be seriously injured or ill, go on to the next step to check the victim further before calling 9-1-1—and then call 9-1-1 or a healthcare provider if needed.

Always call 9-1-1 when:

- The victim may have a life-threatening condition
- The victim is unresponsive (not talking, moving, or responding to you)
- The victim's condition may become life threatening
- Moving the victim could make his or her condition worse

Box 1-2 lists serious conditions for which to call 9-1-1. Later chapters on first aid also describe when to call 9-1-1 for other specific problems.

---

*The term **sudden illness** is generally used to describe medical conditions that occur suddenly and require first aid until the person can be seen by a medical professional. This term will be used throughout this text. "Sudden" illness is generally different from other illness situations in which the sick person is already under the care of a healthcare professional or has time to see a

healthcare professional for a nonemergency condition. Note that in some cases a person with a nonemergency chronic illness, such as diabetes or asthma, may suddenly experience an emergency situation as a result of that illness. If so, that immediate emergency situation, such as a person with asthma having an attack and not being able to breathe, is then called sudden illness.

Box 1-1 EMS Professionals

Dispatcher

A 9-1-1 call for help is usually received by an EMS dispatcher. This person is trained in obtaining information and determining what emergency personnel and equipment will likely be needed. The EMS dispatcher then sends the appropriate EMS unit to the scene.

Emergency Responders

Usually the first person to arrive at the scene is a first responder. First responders include police officers, firefighters, industrial safety officers, athletic trainers, lifeguards, ski patrollers, and similar professionals who are often close to the scene. The first responder often takes over care of the victim from those giving first aid. The first responder also gathers any information concerning the victim, controls the scene, and prepares for the arrival of more advanced medical help. Emergency medical technicians (EMTs) usually arrive next in an ambulance. They have a higher level of training and licensure and take over the medical care of the victim, give necessary medical care at the scene, and transport the victim for advanced medical care. Paramedics are EMTs with the highest level of training. EMTs can communicate with a physician as needed to provide the best prehospital care.

Hospital Centers

Emergency responders provide prehospital care before and during the transport of the victim to a hospital. Depending on the medical care needed and facilities in the area, the victim receives care from physicians in a hospital emergency department or a specialized center within a hospital.

Note that victims may say their condition is not all that serious. For example, heart attack victims often say they just have "indigestion" even when they have clear heart attack signs and symptoms.

You should call 9-1-1 anyway and let the dispatcher decide when the situation is an emergency.

In addition to calling 9-1-1 for injury or illness, call in these situations:

- Fire, explosion
- Vehicle crash
- Downed electrical wire
- Chemical spill, gas leak, or the presence of any unknown substances
- Swiftly moving or rapidly rising water

How to Call EMS

When you call 9-1-1 or your local emergency number, be ready to give the following information. If, however, this information is not readily available, do not delay making the call:

- Your name
- The phone number you are using
- The location and number of victims—specific enough for the arriving crew to be able to find them
- What happened to the victim(s) and any special circumstances or conditions that may require special rescue or medical equipment

Box 1-2 When to Call 9-1-1

- Unresponsiveness or altered mental status (dizzy, confused, disoriented, etc.)
- Not breathing, difficulty breathing
- Chest pain or pressure that does not go away
- Severe bleeding
- Head or spine injuries
- Poisoning, drug overdose
- Vomiting blood
- Seizures
- Severe burn
- Drowning or near drowning
- Threatened suicide
- Imminent childbirth

- The victim's condition. For example, is the victim responsive? Breathing? Bleeding?
- The victim's approximate age and sex
- What is being done for the victim(s). For example, is anyone on the scene able and willing to give CPR, is an AED present, etc.

It is important not to hang up until the dispatcher instructs you to do so because you may be given advice on how to care for the victim.

If another responsible person is present, tell him or her to call 9-1-1 while you go on to check the victim and give first aid **(Figure 1-7)**. Tell the other person to give the dispatcher the information listed previously.

Many communities have an **enhanced 9-1-1** system that automatically provides the dispatcher with the caller's phone number and the location of land telephone lines. This information can be lifesaving if the call is interrupted, but do not depend on the dispatcher already knowing your location. The location of a cellular telephone may not be known, and even when using a land telephone line you may need to specify more exactly where you are (such as to say you are with the victim in the yard behind the house, to prevent the loss of precious time while EMTs knock at the front door).

If 9-1-1 is not used as the emergency number in your community, post your local emergency telephone number by all telephones and keep the number with you if you travel with a cell phone. Having to find a telephone directory to look up a number will consume critical time. **Box 1-3** describes other issues you may encounter with telephones.

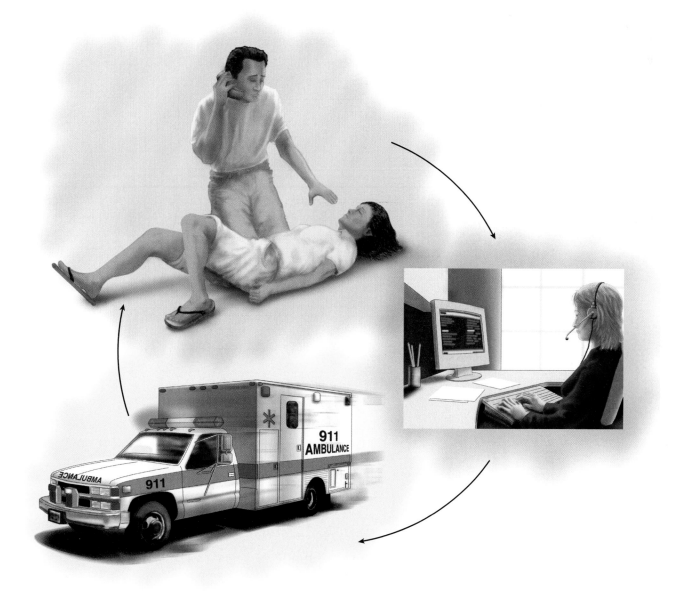

Figure 1-7 Call 9-1-1 to start emergency help on its way to the victim.

Box 1-3 Telephone Issues

Internet telephone services, commonly called VoIP (voice over Internet) services, have become increasingly popular for computer users with broadband Internet service because of lower costs. In 2005, after incidents in which people were unable to call 9-1-1 on their computer phones, the FCC ruled that all VoIP telephone services must allow a connection to EMS through the 9-1-1 number. Many VoIP telephone users do not realize, however, that their telephone will work only as long as their computer and cable line are functioning. In a power outage, for example, a VoIP telephone connected to a computer without an independent power source may stop working, potentially leaving the user no way to call 9-1-1.

Similarly, many people do not realize that most cordless telephones also require electrical power. In a power failure, a wired land telephone should still work, being powered by the telephone line rather than the power circuit, but most cordless telephones will not, even if connected to a land telephone line. Cell phones are not affected by local power outages but may not have a strong signal in all locales.

By one method or another, it is important to ensure that you can always call 9-1-1 in an emergency, even when the power is off.

Note that cell phone users have been encouraged to put a personal contact in their phone directory under the name "ICE" or "In Case of Emergency" so that emergency responders can learn who to call if needed. As a first aider you would not check a victim's telephone or try to contact family members, but you may want to carry your own "in case of emergency" phone number.

Learning Checkpoint 3

1. What number should you call to access EMS?

   a. 9-1-1 if your community uses that number

   b. The local emergency number (if not 9-1-1)

   c. Your company's emergency number (when company policy)

   d. All of the above

2. Call 9-1-1 for

   a. medical problems only.

   b. police and fire services only.

   c. medical problems and fires only.

   d. medical problems and all emergencies.

3. Who usually arrives first at the scene after you have called 9-1-1? _____

   _____

4. List seven things you should be prepared to tell the EMS dispatcher when you call. _____

   _____

In some remote locations, you may not be near a telephone. In these cases you may need to care for the victim for a longer time until the victim receives medical assistance. **Chapter 24** discusses common first aid situations in remote areas. In most other areas, however, your shouts for help will likely attract someone who can reach a telephone quickly to call 9-1-1.

LEGAL CONCEPTS IN FIRST AID

The United States is often said to be a litigious society because lawsuits are common. We hear so much in the media about people being sued that often we are afraid to act—even to help one another—because we worry we might be sued if something goes wrong. Although legal problems very seldom arise in first aid situations, certain legal concepts are important when you interact with another person to give first aid. If you follow certain simple guidelines, you need not be concerned about being sued for giving first aid. If you give first aid as you are trained to do in this course, and do your best, there is little chance of being found legally liable even if the victim does not recover.

To protect yourself, follow these general guidelines:

- Act only as you are trained to act.
- Get a victim's consent before giving first aid.
- Do not move a victim unnecessarily.
- Call for professional help.
- Keep giving care until help arrives.

Good Samaritan Laws

Most states have laws called **Good Samaritan laws** designed to encourage people to help others in an emergency without having to worry about being sued. These laws vary somewhat from state to state, but in general they are designed to protect people who give first aid in an emergency.

These laws do not provide blanket protection, however, regardless of the person's actions. In general, first aiders are legally protected only:

- when acting in an emergency, voluntarily and without compensation.
- when acting as a reasonable, prudent person with the same training would act.
- when performing first aid techniques as trained.
- when *not* doing something outside their training.
- when *not* abandoning a victim after starting to give care.

Ask your instructor about the specific Good Samaritan laws in your area. Remember, however, that regardless of specific laws, first aiders who act with good intentions and as they have been trained will very rarely face any legal issues.

Must You Give First Aid?

In most places private citizens or bystanders at the scene of an emergency have no legal obligation to give first aid. Many people feel an ethical or moral obligation to help others in need, but this is different from a legal obligation.

Because laws do vary in different areas, however, ask your instructor about the law in your area.

There are three important exceptions to the principle that you are not legally required to give first aid. First, once you begin giving first aid in an emergency, you are obligated to continue giving care if you can and to remain with the victim. By beginning to give care you accept and take on an obligation to continue giving care in an emergency. Abandoning a victim in this situation could lead to the worsening of an injury or illness, to disability, or to death.

The second exception is that some people are required to give first aid as a job responsibility. As a paid employee with this job requirement, you then are legally obligated. This is called a **duty to act,** and you may be held liable for failing to act or for acting inappropriately. Off the job, however, depending on your state's laws, you are usually not legally required to give first aid except in special cases.

The final exception is a parent or guardian who is responsible for a child, who has the duty to give the child adequate care. Federal and state laws against child abuse and neglect require parents and guardians to prevent harm and provide medical treatment (**see Chapter 22**).

Consent

Before you give first aid, you must have the victim's **consent.** This means that the victim gives you permission to help him or her using first aid techniques. Touching another person without consent is a criminal action called battery. Consent may be either expressed or implied.

Expressed consent means the victim explicitly gives you permission to give first aid. To ask for consent, first tell the victim who you are and that you have had first aid training, and say what you want to do to help. The victim should understand that you are *asking* for consent, not stating what you plan to do regardless of what the victim wishes. A victim who is responsive (awake and alert) and able to communicate must give you expressed consent before you can give first aid. The victim may give consent by telling you it is okay or by nodding agreement. With an injured or ill child, a parent or guardian present must give expressed consent (**Figure 1-8**).

If the victim is unresponsive, however, or a child's parent or guardian is not present and cannot be reached quickly enough for consent, then you have **implied consent** to give first aid in an emergency. In this case you can assume, unless there is some evidence to the contrary, that the person would, if able, consent to receiving care for a life-threatening condition. Similarly, if a person who initially refused consent becomes unresponsive, consent for care is now implied.

Refusing Consent

Most competent victims of a medical emergency will give consent for first aid when they understand the importance of this first aid. **Competent** means the person is able to understand what is happening and the implications of his or her decision about receiving first aid. A victim may not be competent because of intoxication, the influence of a drug, or altered mental status caused by a severe injury.

Rarely, however, a competent victim may refuse your care when you seek consent. The person may have religious reasons, may be afraid, may not trust you, or may have some other reason. A competent adult has the right to refuse medical care, even care that has already begun, and you must not try to force care on this person. Refusal may be expressed through words, by shaking the head or signaling you to stop, or by trying to push you away. If this happens, follow these guidelines:

- Make sure 9-1-1 has been called even though the victim may seem to refuse all care. The victim may accept treatment from a medical professional.
- Do not try to argue with the victim, especially about personal beliefs. Keep talking to the victim, who may change his or her mind. Explain that you respect his or her right to refuse care but ask the person to reconsider. Explain what may happen if the victim does not receive care.
- To protect yourself legally, make sure someone else at the scene sees or hears the victim's refusal to accept your care.

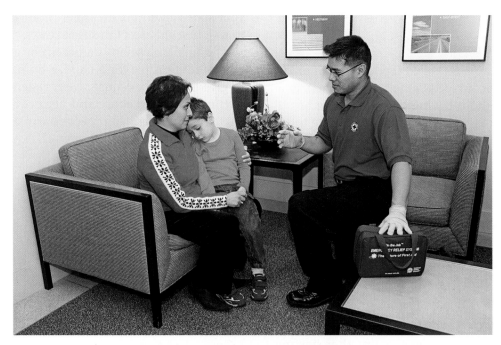

Figure 1-8 A parent or guardian present at the scene must give consent for first aid for a child.

Scope of Care

As noted earlier, first aiders should perform first aid only as they have been trained. The set of first aid techniques one learns in a first aid course is called the **scope of care.** Acting outside your scope of care as a first aider, such as trying to do something you have heard about but have not been trained to do, may make you legally liable for the results of your actions.

Standard of Care

While scope of care refers to *what* you do, **standard of care** refers generally to *how* you perform first aid. Standard of care refers to what others with the same training would do in a similar situation. It is important to give first aid only as you are trained. Any other actions could result in the injury or illness becoming worse.

Negligence

Legally, you may be liable for the results of your actions if you do not follow accepted standards of care when providing first aid; this is called **negligence.** If you are negligent, an injured party may sue you to recover financial damages for the result of your actions. For you to be found guilty of negligence three conditions must be met:

1. You had a duty to act (for example, first aid is your job responsibility).

Learning
Checkpoint ④

1. True or False: The best thing to do in any emergency is to move the victim to your car and rush to an emergency department.

2. You have a duty to act when

    a. you stop at the scene of an emergency.

    b. you have taken a first aid course.

    c. you have a first aid kit with you.

    d. your job requires you to give first aid when needed.

3. To which of the following victims do you have consent to give first aid? (Check all that apply.)

    _____ An unresponsive victim

    _____ A child without parent or guardian present

    _____ All victims, all of the time

    _____ A victim who nods when you ask if it is okay to give him or her first aid

    _____ A child whose parent or guardian gives consent for him or her

4. Check off things you should always do when giving first aid.

    _____ Move the victim.

    _____ Do what you have been trained to do.

    _____ Try any first aid technique you have read or heard about.

    _____ Ask for the victim's consent.

    _____ Stay with the victim until another trained person takes over.

    _____ Transport all victims to the emergency department in your vehicle.

2. You breached that duty (by not acting or by acting incorrectly).
3. Your actions or inaction caused injury or damages (including such things as physical injury or pain).

Examples of negligent actions could include moving a victim unnecessarily, doing something you have not been trained to do, or failing to give first aid as you have been trained.

Abandonment

Once you begin giving first aid in an emergency, do not stop until another trained person takes over. Stay with the victim until help arrives or someone with equal or greater training takes over. If you leave the victim and the injury or illness becomes worse, this is called **abandonment,** a type of negligence. Note that abandonment is different from justified instances of stopping care, such as that you are exhausted and unable to continue or you are in imminent danger because of hazards at the scene.

Confidentiality

When giving first aid you may learn private information about the victim, and that information should not be shared with anyone other than EMS professionals arriving at the scene to take over care of the victim. Although laws vary in terms of precise definitions regarding violation of privacy, **confidentiality** is the general principle that you should not give out any private information about a victim to anyone except for those caring for the victim.

Concluding Thoughts

How often have you heard people say something like "It can't happen to me?" No one ever expects to be injured seriously or experience a sudden crisis of illness, yet it happens to tens of millions of us every year. In fact, it is almost inevitable that eventually you or someone close to you, perhaps a family member or loved one, will need first aid—and you can be the one who makes the difference. The following chapters will help you to be prepared.

Learning Outcomes

You should now be able to do the following:

1. List the four primary goals of first aid.
2. Explain why there is a need for first aid training.
3. Decide to help in an emergency.
4. Describe how to stay prepared for emergencies.
5. Describe the EMS system and the different types of EMS professionals.
6. Explain when to call 9-1-1 and what information to give the dispatcher.
7. Explain what first aiders need to understand about legal issues related to first aid.

Review Questions

1. The goals of first aid include
   a. keeping the victim alive until he or she receives medical care.
   b. preventing the victim's condition from getting worse.
   c. ensuring the victim receives appropriate medical care.
   d. All of the above

2. If you are in a crowd of people when someone is suddenly injured, it is best to
   a. wait to see if someone steps forward to help the victim.
   b. be confident and do not hesitate to offer your help.
   c. offer your cell phone to anyone who wants to call for help.
   d. stay nearby and wait to see if the victim asks for help.

3. Most nonfatal injuries occur in
   a. workplaces.
   b. homes.
   c. public places.
   d. schools.

4. Your primary role in the EMS system is to
   a. call 9-1-1 in an emergency.
   b. assist the EMS crew in caring for a victim.
   c. diagnose the victim's condition to determine which EMS personnel should come.
   d. advise the dispatcher how many emergency responders to send.

5. Before calling 9-1-1, you should know
   a. where you are.
   b. the telephone number you are calling from.
   c. whether the victim is reponsive.
   d. All of the above

6. For which conditions should you call 9-1-1?
   a. Not breathing, difficulty breathing
   b. Poisoning, drug overdose
   c. Vomiting blood, seizures
   d. All of the above

7. You are obligated to give first aid when
   a. any person who is alone needs it.
   b. the victim is seriously injured.
   c. you have already begun voluntarily giving it.
   d. All of the above

8. You usually automatically have consent to give first aid to
   a. all victims.
   b. all responsive victims.
   c. all unresponsive victims.
   d. all child victims.

9. If a responsive, competent adult refuses your first aid, what should you do?
   a. Give first aid anyway.
   b. Ask the person's spouse for consent to give the first aid.
   c. Walk away.
   d. Call 9-1-1 and keep talking to the victim.

10. Standard of care refers to
    a. what others with your training would do in a similar situation.
    b. the standard duty to act.
    c. having a written authorization to give first aid.
    d. guidelines published by the government.

References and Resources

Bureau of Labor Statistics, U.S. Department of Labor. www.bls.gov

Bureau of Labor Statistics, U.S. Department of Labor. Census of fatal occupational injuries. 2002. www.bls.gov

Bureau of Labor Statistics, U.S. Department of Labor. Survey of occupational injuries and illnesses. 2001. www.bls.gov

National Academies of Emergency Dispatch. Medical emergencies: When to call and what to expect when you dial 9-1-1. ASHI/NAED; 2002.

National Center for Health Statistics. www.cdc.gov/nchs/

National Safety Council. www.nsc.org

National Safety Council. Injury facts 2005. Published by National Safety Council, Chicago, IL.

Chapter 2
Acting in an Emergency

Chapter Preview

- Preventing Disease Transmission

- Responding to Emergencies

- After an Emergency

You are driving home from work when you see a vehicle a block ahead swerve off the road. It strikes a telephone pole, which breaks off, and a power line falls down on top of the vehicle. You pull to a stop some distance back. You can see the driver inside, and he is not moving. What should you do?

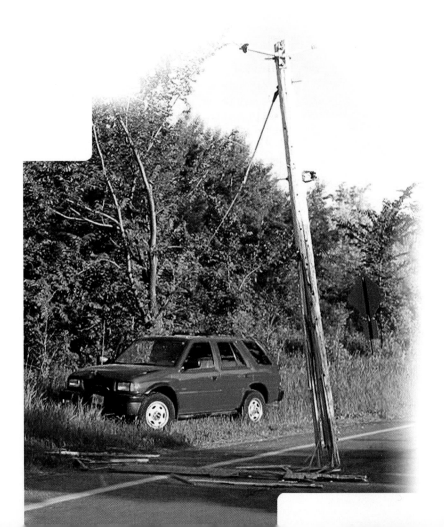

A medical emergency caused by injury or sudden illness can occur at any time in any place. Emergencies vary in many different ways. These may include:

- The nature of the injury or illness
- The severity of the injury or illness
- The presence of other injuries or factors affecting the victim's well-being
- The scene of the emergency (indoors, outdoors, potential hazards present, etc.)
- The victim (child, adult, elderly, friend, stranger, etc.)

Because of these and other factors, no two emergency situations are identical. Yet certain key principles apply to all emergencies. In all emergencies involving injury or illness you should always follow the same basic steps outlined in this chapter.

PREVENTING DISEASE TRANSMISSION

In any emergency situation there is some risk of a first aider getting an infectious disease from a victim who has a disease. That risk is very low, however, and taking steps to avoid being infected greatly reduces that risk.

How Are Infectious Diseases Transmitted?

The transmission of infectious disease occurs through a process involving four stages **(Figure 2-1)**:

1. The process begins with *someone or something having the infection.*
2. *The infectious pathogen (disease-causing bacteria, virus, fungus, or parasite) leaves the infected person's body.* For example:

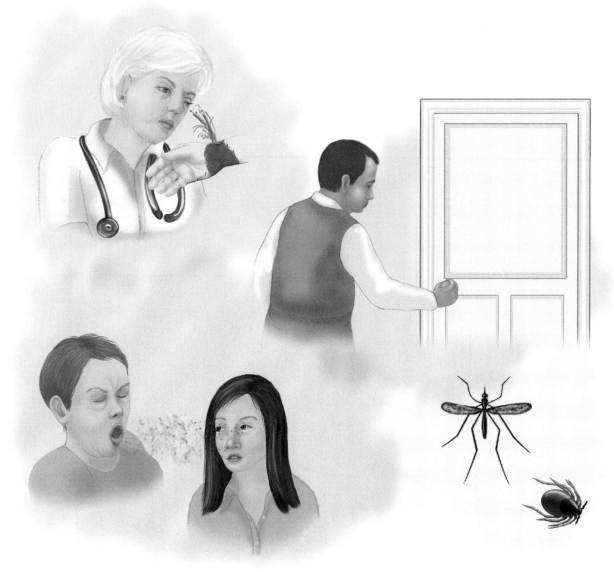

Figure 2-1 Different modes of disease transmission.

- The person may bleed from a cut, and in that person's blood is the pathogen.
- The person may sneeze out little droplets carrying the pathogen.

3. *The infectious pathogen reaches another person and enters his or her body.* This can happen in a number of ways:

- The person may come into contact with the infected person's blood, other body fluid, or infectious material in a way that the pathogen enters his or her body through mucous membranes or nonintact skin (**bloodborne transmission**).
- The person may inhale the pathogen in tiny droplets from the air (**airborne transmission**).
- The person may be bitten by an insect, such as a tick or mosquito, carrying the pathogen (**vector transmission** of bloodborne pathogen).

The transmission of a pathogen from one person to another is said to occur through direct or indirect contact:

- **Direct contact** occurs from contact with an infected person or with fluids or substances from that person.
- **Indirect contact** occurs from contact with contaminated objects, food or drink, droplets in the air, or vectors such as insects.

4. *The second person develops the infection.* Just having the pathogen enter the body does not automatically mean a person will become ill. If vaccinated against the disease, the body will kill the pathogen before it can cause disease. A person's immune system may be able to kill some pathogens and thereby prevent illness. If it does not, a person may become infected. The process then starts all over again.

Bloodborne Disease

Several serious diseases can be transmitted from one person to another through contact with the infected person's blood. These are called **bloodborne diseases.** Bacteria or viruses that cause such diseases, called pathogens, are also present in some other body fluids, such as semen, vaginal secretions, and bloody saliva or vomit. Other body fluids such as nasal secretions, sweat, tears, and urine do not normally transmit pathogens. Three serious bloodborne infections are HIV, hepatitis B, and hepatitis C (**Table 2-1**).

Protection Against Bloodborne Disease

Because these bloodborne diseases cannot be cured, they should be prevented. The best prevention is to avoid contact with *all* victims' blood and body fluids. You cannot know whether a victim (even a close friend) is infected as often these diseases do not produce signs and symptoms. Even victims may not know that they are infected.

The Centers for Disease Control and Prevention (CDC) therefore recommends taking **standard precautions** whenever you give first aid. The term **universal precautions** is also used to describe measures to prevent infection (**Box 2-1**). Take these precautions for all victims, all the time, and always assume that blood and other body fluids may be infected. Follow these recommendations to avoid coming into contact with a victim's blood or body fluids:

- Use personal protective equipment.
- If you do not have medical exam gloves with you, put your hands in plastic bags or have the victim dress his or her own wound.
- Wash your hands with soap and water before and after giving first aid.
- Keep a barrier (such as gloves or a dry cloth) between body fluids and yourself.
- Cover any cuts or scrapes on your skin with protective clothing or gloves.
- Do not touch your mouth, nose, or eyes when giving first aid (e.g., do not eat, drink, or smoke).
- Do not touch objects soiled with blood or body fluids.
- Be careful to avoid being cut by anything sharp at the emergency scene, such as broken glass or torn metal.
- Use absorbent material to soak up spilled blood or body fluids, and dispose of it appropriately. Clean the area with a commercial **disinfectant** or a freshly made 10% bleach solution.
- If you are exposed to a victim's blood or body fluid, wash immediately with soap and water and call your healthcare provider. At work, report the situation to your supervisor.

Handwashing

Effective handwashing is essential for preventing disease transmission. Follow these guidelines (see Skill "Handwashing"):

- Wash any exposed skin, ideally with antibacterial soap, as soon after an exposure as possible.

Box 2-1 Infection Control Terminology

Because of changes in infection control terminology over the last two decades, there has been some confusion about the exact meanings and applications of the terms *universal precautions, standard precautions,* and *body substance isolation.*

Universal precautions is the term CDC originally promoted in 1987 for actions to protect providers of first aid and healthcare from exposure to bloodborne pathogens. Universal precautions apply to all people's blood, semen, vaginal secretions, and other body fluids containing visible blood or to any objects potentially contaminated with any of these. In its 1991 Bloodborne Pathogens Standard, OSHA required the use of universal precautions, which it defined as "an approach to infection control. According to the concept of Universal Precautions, all human blood and certain human body fluids are treated as if known to be infectious for HIV, HBV, and other bloodborne pathogens." Many healthcare and first aid providers continue to use the term universal precautions, in part because this is the term used in federal and many state laws.

At the same time, many healthcare institutions were following principles of **body sub-stance isolation (BSI),** an infection control concept that originated in efforts to control all infections (not just bloodborne pathogens) that occur within healthcare facilities. BSI precautions assume that *any* body fluid or moist body tissue is potentially infectious.

In 1996 CDC published new guidelines called **standard precautions** intended primarily for infectious disease control within healthcare facilities. Standard precautions combine the major features of universal precautions and BSI precautions. Although some providers feel that standard precautions have replaced universal precautions, CDC states: "Standard precautions were developed for use in hospitals and may not necessarily be indicated in other settings where universal precautions are used, such as child care settings and schools." (*Source: http://www.cdc. gov/ncidod/hip/Blood/UNIVERSA.HTM*)

Because standard precautions are more rigorous than universal precautions, this text will use the term standard precautions. Recognize, however, that in many first aid situations universal precautions are appropriate.

- While washing, be gentle with any scabs or sores.
- Wash all surfaces, including the backs of hands, wrists, between the fingers, and under fingernails.
- Wash hands immediately after removing gloves or other personal protective equipment.
- Before handling any potentially infectious materials, know where the nearest handwashing facility is. You can use facilities such as restrooms, janitor closets, and laboratory sinks, as long as soap is available.
- Do not use sinks in areas where food is prepared.
- Merely wetting the hands will not prevent infection.
- If antiseptic towelettes or antibacterial

handwashing liquid is used without water for the initial cleaning after an exposure, a thorough scrubbing with soap and water is still needed as soon as possible **(Figure 2-2).**

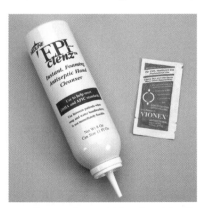

Figure 2-2 Waterless antibacterial handwashing liquid and towelette.

Table 2-1

Bloodborne Disease

Disease	Prevalence	Modes of Transmission	Signs and Symptoms	Testing	Prevention
Acquired immunodeficiency syndrome (AIDS), caused by human immunodeficiency virus (HIV). Eventually fatal.	Almost one million HIV-positive people in the U.S., one-fourth of whom are unaware of their infection	Through infected person's body fluids, including: - Blood - Semen - Vaginal secretions - Breast milk Other body fluids if blood is present. Not by casual contact.	HIV often has no symptoms. AIDS symptoms may include: - Loss of appetite - Weight loss - Fever - Skin rashes - Swollen lymph nodes - Diarrhea - Tiredness - Night sweats - Inability to fight off infection	Blood test Recommended after a potential exposure. Generally positive 12 weeks after exposure. Confirmation test recommended 6 months after an exposure.	No vaccine currently available. Safe first aid practices significantly reduce the risk of contracting HIV or other infectious diseases. - Regular handwashing - Use of barriers - Standard precautions
Hepatitis B (serum hepatitis) Caused by the hepatitis B virus (HBV). Major cause of liver damage, cirrhosis, and liver cancer.	About 80,000 new infections yearly. 1.25 million chronic carriers. 5000 people die of liver problems associated with HBV infection every year.	Transmitted by blood and materials contaminated with blood or body fluids. Blood and semen are the most infectious. - By injection (**needlesticks** or puncture wounds) - Through mucous membranes (blood contamination through eye or mouth) and nonintact skin - Through sexual activity - From infected mother to newborn at birth. Virus may survive for several days in dried body fluids on surfaces.	Often no symptoms. Symptoms usually appear gradually: - Loss of appetite - Nausea - Fatigue - Muscle or joint aches - Mild fever - Stomach pain - Occasionally jaundice (yellow tint to whites of eyes or skin)	Blood test.	Use same precautions as with HIV. Vaccine is available and recommended for healthcare workers and professional rescuers. Employees at risk must be offered free vaccinations by employer. Vaccine also recommended for: - Those having unprotected sex with a partner with HBV or with multiple partners. - Those having anal sex - Those using intravenous drugs - Those with hemophilia - Those who frequently work in countries where HBV is common - Those who live with someone with chronic HBV

Table 2-1 (Continued)

Bloodborne Disease

Disease	Prevalence	Modes of Transmission	Signs and Symptoms	Testing	Prevention
Hepatitis C Caused by the hepatitis C virus (HCV). Causes liver disease; may result in eventual liver failure.	About 25,000 new infections each year. 2.7 million people in the U.S. have chronic HCV infection.	Spread most often through drug injections with contaminated needles. May result from unclean tattoo or body piercing tools or from any item contaminated with blood. Spread through any direct contact with infectious blood.	Usually no symptoms. Occasionally one or more of the following symptoms: - Fatigue - Loss of appetite - Nausea - Anxiety - Weight loss - Alcohol intolerance - Abdominal pain - Loss of concentration - Jaundice	Blood test. Anyone testing positive should have follow-up test. Testing recommended for: - Healthcare workers exposed to HCV-positive blood - Anyone who has used intravenous recreational drugs - Anyone receiving a blood transfusion, organ transplant, or kidney dialysis before 1992 - Anyone treated with a blood product prior to 1987 - Anyone with signs of liver disease	No vaccine available. Use same precautions as with HIV: - Follow barrier practices to prevent contact with blood. - Avoid recreational intravenous drug use. - Do not share toothbrushes, razors, or other items that may be contaminated with blood. - Remember health risks associated with tattoos and body piercing if sanitary practices are not followed.

Personal Protective Equipment

Personal protective equipment (PPE) is any equipment used to protect yourself from contact with blood or other body fluids. PPE includes gloves, barrier devices, and other devices.

Gloves

Most important, keep **medical exam gloves** in your first aid kit and wear them in most first aid situations (**Figure 2-3**). Gloves are a type of barrier; like other barriers, they separate you from potentially

Skill   Handwashing

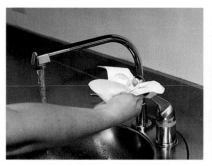

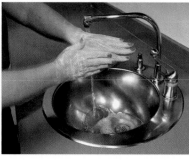

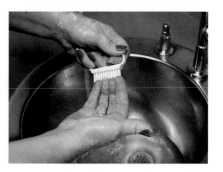

1 Remove any jewelry and your watch. Use a paper towel to turn on water, and adjust the temperature to warm.

2 Wet your hands to above the wrists and lather up with soap. Keep your hands below your elbows throughout the handwashing.

3 Wash all areas of your hands and wrists. Interlace fingers to scrub between them. If your hands were exposed to infectious material, scrub beneath fingernails with a nail brush or nail stick.

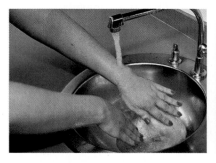

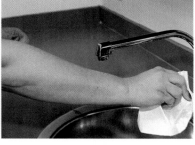

4 Rinse wrists and hands well. (Repeat soaping and washing if your hands were exposed to infectious material.)

5 Dry hands thoroughly with paper towel, and dispose of it properly. Use a new dry paper towel to turn off the water faucet and open the door, and dispose of it properly.

---

infectious materials (see Skill: "Putting on Gloves" and Skill: "Removing Contaminated Gloves"). Medical exam gloves suitable for protection from bloodborne pathogens are made of nitrile, vinyl, **latex,** or other waterproof materials **(Box 2-2)**. For added barrier protection, two pairs of gloves may be worn together in some situations.

When using gloves it is important to remember the following:

- *Check that your gloves are intact.* Check before you put them on and periodically

afterwards. If a hole or tear is present, replace the glove immediately with a new one.
- *Do not use petroleum-based hand lotions.* These lotions may cause latex gloves to disintegrate.
- *Remove contaminated gloves carefully.* Do not touch any part of the contaminated outside of the gloves.
- *Dispose of gloves properly.* After working with any material that may be infected by bloodborne

Box 2-2 Latex Glove Allergy

Medical exam gloves are often made of latex rubber, to which some people are allergic. Signs and symptoms of latex allergy may include skin rashes, hives, itching eyes or skin, flushing, watery or swollen eyes, runny nose, or an asthmatic reaction. Use gloves made of vinyl or other material if you have any of these symptoms or if you work with patients who may have latex allergy.

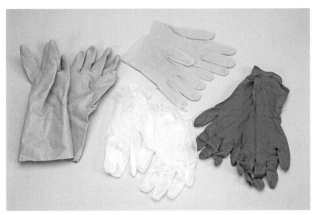

Figure 2-3 Wear gloves to protect yourself from contact with blood or other body fluids.

pathogens, dispose of your gloves in a container clearly marked for biohazardous waste.

- *Handle sharp objects carefully.* Gloves protect against infectious substances but not against sharp objects such as needles that may also transmit infection.

Barrier Devices

A **barrier device** is a pocket face mask or face shield used when giving rescue breaths during cardiopulmonary resuscitation (CPR). This device should be in the first aid kit, and you should always use it for added protection. Because giving rescue breaths with a barrier device can greatly reduce the chance of an infectious disease being transmitted from or to a victim, the use of a barrier device is always recommended **(Figure 2-4)**. **Chapter 5** discusses uses of airway barrier devices more fully.

Other PPE Devices

Other PPE devices include eye protection, masks, and gowns or aprons. These are not required in most first aid situations, although OSHA requires such protections be available in some workplaces. In such cases, OSHA requires employees to be trained in the use of this PPE. Healthcare workers, for example, are required to wear masks and protective eyewear or face shields during procedures that are likely to generate droplets of blood or body fluids, and gowns or aprons when blood or body fluid may be splashed.

Disposal and Disinfection of Supplies and Equipment

Preventing disease transmission also involves correct disposal or disinfection of used first aid supplies and equipment after caring for a victim. First aid kits include many disposable supplies, such as dressings and bandages, that may become soiled by a victim's blood or other body fluids. These must be appropriately disposed of since such items may remain infectious for some time after use. Never reuse any equipment or supplies that are meant to be disposable. Other equipment, such as tweezers used to remove debris from a wound, require disinfection after use.

If EMS arrives to care for a victim of an emergency, they will usually manage the disposal

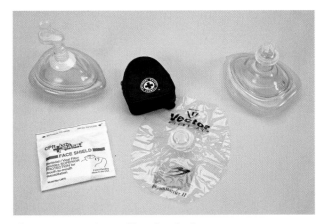

Figure 2-4 Variety of barrier devices.

Skill   Putting on Gloves

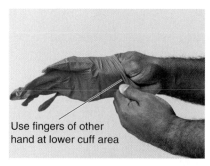

Use fingers of other
hand at lower cuff area

1 Pull glove onto one hand.

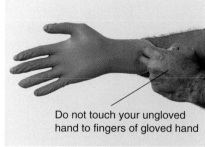

Do not touch your ungloved
hand to fingers of gloved hand

2 Pull glove tight.

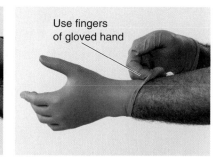

Use fingers
of gloved hand

3 Put on other glove.

Skill   Removing Contaminated Gloves

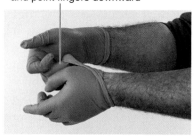

Hold hands away from body
and point fingers downward

1 With one hand, grasp your
other glove at the wrist or
palm and pull it away from
your hand.

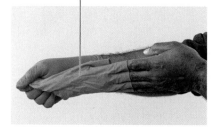

Remove the glove
inside out

2 Pull the glove the rest of the
way off.

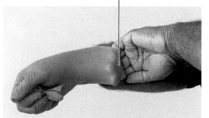

Do not touch the contaminated
outer surface of the glove

3 Holding the removed glove
balled up in the palm of
your gloved hand, insert two
fingers under the cuff of the
remaining glove.

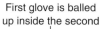

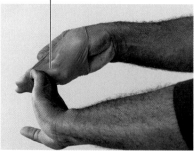

First glove is balled
up inside the second

4 Remove the glove by stretching it up and away from the
hand and turning it inside out
as you pull it off.

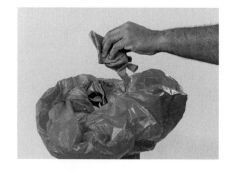

5 Dispose of gloves in a bio-
hazard container and wash
your hands.

Learning
Checkpoint (1)

1. True or False: Bloodborne diseases are transmitted only through contact with an infected person's blood.

2. True or False: The risk of getting a serious infectious disease by giving first aid is greatly reduced when you take precautions.

3. Standard precautions include:

    a. Treat all victims as if their body fluids were infected.

    b. Always wear gloves if blood may be present.

    c. Do not touch your mouth, nose, or eyes when giving first aid.

    d. All of the above

4. Check off which of the following situations could lead to your getting an infectious disease.

    _____ a. Touching a bloody bandage in a trash can

    _____ b. Shaking hands with a person infected with HIV

    _____ c. Receiving a hepatitis B vaccination

    _____ d. Not wearing gloves and giving first aid if you have a cut on your finger

    _____ e. Being near a person with hepatitis C who is coughing

    _____ f. Contact with an unresponsive victim's urine

5. List at least three symptoms of a latex glove allergy. _____

_____

---

of any soiled or infectious materials resulting from first aid care you have given. When professional rescuers are not involved, however, you need to ensure that soiled materials do not come into contact with other people. Many workplaces have a system in place for disposing of hazardous wastes; follow your company's policy. In the home, soiled supplies should be sealed inside a heavy plastic bag that is then sealed inside a second bag before being put in the trash. Make sure others do not come into contact with this trash. For contaminated **sharps** such as needles used for insulin injections or lancets used to draw blood for glucose testing, special containers are required to prevent risks to those handling the trash; talk with your healthcare provider about how to properly dispose of these objects.

To disinfect equipment or surfaces that are soiled by blood or other body fluids, use a 10% solution of household bleach in water. Wear gloves and clean the items or area thoroughly. If clothing or other fabrics are soiled, wash them by themselves in hot, soapy water for at least 25 minutes. Be sure to take a shower and wash well because your skin may have been contaminated through the clothing.

RESPONDING TO EMERGENCIES

There are six basic steps to follow in any emergency:

1. Recognize the emergency.
2. Check the scene.
3. Call 9-1-1 (when appropriate).
4. Check the victim.
5. Give first aid.
6. Have the victim seek medical attention (when appropriate).

Recognize the Emergency

You usually know there is an emergency when you see one. You see an injured or ill victim, or someone acting strangely. You may hear signs of an emergency and realize that someone may be hurt. For example, you might look in the door of a co-worker's office and see a coffee cup overturned on the desk and the telephone receiver off the hook—and then see the man collapsed on the other side of the desk. You may see a crushed bicycle unattended alongside the road—and after checking further see a child lying in the ditch. In situations like this the victim's life may depend on someone recognizing the signs that there is something wrong and taking the time to investigate.

Check the Scene

Once you realize there is an emergency and someone is injured or ill, before going to the victim look to see if there may be other victims. You may need to call immediately for help for multiple victims. Look for any clues that may help you to determine what happened and what first aid may be needed. Also, look for bystanders who may be able to help give first aid or go to a telephone to call 9-1-1.

When we see that someone needs our help, our first tendency is often to rush in to help. In many emergency situations, however, hazards may be present in the scene. For example, if you saw smoke coming out of a window of a house where you know an elderly man lives, your first thought might be to rush inside to rescue him. Consider, however, that you too might be overcome by smoke. Not only would you not have helped the original victim, but you would have become a second victim yourself for others to rescue and care for.

Therefore it is important, when you recognize that an emergency has occurred, to always check the scene before approaching a victim. Remember that you must be safe yourself if you are to help another. Look for any hazards such as the following:

- Smoke, flames
- Spilled gasoline or chemicals, fumes
- Downed electrical wires
- Risk of explosion, building collapse
- Roadside dangers, high-speed traffic
- Deep water, ice
- Potential for violence from someone present in the scene

If the scene is dangerous and you cannot safely approach the victim, *stay away and call for help.* Remember that help is usually only minutes away. The 9-1-1 dispatcher will send a crew with the appropriate training and equipment to safely reach and care for the victim. You may be able to monitor the scene from a safe distance and provide responding EMS personnel with critical information such as the location of the victim. **Box 2-3** describes some specific examples of hazardous situations.

Scene safety also includes protecting yourself from exposure to potentially infectious body fluids or other materials. As you approach a victim, for example, consider the need for using PPE as discussed earlier in this chapter.

Call 9-1-1

Call 9-1-1 (or your local or company emergency number) immediately if you recognize a life-threatening injury or illness. Do not try to transport a victim to the emergency department yourself in such cases. In some exceptional circumstances you may give about two minutes of care before calling 9-1-1.

If the victim is responsive and may not be seriously injured or ill, go on to the next step to check the victim further before calling 9-1-1—and then call 9-1-1 or a healthcare provider if needed.

Check the Victim

When you reach the victim, first check for life-threatening conditions requiring immediate first aid. These include being unresponsive or any threat to the victim's breathing or circulation. If the victim does not have a life-threatening condition, you then go on to look for lesser conditions requiring first aid. **Chapter 4** describes in detail both of these assessments. Unless the scene is dangerous or it is necessary to care for a life-threatening problem, do not move the victim. **Chapter 25** describes how to move a victim when necessary.

Give First Aid

Give first aid once you have checked the victim and know his or her condition. Later chapters describe the first aid steps for the conditions you are likely to find. **Basic life support** is first aid given to a victim with a life-threatening problem of breathing or circulation. Generally you provide basic life support to keep the victim alive until advanced help arrives. In most cases, however, the victim's condition is not

Box 2-3 Hazardous Scenes

Traffic Accidents

Vehicle crash scenes can be extremely dangerous for rescuers because of the risks from passing vehicles, downed electrical wires, fire or explosion, vehicle instability, or other conditions. Rescuers have also been injured by accidentally setting off an automatic airbag when attempting to reach a victim pinned inside a vehicle. For all these reasons it is crucial to ensure that the scene is safe before approaching the vehicle. Do not try to stabilize the vehicle unless you have special training. Never try to remove a victim trapped inside a vehicle, but wait for professional rescuers. You may be able to provide some first aid through an open window or from the back seat.

Fire Scenes

Never enter a burning or smoky building unless you have special training and are functioning as a part of a fire department. Firefighters are highly trained and use special equipment that protects against fire and smoke. Do not let others enter or approach a fire scene. Make sure 9-1-1 has been called, and then try to gather information for responding fire and EMS units, such as the possible number and location of victims, the cause of the fire, the presence of any explosives or chemicals, and other relevant facts.

Electricity

Downed electrical lines at an emergency scene are a major hazard to both the victim and rescuers. Never try to move downed wires, but call 9-1-1 immediately. If downed wires are across a vehicle, do not touch the vehicle. If there are victims in the vehicle, tell them to remain still and not exit the vehicle. Never attempt to remove a victim from a vehicle with a downed wire across it, no matter how seriously injured the victim may be. If there are downed wires across a chain link fence, metal structure, or body of water, do not approach the scene.

Water and Ice Hazards

Water and ice create several hazards. Never enter deep water to reach a victim unless you have been properly trained, and then do so only as a last resort. Instead, try to get a flotation device or rope to the victim **(See Chapter 25)**. Fast-flowing water is a common hazard following natural disasters such as floods and hurricanes. Never enter moving water but wait for trained rescue personnel. A fast water rescue requires careful planning, proper equipment, and training. Ice is also treacherous. Cold-water immersion is very serious and can quickly doom even the best swimmers. Ice rescue should be left for specially trained personnel who have the necessary safety equipment.

Natural Disasters

Natural disasters include such events as tornados, hurricanes, earthquakes, forest and range fires, and floods. Rescue efforts after a natural disaster are usually coordinated through a governmental agency such as the federal or state emergency management agency. If you find yourself in a natural disaster, make personal safety your highest priority. Natural disasters often involve more hazards than you might think, including electrical risks, hazardous materials, and fast-moving water **(See Appendices C, D, E, and F)**.

Hazardous Materials

A hazardous material is any substance, liquid or solid, that is highly flammable, explosive, caustic, toxic, radioactive, or otherwise dangerous. Hazardous materials are usually marked with warning placards **(Figure 2-5)**, but treat any unknown substance as a hazard until proven otherwise. Avoid any spilled liquid or powder as well as possible fumes. Especially dangerous is a vehicular collision involving a truck carrying hazardous materials. Stay well out of the area of a hazardous material spill and keep bystanders away. Call 9-1-1 and let trained **hazmat** professionals handle the emergency.

(continued)

Box 2-3 Hazardous Scenes (continued)

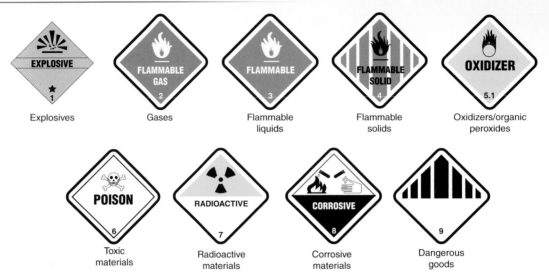

Figure 2-5 A variety of hazardous materials placards.

Hazardous materials are not limited to industrial sites and transportation. There are many potential hazards in the home, including natural gas, gasoline, kerosene, pesticides, and many others. Many hazardous materials are odorless and not easily detected. Some hazardous materials, such as natural gas, are explosion hazards. A seemingly harmless action such as turning on a light switch or using a cell phone may make a spark and set off an explosion.

Unsafe Buildings/Structures

Buildings and other structures may be unsafe because of fire, an explosion, a natural disaster, or deterioration. Never enter an unsafe building alone because of the risk of collapsing structures, hazardous materials, fire, and so on. Call 9-1-1 and let properly trained and equipped professionals manage the rescue.

Wreckage

Wreckage at the scene from an automobile, aircraft, or machinery is hazardous because of the presence of sharp pieces of metal, glass, fuel, and moving parts. The wreckage may also be unstable. Stay out of the scene and call 9-1-1.

Suicide

If a person is threatening suicide and has a weapon, do not enter the scene but call 9-1-1 or law enforcement personnel. **Chapter 22** discusses behavioral emergencies such as suicidal or potentially violent victims.

Hostile Victim/Family

Occasionally a victim or family member may be hostile when you approach or offer first aid. Rage or hostility in a victim may be due to the injury or illness or to emotional factors. Many emergency victims are afraid of losing control, and their fear may become anger. Drug or alcohol abuse may also cause hostile behavior. If a victim seems hostile, first try to quietly explain who you are and that you are there to help them. Often after the victim realizes that you are not a threat but are there to help, the hostility will dissipate. But if the victim refuses your care or threatens you, retreat from the scene and call 9-1-1. Never try to restrain, argue with, or force care upon a victim. **Chapter 22** discusses how to deal with behavioral emergencies such as violent people.

Hostile family members too can be a problem, usually because they are fearful. Listen to what they have to say and act accordingly. If the situation remains hostile, retreat to a safe distance and wait for police officers and other EMS personnel. If at any time your personal safety appears threatened, leave the scene immediately.

life threatening, and your first aid consists of simple actions you can take to help the victim.

Note that first aiders do not administer medications, even aspirin, to victims because of the risks of allergy or other complications. In some cases first aiders may help victims to take their own medications if needed.

Have the Victim Seek Medical Attention

As noted earlier, call 9-1-1 immediately for any emergency (life-threatening) condition. In many cases the injury or sudden illness is not an emergency and you do not need to call 9-1-1, but the victim still needs to see a healthcare provider. For example, a victim may have a serious cut on the arm that stops bleeding quickly when you give first aid. Because of the risk of infection, or because the cut may need stitches to heal well, the victim needs medical attention and should be transported to a hospital emergency department or his or her healthcare provider. Later chapters about specific injuries and problems describe when a victim needs to go to the emergency department or see a healthcare provider. When in doubt, at least call a healthcare provider to see if medical care may be needed.

AFTER AN EMERGENCY

Arriving EMS professionals will take over the care of the victim (**Figure 2-6**). Continue giving first aid

until EMS personnel ask you to stop, as it may take a few minutes for emergency responders to prepare equipment and take over. Then you may still assist with crowd control, obtaining information from bystanders, or assisting the emergency responders in other ways. Depending on the situation, you may have other follow-up activities. If the emergency was traumatic or especially stressful, you may also need help coping with the effects of stress.

After giving first aid, be sure to wash your hands and clean the area well. If the emergency involved bleeding or contamination of the area with other body fluids, disinfect surfaces using a bleach solution or other approved disinfectant. Dispose of all potentially contaminated materials appropriately. If you were in contact with any of the victim's body fluids, report this to the emergency responders so that they can take appropriate action.

Follow-Up Activities

Arriving EMS professionals who take over the care of the victim will ask you questions about what happened, what you observed about the victim, and what first aid you gave. Answer as fully as you can, because the details you provide may be important for the victim's medical care. Review the entire experience in your mind to make sure you have not forgotten to relay some

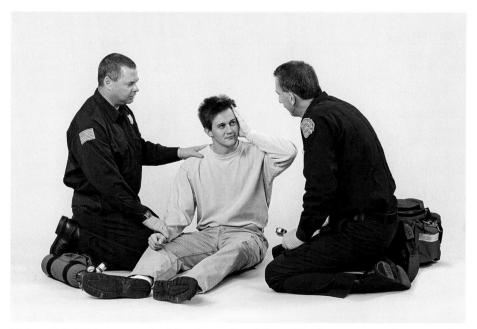

Figure 2-6 EMS personnel with advanced training will take over care of an injured or ill victim after 9-1-1 is called.

important piece of information. For example, a victim who became unresponsive while you were giving him first aid may have experienced a poisoning, and anything the victim said or did when you first saw him may offer medical workers a clue about his condition.

Your descriptions to EMS personnel of what happened and what you did may be, in some situations, a form of legal documentation of actions. If you have any reason to think you may be questioned in the future about your actions, it may be helpful to write down what happened and exactly what you did.

Some emergencies may be related to a crime, such as injuries resulting from an assault or abuse. In such cases the first responders to the scene will help ensure that possible evidence is not destroyed or altered, and law enforcement officials will arrive to preserve and investigate the scene. If you gave first aid to the victim of a crime, your descriptions of what you witnessed may become legal evidence. It is important to cooperate fully with police officers and, again, be as detailed as possible in recounting your observations.

Coping with a Traumatic Event

Emergencies are stressful, especially when the victim does not survive. Not even medical professionals can save every victim. Injuries, illness, or circumstances are often beyond our control. Particularly stressful emergencies include those that involve multiple victims, children, victims of abuse or neglect, and death or injury of a co-worker or friend.

It is normal to have a strong emotional reaction during and immediately after a stressful emergency. Often this reaction gradually diminishes with time, but in some cases the stress remains and problems may result. Stress can cause irritability when interacting with others, difficulty sleeping, problems concentrating, general anxiety or depression, and even physical symptoms. If you recognize that you are feeling or behaving differently after experiencing a traumatic emergency, you may need help coping.

- Talk to others: family members, co-workers, local emergency responders, or your own healthcare provider (without breaching the confidentiality of the victim).
- Remind yourself that your reaction is normal, that we all need help sometimes.
- Do not be afraid or reluctant to seek professional help. Students should ask at the student health center, and employees should check with their human resource department about an employee assistance program or member assistance program. Your healthcare provider can also make a referral.

Learning
Checkpoint ②

1. True or False: If you see someone injured in an emergency, the first thing to do is get to him or her quickly and check his or her condition.

2. When you encounter an injured victim, you should

   a. give first aid until help arrives.

   b. help a victim only if the scene is safe.

   c. call 9-1-1 for life-threatening injuries.

   d. All of the above

3. Which of the following scenes are unsafe?

   _____ Spilled hazardous materials   _____ Structure fires

   _____ Downed electrical wires   _____ Hostile person with a weapon

Concluding Thoughts

Emergency situations vary widely, but in all cases you respond to the emergency in the same basic way: Make sure the scene is safe, check the victim for life-threatening conditions and call 9-1-1, and give the appropriate first aid using standard precautions to minimize your exposure to infectious disease. These principles for acting in an emergency not only guide your response but also ensure your safety while you give the most effective care to someone in need.

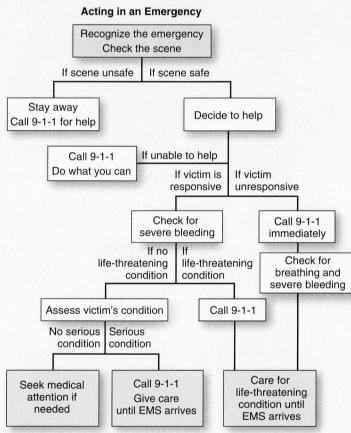

Acting in an Emergency

Learning Outcomes

You should now be able to do the following:

1. Explain how bloodborne pathogens may be transmitted from an infected person to someone else.
2. List several common serious bloodborne diseases.
3. Describe standard precautions to take when giving first aid to prevent disease transmission.

4. Describe the step-by-step actions to take whenever you recognize an emergency.
5. List 8 to 10 types of dangerous emergency scenes you should not enter.
6. List signs of stress that may occur after an emergency and describe how one can get help if needed.

Review Questions

1. A bloodborne pathogen can enter your body through
    a. any break in your skin.
    b. food cooked by someone else.
    c. the municipal water supply.
    d. any physical touching of the victim's skin.

2. Bloodborne pathogens may also be transmitted in
    a. semen.
    b. vaginal secretions.
    c. bloody vomit.
    d. All of the above

3. HIV infection can be prevented when giving first aid by
    a. avoiding all contact with known HIV-positive individuals.
    b. following standard precautions.
    c. getting vaccinated.
    d. wearing a face mask.

4. An effective way to avoid becoming infected when giving first aid is to
    a. ask the victim what diseases he or she may have before giving first aid.
    b. check an unresponsive victim for a medical alert bracelet or necklace.
    c. use barriers to prevent contact with any blood or body fluid.
    d. never touch the victim.

5. Standard precautions include
    a. wearing a face mask with all victims.
    b. using personal protective equipment.
    c. asking a victim about any communicable diseases before giving first aid.
    d. checking a victim's medical record after giving first aid.

6. If you think someone may be inside a house where you see smoke coming from a window, you should

    a. enter only the first floor if you see smoke from an upstairs window.

    b. take a deep breath and hold it while you run inside to look; try not to breathe once inside.

    c. search the house, staying low to the floor on hands and knees.

    d. not go inside but call 9-1-1 immediately.

7. You witness a low-speed car crash into a telephone pole. The driver has no obvious wounds and says he is okay. But he has not moved from behind the wheel, and he looks pale and shaky. What should you do?

    a. Call 9-1-1 and let the dispatcher decide what help may be needed.

    b. Call 9-1-1 only if the driver first gives his consent for you to call.

    c. Ask the driver to get into your vehicle so you can drive him to the nearest hospital.

    d. Wait for a police car to stop; the officer will decide whether help is needed.

8. When you have given first aid to a victim, you should tell arriving EMS personnel

    a. what happened.

    b. what you observed about the victim.

    c. what first aid you gave.

    d. All of the above

References and Resources

Centers for Disease Control and Prevention. Universal precautions for prevention of transmission of HIV and other bloodborne infections. 2004. Available from: www.cdc.gov

National Center for Infectious Diseases. Viral Hepatitis A fact sheet. Centers for Disease Control and Prevention. 2004. Available from: www.cdc.gov

National Center for Infectious Diseases. Viral Hepatitis B fact sheet. Centers for Disease Control and Prevention. 2004. Available from: www.cdc.gov

National Center for Infectious Diseases. Viral Hepatitis C frequently asked questions. Centers for Disease Control and Prevention. 2004. Available from: www.cdc.gov

National Institute for Occupational Safety and Health. Latex allergy: a prevention guide. Centers for Disease Control and Prevention. 2004. Available from: www.cdc.gov

National Safety Council. www.nsc.org

Occupational Safety and Health Administration. Bloodborne facts: personal protective equipment cuts risk. U.S. Department of Labor; 2004.

Occupational Safety and Health Administration. Bloodborne facts: holding the line on contamination. U.S. Department of Labor; 2004.

Occupational Safety and Health Administration. OSHA factsheet: bloodborne pathogens. 2004. Available from: www.osha.gov

Occupational Safety and Health Administration. www.osha.gov

Chapter 3

The Human Body

Chapter Preview

You are called to the storage area at the back of the warehouse where an employee has just been found lying on the floor. As you approach, you think that she may have fallen from the stepladder or a higher shelf, but you do not immediately see what is wrong.

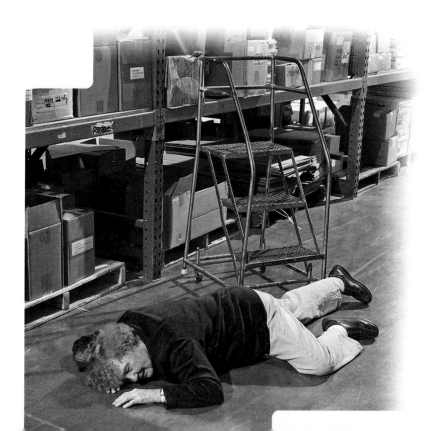

The human body is composed of many different organs and tissues, all working together to sustain life and allow for activity. In health, each organ performs its functions in concert with other body parts and organs. With injury or illness, however, one or more parts of the body are damaged or functioning less effectively. A minor injury may damage only a specific body part or function, but a serious injury or sudden illness can threaten body functions that are necessary for life. Understanding the human body will help you recognize the effects of injuries and illnesses and give effective first aid until the victim receives medical attention.

PRIMARY AREAS OF THE BODY

A detailed understanding of medical language is not necessary for giving first aid and communicating with medical professionals, as when speaking with the 9-1-1 dispatcher. It is helpful, however, to understand the general areas of the body when describing an injury or the victim's signs and symptoms of illness. Following are key terms referring to body areas **(Figure 3-1)**:

- *Extremities.* This refers to both the arms and the legs. Many first aid principles are the same for all the extremities, so this term is often used rather than saying "arms and legs."

- *Thorax.* This refers to the chest area enclosed by the ribs (including the back of the body). The thoracic cavity is the area inside the chest where the heart and lungs are located.

- *Abdomen.* This refers to the area immediately below the thoracic cavity. The stomach, intestines, and other organs are located in the abdominal cavity. For the purposes of describing the location of injuries or signs and symptoms, the abdomen is often divided into quadrants based on the body's midline and an imaginary horizontal line through the umbilicus (navel) **(Figure 3-2)**. The **diaphragm,** a muscle used in breathing, is located between the thoracic cavity and the abdominal cavity.

- *Pelvis.* This refers generally to the area below the abdomen and specifically to the pelvic bones between the hip and the lower spine. In the pelvic cavity are located the bladder and reproductive organs.

- *Spine (spinal column).* This refers to the bones **(vertebrae)** of the back and neck extending

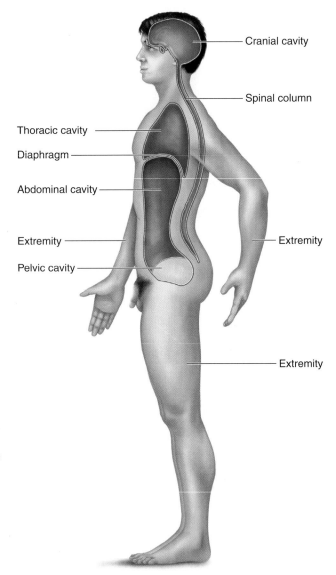

Figure 3-1 Major areas of the body.

from the base of the brain to the *tailbone,* as well as to the nerves, or **spinal cord,** running through the vertebrae. *Spine* is generally used in first aid to refer to injuries to these bones or nerves rather than the less specific words *neck* or *back.*

With these terms you can generally describe the location of injuries and symptoms. Although healthcare professionals use a variety of directional and spatial terms to pinpoint exact locations in the body, first aiders can successfully communicate locations with general words such as *above* or *below, left* and *right,* and so on. Remember that *left* and *right* refer to the *victim's* left and right sides—not yours when facing the victim.

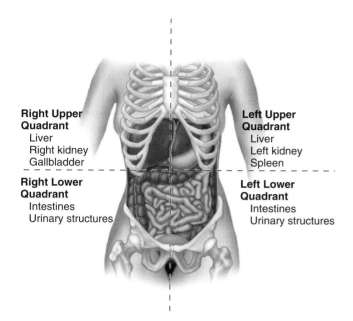

Right Upper Quadrant
Liver
Right kidney
Gallbladder

Left Upper Quadrant
Liver
Left kidney
Spleen

Right Lower Quadrant
Intestines
Urinary structures

Left Lower Quadrant
Intestines
Urinary structures

Figure 3-2 Abdominal quadrants.

BODY SYSTEMS

Life depends on the body carrying out a number of important functions, such as taking oxygen from the air and transporting it to all body cells, extracting nutrients from food, removing wastes, and managing the growth and repair of injured cells. An **organ** is a body part that accomplishes one or more specific functions. In most cases, several organs work together to achieve a larger body function. For example, the stomach and intestines accomplish much of the digestive process, but the gallbladder, pancreas, and liver also have important roles in digestion. The combination of organs that work together to perform a major body function is called a **body system.** Following are brief descriptions of some of the primary functions of the different body systems. Each is described more fully later in this chapter along with its relevance for first aid.

- *Respiratory system.* Provides the oxygen needed by body cells and removes the waste product carbon dioxide.
- *Cardiovascular system.* Moves the blood, which transports both oxygen and nutrients, throughout the body to supply cells and remove wastes.
- *Nervous system.* Controls all body functions and movement and allows for sensory perception and consciousness.

- *Musculoskeletal system.* Gives the body shape and strength and makes movement possible.
- *Integumentary system (skin and related structures).* Protects the body from the environment and germs and helps regulate body temperature.
- *Gastrointestinal system.* Extracts nutrients from food to meet the body's needs for energy and eliminates solid wastes.
- *Immune system.* Helps fight disease.
- *Endocrine system.* Produces hormones that help regulate many body functions.
- *Urinary system.* Removes liquid wastes from the body and helps maintain the body's water balance.
- *Reproductive system.* Makes human reproduction possible.

Although we sometimes talk about each system as if it were separate from others, body systems are closely interrelated and work together to perform many functions. For example, blood is part of the cardiovascular system, which pumps it to all areas of the body. Blood carries oxygen from the lungs (respiratory system) to the body cells, all of which need a continual supply of oxygen to stay alive. Nerve sensors (nervous system) detect the amount of oxygen and carbon dioxide in the blood and speed up or slow down the heartbeat and breathing rate to control the oxygen level. If body temperature drops, muscles of the extremities (musculoskeletal system) may start shivering to produce heat, which is carried by the blood to vital organs. The kidneys (urinary system) filter the blood to remove waste products, which leave the body in the urine. These are just a few examples of the many complex ways body systems work together.

As you learn about different kinds of first aid throughout this text, remember that different parts of the body are often closely related. This will help you understand what is happening in the body during periods of injury and illness so that you can provide first aid most effectively. For example, in someone with asthma, inhaling a substance such as smoke may cause muscles in the airway to spasm and swell, making breathing difficult. As oxygen levels in the blood reaching the brain drop, the person feels dizzy. Changes then occur in the respiratory, cardiovascular, and nervous systems. In this case, understanding how a breathing problem can affect a victim's mental status (responsiveness) can help you focus on correcting the cause.

As you will learn in later chapters, life-threatening injuries and illnesses most often affect the respiratory, circulatory, and nervous systems. Problems affecting these systems may impair the essential delivery of oxygen to body tissues, leading to death. First aiders, therefore, must first assess a victim for problems related to breathing and circulation, and then assess problems related to other body systems.

THE RESPIRATORY SYSTEM

The primary organs of the respiratory system are the structures of the airway and the lungs **(Figure 3-3).** The **airway** is the path air takes from the nose and mouth to the lungs. Air entering the nose or mouth passes through the **pharynx** (throat) to the **trachea** (windpipe). The trachea branches into the left and right **bronchi** (singular: bronchus), the passageways into the lungs. The bronchi branch into smaller tubular passages in the lungs and eventually end in the **alveoli,** the tiny air sacs where oxygen and carbon dioxide pass into and out of small blood vessels called capillaries.

Since the pharynx also leads to the **esophagus,** the tube that carries food to the stomach, another structure, called the epiglottis, is very important for breathing. The **epiglottis** is a tissue flap that prevents solids and liquids from entering the trachea and blocking the airway or reaching the lungs. The epiglottis directs food and drink to pass from the throat to the esophagus and stomach.

Breathing depends on muscular movements that are under the control of the nervous system. When the **diaphragm** (the large muscle below the lungs) contracts, the thoracic cavity and lungs expand, pulling air into the lungs from which oxygen can move into the blood. When the diaphragm relaxes, the size of the thoracic cavity is reduced, and air carrying out carbon dioxide flows back out of the lungs. **Table 3-1** provides some normal reference values for breathing.

The main function of the respiratory system is to allow oxygen to enter the blood from air that is breathed in (inhaled) and to remove carbon dioxide, a waste product of respiration, from the blood into air that is breathed out (exhaled). This is called **external respiration. Internal respiration** is the process of oxygen and carbon dioxide moving into and out of the blood within internal body tissues.

Emergencies Related to the Respiratory System

Respiration is one of the most vital functions in the body, and many different injuries and illnesses can affect it. Any factor that impedes

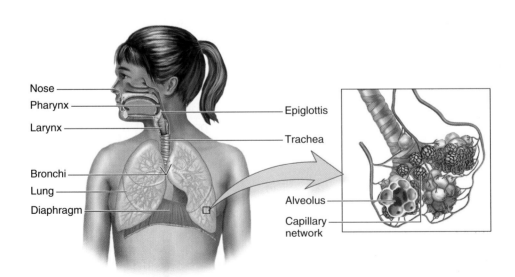

Nose
Pharynx
Larynx
Bronchi
Lung
Diaphragm
Epiglottis
Trachea
Alveolus
Capillary network

Figure 3-3 The respiratory system.

Table 3-1

Normal Reference Values for Breathing Rate

	Breaths per minute
Adult	12–20
Child	15–30
Infant	25–50

the flow of air into and out of the lungs can affect respiration and become life threatening. An **airway obstruction** is a physical blockage of the airway that prevents the flow of air. For example, a person who is eating may have a piece of food lodged in the pharynx, a condition called **choking.** In an unconscious person lying on his or her back, the tongue may block the opening into the pharynx. An injury to the head or neck may also cause the soft tissues of the upper airway to swell and obstruct the airway. All of these are life-threatening situations.

Another potential problem with the airway is a failure of the epiglottis to prevent substances from entering the trachea. The swallowing reflex normally prevents this, but in an unconscious person this reflex may not be functioning. This can result in liquids or solids entering the trachea and lungs. An unconscious person lying on his or her back, for example, may vomit, and the vomit may flow back down the throat and into the trachea and lungs, impeding respiration and possibly causing a severe lung infection. This is one reason why an unresponsive victim is never given anything to drink, because the fluid may flow into the lungs.

Chest injuries may also affect respiration. A broken rib may puncture a lung, making breathing ineffective. A penetrating injury into the lungs from the outside, such as that caused by a bullet or sharp object, may alter the lung pressures needed for inhaling and keep the lungs from filling with air.

Since breathing is controlled by the brain, other factors that affect the nervous system may also cause respiratory emergencies. A poisoning or drug overdose, for example, may severely depress nervous system functions, slowing breathing to the point where the body is not getting enough oxygen. An electrical shock may interrupt the normal nervous system control of respiration and cause breathing to stop.

Finally, some illnesses also cause breathing difficulties. Asthma is a common condition, especially in children, in which airway tissues swell and make it hard for the person to breathe. Chronic lung diseases, more common in the elderly and in smokers, may reduce lung functioning so much that the person struggles to catch a breath.

If the body is not receiving enough oxygen, other organs will begin to fail. The heart will soon stop, and brain cells will begin to die within minutes. In **Chapter 5** you will learn how to recognize breathing emergencies and the appropriate first aid to give victims depending on the cause.

THE CARDIOVASCULAR SYSTEM

The cardiovascular system consists of the heart, blood, and blood vessels (**Figure 3-4**). The primary functions of the cardiovascular system are to

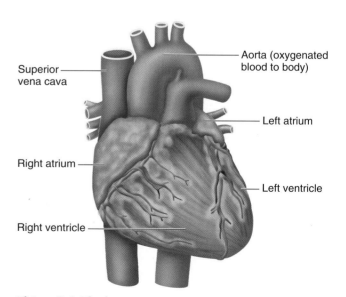

Superior vena cava

Aorta (oxygenated blood to body)

Left atrium

Right atrium

Left ventricle

Right ventricle

Figure 3-4 The heart.

transport oxygen and nutrients in the blood to all parts of the body and to remove carbon dioxide and other wastes from tissues. Other functions include transporting hormones that regulate other body functions, helping regulate body temperature, transporting cells and substances that fight infection, and helping maintain the body's fluid balance.

The heart has four chambers, the left and right atria and the left and right ventricles. The **ventricles** pump the blood through two loops or cycles in the body. First, blood is pumped to the lungs to pick up oxygen and release carbon dioxide. The blood returns to the heart, which pumps it to all areas of the body, releasing oxygen for use by body cells and picking up carbon dioxide for removal. The term **cardiac** refers to the heart. The heart is also part of the body's muscular system, as the heart is composed of a unique kind of muscle (**myocardium**) that contracts to make the pumping action. This pumping action, called **contraction,** is controlled by electrical signals that are in turn controlled by the nervous system.

The blood flows from the heart to body areas through an extensive network of **arteries (Figure 3-5)**. With the heartbeat, pulsing **blood pressure** changes occur in the arteries that can be felt in certain body locations as the **pulse.** Arteries progressively branch into smaller vessels that eventually reach **capillaries,** which are very small blood vessels with thin walls where oxygen and carbon dioxide are exchanged with body cells. From the capillaries the blood drains back to the heart through an equally extensive system of **veins.** Blood flows more evenly through veins, which do not have a pulse. Arteries are generally deeper in the body than veins and are therefore more protected and less likely to be damaged by injuries.

The heart rate, which can be measured as the pulse, is affected by many factors. With exercise, fever, or emotional excitement, the heart rate increases to meet the body's greater need for oxygen. Various injuries and illnesses may either increase or decrease the heart rate. **Table 3-2** provides some normal reference values for heart rate.

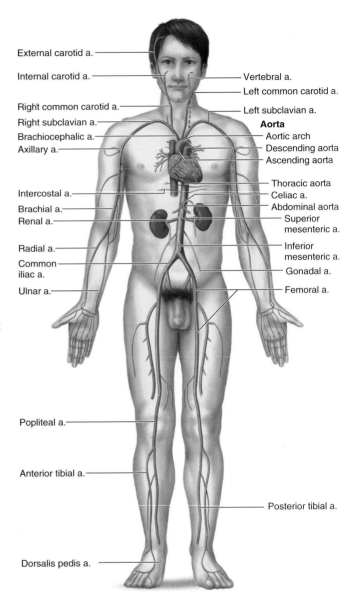

Figure 3-5 Major arteries of the body.

Emergencies Related to the Cardiovascular System

Like the respiratory system, the cardiovascular system's functions are vital for life, health, and well-being. The most vital function is carrying oxygen to the body's tissues. As noted earlier, cells begin to die in vital organs such as the brain after only a few minutes without oxygen. Any injury or illness that affects respiration, therefore, also diminishes the ability of the cardiovascular system to deliver oxygen to the body.

Table 3-2

Normal Reference Values for Heart Rate

	Beats per minute
Adult	60–100
Child	60–150
Infant	120–150

Blood vessel problems may also affect cardiovascular functioning. Bleeding, which often occurs with injuries, may be so severe that not enough blood is left in circulation to adequately provide the oxygen the body needs.

Arterial bleeding is most severe because the blood may spurt out under pressure, leading within minutes to the life-threatening condition called shock. **Shock** occurs when vital body organs are not receiving enough oxygen (see **Chapter 10**).

Bleeding from veins is generally slower but can still be serious or life threatening if it continues. Capillary bleeding is generally minor and usually stops by itself as the blood clots. **Chapter 9** describes the first aid techniques to control bleeding.

Stroke is another type of blood vessel problem involving arteries in the brain. A blood clot or bleeding in the brain may reduce circulation to a part of the brain, causing mental and physical impairments. **Chapter 17** describes the first aid for stroke.

Problems involving the heart can also affect tissue oxygenation. Some conditions,

Learning Checkpoint ①

1. Name two organs inside the thoracic cavity.

2. Which of the following is a function of the respiratory system?

   a. Inhaling and exhaling

   b. Moving oxygen into the blood

   c. Moving carbon dioxide out of body tissues

   d. All of the above

3. At what structure is an airway obstruction most likely to occur?

4. The heart pumps blood to all body tissues through which blood vessels?

   a. Arteries

   b. Veins

   c. Capillaries

   d. All of the above

5. Check off which cardiac problems can affect tissue oxygenation.

   _____ Cardiac arrest

   _____ Kidney failure

   _____ Asthma

   _____ Dysrhythmia

   _____ Diabetes

   _____ Myocardial infarction

   _____ Tetanus infection

such as congestive heart failure, reduce the heart's ability to pump to effectively meet the body's needs. If the heart muscle itself does not receive enough oxygenated blood because of blocked cardiac arteries, part of the heart muscle may die. This is called a heart attack or **myocardial infarction.** The heart may also stop (**cardiac arrest**), in which case the person needs cardiopulmonary resuscitation (CPR), as described in **Chapter 6. Dysrhythmia,** or an abnormal heartbeat, is another type of heart problem that may reduce the heart's pumping effectiveness.

THE NERVOUS SYSTEM

The nervous system has three general sets of functions:

1. Sensory receptors in the skin, eyes, ears, nose, and mouth as well as throughout the body gather information about the internal and external environment and send this information to the brain.

2. The brain integrates and analyzes information, both consciously and automatically, for immediate and future uses.

3. Nerve signals from the brain lead to movements and other actions throughout the body to accomplish specific tasks or to maintain **homeostasis,** a balanced state within the body necessary for effective functioning.

The nervous system controls the actions of most other body systems. For example, when nervous system receptors detect a low level of oxygen in the blood, the brain directs the muscles of breathing to speed up the respiratory rate and the heart to beat faster to ensure that the body gets enough oxygen.

The brain controls the nervous system (**Figure 3-6**). Specific areas in the brain control different functions, such as controlling heart rate, storing memories, creating visual images, and directing muscle movements. The brain connects directly with the spinal cord, the pathway to and from nerves throughout the body. The brain and spinal cord form the **central nervous system.** After leaving the skull the spinal cord is encased inside vertebrae, the bones of the spine (**Figure 3-7**). Nerves project out from the spinal cord between the

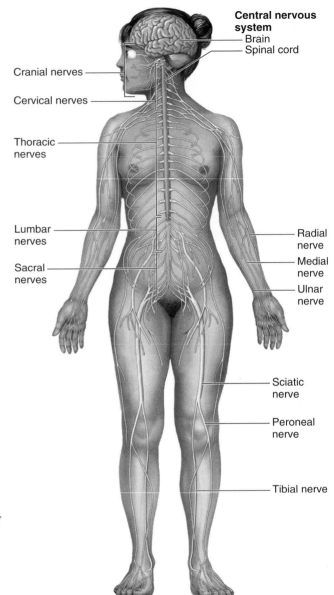

Figure 3-6 The nervous system.

vertebrae of the neck and back and extend throughout the body. Generally, nerves exiting the spinal cord nearer the top control movement and other functions higher in the body, and nerves from the spinal cord nearer the bottom control functions lower in the body.

Emergencies Related to the Nervous System

Injury or illness affecting the nervous system can have general or very specific effects on the body. Head and spinal injuries can have serious or life-

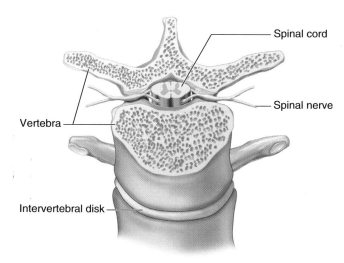

Figure 3-7 The spinal cord.

Spinal cord

Spinal nerve

Vertebra

Intervertebral disk

threatening effects. An injury to a part of the brain, or a disease process such as a stroke that damages a particular brain area, may destroy or impair the function of that brain tissue. If the respiratory center in the brain is damaged, the person may stop breathing. If a muscle control center is damaged, a part of the body may be paralyzed. Head injuries may also cause bleeding or swelling of the brain. Because the brain is tightly encased in the skull, bleeding or swelling puts pressure on the brain and may cause more widespread effects.

Brain functions can also be more generally affected by injury or illness. **Altered mental status** is a phrase used to describe changes in a person's responsiveness, such as becoming confused, disoriented, lethargic, or comatose. Altered mental status may result from such things as head injuries, any injury causing reduced oxygenation, and sudden illness such as stroke, seizure, diabetic emergencies, severe infection, high fever, poisoning, or drug overdose. **Chapter 17** describes the first aid for such emergencies.

Damage to the spinal cord may occur at any level between the base of the skull and the lower back. Significant damage to the cord, such as complete severing caused by a neck or back fracture, often results in a complete loss of function in body areas controlled by nerves exiting the spine below that level. A lower back injury may result in a loss of feeling in the legs and inability to move the legs (**paralysis**). A similar injury to the spinal cord in the neck area may result in

paralysis and loss of feeling in the entire body below the neck. The neck is a particularly vulnerable area because any trauma to the head, such as the head being snapped forward in a vehicle crash or striking a hard object after diving in shallow water, may injure neck vertebrae and the spinal cord. **Chapter 13** describes how to assess an injured victim for a possible head or spine injury and how to protect the spinal cord from additional injury caused by movement.

In addition to head and spinal injuries, injuries elsewhere in the body, as well as some illnesses, also affect the nervous system. Pain will result from damage to nerve fibers in many areas of the body, and therefore pain is always assessed as a symptom that may reveal something about a victim's injury or illness. The pain caused by injured nerves in a cut finger is obvious, but pain within the body is not always so clear-cut. A crushing pain in the chest that extends into the left arm may be caused by a heart attack. Abdominal pain that begins in the area of the umbilicus (navel) and then settles into the lower abdomen on the right side may be a sign of appendicitis. Although pain is not always present with serious conditions, pain should be taken seriously whenever it occurs. The level of pain, however, should not be taken as an indicator of the severity of an injury or illness.

THE MUSCULOSKELETAL SYSTEM

The musculoskeletal system combines two closely related body systems and is composed of bones, muscles, and the structures that join them (ligaments and tendons). The bones of the body have several functions (**Figure 3-8**):

- The skeleton provides shape and support for the body as a whole.
- Groups of bones protect vital internal organs (i.e., the ribs protect the heart and lungs, the skull protects the brain, the vertebrae protect the spinal cord).
- Bone marrow inside certain bones produces blood cells.
- Bones store calcium for use by the rest of the body when needed.
- Bones act as levers to allow movement at joints when muscles act on them.

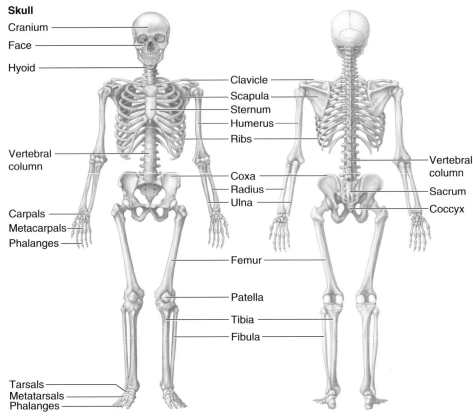

Skull
- Cranium
- Face
- Hyoid

Clavicle
Scapula
Sternum
Humerus
Ribs

Vertebral column

Coxa
Radius
Ulna

Carpals
Metacarpals
Phalanges

Femur

Patella

Tibia

Fibula

Tarsals
Metatarsals
Phalanges

Vertebral column

Sacrum

Coccyx

Figure 3-8 Major bones of the body.

Skeletal muscles attach to bones to create body movements **(Figure 3-9)**. Another function is to produce body heat with movement or shivering. The phrase *musculoskeletal* usually refers to skeletal (voluntary) muscles, but the body also has other kinds of muscle tissue with special functions (called involuntary muscle tissue). As noted earlier, the heart's muscle tissue provides its beating force. The esophagus is a muscular tube with special movements that aid in swallowing and moving food to the stomach. Muscle tissue throughout the gastrointestinal system keeps the products of digestion moving through the digestive tract. The diaphragm is a thin muscle below the lungs that does the primary work of breathing. Muscle tissue inside blood vessels helps keep blood moving through the body. All muscle activity is controlled by the nervous system.

Tendons are fibrous tissues that connect muscles to bones. **Ligaments** are tough bands of tissue that join bones together at joints.

Emergencies Related to the Musculoskeletal System

Musculoskeletal injuries include fractures, dislocations, sprains, and strains. A **fracture** is a broken bone. Although fractures can be serious injuries, particularly when nearby organs or blood vessels are damaged by the broken bone ends, most fractures are not life threatening. Dislocations and sprains are both joint injuries. In a **dislocation,** one or more bones move out of their normal position in a joint, preventing the joint from functioning as usual. Shoulder dislocations are among the most common dislocations. A **sprain** is damage to ligaments and other structures in a joint; the ankle and wrist are commonly sprained by forces on these joints.

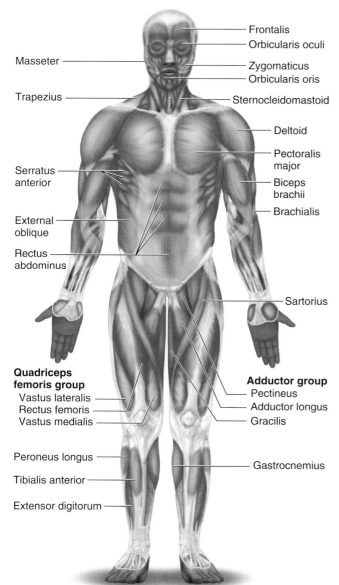

Frontalis
Orbicularis oculi
Masseter
Zygomaticus
Orbicularis oris
Trapezius
Sternocleidomastoid
Deltoid
Pectoralis
major
Serratus
anterior
Biceps
brachii
Brachialis
External
oblique
Rectus
abdominus
Sartorius
**Quadriceps
femoris group**
Vastus lateralis
Rectus femoris
Vastus medialis
Adductor group
Pectineus
Adductor longus
Gracilis
Peroneus longus
Tibialis anterior
Gastrocnemius
Extensor digitorum

Figure 3-9 Major muscles of the body.

A **strain** is a tearing of muscle or tendon tissue usually caused by overexertion of the muscle. All of these injuries require first aid, as you'll learn in **Chapter 15.**

Musculoskeletal injuries are often associated with other injuries. Vertebral fractures are likely to injure the spinal cord and cause nervous system damage. Fractures of the **femur,** the long bone in the thigh, often cause much soft tissue damage and bleeding. A fracture of the pelvis may damage the bladder or other organs in the pelvic cavity. A skull fracture may cause brain damage.

The musculoskeletal system is also affected by illnesses, although most of these do not occur suddenly and therefore seldom require first aid. Arthritis (chronic joint inflammation causing pain and restricted motion), muscular dystrophy (disorders of progressive degeneration of muscles), and osteoarthritis (weakening of bones, usually with aging) are all common musculoskeletal system diseases.

THE INTEGUMENTARY SYSTEM

The integumentary system consists of the skin, nails, hair, and accessory structures such as sweat and oil glands **(Figure 3-10)**. The primary function of the skin is to protect the body from the external environment (temperature extremes, pathogens, and other substances). Other functions include:

- *Regulating body temperature.* When the body is hot, blood vessels in the skin widen to bring heat to the surface to dissipate; sweating also helps cool the skin. When the body is cold, blood vessels constrict to conserve heat, and muscle movements occur such as shivering and "goose bumps" (tiny muscle reactions in the hair follicles).
- *Preventing water loss from the body.* The skin acts as a barrier to prevent water loss.
- *Waste removal.* Through sweating, the skin removes some body wastes.
- *Vitamin production.* Skin cells produce vitamin D.
- *Sensation.* Nerve sensors in the skin react to touch, pressure, pain, and temperature.

Emergencies Related to the Integumentary System

Because skin is the organ most exposed to the environment, it is frequently damaged by traumatic injuries. Cuts and scrapes are common causes of bleeding. The blood vessels in the skin are relatively small, and bleeding from the skin seldom involves as much blood loss as from deeper blood vessels. Any openings in the skin, however, may allow pathogens into the body. As described in **Chapter 2, pathogens** are germs capable of causing disease, including bloodborne pathogens that can cause serious illnesses. Take precautions if you will be exposed to a victim's body fluids.

Exposure to temperature extremes can damage the skin. Skin exposed to freezing temperatures

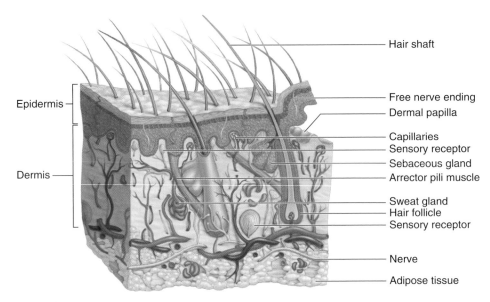

Figure 3-10 Anatomy of the skin.

may get **frostbite,** in which tissue freezes and dies. Very high temperatures and many chemicals cause skin **burns,** which destroy tissue and may allow loss of body heat and body fluid (**See Chapter 12**). Because sunburn damages skin in a way that makes skin cancer more likely later on, pre-

Learning
Checkpoint ②

1. Check off injuries and illnesses that may cause altered mental status.

_____ Head injuries   _____ Stroke

_____ Seizure   _____ Diabetic emergencies

_____ High fever   _____ Poisoning

_____ Drug overdose   _____ Severe infection

2. A spinal injury may result in

  a. myocardial infarction.   **c.** paralysis.

  b. lung infection.   **d.** All of the above

3. Define a dislocation. _____

4. Why might a fractured femur be life threatening?

  a. Loss of calcium stored in the bone   **c.** Injury to soft tissues of the leg

  b. Severe bleeding   **d.** All of the above

5. In what situation can even a small skin cut be very serious?

_____

cautions should be taken to protect the skin from sun exposure.

Although skin functions help regulate body temperature, when a person is exposed to cold or heat, regulatory mechanisms may not be able to keep the body at its normal temperature. The skin of a victim of hypothermia (whole body cooling) often looks pale and cool. In heatstroke, a life-threatening condition in which the body becomes overheated, sweating stops and the skin is flushed and very hot to the touch. **Chapter 21** describes the first aid for heat and cold emergencies.

The skin often reveals important information about the condition of the body. For example, when blood oxygen levels are low, the skin may look bluish, especially at the lips, under the nails, and around mucous membranes. This skin color is called cyanosis. The skin of a victim in shock is often cool, clammy or sweating, and pale or bluish. Sweating and pale skin are also signs of a possible heart attack. Many sudden illnesses also cause sweating and skin color changes (flushed or pale). In dark-skinned individuals, the skin color generally becomes ashen rather than pale.

Because skin condition is a sensitive indicator of circulatory status, the skin can also help you monitor the effects of some first aid techniques. For example, when a victim's fractured arm or leg is splinted, the skin of the fingers or toes is periodically checked to ensure that circulation to the extremity has not been cut off.

THE GASTROINTESTINAL SYSTEM

The primary function of the gastrointestinal system is to digest food and extract nutrients to meet the body's needs for energy and specific dietary substances. Food and fluids pass through the esophagus to the stomach and then to the small and large intestines, where nutrients are absorbed into the blood to be transported to body cells **(Figure 3-11)**. Wastes are eliminated through the anus.

Accessory organs of digestion include the pancreas and liver, which produce substances that aid in digestion, and the gallbladder, which stores bile made by the liver. The liver has several other important functions.

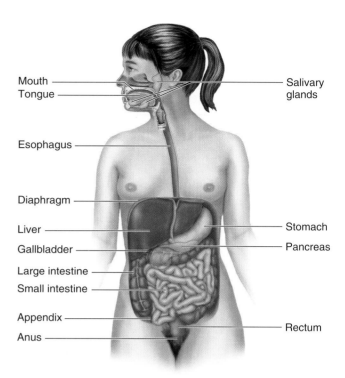

Figure 3-11 The gastrointestinal system.

Emergencies Related to the Gastrointestinal System

Since the abdominal cavity is not protected by bones, gastrointestinal organs can be easily injured by traumatic forces. In a closed abdominal injury the skin is not broken, but pain or tenderness along with a swollen or rigid abdomen may suggest an internal injury. In an open abdominal wound, internal organs may be exposed to the outside, raising the risk of infection. **Chapter 14** describes first aid for abdominal injuries.

The gastrointestinal system may also be involved in a number of sudden illnesses and conditions. An ingested poison is absorbed in the same manner as nutrients from food and once in the blood can affect the entire body.

Various illnesses can cause vomiting or diarrhea. If either continues for a prolonged period, the victim may become dehydrated, a serious condition in which the body loses needed water. Infants, especially, can lose significant amounts of body fluid from diarrhea, which quickly becomes a medical emergency. Vomiting blood is likely a sign of serious illness.

The liver too is affected by many illnesses as well as by chronic alcohol use. As noted in **Chapter 2,** hepatitis is a bloodborne disease that frequently causes liver damage. Because the liver is a vital organ whose functions are necessary for life, it is critical to take appropriate precautions to prevent the transmission of hepatitis in first aid situations.

THE LYMPHATIC AND IMMUNE SYSTEMS

The lymphatic system consists of the lymph nodes and lymphatic vessels located throughout the body, along with other organs (**Figure 3-12**).

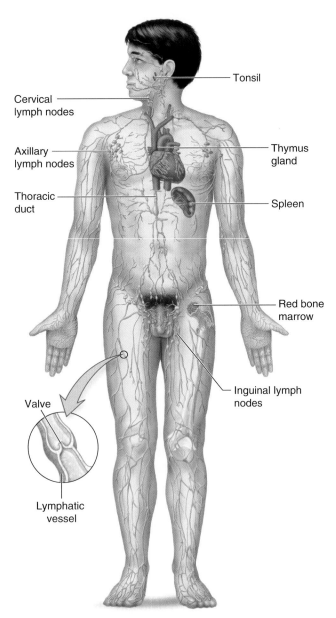

Tonsil

Cervical lymph nodes

Axillary lymph nodes

Thoracic duct

Thymus gland

Spleen

Red bone marrow

Inguinal lymph nodes

Valve

Lymphatic vessel

Figure 3-12 The lymphatic system.

The lymphatic system helps the body to absorb fats and maintain a fluid balance, but its primary function is to help defend against disease as part of the immune system. Lymphocytes, a type of white blood cell, help fight infection. Other organs and the cells of the immune system work together with the lymphatic system to provide defense mechanisms against pathogens and foreign substances that enter the body.

Emergencies Related to the Immune System

Although many illnesses and other health problems may result from problems in the immune system, seldom do these occur suddenly and require first aid or immediate treatment. A wound that is not properly cared for, however, may develop an infection if the body's immune system does not eliminate pathogens that may enter the body through the wound. As described in **Chapter 2**, HIV, an infection attacking the immune system and causing AIDS, may also enter the first aid provider's body as a result of exposure to an infected victim's body fluids. Taking precautions against infection is necessary in all emergencies.

The related concept of **immunity** is also important in first aid. A **vaccine** is a form of preventive care that bolsters the body's immune system to prevent the vaccinated person from becoming infected by a specific pathogen. A vaccine is available for hepatitis B, for example, which healthcare workers and professional rescuers often receive because of the risk of acquiring this bloodborne infection when caring for victims of injury. Tetanus vaccine similarly gives protection against wounds being infected by the deadly tetanus bacterium, which is commonly present in the environment.

THE ENDOCRINE SYSTEM

The endocrine system includes a series of glands in various body areas that produce hormones. **Hormones** are chemical messengers that are carried in the blood and affect the functioning of organs throughout the body. More than two dozen hormones are produced in the body, each with specific functions and effects. For example, the thyroid gland produces hormones that regulate growth and development. The gonads (testes in men, ovaries in women) produce steroid hormones that stimulate the development of male and female sex characteristics and allow reproductive functions. The pancreas secretes a hormone called **insulin** that helps regulate blood sugar levels.

Emergencies Related to the Endocrine System

All hormones affect a person's health, and the over- or underproduction of each can cause disease. Most of these problems develop more slowly, however, and are seldom issues for first aid—with one major exception. **Diabetes** is a metabolic disorder affecting over 16 million people in the United States. Diabetics either do not produce enough insulin or have developed resistance to the effects of insulin. A person with diabetes may suddenly become very ill because of very high or very low blood sugar levels related to this insulin problem. Without treatment or first aid, a diabetic crisis can quickly progress to a medical emergency (see **Chapter 17**).

THE URINARY SYSTEM

The urinary system removes dissolved metabolic wastes from the body through the urine and helps the body maintain fluid and electrolyte balances. Metabolic wastes result from cellular functions within the body. The blood transports these wastes to the **kidneys,** which filter them out and produce urine (**Figure 3-13**). Urine is transported to the **bladder,** which stores urine until it is passed to the outside.

Emergencies Related to the Urinary System

Traumatic injury may damage the bladder or kidneys, possibly resulting in blood in the urine. Blood in the urine is always a sign of a problem requiring medical attention.

Many medical problems affecting the urinary system do not develop suddenly and therefore are usually not first aid issues.

Since the frequency and amount of urine passed depends in part on how much water is present in the body, changes in urination may

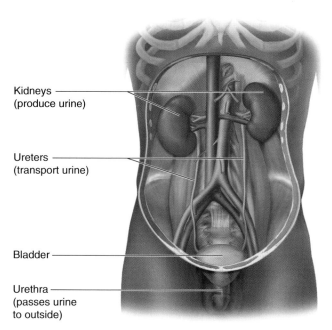

Kidneys (produce urine)

Ureters (transport urine)

Bladder

Urethra (passes urine to outside)

Figure 3-13 The urinary system.

indicate the presence of a health problem. A long period without urination in an infant, for example, may be a sign of dehydration, a medical emergency.

THE REPRODUCTIVE SYSTEM

Unlike other body systems that are identical or similar in males and females, the reproductive system involves different organs in males and females. The reproductive system in males produces sperm, the male reproductive cell, and transports the sperm for delivery into the female vagina. In females the system produces eggs, the female reproductive cells, and supports and nurtures in the uterus an egg fertilized by sperm as it develops into a fetus; other functions relate to childbirth and lactation (producing milk for breastfeeding infant). The term **genitals** refers to the male and female sex organs (penis and testicles in males; the labia, clitoris, and vagina in females).

Emergencies Related to the Reproductive System

Abdominal injuries may damage the genitals or reproductive organs, and such wounds may require special first aid (see **Chapter 11**). Because our culture views the genitals as a very private body area, care for these injuries should include concern for the victim's privacy and be performed with sensitivity.

In rare situations a pregnant woman may develop complications. Occasionally childbirth may occur without the pregnant woman being attended by a doctor, midwife, or other person trained in childbirth. In such cases a first aider may need to assist the pregnant woman. Childbirth is usually a normal, natural process that takes place without problems or complications. Sometimes, however, a medical emergency may occur. **Chapter 23** describes first aid in pregnancy and childbirth.

Learning Checkpoint ③

1. What is important about vomiting?

    a. It can lead to dehydration.

    b. It may be a sign of serious illness.

    c. Vomiting blood often indicates a serious illness.

    d. All of the above

2. Name a vaccination *all* people should have periodically throughout their lives.

_____

3. Diabetes involves a problem in the body with which hormone?

    a. Insulin

    b. Bile

    c. Steroids

    d. Any of the above

4. Blood present in the urine always means

    a. a sexually transmitted disease is present.

    b. the person has a yeast infection.

    c. the person should seek medical attention.

    d. the person needs to restore electrolyte balance.

Concluding Thoughts

When you encounter a victim in need of first aid, the nature of the problem may be obvious or it may be difficult to judge. A simple cut that is bleeding, for example, does not require knowledge of the cardiovascular system before you can give first aid. With many injuries and illnesses, however, understanding what is going on in the body will help you assess the problem and remember what first aid to give. Understanding how a breathing problem can cause altered mental status, for example, or how a person with diabetes may experience a sudden emergency, can help you to know what actions to take. The general principles described in this chapter will become more meaningful as you learn about specific injuries and illnesses throughout the rest of this text.

Learning Outcomes

You should now be able to do the following:

1. Describe the primary areas of the body.
2. List the 10 body systems and explain a key function of each.
3. For each body system, describe at least one injury or illness that affects the functioning of that system.

Review Questions

1. The main function of the respiratory system is to
   a. filter the blood.
   b. transport nutrients to body tissues.
   c. protect the body from pathogens.
   d. provide oxygen for body tissues.

2. A problem in one body system
   a. can affect the functioning of other body systems, too.
   b. affects only that system.
   c. affects only that system plus the nervous system.
   d. affects every system in the body.

3. A person who is choking is said to have
   a. altered mental status.
   b. an airway obstruction.
   c. a dysrhythmia.
   d. a metabolic disorder.

4. What life-threatening problem occurs when vital organs are not receiving enough oxygen?
   a. Diabetes
   b. Hypothermia
   c. Shock
   d. Seizures

5. Inside the vertebrae is the
   a. central nervous system.
   b. spinal cord.
   c. spinal ligament.
   d. peripheral nervous system.

6. Heart attack may cause
   a. crushing pain in the chest.
   b. severe bleeding.
   c. seizures.
   d. airway obstruction.

7. The functions of the musculoskeletal system include
   a. protecting internal organs.
   b. producing lymph.
   c. circulating blood.
   d. regulating hormones.

8. Skin changes may help you determine when a victim has
   a. hypothermia.
   b. heatstroke.
   c. sudden illness.
   d. All of the above

9. A sign of an internal abdominal injury is
   a. sweating.
   b. seizures.
   c. a swollen or rigid abdomen.
   d. All of the above

10. A person with diabetes may have an emergency caused by
    a. very high blood sugar levels.
    b. very low blood sugar levels.
    c. either very high or very low blood sugar levels.
    d. a fluid balance problem.

References and Resources

BodySmart: An Online Examination of Human Anatomy and Physiology. Available from: www.getbodysmart.com

National Institutes of Health. Anatomy & Physiology. Available from: http://training.seer.cancer.gov/module_anatomy/anatomy_physiology_home.html

National Safety Council. www.nsc.org

Saladin KS. Anatomy and physiology: the unity of form and function. 3rd ed. New York: McGraw-Hill; 2004.

Chapter 4

Assessing the Victim

Chapter Preview

- The Initial Assessment
- The Recovery Position
- The Secondary Assessment
- Monitor the Victim

Late in the afternoon you stop by your supervisor's office to drop off a report. When you knock on the door it swings open. You look inside and see him slumped over his desk. You call his name as you approach, but he doesn't respond, so you tap him on the shoulder and ask if he's okay. He still does not respond. What do you do now?

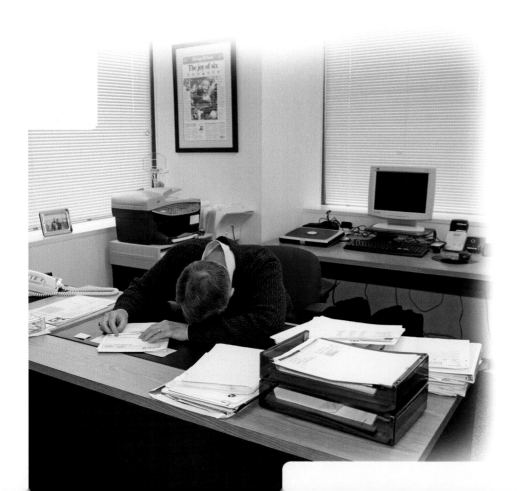

As described in **Chapter 2**, after you recognize the emergency and check the scene for safety, you then check the victim to see what problems may need first aid. This check, called an **assessment,** has two primary steps:

1. In the **initial assessment,** check for immediate life-threatening conditions. Check for responsiveness and breathing.
2. In the **secondary assessment,** get the victim's history (find out what happened and what may have contributed to the emergency), and perform a physical examination of a responsive victim to check for any injuries or other signs of sudden illness.

Then while giving first aid for any injuries you find, and while waiting for help to arrive, continue with a third step:

3. Monitor the victim for any changes.

Always perform these steps in this order. If you find a life-threatening problem, such as the absence of breathing, the victim needs immediate help. This victim could die if you first spend time looking for broken bones or asking bystanders what happened. **Always remember to do the initial assessment first.**

THE INITIAL ASSESSMENT

In the initial assessment you check the victim for life-threatening conditions. The key conditions to look for immediately are unresponsiveness, lack of normal breathing, and severe bleeding. The entire initial assessment should take less than a minute.

Because of the risk of aggravating a spine injury, do not move the victim to perform this assessment except when absolutely necessary for two circumstances:

1. The patient faces an immediate danger if not moved, because
   - fire is present or likely to occur.
   - explosives are present or there is a danger of explosion (e.g., a natural gas leak).
   - the patient cannot be protected from other hazards at the scene.
   - you are unable to gain access to other patients who need lifesaving care.
   - you cannot make the scene safe (e.g., a structure about to collapse).

2. You cannot give lifesaving care because of the patient's location or position (e.g., a victim who needs CPR is sitting in a chair or lying on a bed).

Check for Responsiveness

As you approach, you may notice immediately whether the victim is responsive. Responsive means a person is conscious and awake. A victim who is speaking, coughing, crying, or moving is responsive. Even if the victim cannot talk because of an injury, he or she may be able to move and thereby signal responsiveness. A victim who cannot talk or move may be paralyzed but may still be able to respond through purposeful eye movements or other signs. This is why we say *responsive* rather than *conscious:* we cannot always know whether a person is conscious or unconscious, but we do know whether that person responds to us.

Just knowing the victim is responsive is not enough, however. Any victim who can talk is obviously responsive, and is able to breathe—but the victim may have severe bleeding, a life-threatening condition. A victim who moves is responsive, but if this person is not speaking, crying, or coughing, the victim may be unable to breathe because of an obstructed airway (choking) or other breathing problem. Therefore, even with a responsive victim, you must still continue to check for breathing and severe bleeding.

If the victim is not speaking, making other sounds, or moving, tap the person gently on the shoulder and ask, "Are you okay?" **(Figure 4-1)**. Be careful not to move the victim in any way when assessing responsiveness. Do not shake the victim's shoulder or touch the head or neck, because the victim may have a spinal injury that any movement could worsen. If the victim still does not respond, this is a life-threatening emergency, and you must act quickly. If someone else is present, have that person call 9-1-1 while you continue to check the unresponsive victim.

Unresponsiveness may be a sign of an urgent, life-threatening problem (such as not breathing) or it may result from a less urgent problem. Since you cannot yet know, you must continue to check the victim. Regardless of its cause, and regardless of whether other life-threatening problems are present, *unresponsiveness in itself is considered an emergency.* For example, if the victim is on his or her back, the tongue may move back in the throat and block the airway, preventing breathing.

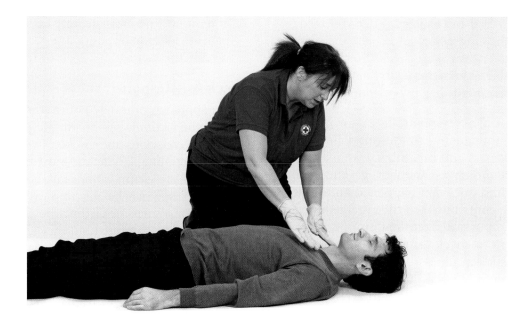

Figure 4-1 Check the victim for responsiveness by tapping the shoulder and asking, "Are you okay?"

The degree of a victim's responsiveness is frequently assessed using the AVPU scale (**Box 4-1**). This scale is useful for noting changes in a victim's responsiveness during the time you are providing care and for communicating this information to arriving EMS professionals.

Check for Breathing

After checking for responsiveness, check next for normal breathing. If the victim can speak or cough, then he or she is breathing. In an unresponsive victim, to check breathing, you must ensure the airway is open.

The airway is the route air moves from the mouth and nose through the throat (pharynx) and down to the lungs. The airway may be blocked by something stuck in the throat, by swollen airway tissues in a victim with a severe allergic reaction or a neck injury, or by an unresponsive victim's own tongue.

If a responsive victim is talking, crying, or coughing, the airway is open. In some cases, described in **Chapter 5** on breathing problems, a victim with a very weak, wheezing cough may have a partially blocked airway and may not be breathing normally, which also is an emergency.

In an unresponsive victim, you may need to open the airway. If the victim is lying on his or her back, you must prevent the tongue from obstructing the airway by positioning the victim's head to open the airway. This is done by tilting the head back and lifting the chin as shown in **Figure 4-2**. This is called the head tilt-chin lift. This position moves the tongue away from the opening into the throat to allow air to pass through the airway.

If you find an unresponsive person in a position other than lying on his or her back, do not immediately roll the victim onto his or her back to open the airway. Moving a victim unnecessarily may cause additional injury, especially if the victim may have a spinal injury. In this case, try to determine whether the victim's airway is open by looking, listening, and feeling for breathing through the nose or mouth without moving the victim. Put your ear close to the victim's mouth and listen and feel for breaths while watching the chest for the rise and fall of breathing. A victim who is clearly breathing obviously has an open airway, and you should not move this victim unless it is necessary for providing other care.

Box 4-1 The AVPU Scale

A = **Alert.** The victim is aware of the time and where he or she is.

V = Responds to **Verbal** stimuli. The victim is not clearly oriented to time and place but responds when spoken to.

P = Responds to **Painful** stimuli. The victim does not respond when spoken to but moves or responds to pain, as when pinched between the neck and shoulder.

U = **Unresponsive** to all stimuli. The victim's eyes are closed and there is no movement or other response to painful stimuli.

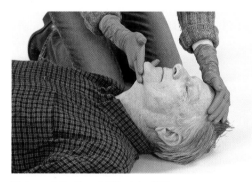

Figure 4-2 Head tilt-chin lift.

If you are unable to determine whether an unresponsive victim is breathing, you will need to move the victim into a face-up position to open the airway and check for breathing (**Figure 4-3**). With the help of others if possible, carefully roll the victim onto his or her back, keeping the head in line with the body as described in **Chapter 13**. Then open the airway.

The maneuvers just described for checking the airway are used for an unresponsive victim. A responsive victim may have a blocked airway,

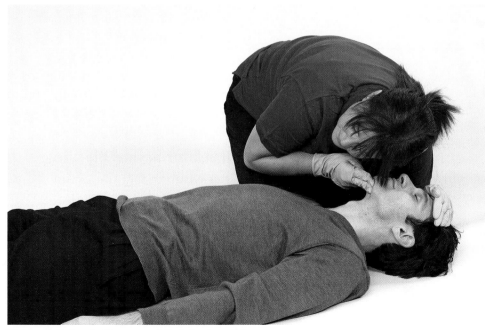

Figure 4-3 Look, listen, and feel for breathing.

Skill Initial Assessment

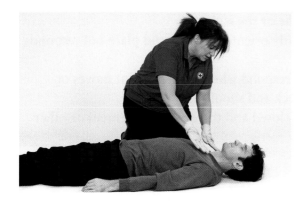

1 Check responsiveness.

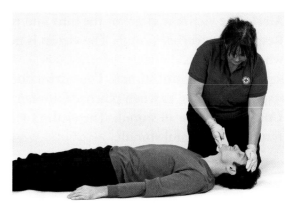

2 Open the airway with the head tilt-chin lift.

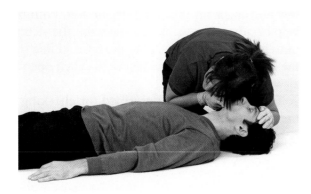

3 Check for breathing.

4 Check for severe bleeding.

---

too, usually caused by choking on some object lodged in the throat. This victim will be unable to speak or make other sounds and typically signals an inability to breathe by clutching at the neck. A choking victim needs immediate first aid to clear the airway, as described in **Chapter 7**.

After positioning an unresponsive victim to open the airway, check immediately for normal breathing. Regular, unobstructed breathing is necessary to sustain life. To check, lean over with your ear close to the person's mouth and nose and *look* at the victim's chest to see if it rises and falls with breathing. *Listen* for any sounds of breathing and *feel* for breath on your cheek. If you do not detect any signs of breathing within 10 seconds, assume the person is not breathing. Lack of breathing may be caused by

an obstructed airway (choking) or other causes. If the victim is not breathing, you must immediately give rescue breaths and start CPR as described in **Chapters 5 and 6**.

Check for Severe Bleeding

After ensuring that the victim is breathing, next check for severe bleeding. If the victim is bleeding profusely, vital organs are not receiving enough oxygen to sustain life.

Check for severe bleeding by quickly looking over the victim's body for obvious blood. Check for blood-saturated clothing or blood pooled under the body. Control any severe bleeding with direct pressure (see **Chapter 9**).

This step completes the initial assessment (see Skill: "Initial Assessment"). As described in the fol-

Helmet Removal

Helmets are worn by people in a variety of activities: bicycle riders, motorcycle riders, athletes playing sports such as football, and construction site workers. If an injured victim is wearing a helmet, it should be removed only if absolutely necessary to care for a life-threatening condition, because removal involves the risk of moving the victim's head or neck and possibly worsening a spinal or head injury. Leave the helmet in place for arriving EMS professionals, unless a full-face helmet absolutely must be removed to perform CPR. With many sports helmets, the face guard can be removed so that the helmet can be left on while CPR is given.

lowing chapters on basic life support, if the initial assessment reveals a life-threatening condition, you immediately begin to provide care for it. Only if it is clear that the victim is breathing and not bleeding severely do you move on to the secondary assessment to check for additional injuries or signs of a sudden illness requiring care. An unresponsive victim should be positioned on his or her side in the recovery position following the initial assessment.

THE RECOVERY POSITION

An unresponsive victim who is breathing, and who is not suspected of having a spinal injury, should be put in the **recovery position (Figure 4-4)**. This position is used for several reasons:

- It helps keep the airway open so that you do not need to maintain the head tilt-chin lift position.

- It allows fluids to drain from the mouth so that the victim does not choke on blood, vomit, or other fluids.
- It prevents the victim from inhaling stomach contents if the victim vomits.

If possible, unless this could worsen the victim's injury, put the victim on his or her left side. Because of anatomical differences inside the body, the left side reduces the chances of the victim vomiting. The modified HAINES (High Arm IN Endangered Spine) position is recommended because it reduces movement of the neck in case of potential spinal injury (see Skill: "Recovery Position: Modified HAINES").

For an unresponsive, breathing infant, hold the infant face down over your arm with his or

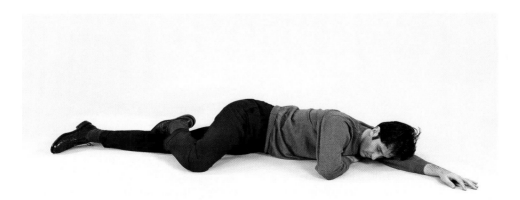

Figure 4-4 The recovery position.

Skill   Recovery Position: Modified HAINES

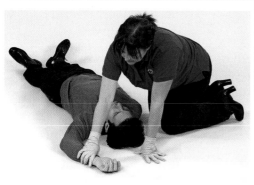

1 Extend the victim's arm that is farther from you above the victim's head.

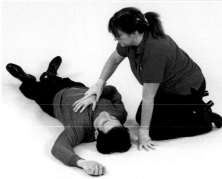

2 Position the victim's other arm across the chest.

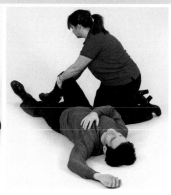

3 Bend the victim's nearer leg at the knee.

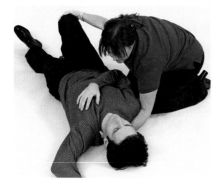

4 Put your forearm that is nearer the victim's head under the victim's nearer shoulder with your hand under the hollow of the neck.

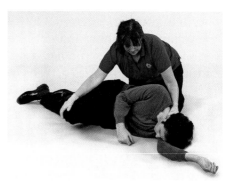

5 Carefully roll the victim away from you by pushing on the victim's flexed knee and lifting with your forearm while your hand stabilizes the head and neck. The victim's head is now supported on the raised arm.

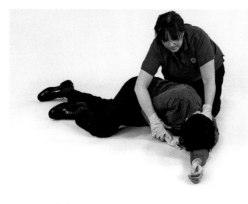

6 While continuing to support the head and neck, position the victim's hand palm down with fingers under the armpit of the raised arm, with forearm flat on the surface at 90 degrees to the body.

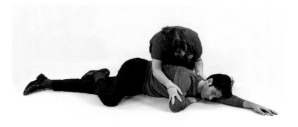

7 With victim now in position, check the airway and open the mouth to allow drainage.

her head slightly lower than the body (**Figure 4-5**). Support the head and neck with your hand and keep the nose and mouth clear.

Once the victim is in the recovery position, continue to monitor breathing while waiting for advanced help to arrive, and observe the victim for bleeding, medical alert bracelets or insignia, and any deformities that may indicate a serious injury. Give this information to responding EMS professionals.

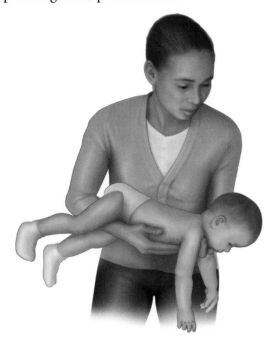

Figure 4-5 Infant recovery position.

THE SECONDARY ASSESSMENT

Remember that the secondary assessment is performed only for victims without life-threatening conditions. Do not interrupt care for a serious problem in order to carry out a secondary assessment. But if the victim's condition seems stable and no threats to life require your attention, then the secondary assessment can provide additional information about the injury or illness. That information may help you care for the victim and may be of value to arriving EMS professionals. The secondary assessment can usually be performed with responsive victims of injury or sudden illness who are not experiencing a breathing problem. Some aspects of the secondary assessment may be performed with unresponsive victims.

The secondary assessment has two primary parts: the history and the physical examination. In both parts, focus your attention primarily on the injured area, taking into account the cause and nature of the injury (often called the "mechanism of injury").

Get the Victim's History

After the initial assessment, get the victim's **history** to try to find out more about what happened and the victim's condition. Talk to a responsive victim.

Learning
Checkpoint (1)

1. You first encounter a victim lying quietly on the floor. Number the following actions in the correct order.

_____ **a.** Listen near victim's mouth for breathing sounds.

_____ **b.** Check to see if victim responds to your voice or touch.

_____ **c.** Open the airway if needed.

2. Describe three ways you can detect if a victim is breathing.

_____

3. True or False: If you hear a victim coughing, you can assume he or she is breathing.

With an unresponsive victim, ask bystanders about what they know or saw. With a potentially serious injury, try to assess the forces involved. For example, a victim who fell from a height or was struck in the head by a heavy object is at greater risk of having a spinal injury, and you must be careful not to move this victim during your assessment or when giving first aid.

When taking the history of a responsive victim of sudden illness, ask fully about the victim's situation to learn possible causes. For example, in a case of poisoning the victim may not immediately associate present symptoms with something ingested an hour or more ago. Or a victim could be experiencing the effects of carbon monoxide breathed inside a building, even though you encountered the victim outside.

Use the **SAMPLE** format to ensure that you cover the victim's full history:

S = **Signs and symptoms.** What can you observe about the victim (**signs**)? Ask the victim how he or she feels (**symptoms**), and ask for a description of any pain felt.

A = **Allergies.** Ask the victim if he or she has any allergies to foods, medicines, insect stings, or other substances. Look for a medical alert ID.

M = **Medications.** Ask the victim if he or she is taking any prescribed medications or over-the-counter products, including vitamins, supplements, and herbal remedies.

P = **Previous problems.** Ask the victim if he or she has had anything like this before or if he or she has any other illnesses. Again, a medical alert ID may indicate the victim has a condition such as diabetes or epilepsy.

L = **Last food or drink.** Ask the victim what he or she last ate and when.

E = **Events.** Ask the victim what happened, and try to identify the events that led to the current situation. When did the victim first begin to experience the problem?

If the victim is unresponsive, ask family members or bystanders whether they know the answers to these questions. Also check the scene for clues to what may have happened.

The victim may have just taken a medication, for example, or you may see something like a syringe that could indicate possible drug abuse. A nearby container of a poisonous household product could indicate a possible poisoning. Consider the environment: a very cold or hot environment may produce a temperature-related emergency or contribute to sudden illness. Finally, consider the victim's age. A younger person who slips on ice and falls may have only a bruise, whereas an elderly woman who falls is more likely to have broken her hip.

The information from the SAMPLE history may help you to give the right first aid. When help arrives, give the information you gathered to the EMS professionals. It will help them to provide the appropriate medical care.

Physical Examination

The secondary assessment of an injured or ill victim who is responsive also includes a **physical examination.** With this examination you may find other injuries that need first aid or additional clues to the victim's condition. Remember that you do not stop giving first aid for a serious condition just to do or complete this examination. Instead, keep the victim still and calm and wait for EMS professionals.

Remember that an unresponsive victim should be kept in the recovery position until EMS professionals arrive. Continue to monitor the victim's breathing, and observe the victim for bleeding and other signs of serious injury.

Allow a responsive victim to remain in the position he or she finds most comfortable while conducting the physical examination. The victim does not need to be moved to lie on his or her back as shown in the illustrations.

Ask a responsive victim for consent to do a physical examination, like any other first aid, and describe what you are about to do before touching the victim. Keep away from any body area the victim tells you is very painful. Watch for a victim's facial expression or stiffening of a body part, which may reveal pain or tenderness the victim does not tell you about.

Focus on the area the victim knows is injured. You do not need to touch every body area, for example, if the victim has only an injured arm and the nature of the injury does not suggest other body areas may be injured.

The physical examination of a responsive adult includes examining the victim from head to toe looking for anything out of the ordinary (**Box 4-2**). You begin at the head because injuries here are more likely to be serious than injuries in the extremities or lower in the body. As a general rule, look for the following signs and symptoms of injury or illness throughout the body, comparing one side of the body to the other:

- Pain when an area moves or is touched
- Bleeding or other wounds
- An area that is swollen or deformed from its usual appearance
- Skin color (flushed, pale, or ashen), temperature (hot or cold), moisture (dry, sweating, clammy)
- Abnormal sensation or inability to move the area

While performing the examination, watch for changes in the victim's condition. For example, the victim may at first be fully responsive and alert, but as you continue to check different body areas, the victim may become disoriented or dizzy, suggested changing mental status. The victim's breathing may change or stop. Call 9-1-1 if the victim's condition becomes more serious and the call was not made earlier.

You may have to remove some of the victim's clothing to examine an injured body area. Remove clothing or shoes only when necessary, such as to apply pressure on a wound to control bleeding, because moving the body part could cause additional injury. Protect the victim's privacy and prevent exposure to the cold. Follow these guidelines for removing clothing:

- Carefully roll or fold up a sleeve to expose an arm.
- To remove a jacket or shirt when an arm is injured, remove the uninjured arm from its sleeve first and then carefully work the jacket or shirt around the body and down off the injured arm while supporting it.
- Gently pull up a pants leg to expose the calf or knee. With scissors, carefully cut along the seam to expose the thigh.

Box 4-2 Signs and Symptoms of Injury and Illness

The victim may tell you about:
- Pain, tenderness
- Dizziness, feeling faint
- Nausea
- Tingling or abnormal sensation, no sensation
- Thirst
- Hot, cold

You may see:
- Painful expression, guarding against movement
- Bleeding, wound, bruise, swelling
- Abnormal skin color
- Deformity, inability to move part
- Unusual chest movement
- Vomit, incontinence

You may feel:
- Damp skin
- Hot or cold skin
- Swelling
- Deformity

You may hear:
- Noisy breathing
- Groaning, sounds of pain
- Stress in victim's voice
- Sucking chest wound

You may smell:
- Odor of a drug used
- Odor of poisonous or hazardous substance
- Fruity smelling breath (diabetic emergency)

- Support the victim's ankle when removing a shoe. Leave long boots on.
- If you cannot easily slide off a tight sock, lift it gently with your fingers and cut it open with scissors.

Check the Head and Neck

Do not move the head or neck during the examination. Gently feel the skull for bleeding, bumps, or depressions. Check the ears and nose for blood or a clear fluid. Check the pupils of both eyes, which should be of equal size and should respond to light when you cover and uncover the eyes with your hand. Check the victim's breathing for ease of breathing and regularity, and note any unusual breath odor. Check the mouth for burned areas. Check the neck for a medical alert necklace, deformity or swelling, bleeding, and pain. Observe the skin of the head and neck for color, temperature, and moisture.

Check the Torso

Check the chest and sides, feeling for deformity, wounds, or tender areas. Look for blood in any area. Ask the victim to take a deep breath and feel and look for easy, symmetrical expansion of the chest with breathing or for signs of pain on breathing. Gently feel along the collarbones and shoulders for deformity, swelling, or pain.

If you suspect a problem in the abdominal or pelvic areas, gently check the abdomen for rigidity, pain, or bleeding, and gently feel both sides of the hips and pelvis to check for pain or deformity.

Check the Extremities

Check the arms for bleeding, deformity, and pain. Ask the victim to bend his or her elbows, wrists, and fingers. Look for a medical alert bracelet. Touch the fingers and ask if the sensation feels normal to the victim. Check the skin color and temperature of the hand to detect impaired circulation. Ask the victim to shrug the shoulders.

Check the legs for bleeding, deformity, and pain. Unless you suspect a back, abdomen, or pelvic injury, ask the victim to point and wiggle the toes. Check the skin temperature and color of the feet. Touch the feet and ask if the sensation feels normal to the victim.

If you find anything unusual in the extremities, compare that extremity with the opposite side and note differences (see Skill: "Physical Examination").

Examining a Child or Infant

The assessment of a child or infant is similar to that of an adult, taking into account physical differences and the child's different language skills and emotional state. Use simple questions to gather the history, such as, "Where does it hurt?" Talk with the child's parents or guardians, if possible, and involve them in the physical examination (**Figure 4-6**). Allow a parent or guardian holding an infant or young child to continue to hold the victim during the examination. With a young child it is often better to perform the physical examination from toe to head rather than from the head first, to allow the child to get used to you in a more nonthreatening manner. Since a child is more likely to become upset or anxious, talk to him or her calmly and soothingly before starting the examination, and look for signs of anything unusual before touching the child. A child who is upset often reacts with physical changes that may mask or confuse the signs of injury.

MONITOR THE VICTIM

Give first aid for injuries or illness you discover in your assessment, as described in the following chapters. With very minor conditions the victim may need no more than your first aid. In other situations the victim may need to see a healthcare provider or go to the emergency department. With all life-threatening or serious conditions, you should have called 9-1-1 and will now be awaiting the arrival of help.

While waiting, monitor the victim to make sure his or her condition does not worsen. With an unresponsive victim or a victim with a serious injury, repeat your assessment of breathing at least every five minutes.

If you find any problems in any body area, do not let the victim move. Wait for help.

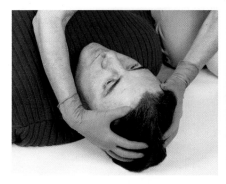

1 Being careful not to move the victim's head or neck, check the head.

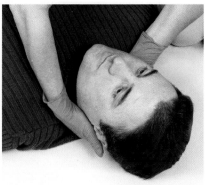

2 Check neck area for medical alert necklace, deformity or swelling, and pain. Do not move the neck.

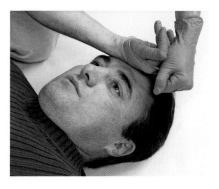

3 Check skin appearance, temperature, moisture.

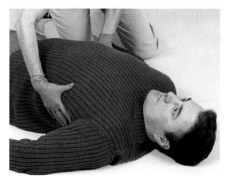

4 Check chest. Ask victim to breathe deeply.

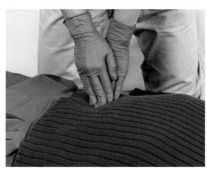

5 Check abdomen.

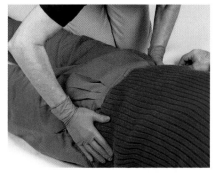

6 Check pelvis and hips.

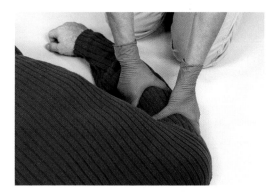

7 Check upper extremities. Look for medical alert bracelet.

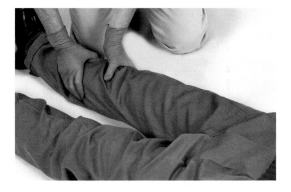

8 Check lower extremities.

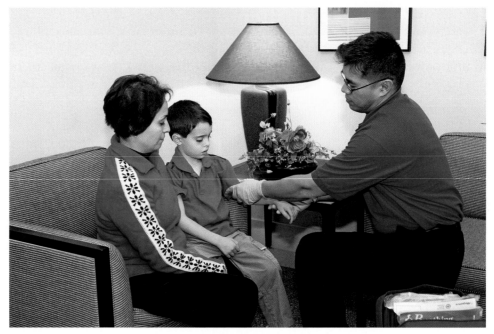

Figure 4-6 Involve the child's parent or guardian in the history and physical examination.

Learning
Checkpoint ②

1. When is the secondary assessment performed?

   a. Immediately before giving CPR when needed

   b. In all victims, right after the initial assessment

   c. After checking for responsiveness

   d. After determining that there are no life-threatening conditions

2. Write what each letter in the SAMPLE history stands for

   S = _____   **P** = _____

   A = _____   **L** = _____

   M = _____   **E** = _____

3. Describe what signs and symptoms of injury you are looking for as you examine each part of a victim's body.

   _____

   _____

Concluding Thoughts

You can see why a victim of injury or sudden illness is assessed in two stages: if the initial assessment reveals a life-threatening problem, then you must provide basic life support immediately without going on to the history and physical examination. **Chapter 5** is the first of four chapters describing basic life support for life-threatening problems. Remember: a breathing problem is an *immediate* threat to life, requiring action within seconds because body tissues will begin to die within minutes.

Learning Outcomes

You should now be able to do the following:

1. Explain how to check the victim's responsiveness.

2. Demonstrate how to open the airway and check for breathing.

3. Demonstrate how to move a victim into the recovery position and explain when this is done.

4. Explain the importance of each element in the SAMPLE history.

5. Demonstrate how to perform a physical examination of a responsive victim without a life-threatening problem.

Review Questions

1. The initial assessment checks the victim for
   a. bone fractures.
   b. severe bleeding.
   c. severe allergies.
   d. spinal injuries.

2. Assess a victim for responsiveness by
   a. tapping the shoulder and asking if he or she is okay.
   b. pinching the cheek between thumb and forefinger.
   c. checking for pupil reactions to light.
   d. checking skin for normal color and temperature.

3. If a victim can talk to you, you can be sure he or she
   a. does not have a life-threatening condition.
   b. does not have a spinal injury.
   c. is breathing.
   d. All of the above

4. To open the airway of an unresponsive victim
   a. tilt the head back and lift the chin.
   b. pry open the mouth with both hands.
   c. tilt the head back while prying open the mouth.
   d. do not tilt the head back but hold the chin down.

5. How long should you check an unresponsive victim for breathing before concluding he or she is not breathing?
   a. About two seconds
   b. No more than 10 seconds
   c. About 20 to 30 seconds
   d. About one minute

6. Advantages of the recovery position include which of the following?
   a. It lowers the victim's blood pressure.
   b. It allows fluids to drain from the mouth.
   c. It helps reduce shock.
   d. It helps ensure that the brain receives sufficient oxygen.

7. When gathering a SAMPLE history from a suddenly ill victim, which should you ask about?
   a. Allergies and medications taken
   b. Age and weight
   c. Recent meals and favorite foods
   d. Most recent annual physical exam

8. During the physical examination, what are you looking for?
   a. Bleeding or wounds
   b. A swollen area
   c. Pain upon being touched
   d. All of the above

References and Resources

American Heart Association. Available from: www.american heart.org.

American Heart Association. 2005 International consensus on cardiopulmonary resuscitation (CPR) and emergency cardiovascular care (ECC) science with treatment recommendations. *Circulation,* 112(22). November 29, 2005.

National Safety Council. www.nsc.org

Chapter 5

Basic Life Support 1: Rescue Breaths

Chapter Preview

- Overview of Basic Life Support
- Respiratory Emergencies
- Respiratory Arrest and Respiratory Distress
- Rescue Breaths

It has been an hour since basketball practice ended, but as usual some of the players stayed to practice their shots. As you lock up your office and head down the hall for the exit doors, you notice the gym lights are still on and look in. A player lies crumpled on the floor, and everyone else is gone. He doesn't respond to your voice or touch when you reach his side. What do you do?

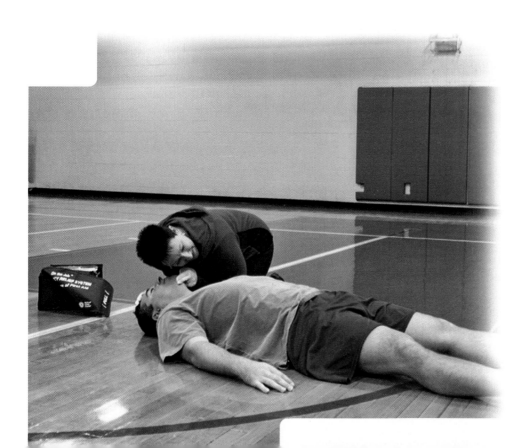

In **Chapter 4** you learned how to check the victim's breathing during the initial assessment. An unresponsive person who is not breathing needs CPR immediately. CPR combines rescue breaths and chest compressions to move oxygenated blood to vital organs. This chapter discusses respiratory emergencies and describes how to give rescue breaths.

OVERVIEW OF BASIC LIFE SUPPORT

Basic life support (BLS) refers to first aid given if the victim's breathing or heart stops. Many things can cause breathing or the heart to stop. Whenever either breathing or the heart stops, the other also stops very soon. BLS is often needed for victims of:

- Heart attack
- Drowning
- Choking
- Other injuries or conditions that affect breathing or the heart

Basic life support consists of several first aid skills, often called **resuscitation.** A victim who is not breathing normally needs rescue breaths and CPR to move oxygen into the body and to circulate blood in the body to keep vital organs alive. A victim who is choking also needs first aid to clear the airway to allow either natural breathing or rescue breaths. A victim whose heart is in a condition called ventricular fibrillation, which is common after heart attacks and other situations, needs an electrical shock given by an automated external defibrillator (AED) to restore a more normal heart rhythm.

This chapter focuses on respiratory emergencies and rescue breaths. The additional skills used in CPR, choking care, and use of an AED are described in the following chapters.

Differences Among Adults, Children, and Infants

Some BLS skills are performed somewhat differently with adults, children, and infants. These differences are based on age and result from anatomical and physiological differences in the human body at different ages. Standard age groups for BLS performed by lay rescuers are defined in the following way. Remember these age categories in reference to all BLS techniques (rescue breaths, CPR, choking care, and AED use):

Infant—birth to 1 year

Child—ages 1 to 8

Adult—over age 8

RESPIRATORY EMERGENCIES

Any illness or injury that causes a victim to stop breathing, or to breathe so ineffectively that the body is not receiving enough oxygen, is a respiratory emergency. The two primary types of breathing emergencies are respiratory arrest and respiratory distress.

All body tissues need a continual supply of oxygen to function and to maintain life. As described in **Chapter 3**, the respiratory system, working primarily with the cardiovascular system, provides this needed oxygen. In the lungs, oxygen moves out of the air into the blood, which is then circulated throughout the body. Carbon dioxide, a waste product of cellular metabolism, is also picked up from the tissues by the blood and eliminated in the lungs. The functioning of the respiratory and cardiovascular systems also depends on the muscles of breathing and nervous system control of breathing and the heart. A problem in any of these areas can result in a respiratory emergency. For example:

- A physical obstruction in the airway, such as food blocking the pharynx, or immersion in water, can make it impossible for air to reach the lungs.
- An injury to the chest can penetrate the lungs and hinder the movement of air into and out of the lungs with breathing.
- Breathing in carbon monoxide from a faulty furnace or smoke from a fire can reduce the availability of oxygen in the lungs and cause less oxygen to be present in the blood for body tissues.
- A heart problem can result in insufficient blood being circulated in the body, reducing the amount of oxygen available for tissues.
- An electrical shock can disrupt the nervous system's control of either breathing or the heartbeat, thereby disrupting the flow of oxygen to the body.
- A drug overdose or poisoning can depress nervous system control of breathing such that insufficient oxygen reaches body tissues.

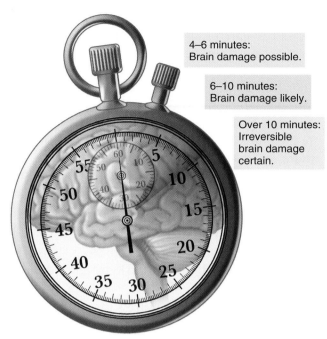

4–6 minutes:
Brain damage possible.

6–10 minutes:
Brain damage likely.

Over 10 minutes:
Irreversible
brain damage
certain.

Figure 5-1 Without oxygen, vital organs soon begin to die.

These are just a few of the many ways in which respiratory emergencies may occur. Regardless of the cause, body cells begin to die soon after losing their oxygen supply. Brain cells are very susceptible to low levels of oxygen and begin to die as soon as four minutes after oxygen is cut off. Within six minutes brain damage is likely (**Figure 5-1**). Death is likely soon after.

RESPIRATORY ARREST AND RESPIRATORY DISTRESS

Respiratory arrest means that breathing has completely stopped. Again, this condition may result from many different causes. You do not need to know the exact cause, however, because the BLS steps for respiratory arrest are the same in all cases.

With **respiratory distress,** on the other hand, the victim is still breathing, but the breathing is difficult and may become so ineffective that the victim's blood oxygen content drops to a life-threatening level. Respiratory distress may occur with different illnesses and injuries. Someone with asthma, for example, may experience great difficulty breathing when tissues of the airway swell and make it difficult to move air into and out of the lungs. A severe allergic reaction may cause a similar problem.

The first aid for victims of respiratory distress is somewhat different because the victim is still breathing. In this case care focuses on easing the breathing crisis and addresses the cause of the problem if possible. Conditions causing respiratory distress are described in **Chapter 17**. Note, however, that respiratory distress can progress to respiratory arrest, in which case the victim needs BLS as described in this chapter.

Prevention of Respiratory Arrest

Respiratory arrest can be prevented by preventing its common causes, including drowning and sudden infant death syndrome (SIDS), as well as all general injury prevention measures. The prevention of choking, a common cause of respiratory arrest, is described in **Chapter 7**. Since breathing stops when the heart stops, preventing cardiac arrest also prevents respiratory arrest; this is discussed in **Chapter 6**.

Preventing Drowning

About 3000 people die each year from drowning in the United States. Roughly two-thirds of these are between 15 and 64 years of age. A little less than one-third are children under age 14 and a much smaller percentage are older adults. About three times this total number of victims receive emergency treatment for near drowning, and many of these have permanent disabilities from brain damage caused by lack of oxygen during submersion or related factors.

Although drowning is the second leading cause of injury-related death for children 1 to 14 years old, most parents say they do not worry about their child drowning. This overconfidence and lack of concern is likely a significant factor in the poor supervision of children around water. Among children, 90% of drownings occur with an adult "supervising" but distracted by other factors.

The prevention of drowning is based on understanding the primary risk factors:

- Most infant victims drown in bathtubs, buckets, or toilets. An infant should never be left unsupervised near water, even to a depth of an inch or two, for even a moment.
- Most victims one to four years old drown in residential swimming pools with one or both parents at home at the time—with the

child usually out of sight for less than five minutes. Never leave a young child alone in or near the water, even if the child has had beginning swimming lessons or promises to stay out of the water in your absence. All children should be supervised by an adult who maintains continuous visual contact and does not engage in distracting activities such as talking on the telephone or reading. Pools should have protective barriers with effective locks. Parents should never trust floating toys, rafts, or inner tubes to keep their children afloat.

- Up to 50% of drowning deaths in the age group with the most drownings, adolescents and adults, are associated with alcohol use during water recreational activities. Alcohol influences balance, coordination, and judgment, which are key factors in situations that lead to drowning. Prevention is simple: do not drink and go into or near the water. Swim with a buddy, never dive into shallow or unknown water, and wear a lifejacket or personal flotation device (PFD) in water sports.

- About 70% of the 750 annual deaths during boating activities result from drowning. Most victims are not wearing life preservers, and in about 40% of cases alcohol is involved. Following safe boating guidelines can help prevent most of these drowning deaths.

Preventing SIDS

Sudden infant death syndrome (SIDS), sometimes also called crib death, is the sudden death of an infant under age one of unexplained causes. It occurs most commonly between two and four months of age and is the most common cause of infant death after one month of age. About 2300 infants die of SIDS in the United States every year, a number that has dropped in recent years with efforts to educate parents and caregivers. Current research suggests that SIDS may result from certain congenital differences that make some infants more susceptible, but evidence also indicates that preventive efforts can prevent SIDS from occurring in most cases. It has also been estimated that as many as 900 of the deaths that are attributed to SIDS may have resulted from simple suffocation because these infants are found in suffocating environments and positions, often lying on the stomach with nose and mouth covered by soft bedding.

To reduce the risk of SIDS and suffocation:

- Place infants on their backs to sleep. This step alone lowers the risk of SIDS by more than 50%.
- Use a firm, flat crib mattress that meets safety standards.
- Remove pillows, comforters, toys, and other soft objects from the crib.
- Do not cover the infant's head during sleep.
- If a blanket must be used, use a thin blanket, tuck it under the edges of the mattress, and keep it at chest level and below to reduce the likelihood of the infant pulling it over his or her face.
- Avoid smoking. When a woman smokes during pregnancy, the infant is three times more likely to have SIDS, and an infant exposed to passive smoke has double the risk.
- Maintain a normal temperature in the infant's room but do not overheat the infant.
- Do not have the infant sleep in a bed shared with siblings or parents. Experts recommend having the infant's crib beside the bed when parents wish to be close and to facilitate breastfeeding.
- Give an infant between 1 and 12 months of age a pacifier at bedtime.

Learning Checkpoint (1)

1. Basic life support helps keep a victim alive when _____ stops.

2. For purposes of basic life support techniques, a child is defined as someone between the ages of _____ and _____ .

RESCUE BREATHS

Giving rescue breaths is a technique of blowing air into a nonbreathing victim's lungs to oxygenate the blood. Rescue breaths are given along with chest compressions, which help circulate the oxygenated blood to vital organs, keeping the victim alive until the victim is resuscitated or EMS personnel arrive to give advanced care.

Rescue breaths are given with the first aider's own air unless special equipment is available. The air around us contains about 21% oxygen, and the breath we exhale contains about 16% oxygen—still enough oxygen to increase the oxygen level in the victim's blood to maintain life. When a first aider blows air into the victim's mouth or nose, this air moves into the lungs in a manner similar to natural breathing. The chest rises as the lungs expand, and oxygen moves into the blood in the small vessels within the lungs. After each breath the chest is allowed to fall and the air is "exhaled" out, then the next breath is given.

Rescue breaths are given along with chest compressions to any victim who is not breathing normally. An unresponsive victim who is occasionally gasping is not breathing and needs CPR. Give two rescue breaths, when you discover the victim is not breathing normally. Then begin CPR.

Also have someone call 9-1-1 immediately. If an AED is available, send someone to get it (see **Chapter 8**).

Techniques for Giving Rescue Breaths

First position the victim on his or her back. Open the airway using the head tilt-chin lift. Use a barrier device to protect against disease transmission if you have one, but do not delay giving rescue breaths to get one. Even without a barrier device the risk of contracting an infectious disease from rescue breathing is very low.

The basic technique is to blow air slowly into the victim while watching the chest rise to make sure your air is going into the lungs. Do not try to rush the air in or blow too forcefully. Do not take a big breath in order to exhale more air into the victim; just take a normal breath. Give each breath over about one second. If the breath does not go in—if you feel resistance or do not see the victim's chest rise—then try again to open the airway. If your breath still does not go in, then the victim

has an airway obstruction and needs care for choking (see **Chapter 7**). If your initial breath does go in, give a second breath over one second and then begin chest compressions as described in **Chapter 6**.

Remember these key points:

- Do not blow harder than is needed to make the victim's chest rise.
- After each breath remember to let the air escape and the chest fall.
- Blowing in too forcefully or for too long is ineffective and may put air in the stomach which may cause vomiting.

Mouth to Barrier

Barrier devices are always recommended for giving rescue breaths and should be kept in the first aid kit (**Figure 5-2**). The two most common types of barrier devices are pocket masks and face shields. Both types of devices offer protection from the victim's saliva and other fluids, as well as from the victim's exhaled air when equipped with a one-way valve. With either device, keep the victim's head positioned to maintain an open airway as you deliver rescue breaths through the device.

A pocket mask is positioned on the victim's face over both the mouth and nose. A one-way valve in the mouthpiece lets your air flow into the victim but directs the victim's exhaled air out another way so that it does not reach you directly during rescue breathing. With a face mask, as with any barrier device, make sure it is well sealed to the victim's face, and watch the victim's chest rise to confirm that your air is going into the victim.

A face shield is also positioned over the victim's mouth as a protective barrier. The victim's nose is pinched closed when giving a rescue breath to prevent the air from coming out the nose instead of entering the lungs.

Mouth to Mouth

If you do not have a barrier device, pinch the victim's nose shut and seal your mouth over the victim's mouth. Blow into the victim's mouth, watching the chest rise to confirm that the air is going in.

Mouth to Nose

If the victim's mouth cannot be opened or is injured, or if you cannot get a good seal with your mouth over the victim's mouth, you can give rescue breaths through the nose. Hold the victim's mouth closed,

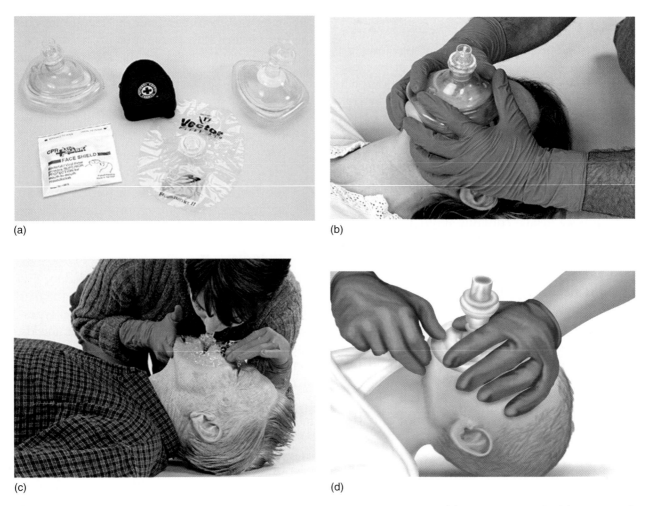

(a)

(b)

(c)

(d)

Figure 5-2 (a) Barrier devices. (b) Position pocket mask over mouth and nose. (c) Position face shield over mouth and pinch nose. (d) Mask used with an infant.

seal your mouth over the nose to blow in, and then allow the mouth to open to let the air escape.

Mouth to Stoma

Because of past illness or injury, some people breathe through a hole in their lower neck called a **stoma** (Figure 5-3). In the initial assessment, check this hole to see if the victim is breathing. To give rescue breaths through a stoma, cup your hand over the victim's nose and mouth to prevent your air from leaving by the nose and mouth instead of going to the lungs. Then seal your mouth over the stoma, and give rescue breaths as usual. Or, you can use a round pediatric face mask if you have one.

Mouth to Nose and Mouth

Because of their smaller size, infants and very small children are generally given rescue breaths through both their mouth and nose. Seal your mouth over both the nose and mouth and give gentle breaths as usual, watching to see the chest rise with each breath.

Potential Problems with Rescue Breaths

Usually it is a straightforward procedure to give rescue breaths. Two special situations that can cause problems are air that enters the stomach and loose dentures.

Remember that in the pharynx, the oral cavity meets both the trachea (which goes to the lungs) and the esophagus (which goes to the stomach). Usually, if the head is positioned correctly to open the airway and rescue breaths are not given too forcefully or too fast, the air will move through the trachea into the lungs rather than down the esophagus to the stomach. In some cases, air does move into the stomach, however.

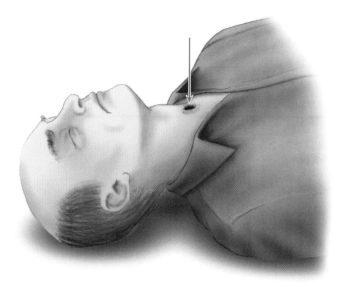

Figure 5-3 Victim with a stoma.

the stomach makes vomiting more likely. Vomiting presents two problems. First, if an unresponsive victim vomits during BLS care, you have to roll the victim onto his or her side to drain the victim's mouth, and then wipe the mouth clean before continuing. Second, when the victim vomits there is a risk of **aspiration,** which is the movement of vomit or other fluids or solids into the lungs, which can cause a serious infection and other problems. For these reasons, when giving rescue breaths be sure to:

- Open the airway first.
- Watch the chest rise as you give breaths.
- Blow slowly and steadily rather than too quickly.
- Stop each breath when the chest rises rather than continuing to blow.
- Let the chest fall between breaths.

If the airway is not sufficiently open, if rescue breaths are given too quickly, or if you continue to blow in air even after the lungs have expanded and the chest has risen, then air may be forced into the stomach. In this situation, not only is the victim possibly not receiving enough air in the lungs to oxygenate the blood, but the air in

If a victim is wearing dentures, they are usually left in place when breaths are given. It is generally easier to give rescue breathing with dentures in their normal position. If they become loose and make it difficult to give breaths or may even fall back in the mouth to block the airway, then remove the dentures before giving rescue breaths.

Learning
Checkpoint ②

1. Rescue breaths are needed to

   a. get oxygen into the victim's blood.

   b. circulate the blood to vital organs.

   c. open the victim's airway.

   d. All of the above

2. True or False: Blow as hard as you can into the victim's mouth during rescue breathing.

3. What is the best way to confirm that your breaths are going into the victim's lungs?

   a. Listen at the victim's mouth for escaping air.

   b. Place one hand on the victim's abdomen to feel movement.

   c. Watch the victim's chest rise and fall.

   d. None of the above

4. When giving rescue breaths, give each breath over _____ second(s).

Concluding Thoughts

Remember to check for normal breathing in any unresponsive victim. If an unresponsive victim is gasping or is not breathing, give two rescue breaths to move oxygen into the victims lungs, and then start chest compressions as you will learn in **Chapter 6**.

Learning Outcomes

You should now be able to do the following:

1. List ways to prevent drowning and SIDS.

2. Describe the age categories for adults, children, and infants related to differences in basic life support skills.

3. Explain how to give rescue breaths via a barrier device, the mouth, the nose, or a stoma, and to an infant.

Review Questions

1. For the purposes of BLS, when does an infant become a child?
   a. At six months
   b. At one year
   c. At 15 pounds
   d. At 25 pounds

2. Rescue breaths are given with the victim in what position?
   a. On the back
   b. On the side
   c. On the back or the side
   d. In the position in which the victim is found

3. How long should it take to deliver one rescue breath?
   a. ½ second
   b. 1 second
   c. 1½ seconds
   d. 2 seconds

4. Why should a barrier device be used with rescue breaths?
   a. To help get more air into the victim
   b. To prevent vomiting
   c. To protect against infectious disease
   d. To prevent air from entering the esophagus

5. Vomiting during rescue breaths may result from
   a. blowing in too forcefully.
   b. blowing in for too long.
   c. blowing in too fast.
   d. All of the above

References and Resources

American Heart Association. www.americanheart.org

First Candle/SIDS Alliance, SIDS Q & A. Available from: www.firstcandle.org

American Heart Association. 2005 International consensus on cardiopulmonary resuscitation (CPR) and emergency cardiovascular care (ECC) science with treatment recommendations. *Circulation*, 112(22). November 29, 2005.

National Center for Injury Prevention and Control. Water-related injuries: fact sheet. Available from: www.cdc.gov/ncipc/factsheets/drown.htm

National Safe Kids Campaign. www.safekids.org

National Safety Council. www.nsc.org

Chapter 6

Basic Life Support 2: CPR

Chapter Preview

- Prevention of Cardiovascular Illness
- Cardiac Chain of Survival
- Call First/Call Fast
- The Use of CPR
- Technique of CPR

You are walking past your neighbor's house when you hear a scream for help. You knock on the door and offer to help. Your neighbor lets you in and you find her husband unresponsive on the floor. "He just collapsed," she tells you. You send her to call 9-1-1 and quickly check to see whether he is breathing. He is not breathing. How do you handle this situation?

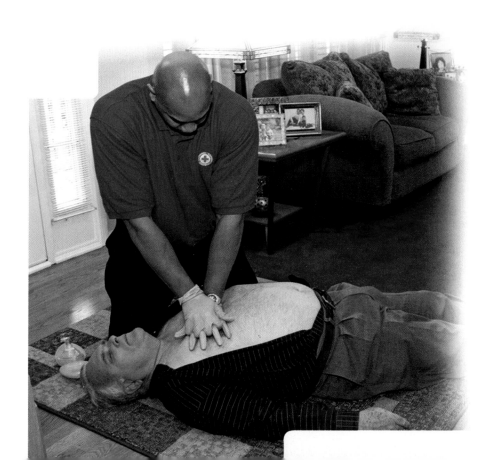

As you learned in **Chapter 5**, rescue breaths are given to oxygenate the blood of someone whose breathing has stopped. In addition, chest compressions are given to circulate the oxygenated blood to vital organs. Rescue breaths combined with chest compressions are called **cardiopulmonary resuscitation (CPR).**

Give CPR to any unresponsive victim who is not breathing normally. The specific steps for CPR vary somewhat for adults, children, and infants. It is important to learn and practice the skills for all age groups.

CPR is most commonly needed by victims in cardiac arrest as a result of a heart attack. Because a heart attack is usually caused by cardiovascular disease, preventing cardiovascular illnesses by maintaining a healthy lifestyle is the most effective way to prevent heart attacks and other cardiovascular emergencies such as stroke.

PREVENTION OF CARDIOVASCULAR ILLNESS

The term *cardiovascular illness* refers to several different diseases involving the heart and blood vessels (**Figure 6-1**). Cardiovascular disease becomes more common as a person ages, but as **Figure 6-2** shows, these diseases are surprisingly common even in young adults. The three most common cardiovascular diseases are:

- Heart disease, such as **coronary heart disease** (blockage of vessels supplying heart muscle with blood, often leading to heart attack)
- **Stroke** (sudden impairment of blood circulation in a part of the brain)
- **Hypertension** (high blood pressure, a very common condition that can lead to both heart attack and stroke)

Until 2002, heart disease was the most common cause of death in Americans under age 85, resulting in about 450,000 deaths a year. The incidence of heart disease has dropped slightly in recent years, and cancer is now the number one killer—but heart disease is still very common. Over 13 million people in the United States have coronary heart disease, and about 700,000 first-time heart attacks occur each year.

Stroke has been and remains the number three cause of death overall. About 700,000 people a year have a stroke, resulting in over 162,000 deaths. Over five million people are living with the effects of stroke, which often include severe disability. Stroke is discussed in **Chapter 17.**

Almost one-third of all people in the United States have high blood pressure—over 65 mil-

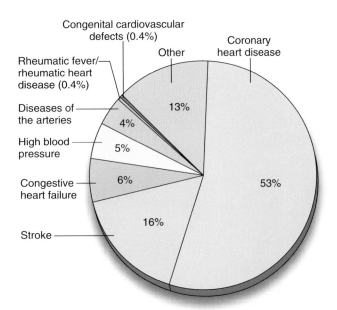

Figure 6-1 Percentage breakdown of deaths from cardiovascular disease.

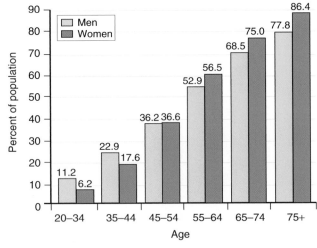

Figure 6-2 Prevalence of cardiovascular diseases in Americans age 20 and older by age and sex.

lion people. Although this disease directly results in almost 50,000 deaths a year, hypertension contributes as a risk factor to many more deaths caused by heart attack, stroke, or other diseases.

Taken together, these three cardiovascular diseases along with the others shown in **Figure 6-1** constitute the number one health problem in the United States today. Yet many of the risk factors leading to these diseases can be prevented.

Cardiovascular Risk Factors

A **risk factor** is anything that makes it more likely that a person will develop a particular disease. Some risk factors are beyond our control, but others are lifestyle factors that a person can avoid or change. Following are the known risk factors for cardiovascular disease:

Risk factors that cannot be changed
- Increasing age
- Male gender
- Race
- Hereditary factors

Preventable risk factors
- Smoking
- High cholesterol levels
- High blood pressure
- Physical inactivity
- Obesity and overweight
- Stress

Even though some risk factors cannot be changed, it is important to be aware of them when they increase your risk of cardiovascular disease. In general, the risks of these diseases rise with increasing age. Men are more likely to have cardiovascular disease—although the rates are also high with women, who should not feel immune to heart attacks and other problems. African Americans generally have a higher prevalence of high blood pressure than Caucasians and therefore have a greater risk for cardiovascular disease. Hereditary factors such as a family history of heart disease also can increase one's risk.

If you know your risk for cardiovascular disease is high because of risk factors beyond your control, it is all the more important to focus on those risk factors you *can* control. Risk factors often have an additive effect: the more risk factors you have, the higher your danger overall for developing disease.

Prevention of cardiovascular disease, therefore, involves eliminating risk factors by living a healthy lifestyle. In general, this means:

- Not using tobacco
- Eating healthy foods to prevent overweight, to help lower cholesterol levels and blood pressure, and to help prevent diabetes
- Maintaining low cholesterol levels, with medication when appropriate
- Controlling high blood pressure with diet, exercise, weight control, and medication if needed
- Getting sufficient regular exercise to help prevent overweight, high blood pressure, diabetes, and stress
- Preventing or managing stress

You should notice how these risk factors are interrelated. For example, inactivity puts one at risk for being overweight, and weight control helps prevent hypertension as well as helping one manage stress. Eating well also helps prevent overweight and helps to control blood pressure. These interrelated risk factors are sometimes referred to as a *constellation* of factors. To maintain good cardiovascular health, we should focus not on one or two factors but on a whole constellation of healthy choices that together result in a healthy lifestyle.

Maintaining Cardiovascular Health

Cardiovascular health can be attained and maintained with a lifestyle that includes good diet, exercise, weight and blood pressure control, and stress management.

All of these factors involve behavioral habits that typically begin in childhood, although they may also develop later in life. Adults who understand that they need to eat healthily and get exercise, for example, may have difficulty doing so if they have habitually behaved otherwise. The following sections, therefore, focus on establishing good habits early in childhood as well as developing them later in life when needed.

In recent years more media attention has been given to the cardiovascular health of children. The problems of childhood obesity, high cholesterol levels, poor diet, and lack of exercise are now recognized. Although few children actually experience heart disease other than rare congenital problems, from a very early age they form habits that often stay with them for life.

Smoking

Smoking and other use of tobacco contribute to poor cardiovascular health. Smokers have a risk two to four times higher for cardiovascular disease than nonsmokers. Children learn about smoking at a very early age by observing adults. About 80% of adults who use tobacco began before age 18, most starting at age 14 to 15. Do not smoke around children, both because of the risks of secondhand smoke and because you as an adult caregiver are a role model and would be implicitly teaching children it is okay to smoke. Support the efforts of schools and other organizations to teach children that all tobacco use is unhealthy.

Most adults who smoke know that it is an unhealthful habit yet still have difficulty quitting. Over 22% of the population still smokes. Many smoking cessation programs have been developed and have proved effective when one is motivated to stop. For information, contact the American Cancer Society, American Lung Association, or American Heart Association. The U.S. Surgeon General states that a program for quitting smoking is most effective if it includes these five steps:

1. Get ready.
2. Get support.
3. Learn new skills and behaviors.
4. Get medication and use it correctly.
5. Be prepared for relapse or difficult situations.

Admittedly, it is not easy to quit smoking, as nicotine is a highly addictive substance. But a commitment to quitting along with a realistic attitude and plan has led to millions of adults successfully breaking the habit. Your cardiovascular health and risk for cancer begin to improve the day you quit.

Diet

Good nutrition affects a child's health in the present and influences habits that will affect cardiovascular health later on. Children's food preferences are influenced by many factors, such as what the family eats at home, what they see other children eat at childcare or at school, and what television commercials "teach" them to eat. You cannot counteract all of these influences, of course, but encouraging a good diet is the responsibility of all adult caregivers.

Most current nutritional research continues to support what we have known for some time: high-fat and high-sugar foods are unhealthy, and eating a variety of foods with an emphasis on fruits, vegetables, and whole grains and cereals is healthy and promotes a normal weight. In 2005 a federal government panel reviewed previous dietary recommendations and issued the revised guidelines for adults and children over age two listed in **Box 6-1**. In addition, certain dietary changes are recommended for specific population groups, such as older adults, pregnant women, overweight adults, and others. Talk to your healthcare provider about changes that may be important for you.

In almost all instances, healthy alternatives to unhealthy foods and snacks are available that taste just as good. Choose low-fat frozen yogurt or frozen fruit bars rather than ice cream, skim or low-fat milk rather than whole milk, whole wheat bread rather than white bread, and so on. In all these ways you will help set the stage for a lifetime of cardiovascular health.

Cholesterol

Cholesterol is a fatty substance the body needs to carry out important functions. Cholesterol is taken into the body from the diet, especially from foods high in animal fats, and it is manufactured in the liver. Hereditary factors also affect your cholesterol level. Because of these factors outside your control, you cannot assume you have a low blood level of cholesterol just because you eat well.

High cholesterol levels are very common in the United States. About 95 million people, or 45% of the population, have borderline-high or high levels of low-density lipoprotein (LDL), the *bad* type of cholesterol. This is due in part to a generally poor diet and lack of exercise. Cholesterol affects cardiovascular health because it is deposited in the arteries along

Box 6-1 Federal Dietary Guidelines

- Consume a variety of nutrient-dense foods and beverages within and among the basic food groups while choosing foods that limit the intake of saturated and trans fats, cholesterol, added sugars, salt, and alcohol.
- Meet recommended intakes within energy (calorie) needs by adopting a balanced eating pattern.
- Consume a sufficient amount of fruits and vegetables while staying within energy needs. Two cups of fruit and two and one-half cups of vegetables per day are recommended for a reference 2000-calorie intake, with higher or lower amounts depending on the calorie level.
- Choose a variety of fruits and vegetables each day. In particular, select from all five vegetable subgroups (dark green, orange, legumes, starchy vegetables, and other vegetables) several times a week.
- Consume three or more ounce-equivalents of whole-grain products per day, with the rest of the recommended grains coming from enriched or whole-grain products. In general, at least half the grains should come from whole grains.
- Consume three cups per day of fat-free or low-fat milk or equivalent milk products.
- Consume less than 10% of calories from saturated fatty acids and less than 300 mg/day of cholesterol, and keep trans fatty acid consumption as low as possible.
- Keep total fat intake between 20% and 35% of calories, with most fats coming from sources of polyunsaturated and monounsaturated fatty acids, such as fish, nuts, and vegetable oils.

- When selecting and preparing meat, poultry, dry beans, and milk or milk products, make choices that are lean, low-fat, or fat-free.
- Limit intake of fats and oils high in saturated and/or trans fatty acids, and choose products low in such fats and oils.
- Choose and prepare foods and beverages with little added sugars or caloric sweeteners.
- Reduce the incidence of dental cavities by practicing good oral hygiene and consuming sugar- and starch-containing foods and beverages less frequently.
- Consume less than 2300 mg (approximately 1 tsp of salt) of sodium per day.
- Choose and prepare foods with little salt. At the same time, consume potassium-rich foods, such as fruits and vegetables.
- Those who choose to drink alcoholic beverages should do so sensibly and in moderation—defined as the consumption of up to one drink per day for women and up to two drinks per day for men.
- Alcoholic beverages should not be consumed by some individuals, including those who cannot restrict their alcohol intake, women of childbearing age who may become pregnant, pregnant and lactating women, children and adolescents, individuals taking medications that can interact with alcohol, and those with specific medical conditions.
- Alcoholic beverages should be avoided by individuals engaging in activities that require attention, skill, or coordination, such as driving or operating machinery.

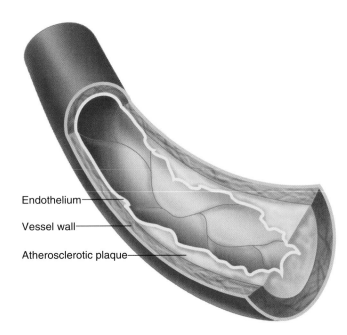

Endothelium

Vessel wall

Atherosclerotic plaque

Figure 6-3 High blood cholesterol levels contribute to buildup of plaque inside arteries.

with other substances as **plaque (Figure 6-3)**. A buildup of plaque leads to the condition called **atherosclerosis,** a narrowing and "hardening" of the arteries. Atherosclerosis in coronary arteries can cause a heart attack and in arteries in the brain can cause a stroke.

Because high cholesterol levels are a risk factor for cardiovascular disease, adults need regular testing. Increasingly pediatricians are testing children as well. Only a blood test can determine your cholesterol level.

If you are found to have high blood levels of LDL, you can take several steps to control this risk factor:

- Avoid high-cholesterol foods such as animal fats.
- Maintain a healthy weight (cholesterol levels rise in overweight people).
- Get more exercise (cholesterol levels generally rise with inactivity). Make it your goal to get 30 to 60 minutes of exercise on most or all days of the week.
- Talk with your healthcare provider about whether a cholesterol-lowering medication is appropriate for you. If you do take a medication, do so consistently. For a variety of reasons, only 30% to 40% of those prescribed

these medications are still taking them a year later even though they still need them—perhaps because they feel fine. Remember that usually you can't feel the results of plaque building up in your arteries and threatening your health.

Exercise

It has become a cliché but is nonetheless true: most children and adults do not get enough exercise. Almost 40% of the population reports no leisure-time physical activity at all, with many more not engaging in any activity regularly. Television, computer games, and the Internet have contributed to children becoming more sedentary than decades ago. Adults often say they are too busy with work and family responsibilities to engage in activities that provide exercise.

Exercise is good not only for the muscles but for the heart, lungs, and blood vessels. Like diet, exercise helps both adults and children be healthier now while building a foundation for future cardiovascular health and a longer, healthier, happier life. Following are the 2005 federal recommendations for physical activity for children and adults:

- Engage in regular physical activity and reduce sedentary activities to promote health, psychological well-being, and a healthy body weight.
- *To reduce the risk of chronic disease in adulthood:* Engage in at least 30 minutes of moderate-intensity physical activity at work or home on most days of the week.
- *For most people,* greater health benefits can be obtained by engaging in physical activity of more vigorous intensity or longer duration.
- *To help manage body weight and prevent gradual, unhealthy body weight gain in adulthood:* Engage in approximately 60 minutes of moderate- to vigorous-intensity activity on most days of the week while not exceeding caloric intake requirements.
- *To sustain weight loss in adulthood:* Participate in at least 60 to 90 minutes of daily moderate-intensity physical activity while not exceeding caloric intake requirements. Some people may need to consult with a health-

care provider before participating in this level of activity.

- *Achieve physical fitness* by including cardiovascular conditioning, stretching exercises for flexibility, and resistance exercises or calisthenics for muscle strength and endurance.
- *Children and adolescents:* Engage in at least 60 minutes of physical activity on most, preferably all, days of the week.
- *Pregnant women:* In the absence of medical or obstetric complications, incorporate 30 minutes or more of moderate-intensity physical activity on most, if not all, days of the week. Avoid activities with a high risk of falling or abdominal trauma.
- *Breastfeeding women:* Be aware that neither acute nor regular exercise adversely affects the mother's ability to successfully breastfeed.
- *Older adults:* Participate in regular physical activity to reduce functional declines associated with aging and to achieve the other benefits of physical activity identified for all adults.

Both children and adults get more exercise if it is fun. Almost all age-appropriate sports and energetic activities that children enjoy are good forms of cardiovascular exercise. Adults can choose from a full range of exercise programs developed for use at home or at a fitness center. Even brisk walking counts.

Adults who are presently out of shape, especially those over age 50 who have become sedentary, should talk to their healthcare provider before beginning an exercise program. Often it is best to begin slowly and gradually increase your workouts to a comfortable yet effective level.

As with other lifestyle changes, it is important to have a realistic attitude when beginning an exercise or fitness program. People often join a fitness club or purchase exercise equipment for home use, begin strenuously, and soon quit. A long-term commitment is needed, developing a plan that realistically fits your lifestyle and personal interests.

Make physical activity a routine part of the day, not a special requirement at certain times. Everyone needs to think of physical activity as being as "normal" in their life as eating or sleeping, not something special to be done just when you feel

like it or only to meet a specific weight goal. It is important to help children to develop this attitude, too.

Weight Control

About 30% of adults in the United States are obese by current standards, and another 35% are overweight. Overweight and obesity contribute to many other diseases in addition to cardiovascular disease.

Overweight and obesity are categorized in relation to a person's **body mass index (BMI),** a measure of weight in relation to a person's height. The higher the BMI number, the greater the percentage of fat in a person's body. Overweight is defined as a BMI of 25 to 30, and obesity is a BMI of 30 or higher. The chart in **Figure 6-4** provides an approximate BMI for adults based on height and weight.

The habits that lead to overweight start early in life. Prevention is a better approach than having to lose weight later on and keep it off. The earlier recommendations for diet and exercise, while promoting good health generally, are also the keys to preventing a weight problem from developing.

The cornerstones of all effective weight-loss programs combine a healthy diet with adequate physical activity, as detailed in the previous section. Many different programs have been developed, including a large number of programs that involve fad diets or dietary supplements that promise to burn off the fat. Research shows, however, that controlling caloric intake and getting exercise are the only factors that result in successfully losing weight and keeping it off. Like other major lifestyle changes, such as quitting smoking, weight control requires commitment, a realistic attitude and plan, and time and effort. An excellent starting point is talking with your healthcare provider to learn what kind of program will work best for you.

High Blood Pressure

As noted earlier, over 65 million people in the United States have high blood pressure—and in many this condition is not controlled. Hypertension is often called the *silent killer* because in most people it causes no symptoms and the person can be completely unaware of having it. Yet

Body Mass Index (BMI) Table

BMI	19	20	21	22	23	24	25	26	27	28	29	30	31	32	33	34	35
Height	Weight (in pounds)																
4'10" (58")	91	96	100	105	110	115	119	124	129	134	138	143	148	153	158	162	167
4'11" (59")	94	99	104	109	114	119	129	128	133	138	143	148	153	158	163	168	173
5' (60")	97	102	107	112	118	123	128	133	138	143	148	153	158	163	168	174	179
5'1" (61")	100	106	111	116	122	127	132	137	143	148	153	158	164	169	174	180	185
5'2" (62")	104	109	115	120	126	131	136	142	147	153	158	164	169	175	180	186	191
5'3" (63")	107	113	118	124	130	135	141	146	152	158	163	169	175	180	186	191	197
5'4" (64")	110	116	122	128	134	140	145	151	157	163	169	174	180	186	192	197	204
5'5" (65")	114	120	126	132	138	144	150	156	162	168	174	180	186	192	198	204	210
5'6" (66")	118	124	130	136	142	148	155	161	167	173	179	186	192	198	204	210	216
5'7" (67")	121	127	134	140	146	153	159	166	172	178	185	191	198	204	211	217	223
5'8" (68")	125	131	138	144	151	158	164	171	177	184	190	197	203	210	216	223	230
5'9" (69")	128	135	142	149	155	167	169	176	182	189	196	203	209	216	223	230	236
5'10" (70")	132	139	146	153	160	167	174	181	188	195	202	209	216	222	229	236	243
5'11" (71")	136	143	150	157	165	172	179	186	193	200	208	215	222	229	236	243	250
6' (72")	140	147	154	162	169	177	184	191	199	206	213	221	228	235	242	250	258
6"1" (73")	144	151	159	166	174	182	189	197	204	212	219	227	235	242	250	257	265
6'2" (74")	148	155	163	171	179	186	194	202	210	218	225	233	241	249	256	264	272
6'3" (75")	152	160	168	176	184	192	200	208	216	224	232	240	248	256	264	272	279

Source: Evidence Report of Clinical Guidelines on the Identification, Evaluation, and Treatment of Overweight and Obesity in Adults, 1998. NIH/National Heart, Lung, and Blood Institute (NHLBI).

Figure 6-4 Body mass index.

hypertension is linked to high death rates caused by heart attack, stroke, or other diseases.

Although in some cases hypertension is caused by an underlying condition that may be treated, in the great majority of cases it exists without a specific known cause that can be addressed. Hypertension is diagnosed by regular blood pressure tests. The current standards classify different levels of hypertension according to seriousness. Prehypertension is a systolic blood pressure of 120 to 139, stage 1 hypertension is 140 to 159, and stage 2 hypertension is 160+. By these standards, even those in the prehypertension category are at some risk and should take steps to control their blood pressure. Because blood pressure generally rises with age, it is now estimated that by age 55, adults have a 90% chance of being hypertensive.

Recommendations for controlling blood pressure involve both lifestyle changes and medications. For those with prehypertension, lifestyle changes alone are generally sufficient:

- Maintain a normal weight.
- Get more physical activity.
- Reduce salt intake.

Many individuals with stage 1 or 2 hypertension will also need medication to lower their blood pressure. The risks of hypertension are among the reasons that everyone should have periodic physical examinations by their healthcare providers, who will give appropriate recommendations for controlling high blood pressure.

Stress

Stress is an emotional or mental state that is generally considered a risk factor for cardio-vascular disease. Long-term, frequent stress is thought to have various negative effects on a person's physical health, although it is difficult for research studies to study the exact effects of stress because of issues of quantifying and measuring stress and separating this factor from other risk factors. Nonetheless, there is some evidence that excessive stress lowers the body's immune functions and has other negative effects, and that stress reduction in some cases has a positive benefit. Interestingly, some of the other healthy lifestyle decisions described previously also help one to control or reduce stress, such as exercise and a good diet. Those who frequently feel stressed, however, would gain from talking to their healthcare provider about programs for stress reduction.

CARDIAC CHAIN OF SURVIVAL

Cardiac arrest victims need BLS. **Cardiac arrest** refers to a sudden stop in the beating of the heart.

To recognize the urgent need for quick actions to save the lives of cardiac arrest victims, the Citizen CPR Foundation created the concept of the cardiac **chain of survival (Figure 6-5)**. This chain has four crucial links:

1. **Early Recognition and Access to EMS.** *Recognize that a victim whose heart has stopped needs help immediately!* It is also important that you recognize the signs and symptoms of a potential life-threatening condition such as a heart attack or a stroke in a responsive person (see **Chapter 17**). Do not wait until a person becomes unresponsive to start the chain of events needed to keep him or her alive. Call 9-1-1 and get help on the way.

The victim needs early access to advanced medical care.

2. **Early Bystander CPR.** For a nonbreathing, unresponsive victim, start cardiopulmonary resuscitation (CPR) immediately. This helps keep the brain and other vital organs supplied with oxygen until the automated external defibrillator (AED) arrives.

3. **Early Defibrillation.** An AED, now present in many public and work places, can help get the heart beating normally again after a cardiac arrest. Send someone right away to get the AED.

4. **Early Advanced Care.** The sooner the victim is treated by emergency care professionals, the better the chance for survival. You can help make sure the victim reaches this last link in the chain by acting immediately with the earlier links.

CALL FIRST/CALL FAST

In any situation in which you recognize that a victim of injury or illness is unresponsive, if someone else is present at the scene, have that person call 9-1-1 immediately. Shout for anyone who may hear you, and have them call 9-1-1 and go for an AED.

When you are alone, however, you need to decide whether to call immediately or to first begin to provide care for the victim. The rule that lay rescuers should follow depends on the victim's age. An adult who is found unresponsive is more likely to be the victim of a heart attack and therefore needs defibrillation urgently. For an adult, therefore, if you are alone with the victim, call 9-1-1 immediately and then return to provide CPR. **Remember: Call first.**

An infant or child who is found unresponsive, however, is more likely to be experiencing an

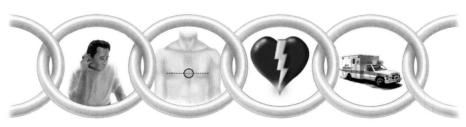

Figure 6-5 Cardiac Chain of Survival.

airway or breathing problem and less likely to need defibrillation. For an infant or child, therefore, if you are alone with the victim and no one hears your shouts for help, you should give 5 cycles of chest compressions and rescue breaths (about 2 minutes of CPR) before pausing to call 9-1-1 and then continuing to provide CPR. **Remember: Start CPR first but call fast.**

THE USE OF CPR

CPR is used for all unresponsive victims who are not breathing. Remember that airway and respiratory problems cause breathing, and then the heart, to stop, as described in **Chapter 5**. Cardiac arrest is also commonly caused by:

- Heart attack or other heart disease
- Drowning
- Suffocation
- Stroke
- Allergic reaction
- Diabetic emergency
- Prolonged seizures
- Drug overdose
- Electric shock
- Certain injuries

You do not need to know the cause of respiratory arrest, however, before starting CPR. The techniques for CPR are the same regardless of cause.

CPR helps keep the victim alive by circulating some oxygenated blood to vital organs. Rescue breaths move oxygen into the lungs where it is picked up by the blood. Compressions on the **sternum** (breastbone) increase pressure

Learning
Checkpoint ①

1. CPR stands for

   a. cardiac position for recovery.

   b. cardiopulmonary resuscitation.

   c. chest pump rescue.

   d. None of the above

2. Put a check mark next to risk factors for cardiovascular disease.

   _____ Smoking   _____ High cholesterol levels

   _____ Regular aspirin use   _____ Inactivity

   _____ High blood pressure   _____ Family history of heart disease

   _____ Growing older   _____ Working full-time

3. The first crucial link in the cardiac chain of survival is

   _____

4. *Call first* (before starting CPR) for which of these victims? (Check all that apply.)

   _____ Unresponsive nonbreathing adult victim

   _____ Unresponsive nonbreathing infant

   _____ Unresponsive nonbreathing child

inside the chest, which moves some blood to the brain and other tissues. The circulation of blood resulting from CPR is not nearly as strong as the circulation from a heartbeat, but it can help keep brain and other tissues alive until a more normal heart rhythm is restored. Often an electric shock from an AED or other medical procedures called **advanced cardiac life support (ACLS)** are needed to restore a heart-beat—and CPR can keep the victim alive until then. In some instances, breathing and a more normal heart rhythm may return spontaneously with CPR.

CPR has clearly been demonstrated to save lives in many circumstances. With the most common cause of cardiac arrest, a heart attack, CPR and defibrillation within three to five minutes after the victim collapses can save over 50% of victims. Given that sudden cardiac arrest occurs in more than 900 people with heart disease *every day,* you can see that CPR followed by AED can save many thousands of lives every year. The exact number of lives saved is unknown because no agency collects all national data on CPR use in all circum-stances. Remember that CPR is only one step in the cardiac chain of survival, however. In most cases CPR serves only to keep the victim alive until an AED and/or EMS professionals arrive at the scene.

TECHNIQUE OF CPR

The general technique of CPR involves alternat-ing chest compressions and rescue breaths. After checking the victim and determining the absence of normal breathing, start chest compressions immediately after giving the initial two rescue breaths. For a victim of any age, these are the general steps of CPR:

1. Find the correct hand position on the lower half of the breastbone midway between the nipples in adults and children, or just below this line in infants, as shown in **Figure 6-6**.
2. Compress the chest hard and fast at a rate of 100 compressions per minute. Note that this is the *rate, or speed, for giving compressions*—not the number of compressions actually given—since it is necessary to stop compres-sions to give rescue breaths. Compressions in

an adult should be 1½ to 2 inches deep. In an infant or child, compressions should be ⅓ to ½ the depth of the chest. Release completely between compressions to let the chest return to its normal height, but do not take your hands or fingers from the chest.
3. Alternate 30 chest compressions and 2 rescue breaths. Give each breath over one second.

For the detailed CPR steps, see the Skill: "CPR." Appendix A describes how more highly trained healthcare providers give CPR and how two trained rescuers can work together to give CPR.

Compression-Only CPR

A nonbreathing unresponsive victim needs both rescue breaths and chest compressions to move oxygenated blood to vital organs. However, if for any reason you cannot or will not give rescue breaths, you should still give the victim chest compressions. This gives the victim a better chance for survival than doing nothing.

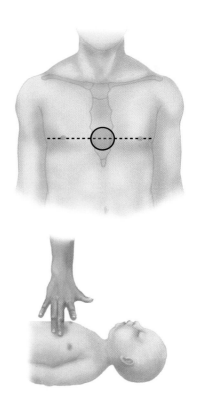

Figure 6-6 Proper placement for compressions.

Skill   **CPR**

1 Open airway and determine if the victim is not breathing normally.

2 Give 2 rescue breaths, each lasting 1 second. (If the first breath does not go in, reposition the head and try again; if the second breath still does not go in, give choking care—see **Chapter 7**.)

3 Put hand(s) in correct position for chest compressions.

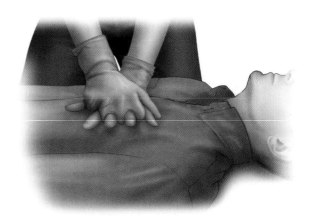

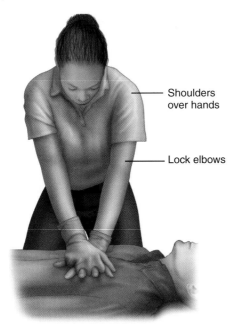

Shoulders over hands

Lock elbows

4 Give 30 chest compressions at rate of 100 per minute. Count aloud for a steady, fast rate: "One, two, three . . . ." Then give 2 breaths.

5 Continue cycles of 30 compressions and 2 breaths.

6 Continue CPR until:
- Victim begins to move
- An AED is brought to the scene and is ready to use
- Professional help arrives and takes over
- You are too exhausted to continue

7 a. If the victim starts moving check for normal breathing. If the victim is breathing normally, put him or her in the recovery position and monitor breathing.
  b. When an AED arrives, start the AED sequence.

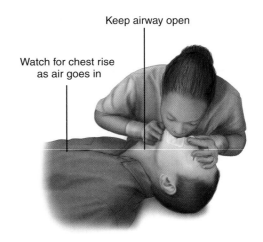

Keep airway open

Watch for chest rise as air goes in

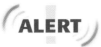

ALERT

Chest Compressions

- Be careful with your hand position for chest comsions. Keep fingers off the chest.

- Do not give compressions over the bottom tip of breastbone.

- When compressing, keep your elbows straight an keep your hands in contact with the chest at all ti

- Remember to compress the chest hard and fast, b the chest recoil completely between compression

- Minimize the amount of time used giving rescue breaths between sets of compressions.

Box 6-2 Problems with CPR Technique

It is well known that CPR saves lives and that CPR training is needed to effectively use this procedure. CPR is taught in the classroom using manikins, of course, and thus the skill is typically learned in ideal circumstances rather than real-life situations, which may be very different. It is often difficult to evaluate the effectiveness of CPR given in the field because of the many variables that determine victim outcome.

A study reported in 2005, however, demonstrated that CPR even when given by professional paramedics is often ineffective because of poor technique. This study used a specially designed and equipped AED that recorded factors related to the depth and rate of chest compressions administered. The study analyzed data generated from victims experiencing cardiac arrest resulting from cardiac disease.

This study showed two key problems in the chest compression technique of many of these rescuers. Compressions were not delivered steadily and constantly at all times during the resuscitation efforts (not counting the "time-out" periods when the AED is analyzing the victim's heart rhythm or administering a shock). Equally important, more than half of the compressions given were too shallow, resulting in ineffective blood flow. In addition, many rescuers gave compressions at too fast a rate, which does not allow chest pressures to drop sufficiently between compressions to maximize blood flow.

Other studies have also shown that only good-quality CPR improves the victim's chances of survival. The quality depends mostly on giving chest compressions at the correct rate and depth.

More research is likely needed before it is clearly understood why CPR skills seem to deteriorate soon after a rescuer learns or refreshes them, as well as how to correct this problem. The evidence clearly indicates, however, the importance of performing CPR as learned— especially the depth and rate of chest compressions. Perhaps even the knowledge that one is likely to give compressions too shallowly will help rescuers and first aiders in the future to remember to focus on their technique in order to provide the quality CPR the victim needs to survive.

Learning
Checkpoint (2)

1. When is it appropriate to start CPR?

    a. As soon as you determine the victim is unresponsive.

    b. As soon as you determine the victim is not breathing normally.

    c. As soon as you determine the victim is both unresponsive and not breathing normally.

    d. Only when you have called 9-1-1 and the dispatcher tells you to start CPR.

2. Describe how to find the site for chest compressions in an adult or child victim.

_____

_____

3. Chest compressions in an adult should be _____ to _____ inches deep. In an infant or child, compress to a depth of _____ to _____ of the chest depth.

4. What is the correct ratio of chest compressions to breaths?

    a. 15 to 1   **c.** 30 to 1

    b. 15 to 2   **d.** 30 to 2

5. If you are performing CPR on an adult victim when an AED is brought to the scene and is ready to use, what action should you take?

    a. Use the AED as soon as it is set up.

    b. Continue CPR for at least 15 cycles before using the AED.

    c. Use the AED only if you can feel the victim's heart quivering in his or her chest.

    d. Use the AED only if the victim showed signs and symptoms of having a heart attack; otherwise, do not use it but continue CPR.

Concluding Thoughts

Remember that, as important as CPR is for sustaining life, in many cases of cardiac arrest the victim also needs defibrillation to restore a normal heartbeat. The use of an automated external defibrillator (AED), the final step for lay rescuers in basic life support, is described in **Chapter 7.**

Learning Outcomes

You should now be able to do the following:

    1. List the risk factors for cardiovascular disease.

    2. Explain general principles for maintaining cardiovascular health and preventing cardiovascular disease.

3. List the steps in the cardiac chain of survival.

4. Describe when to call 9-1-1 before starting CPR and when to give 2 minutes of CPR before calling 9-1-1.

5. Demonstrate the procedure for giving CPR.

Review Questions

1. Preventable risk factors for cardiovascular disease include
   a. smoking.
   b. high cholesterol levels.
   c. inactivity.
   d. All of the above

2. Call 9-1-1 first before beginning CPR for
   a. an unresponsive adult victim who is not breathing.
   b. an unresponsive child or infant who is not breathing.
   c. a responsive adult victim.
   d. a responsive child or infant.

3. The hand position for chest compressions depends on
   a. the cause of the victim's cardiac arrest.
   b. the victim's age.
   c. how long the victim has been in cardiac arrest.
   d. the victim's weight.

4. The correct hand position for chest compressions in adults is
   a. on the top of the breastbone below the neck.
   b. on the lower end of the breastbone just above the abdomen.
   c. on the lower half of the breastbone midway between the nipples.
   d. three finger-widths above where the ribs join.

5. The correct ratio of chest compressions to breaths is
   a. 5 to 2.
   b. 10 to 2.
   c. 15 to 2.
   d. 30 to 2.

6. What is the correct position for the first aider's elbows when giving CPR to an adult?
   a. Bent and locked
   b. Straight and locked
   c. Bent and flexible
   d. Straight and flexible

7. If a victim begins breathing after you have given CPR, what do you do?
   a. Put the victim in the recovery position.
   b. Continue chest compressions and rescue breaths.
   c. Continue giving only chest compressions.
   d. Give rescue breaths only.

8. When should you send someone to bring an AED to the scene when you encounter an unresponsive adult?
   a. As soon as you see the victim is unresponsive
   b. As soon as the 9-1-1 dispatcher tells you to
   c. After one minute of CPR
   d. It depends on the cause of the victim's condition

9. It is acceptable to stop CPR when
   a. ten minutes have passed and the victim has not recovered.
   b. twenty minutes have passed and the victim has not recovered.
   c. you are too exhausted to continue.
   d. the victim feels cold all over.

10. Which is the correct way to give chest compressions to an infant between breaths?
    a. Give 15 compressions at a rate of 80 per minute.
    b. Give 15 compressions at a rate of 100 per minute.
    c. Give 30 compressions at a rate of 80 per minute.
    d. Give 30 compressions at a rate of 100 per minute.

References and Resources

American Cancer Society. www.cancer.org

American Heart Association. www.americanheart.org

American Heart Association. 2005 International consensus for cardiopulmonary resuscitation (CPR) and emergency cardio-vascular care (ECC) science with treatment recommendations. *Circulation*, 122(22). November 29, 2005.

American Lung Association. www.lungusa.org

Citizen CPR Foundation. Chain of survival: converting a nation. 2004. Available from: www.citizencpr.org

Flegal KM, et al. Excess deaths associated with underweight, overweight, and obesity. *JAMA.* 2005; 293(15).

National Center for Chronic Disease Prevention and Health Promotion. The importance of physical activity. Available from: www.cdc.gov/nccdphp

National Safety Council. www.nsc.org

U.S. Department of Health and Human Services, Public Health Service. Consumer guide: you can quit smoking. Available from: www.ahrq.gov/consumer/tobacco/quits.htm

U.S. Department of Health and Human Services and the U.S. Department of Agriculture. Dietary guidelines for Americans 2005. Available from: www.health.gov/dietaryguidelines/dga2005/report

Wik L, et al. Quality of cardiopulmonary resuscitation during out-of-hospital cardiac arrest. *JAMA.* 2005; 293(3).

Chapter 7

Basic Life Support 3: Choking Care

Chapter Preview

- Choking Emergencies
- Preventing Choking
- Airway Obstruction

You are having a cup of tea in the lunch room when you see a man at the next table suddenly bring his hands up to his throat. He looks frantic and his mouth is open, but he is not speaking. The others at his table are looking at him but no one has moved to help—they do not seem to know what to do. You approach the man, who you think may be choking. What should you say and do?

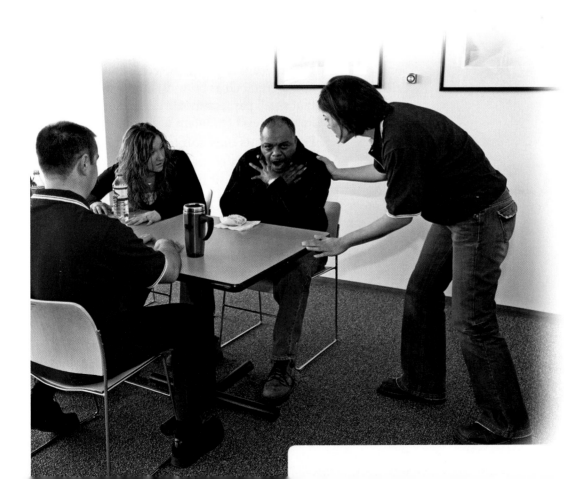

As described in **Chapter 5**, the inability to breathe is a life-threatening emergency, and body cells not receiving oxygen begin to die within minutes. Choking is a common cause of respiratory arrest, the stopping of breathing. Because time is so critical in these emergencies, it is important to be prepared to give immediate care to responsive or unresponsive choking victims.

CHOKING EMERGENCIES

With airway obstructions the victim cannot breathe because the airway is blocked by a foreign object, an anatomical structure such as the tongue, or fluid or vomit. These emergencies require immediate care to clear the obstruction and enable the victim to breathe **(Figure 7-1)**. The inability to breathe because of an airway obstruction is commonly called choking.

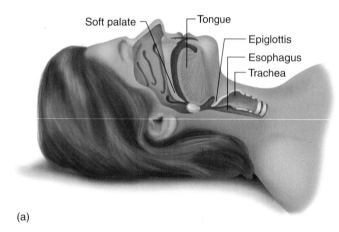

Soft palate — — Tongue
— Epiglottis
— Esophagus
— Trachea

(a)

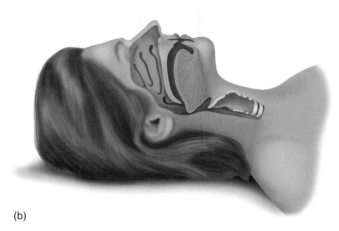

(b)

Figure 7-1 (a) Food lodged in the airway, obstructing breathing. (b) The tongue blocking the airway in an unresponsive victim.

PREVENTING CHOKING

Choking is common in both adults and children. Over 4000 people die from choking each year in the United States. Although people often think of choking as a problem primarily for infants and young children, in fact the age group that experiences choking most frequently is adults 65 and older, who are more than twice as likely to die from choking as younger adults. Perhaps because most parents and caretakers know about the choking risk for younger children, fewer children—about 170 children under age 14—die each year from choking. Yet virtually all of these cases of choking could have been prevented.

In adults, choking often results from trying to swallow large pieces of food that have not been chewed sufficiently, from eating too quickly, or from eating while engaged in other activities. Choking is more common in those under the influence of alcohol or drugs. Choking is also more likely in those wearing dentures, apparently because of a diminished sensation for how well food has been chewed before attempting to swallow.

Choking is a serious threat to infants and children up to three or four years of age and a significant cause of death. An infant or young child may put any small object in his or her mouth, and nonfood items account for about 70% of choking deaths in children. Follow these guidelines to prevent choking in infants and children:

- Do not leave any small objects within reach of an infant (such as buttons, beads, coins). Ensure that small parts cannot break off toys or other items around the infant or young child.
- Feed infants only soft foods that do not require chewing.
- Have children sit in a high chair or at a table to eat. Never let a child move around while eating.
- Teach children not to eat too fast or to talk or laugh while eating.
- Cut up foods a child could choke on, like hot dogs, into small pieces.
- Do not give children under age three foods like these:
  ◦ Peanuts
  ◦ Popcorn
  ◦ Grapes
  ◦ Chunks of raw vegetables or fruits

Learning Checkpoint ①

1. List at least four situations in which choking is a risk for an adult.

_____

2. Put a check mark next to food items that should not be given to a child under age 3.

_____ Popcorn   _____ Grapes

_____ Jell-O   _____ Corn kernels

_____ Marshmallows   _____ Soft bread slices

_____ Spaghetti   _____ Gum

- ◦ Marshmallows
- ◦ Gum
- • Supervise young children while they eat, and be prepared to care for a child who chokes.

AIRWAY OBSTRUCTION

A victim is choking when the airway is obstructed either partially or fully. A victim can choke on:

- • Food or other foreign bodies in the mouth
- • The tongue (in an unresponsive victim lying on his or her back)
- • Teeth or other body tissues resulting from injury
- • Vomit

A complete **airway obstruction** means the victim is getting no air at all and consequently no oxygen in the blood. This victim will soon become unresponsive, and not long after breathing stops, the heart will stop, too. Choking care is urgently needed.

A partial obstruction means that something is partly blocking the airway but that the victim is still getting some air into the lungs around the obstructing object. The victim may be getting enough air to cough out the obstructing object.

Assessing Choking

Most cases of choking in adults occur while eating. Most cases of choking in infants and children occur while eating or playing. Often, therefore, someone is present and recognizes the choking event while the victim is still responsive. Choking may be either mild or severe. With a mild

obstruction the victim is usually coughing forcefully in an attempt to expel the object. The victim is getting some air and may be making wheezing or high-pitched sounds with breaths, along with coughing. Do not interrupt the person's coughing or attempts to expel the object; do not pound the person on the back in an effort to help.

With severe choking, however, the victim is getting very little air or none at all. The person may look frantic and be clutching at the throat **(Figure 7.2)**. You may notice a pale or bluish coloring around the mouth and nail beds. A victim who is coughing very weakly and silently, or not coughing at all, is unlikely to expel the obstructing object. The victim cannot speak. Simply ask the victim if he or she is choking.

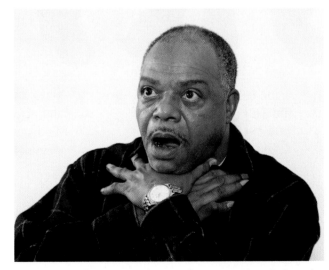

Figure 7-2 The universal sign of a responsive victim who is choking.

Skill Choking Care for Responsive Adult or Child

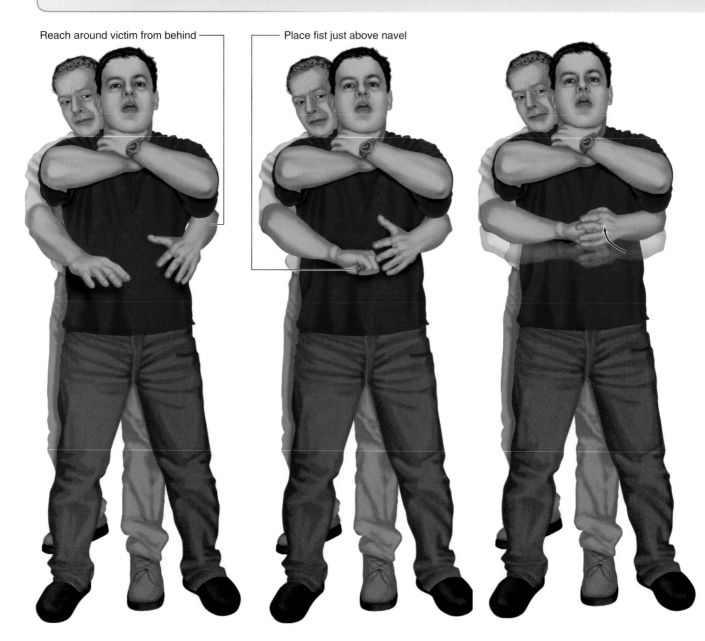

Reach around victim from behind

Place fist just above navel

1 Stand behind an adult victim with one leg forward between the victim's legs. Keep your head slightly to one side. With a small child, kneel behind the child. Reach around the abdomen.

2 Make a fist with one hand and place the thumb side of the fist against the victim's abdomen just above the navel.

3 Grasp your fist with your other hand and thrust inward and upward into the victim's abdomen with quick jerks. Continue abdominal thrusts until the victim can expel the object or becomes unresponsive. If abdominal thrusts do not succeed in clearing the object from the airway, you may try chest thrusts and back blows.

If the victim cannot answer but indicates that he or she is choking, begin choking care for a responsive victim.

An unresponsive victim who may be choking is assessed by checking for breathing as described in **Chapter 4.** If the victim is not breathing, position the head to open the airway and give two rescue breaths. If your first breath does not go into the victim and make the chest rise, make another attempt to open the airway and give a second breath. If it does not go in, assume that the victim has an obstructed airway and needs choking care.

Care for Choking Adults and Children

Choking care depends on whether the victim is responsive or unresponsive and whether, in an unresponsive victim, the obstruction is mild or severe:

- For a **responsive choking victim who is coughing,** encourage the coughing to clear the object. Stay with the victim and call 9-1-1 if the object is not immediately expelled.
- For a **responsive choking victim who cannot speak or cough forcefully** give abdominal thrusts as described in the Skill: "Choking Care for Responsive Adult or Child."
- For **an unresponsive choking victim,** if your rescue breaths do not go in, immediately call (or have someone call) 9-1-1 and begin CPR.

With a responsive victim, after quickly asking for consent and telling the victim what you intend to do, and having someone else call 9-1-1, stand behind the victim and reach around to the abdomen. Having one leg forward between the victim's legs helps you to brace in case the victim becomes unresponsive and falls. Keep your head slightly to the side in case the victim's head snaps back if the victim becomes unresponsive.

Make a fist with one hand and place the thumb side of the fist against the victim's abdomen just above the navel. Grasp the fist with your other hand and thrust inward and upward into the victim's abdomen with quick jerks. The pressure of each jerk serves to force air from the lungs up the trachea to expel the object. Pause only briefly after each abdominal thrust to see if the victim is able to breathe or cough, and continue with additional thrusts if not.

If you are giving abdominal thrusts to a child or someone much shorter than you, kneel behind the victim. If the victim is much taller than you, ask the victim to kneel or sit because it is

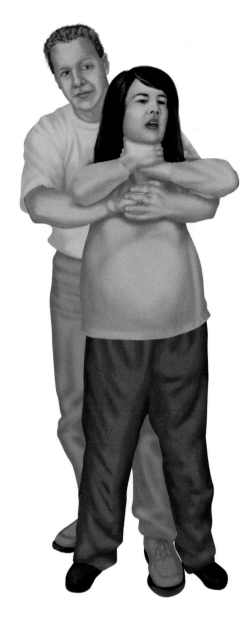

4 For a responsive pregnant victim, or any victim you cannot get your arms around, give chest thrusts in the middle of the breastbone from behind the victim. Take care not to squeeze the ribs with your arms. If chest thrusts do not clear the obstructing object, support the woman's chest with one hand and give back blows with the other.

Skill **Choking Care for Unresponsive Adult or Child**

1 Open airway and determine that the victim is not breathing.

2 Give two rescue breaths, each lasting 1 second. If the first breath does not go in and the chest does not rise, position the head again to open the airway, and try again.

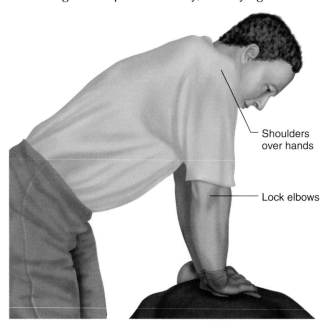

Shoulders over hands

Lock elbows

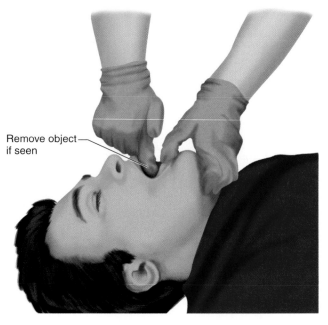

Remove object if seen

3 If breaths still do not go in, give chest compressions. Put hand(s) in correct position for chest compressions.

4 Give 30 chest compressions to at a rate of 100 per minute. Count aloud for a steady, fast rate: "One, two, three . . . ." Then give two breaths. Look inside the mouth when opening the mouth to give breaths, and remove any object you see.

5 Continue CPR until:
- The victim begins to move
- Professional help arrives and takes over
- You are too exhausted to continue

important that your thrusts are upward as well as inward, which is impossible if you have to reach up to the victim's abdomen.

Note that because abdominal thrusts may sometimes cause internal injury, a victim who is treated with abdominal thrusts is recommended to be examined by a healthcare provider.

When a severe airway obstruction is not cleared, the victim will become unresponsive within minutes. You may have found the victim in an unresponsive condition, or the victim may become unresponsive while you are giving abdominal thrusts if the object is not expelled. In the latter case, quickly and carefully lower the victim and lay him or her on his or her back on the floor. Make sure 9-1-1 has

been called. Begin the CPR sequence by opening the airway. When you open the victim's mouth to give a rescue breath, look first for an object in the mouth. If you see an object in the victim's mouth, remove it. If the object is expelled, give two rescue breaths as usual and continue CPR.

If the obstruction remains, the chest compressions of CPR may expel the foreign object. While giving CPR, each time you open the victim's mouth to give breaths, check first to see if an object is visible, and if so, remove it.

Care for Choking Infants

If a responsive choking infant can cry or cough, watch carefully to see if the object

Skill **Choking Care for Responsive Infant**

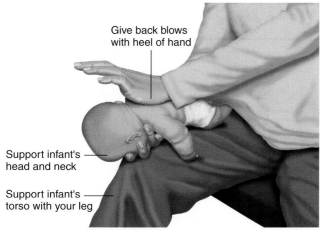

Give back blows with heel of hand

Support infant's head and neck

Support infant's torso with your leg

1 Support the infant's head in one hand, with the torso on your forearm and your thigh. Give up to 5 back blows between the shoulder blades.

2 Check for expelled object. If not present, continue with next step.

Transfer support of head and neck to other hand

3 With other hand on back of infant's head, roll the infant face up.

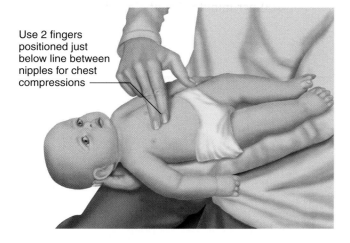

Use 2 fingers positioned just below line between nipples for chest compressions

4 Give up to 5 chest thrusts with two fingers. Check mouth for expelled object.

5 Repeat steps 1 through 4, alternating back blows with chest thrusts and checking the mouth. If alone, call 9-1-1 after one minute. Continue until the object is expelled or the infant becomes unresponsive. If the infant becomes unresponsive, give CPR. Look inside the mouth when opening the mouth to give breaths, and remove any object you see.

comes out. If the infant is responsive but cannot cry or cough, have someone call 9-1-1 and give the infant alternating back blows and chest thrusts in an attempt to expel the object. Support the infant in one hand against your thigh as you sit or stand, keeping the infant's head lower than the body. To prevent spinal injury, be sure to support the infant's head and neck during these maneuvers. The detailed steps for back blows and chest thrusts are described in the Skill: "Choking Care for Responsive Infant."

If an infant to whom you were giving responsive choking care then becomes unresponsive, send someone to call 9-1-1, and give chest compressions. As with an adult or child, the chest compressions may cause the object to be expelled. Check for an object in the mouth before you give a breath, and remove any object you see. Never do a finger sweep of the mouth if you do not see an object, because this could force an object deeper into the throat.

When you encounter an unresponsive infant, first check for breathing as usual. If the infant is not breathing when you have opened the airway, give two breaths. If your first breath does not go in and the infant's chest does not rise, try again after you reposition the head to open the airway. If the second breath does not go in, then the infant has an airway obstruction and you should provide CPR and check the mouth for an object each time you open it to give a rescue breath.

Self-Treating Choking

If you are choking when alone, give yourself abdominal thrusts to try to expel the object. You may try using your hands, or lean over and push your abdomen against the back of a chair or other firm object (**Figure 7-3**).

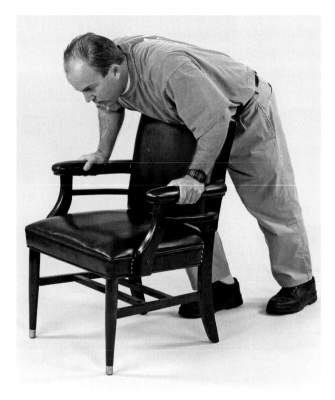

Figure 7-3 Abdominal self-thrusts.

Learning
Checkpoint ②

1. For a responsive adult victim who is choking, you should

   a. start CPR immediately.

   b. alternate back blows and chest thrusts.

   c. give abdominal thrusts.

   d. No first aid action is needed until the victim becomes unresponsive.

2. True or False: A choking victim who is coughing forcefully is still able to breathe and may be able to cough out the foreign body.

3. True or False: A choking victim who is unable to breathe will soon become unresponsive.

4. For a responsive choking infant,

   a. support the head as you position the infant.

   b. alternate back blows and chest thrusts.

   c. check the infant's mouth for an expelled object.

   d. All of the above

5. Explain why CPR is given to a choking victim who becomes unresponsive.

Concluding Thoughts

So far you have learned the basic life support skills of rescue breaths, CPR, and care for choking victims. **Chapter 8** describes the final BLS skill: the use of an automated external defibrillator (AED) for a victim whose heart is not beating normally.

Learning Outcomes

You should now be able to do the following:

1. List ways to prevent choking.

2. Demonstrate choking care for a responsive adult, child, and infant.

3. Demonstrate choking care for an unresponsive adult, child, and infant.

Review Questions

1. What increases the risk of choking in an adult?
   a. Taking high blood pressure medication
   b. Overcooking foods
   c. Having gum disease
   d. Drinking alcohol with meals

2. A victim with a severe airway obstruction
   a. cannot speak or cough forcefully.
   b. cannot speak but can cough forcefully.
   c. can speak and cough weakly.
   d. can speak but only in short sentences.

3. To give abdominal thrusts to a responsive choking adult, what hand position is used?
   a. Both hands together on the bottom edge of the breastbone
   b. Both hands together just above the navel
   c. One hand at the navel and one hand at the "V" where the lower ribs meet
   d. One hand on the bottom rib at each side

4. What is important when giving choking first aid to a responsive infant?
   a. Alternate series of back blows and chest thrusts.
   b. Keep the infant's head raised above the body.
   c. Give CPR in the usual way.
   d. Perform a more gentle version of the adult responsive choking technique.

References and Resources

American Heart Association. www.americanheart.org

American Heart Association. 2005 International consensus on cardiopulmonary resuscitation (CPR) and emergency cardio-vascular care (ECC) science with treatment recommendations. *Circulation*, 112(22). November 29, 2005.

National Safe Kids Campaign. www.safekids.org

National Safety Council. www.nsc.org

Chapter 8

Basic Life Support 4: Automated External Defibrillator (AED)

Chapter Preview

- Public Access to Defibrillation
- The Heart's Electrical System
- How AEDs Work
- Using an AED

- Special Considerations
- Potential AED Problems
- AED Maintenance

You are called to the scene where a man is lying unresponsive on the floor. Someone has already called 9-1-1. You know where an AED is located in the building, and you send someone for it as you check the victim for breathing. The victim is not breathing. You give two breaths and watch his chest rise and fall, and then you begin chest compressions. About one minute later the other person returns with an AED and first aid kit. What series of actions should you now take?

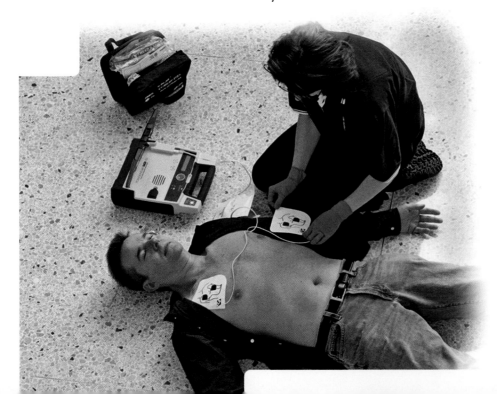

Not every victim who receives BLS needs an automated external defibrillator (AED), but many do. In many cases of cardiac arrest, the victim's heart has an abnormal rhythm that does not circulate the blood, and this rhythm can often be corrected with the AED. Remember the cardiac chain of survival: an AED should be used with any unresponsive victim who is not breathing.

PUBLIC ACCESS TO DEFIBRILLATION

To give a victim of cardiac arrest the best chances for resuscitation, CPR and **defibrillation** must begin as soon as possible. Ideally an AED should reach the victim within minutes (**Box 8-1**). All ambulances and many other emergency responders carry AEDs and reach the scene quickly after 9-1-1 is called, but the availability of AEDs in public places where people may experience heart attacks helps to ensure that a unit is present when needed by a trained first aider or first responder. Public access to defibrillation (PAD) programs have worked to make AEDs available in workplaces, public gathering places, and other facilities for use by trained rescuers and first aiders. Increasingly visible are signs in public places indicating where AEDs are located (**Figure 8-1**).

In many areas a healthcare provider oversees the placement and use of the AED, as well as AED training. For professional rescuers, this is called **medical direction.** Your course instructor will inform you how to meet any legal requirements in your area for using an AED. Note, however, that laws regarding AEDs are changing. In 2004, with FDA approval of non-prescription AEDs for home use, AED units that do not require specific training began appearing in homes and other settings. These

Box 8-1 AEDs Save Lives

Although it is unknown exactly how many lives have been saved by the use of AEDs, because no national agency collects reports, studies show that AEDs used by trained lay rescuers are saving many hundreds of lives every year—a number that is increasing as more lay people are receiving training and more AEDs are put in public places.

The placement of AEDs in areas where people gather and the training of lay rescuers, according to a National Institutes of Health (NIH) study, doubles the survival rate of victims of sudden cardiac arrest, compared to areas where AEDs are not present. Other studies have shown similar or more dramatic results. AED use by nonmedical employees in a study of cardiac arrests occurring in casinos revealed a 74% survival rate when the AED was used within three minutes. A study of cardiac arrests among airline passengers showed that AEDs used by airline employees resulted in a 40% survival rate. In contrast, when an AED is not used within minutes, survival rates of victims in cardiac arrest and ventricular fibrillation are generally under 5%.

Tens of thousands of AEDs have been placed in public places for use by rescuers at the scene. The number grows every year, and success stories from community access programs continue to gain attention. In Austin, Texas, for example, over 200 AEDs have been deployed in public places, and 76 lives were saved in the first four years. The American Heart Association estimates that the widespread availability and use of AEDs could save up to 50,000 people a year in the United States.

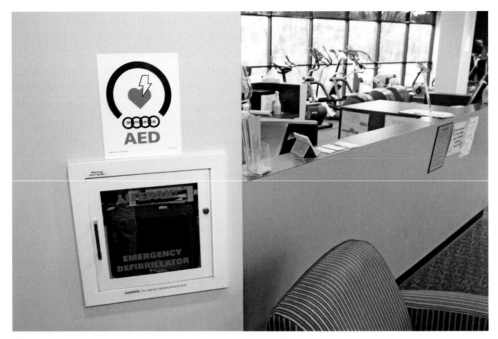

Figure 8-1 AEDs are increasingly common in public places.

devices have been demonstrated to be safe for use by lay people who follow the instructions printed on the device and the device's voice prompts during use. AED training will always offer benefits, but AEDs have become so simple to use that additional changes in AED regulations may be forthcoming.

THE HEART'S ELECTRICAL SYSTEM

The heart pumps blood to the lungs to pick up oxygen and then pumps oxygenated blood to all parts of the body. The heart consists of four chambers called the left atrium, the right atrium, and the left and right ventricles. The ventricles, the lower chambers of the heart, do most of the pumping. The heart's electrical system keeps the four chambers of the heart synchronized and working together. The sinoatrial and atrioventricular (AV) nodes help organize and control the rhythmic electrical impulses that keep the heart beating properly **(Figure 8-2)**.

With a heart attack or other heart problems, this rhythmic electrical control may be disrupted, causing an abnormal heart rhythm such as ventricular fibrillation.

Ventricular Fibrillation

Ventricular fibrillation (V-fib) is an abnormal heart rhythm that commonly occurs with heart attacks and stops circulation of the blood. Although we say a victim in V-fib is in cardiac arrest, the heart is not actually completely still but is beating abnormally. **Fibrillation** means the ventricles of the heart are

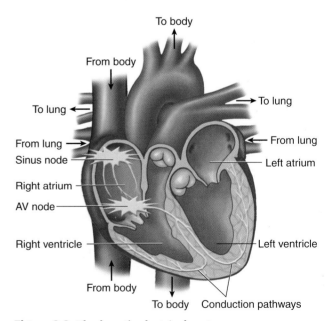

Figure 8-2 The heart's electrical system.

The History of AEDs

Like much medical technology, AED technology began slowly but has advanced rapidly in recent decades with the development of new devices. Animal experiments as early as 1775 revealed that an electrical shock could restore a heartbeat in some instances, although it took until the mid-nineteenth century before ventricular fibrillation was understood. By 1900, further animal experiments demonstrated how a strong shock could correct ventricular fibrillation. In the 1920s, research on the use of defibrillation in humans was funded by the Consolidated Edison electric company—in response to increasing incidents of electrocution as more homes and factories were wired for electricity.

The first successful human defibrillation occurred in 1947 using internal cardiac paddles, and external defibrillation proved successful in 1956. Gradually defibrillators, which then depended on AC electricity sources, were installed in hospitals.

At the same time, coronary heart disease was becoming one of the leading causes of death in Europe and North America, with most coronary deaths occurring, as today, outside the hospital where defibrillation could not be performed. The cardiologist Frank Pantridge sought to solve this problem, and in 1965 he developed the first portable defibrillator. It weighed over 150 lbs. and required automotive batteries—but it could be successfully installed in ambulances.

From that point on, often with the aid of technologies developed in other fields, defibrillators became smaller and lighter and more widely used. Believing that lay people could be trained to use a defibrillator, and that the device should be positioned alongside every fire extinguisher, Dr. Pantridge continued to work through the 1970s and 1980s on improvements that would ensure a shock would not be given to a cardiac arrest victim unless ventricular fibrillation was present. Eventually the automatic external defibrillator was developed to meet this goal, and in 1982 the FDA approved the first clinical trials for AED use by EMTs.

Continued improvements in battery and computer technology have since led to AED devices becoming smaller, lighter, and safer. As the use of AEDs has spread from professional prehospital rescuers to trained citizens, increasing numbers of lives have been saved, and the value of AEDs in public settings has been increasingly recognized.

Social and political advances have followed the technological advances of AEDs. In 2004, the year in which the developer of the first portable defibrillator died, two significant events occurred that will increase the lifesaving capabilities of AEDs still further. The U.S. Congress authorized $30 million in grants to states and communities to place more AEDs in public places and to train more people in their use by passing the Community Access to Emergency Devices Act. A few months later, the FDA approved the first nonprescription AED intended for home use. With these developments, increasing numbers of lives will be saved.

quivering instead of beating rhythmically. Blood is not filling the ventricles and is not being pumped out to the lungs or body as usual.

Since heart attack is the most common cause of cardiac arrest, ventricular fibrillation is a common occurrence. Studies show that in approximately half the cases of cardiac arrest, the victim's heart is in fibrillation and therefore would benefit from a shock delivered by the AED.

How AEDs Work

The AED automatically checks the victim's heart rhythm and advises whether the victim needs a shock. The pads placed on the victim's chest are connected by cables to the main unit, which contains wires through which an electrical current passes. The pads monitor the heart's electrical activity, and the unit determines whether an abnormal rhythm is present for which a shock is needed. If the victim's heart is in V-fib, the machine will advise giving an electric shock to return the heart to a normal rhythm. This is called defibrillation, or stopping the fibrillation of the heart **(Figure 8-3)**.

The AED's **electrodes,** or pads, are placed on the victim's chest (or, with some AED models, on the front and back of the chest of a small child), and when the unit delivers a shock, electricity travels through the cables to the pads and then through the body to the heart and "jolts" the heart's electrical system, often restoring a normal heartbeat. Because electrical current passes through the pads, it is important to position them correctly on the body and to avoid water, metal, and any other substance that conducts electricity.

AEDs are simple to use, but they must be used right away. With every minute that goes by before defibrillation begins, the victim's chances for survival drop by about 10%.

The AED Unit

AEDs are complex inside despite their ease of use. They contain a battery and are portable.

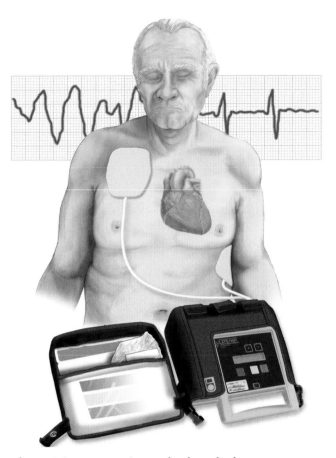

Figure 8-3 An AED gives a shock to the heart.

Some models have a screen that tells you what to do; all models give directions in a clear voice. AED models vary somewhat in other features, but all work in the same basic way **(Figure 8-4)**.

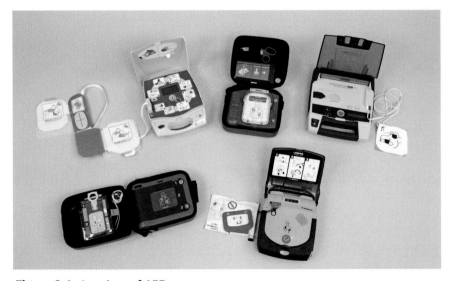

Figure 8-4 A variety of AEDs.

Learning
Checkpoint (1)

1. True or False: An AED works by giving a shock to a heart that is fibrillating to restore it to a normal rhythm.

2. True or False: It is very risky to use an AED because the unit cannot tell whether the victim's heart is beating normally or not.

3. About what percentage of cardiac arrest victims are in fibrillation and require a shock?

USING AN AED

In any situation in which a victim suddenly collapses or is found unresponsive, be thinking about the possibility of cardiac arrest even as you approach. If someone else is present and you know an AED is available nearby, send that person to call 9-1-1 and get the AED. It is better to have it right away and not use it than to need it and have to wait for it.

Determine the Need for AED

As always, with any unresponsive victim, send someone to call 9-1-1 and to get an AED. If the victim is not breathing, you will need to use the AED.

Start CPR

Remember BLS and the chain of survival. Give CPR until the AED arrives at the scene and is ready to use. If you arrive at the victim with an AED, check the victim for breathing and then use the AED immediately before starting CPR. If another rescuer is present, one should begin CPR while the other sets up the device. Continue CPR until the unit is ready to analyze the victim's heart rhythm, and then stop and follow the unit's instructions.

Attach the AED to Victim

Be sure the victim is not in water or in contact with metal. Water or metal conduct electricity that may pose a risk to you or others. Place the AED near the victim's shoulder (on the left side if possible), turn it on, and attach the pads (electrodes) to the victim's chest. Most AED units have a diagram on the pads or the unit itself to remind you where to position them (**Figure 8-5**). Typically the first pad is placed

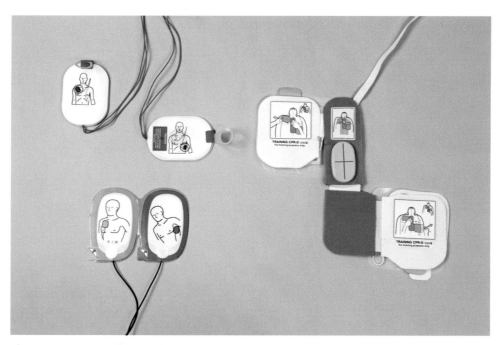

Figure 8-5 AED pads usually include diagrams showing correct pad placement.

Skill   Using an AED

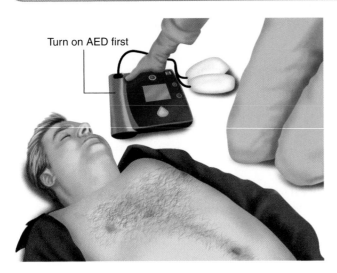

Turn on AED first

Turn on AED first

1   Position victim away from water and metal. Place unit by victim's shoulder and turn it on.

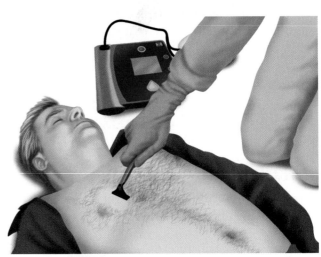

2   Expose victim's chest, and dry or shave the area if necessary.

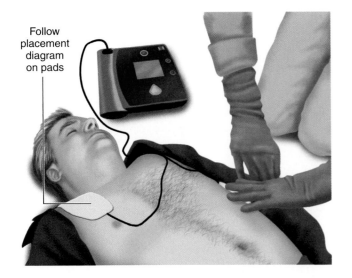

Follow placement diagram on pads

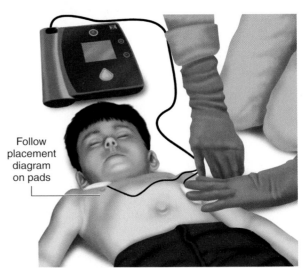

Follow placement diagram on pads

3   Apply pads to victim's chest. If needed, plug the cables into the unit.

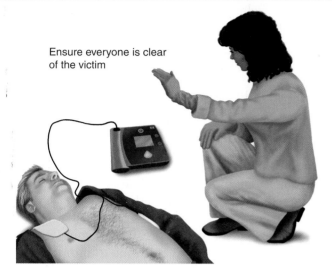

Ensure everyone is clear of the victim

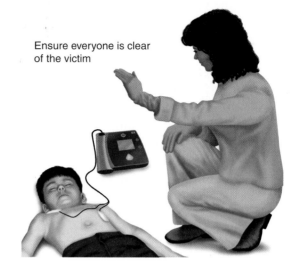

Ensure everyone is clear of the victim

4 Stand clear during rhythm analysis.

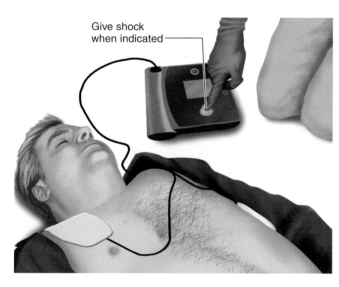

Give shock when indicated

5 Follow prompts from AED unit to (a) press the shock button or (b) do not shock but immediately give CPR with the pads remaining in place, starting with chest compressions.

6 Follow the AED's prompts to analyze the rhythm again after 5 cycles of CPR (about 2 minutes).

7 Continue steps 5 and 6 until the victim moves or professional rescuers arrive and take over.

8 If the victim recovers (moves), check for breathing and put a breathing, unresponsive victim in the recovery position (with pads remaining in place) and continue to monitor breathing.

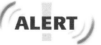 **ALERT**

- Do not use a cell phone or two-way radio within 6 feet of an AED.

on the right side below the collar bone and to the right of the breastbone. The second pad is placed below and to the left of the left nipple and above the lower rib margin.

Attach the AED pads to the victim only if the victim is unresponsive and not breathing. Expose the victim's chest, and dry the skin with a towel or dry clothing (heart attack victims are often sweating). If the victim has heavy chest hair, quickly shave the pad areas. If a razor is not available, use scissors or trauma shears (which should be kept with the AED) to trim the hair and allow skin contact with the pads. Remove the backing from the pads and apply the pads firmly on the victim's chest. If required with your AED model, plug the pad cables into the main unit.

Analyze and Shock

With the pads in place and the AED unit on, most AED models then automatically analyze the victim's heart rhythm. Do not move or touch the victim while it is analyzing. After it analyzes the heart rhythm, the unit will advise you whether to give a shock or to continue CPR. If a shock is advised, be sure no one is touching the victim. Look up and down the victim and say, "Everybody clear!" Once everyone is clear, administer the shock (when advised). After the shock, immediately give CPR for five cycles (about 2 minutes). Then the AED will analyze again and advise another shock if needed, or continuing CPR (with the pads left in place).

Note that different AEDs may use slightly different prompts. Follow the unit's voice and picture prompts through this process. Some units can be programmed to administer the shock automatically rather than prompt the user to push the shock button; in this case always follow the unit's prompts.

If the victim recovers (moves and is breathing), put an unresponsive, breathing victim in the recovery position and continue to monitor his or her breathing. Keep the AED pads in place as some victims may return to V-fib and require defibrillation again.

The AED may also say no shock is indicated. This means the victim's heart will not benefit from defibrillation. If this is so, immediately continue CPR (see Skill: "Using an AED").

Learning Checkpoint ②

1. Which statement is true about the pads (electrodes) of an AED?

   a. The AED has two pads which must be correctly positioned.

   b. The AED has four pads which must be correctly positioned.

   c. The AED has two pads, but only one needs to be put on the victim's chest (the other is a spare).

   d. The pads are used only if a heart rhythm is not detected when the machine is placed in the center of the victim's chest.

2. If the AED unit advises you to give a shock, what do you do next?

   a. Continue CPR while asking someone else to push the shock button.

   b. Place a wet towel over the victim's chest and push the shock button.

   c. Make sure everyone is clear of the victim and then push the shock button.

   d. Wait about one minute for the unit to confirm analysis of a shockable rhythm.

3. When an AED is available, when is CPR given to an unresponsive victim who is not breathing?

SPECIAL CONSIDERATIONS

Some situations involve special considerations in the use of the AED.

Children

Follow the adult guidelines for children over age eight. Although much more rare, sudden cardiac arrest can occur in younger children, too, from causes such as:

- Sudden infant death syndrome
- Poisoning
- Drowning
- Heart problem

In most cases, cardiac arrest in a child is not caused by a heart problem, and in most cases the child's heart is not in V-fib. Therefore, give a child two minutes of CPR *before* using the AED unless the child was witnessed to collapse suddenly. If the child does not recover, then use the AED as usual. This is different from the protocol for adults, in whom cardiac arrest is more likely to be the result of heart attack, therefore requiring the use of the AED as soon as possible.

In recent years the value of defibrillating a young child in sudden cardiac arrest has been recognized, and pediatric AED electrode pads are now available. It is important to use only approved pediatric AED electrode pads, which are smaller than those for adults and produce lower-energy shocks on a child under age eight. Usually the pads have a distinctive appearance to prevent their being confused with adult pads, such as pink connectors and teddybear emblems. If pediatric pads are not available, however, using adult pads is better than not using the AED at all. Pediatric pads should not be used for an adult, however, because the lower energy is insufficient to affect the heart rhythm **(Figure 8-6)**.

Be sure to follow the device's instructions for pad placement on a small child. The AED shown on the right in **Figure 8-6**, for example, uses pad placement on the front and back of the child's chest. Testing has demonstrated that with small children and infants, it can be difficult to position both pads on the front of the chest, and studies have shown placement on the front and back also delivers an effective shock **(Box 8-2)**.

Currently, AED use on both adults and children from ages one to eight is recommended. AED use for infants is not recommended against, but the evidence is considered "indeterminate"

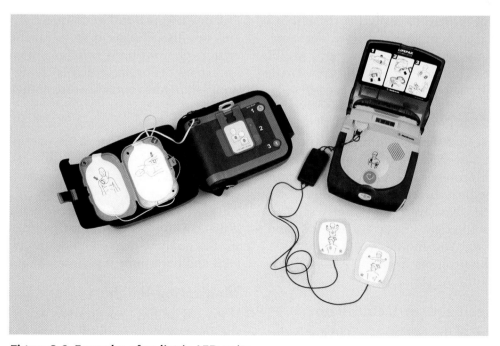

Figure 8-6 Examples of pediatric AED units.

Box 8-2 Changing AED Technology

AEDs were first designed for use on adults and older children and therefore originally had pads that came in one size only. These were placed in the typical manner on the upper right and lower left chest, as described earlier. When research showed the benefit of lower-energy shocks for pediatric victims, newer units were developed that used separate pediatric pads, sometimes placed on the front and back of the chest because of the difficulty of placing both pads far enough apart on a small child's chest. At this time, AED technology continues to evolve, with some new units now able to determine characteristics of the victim and adjust the shock level automatically. Other new units now use the same pads for all victims, regardless of size and weight, but have a separate switch on the unit for pediatric victims. With

such advances, separate pediatric pads may eventually become obsolete.

Up through 2005, most AED units used a protocol that advised a series of up to three "stacked" shocks. With technical improvements in AEDs, however, studies showed that a single shock immediately followed by CPR was more effective, and this became the recommended protocol. It is anticipated that AEDs will be reprogrammed to follow this revised protocol, although older units may remain in some settings for a time. Older AED units may also continue to prompt rescuers to check the victim's pulse or signs or circulation, even though lay rescuers are no longer taught to perform this action before giving CPR immediately to a nonbreathing, unresponsive victim.

regarding the benefit of AED use for infants versus the risks of incorrectly analyzing rhythm or delivering an inappropriate shock level. There are proponents for infant AED use, however, and AED manufacturers claim they are safe and appropriate with the use of the correct pediatric pads.

Traumatic Injury

Cardiac arrest in a severely injured victim is usually caused by the traumatic injury, not by a heart rhythm problem like V-fib. In such cases your local medical direction may specify not to use the AED. However, if the injury seems minor, the victim's cardiac arrest may respond to defibrillation. You should attach the pads and follow the prompts from the AED. When in doubt, use the AED.

Internal Pacemaker or Defibrillator

When you expose the victim's chest to apply the AED pads, you may see a bulge beneath the vic-

tim's skin from an implanted **pacemaker** or defibrillator (**Figure 8-7**). Do not place a pad on this area but instead place it several inches away. If the victim's chest or body is jerking, there may be an implanted defibrillator that is giving shocks; wait until jerking has ended before applying the pads.

Hypothermia

Detecting breathing in a victim of hypothermia (low body temperature) can be difficult. Handle a hypothermic victim very carefully because jarring may cause cardiac arrest. Follow your local guidelines for AED use if you find no signs of breathing. Typically, if the AED finds a shockable rhythm and advises shocks, no more than one shock is given, and then CPR and rewarming is performed until help arrives.

Medication Patches

If the victim has a medication patch or paste on the chest, remove it and wipe the chest before applying the AED pads (**Figure 8-8**).

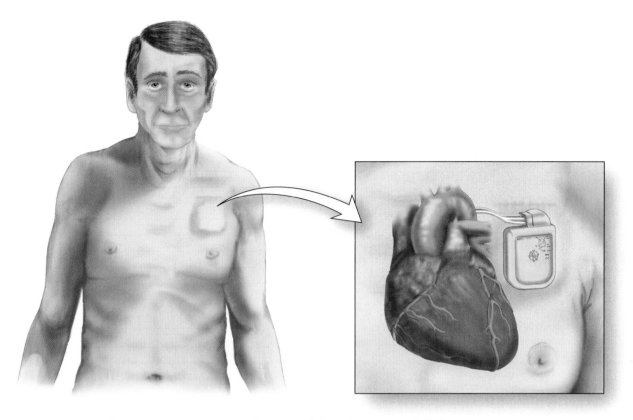

Figure 8-7 Vary AED pad placement if there is an internal device.

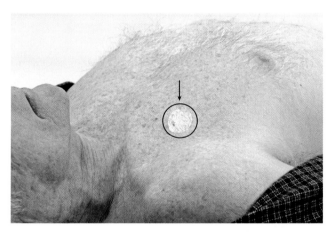

Figure 8-8 Remove medication patches prior to AED use.

POTENTIAL AED PROBLEMS

An AED must be maintained regularly and the battery kept charged. With regular maintenance an AED should not have any problems during use.

The AED may also prompt you to avoid problems. If you get a low battery prompt, change the battery before continuing. Another prompt may advise you to avoid moving the victim if the AED detects motion.

AED MAINTENANCE

AEDs require regular maintenance. Check the manual from the manufacturer for periodic scheduled maintenance and testing of the unit.

A daily inspection of the unit helps ensure that the AED is always ready for use and all needed supplies are present. Professional rescuers usually inspect the unit at the beginning of their shift. Most facilities with an AED use a daily checklist form (**Figure 8-9**). A checklist should always be adapted for the specific AED model, including the manufacturer's daily maintenance guidelines. In addition, many units come with a simulator device to be used to check that the AED is correctly analyzing rhythms and delivering shocks; this may be part of the daily inspection routine.

AED INSPECTION CHECKLIST

Date: _____   Location: _____   AED Model: _____

Inspected by: _____   Signed: _____

Criteria	ok/no	Corrective action/remarks
AED unit		
verify correctly placed	_____	_____
clean, clear of objects	_____	_____
no cracks or damage to case	_____	_____
cables/connectors present and not expired	_____	_____
fully charged battery in place	_____	_____
charged spare battery present	_____	_____
check status/service light indicator	_____	_____
check absence of service alarm	_____	_____
power on, self-test	_____	_____
Supplies		
Two sealed sets of electrode pads	_____	_____
Verify expiration date on pad packages	_____	_____
Razor	_____	_____
Medical exam gloves	_____	_____
Hand towels	_____	_____
Alcohol wipes	_____	_____
Scissors	_____	_____
Pocket mask or face shield	_____	_____

Figure 8-9 Example of an AED checklist.

Learning
Checkpoint ③

1. Name at least one situation in which a young child may experience sudden cardiac arrest and could benefit from the use of a pediatric AED.

   _____

2. Describe where to put the AED pads if you see that a victim has an implanted pacemaker or defibrillator.

   _____

3. What should you do with the AED pads if the victim has a medication patch on his or her chest?

   _____

Table 8-1

Summary of Basic Life Support

Step	Infant (under 1 year)	Child (1–8 years)	Adult (over 8 years)
1. Check for responsiveness	Stimulate to check response	"Are you okay" - Tap shoulder	
2. If unresponsive, call 9-1-1	Send someone to call Give 5 cycles of CPR before calling yourself if alone		Send someone to call Call immediately if alone
3. If unresponsive: Open airway	Head tilt-chin lift (but do not overextend neck)	Head tilt-chin lift	
4. Check breathing	Look, listen, feel for breathing		
5. If not breathing: Give 2 breaths, watch chest rise	Use barrier device or cover mouth, nose or stoma Each breath lasts 1 second		
6. If chest does not rise with first breath: Reposition airway and try again	Each breath lasts 1 second		
7. Start chest compressions	For compressions use 2 fingers just below line between nipples	For compressions use one or two hands midway between nipples	For compressions use both hands, one on top of other, midway between nipples
Compression depth	Compress chest $\frac{1}{3}$ to $\frac{1}{2}$ of chest depth		Compress chest $\frac{1}{2}$–2 inches
Compression rate and ratio of compressions to breaths	Compress at rate of 100/minute-30 compressions per 2 breaths		
8. Continue CPR until AED arrives, victim begins to move, or a professional rescuer takes over	Continue cycles of 30 compressions and two breaths		
9. Use AED when available (if victim is unresponsive and not breathing)	Not recommended	Use pediatric electrode pads if available	Use adult AED electrode pads
10. If victim begins to move and is breathing, put in recovery position	Hold infant in recovery position and monitor breathing	Lay on side in recovery position and monitor breathing	

Concluding Thoughts

This chapter concludes the series of chapters on basic life support. You have learned how rescue breaths, CPR, choking care, and the AED work together in the treatment of victims in respiratory or cardiac arrest. These are crucial skills for first aiders, and they are also skills that need periodic refreshing in order to remain effective. Even as you may now become credentialed in CPR and AED, remember that to use these skills well to save a life, you will need to practice your skills and stay current with refresher courses.

Learning Outcomes

You should now be able to do the following:

1. Explain how AEDs work to correct an abnormal heart rhythm.

2. Describe when an AED should be used and the basic steps for use.

3. Demonstrate how to use an AED with an adult or child victim.

4. List special considerations to be aware of when using an AED with certain types of victims or situations.

Review Questions

1. What is occurring in ventricular fibrillation?
   a. The ventricles of the heart have stopped moving.
   b. The ventricles of the heart are contracting too slowly.
   c. The ventricles of the heart are quivering rather than pumping.
   d. The ventricles of the heart are contracting with opposing rhythms.

2. An AED administers a shock to the victim
   a. whenever you turn it on.
   b. automatically after determining the presence of ventricular fibrillation.
   c. when you push the shock button after being prompted to do so.
   d. about 3 seconds after the pads are applied to the victim.

3. What should you do before using an AED?
   a. Ensure that the victim is not breathing.
   b. Administer CPR until the AED is ready to use.
   c. Place it next to the victim and turn it on.
   d. All of the above

4. The AED pads should be positioned where on the victim?
   a. Where the diagram on the unit indicates placement
   b. Below the nipples on both sides of the chest
   c. Above the nipples on both sides of the chest
   d. One on the chest and the other on the abdomen

5. While the AED is analyzing the victim's heart rhythm,
   a. continue CPR.
   b. do not touch the victim.
   c. push the shock button.
   d. push down on the pads to hold them in place.

6. If the AED indicates no shock is needed, you should then
   a. wait 20 seconds and try again.
   b. give CPR starting with chest compressions.
   c. give a lower-power shock.
   d. take the pads off and reposition them.

7. An AED may be used with a child one to eight years old if
   a. you use special pediatric pads.
   b. you turn the voltage knob to a lower setting.
   c. you put the pads on the legs to lower the voltage through the heart.
   d. you put petroleum jelly between the skin and the pads.

8. When using an AED with a victim of hypothermia,
   a. briskly rub the victim's chest to warm up the skin below the pads.
   b. handle the victim very carefully.
   c. put oil on the pads to provide better conductivity.
   d. wait until you have fully warmed the body before applying the pads.

References and Resources

American College of Emergency Physicians. Automatic external defibrillators. 2004. www.acep.org

American Heart Association. Questions and answers about AEDs and defibrillation. 2001. www.americanheart.org

Hazinski MF, et al. Lay rescuer automated external defibrillator ("public access defibrillation") programs. *Circulation.* 2005; 111.

American Heart Association. 2005 International consensus on cardiopulmonary resuscitation (CPR) and emergency cardiovascular care (ECC) science with treatment recommendations. *Circulation*, 112(22). November 29, 2005.

National Center for Early Defibrillation. AED training. 2003.

National Center for Early Defibrillation. www.early-defib.org

National Safety Council. www.nsc.org

Occupational Safety and Health Administration. Technical information bulletin: cardiac arrest and automated external defibrillators (AEDs). 2004. www.osha.gov

Chapter 9
Controlling Bleeding

Chapter Preview

- Effects of Blood Loss
- External Bleeding
- Internal Bleeding

You receive a call that a worker in the shipping department is injured. You grab the first aid kit and are there within a minute. The injured man is holding a bloody rag wrapped around his hand. He says he was using a box cutter, which slipped and made a gash in his palm. He unwraps the rag to show you, and you see a deep laceration that is still bleeding. What are the important steps you should take?

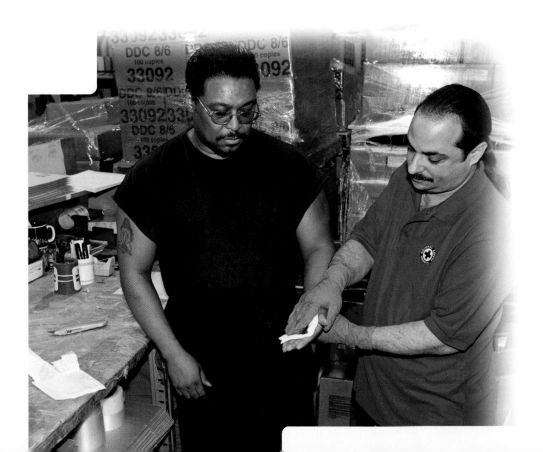

Blood carries oxygen from the lungs to all parts of the body. Many kinds of injuries damage blood vessels and cause external or internal bleeding. Bleeding may be minor or life threatening. Severe loss of blood can threaten the ability of the cardiovascular system to get the needed oxygen to vital organs. Severe bleeding, therefore, can be as great a threat to life as respiratory or cardiac arrest. This is why the victim is examined for severe bleeding in the initial assessment. Fortunately, most external bleeding is not that severe and can be controlled with first aid techniques.

EFFECTS OF BLOOD LOSS

As you learned in **Chapter 3**, the cardiovascular system has several important functions. Of all these, none is more important than transporting oxygen to the body. Without oxygen, vital tissues begin to die within minutes. Although the other functions of blood are also essential for life, the lack of oxygenation resulting from severe blood loss is the most serious first aid issue.

Fortunately, the body can compensate for a small blood loss without ill effects (**Box 9-1**).

Box 9-1 Effects of Blood Loss

Blood loss after an injury may occur quickly with severe bleeding, but usually the body passes through a series of stages as blood volume drops:

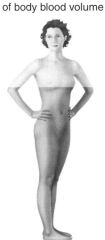

Class 1
Blood loss up to 15% of body blood volume

Class 2
Blood loss of 15–30% of body blood volume

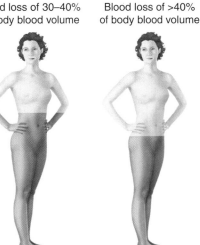

Class 3
Blood loss of 30–40% of body blood volume

Class 4
Blood loss of >40% of body blood volume

With a loss of up to 15% of blood volume, the body can compensate for the loss of volume by constricting (shrinking) blood vessels to maintain blood pressure and can continue to transport oxygen to organs. The victim remains alert, and blood pressure and pulse are close to normal.

With a loss of 15% to 30% of blood volume, constricting blood vessels maintain blood flow to vital organs such as the brain and heart while reducing blood flow to other body areas. The skin looks pale or ashen, cool, and dry. Heart and respiratory rates increase in an attempt to compensate. The victim may feel restless and confused.

With a loss of 30% to 40% of blood volume, the body can no longer compensate. Blood pressure falls, and the victim experiences **shock,** a serious condition in which vital organs are not receiving enough oxygenated blood. The victim is confused or anxious. Without medical treatment soon, vital organs will fail and the victim will die.

With a loss of more than 40% of blood volume, blood pressure falls further and vital organs begin to fail. The victim becomes lethargic, stuporous, and eventually unresponsive. Death occurs when the brain and other vital organs fail from lack of oxygen.

Table 9-1

Lethal Blood Loss

Hemorrhage	Percent of Total Blood Volume Lost	Effects
Class I	Less than 15%	Generally well tolerated
Class II	15% to 30%	Shock occurs, victim needs rapid transport
Class III	30% to 40%	Severe shock occurs, victim needs immediate transfusion
Class IV	Over 40%	Rapidly fatal

Note: A 15% volume loss in a 150 lb. person is about 750 mL. A 30% loss is about 1.5 liters, and a 40% loss is about 2 liters.
Source: National Safety Council, Injury Facts 2005.

This is why it is possible for a healthy person to donate blood periodically without problems. A larger blood loss, however, can have serious effects, potentially leading to death. **Table 9-1** shows the amount of blood loss that causes shock and the loss that becomes lethal if not immediately corrected. Note that in infants and children, severe bleeding becomes critical more quickly than in adults because the same amount of blood lost represents a higher percentage of the body's blood volume.

When a blood vessel is damaged and blood escapes, the body attempts to control the bleeding through three processes:

- **Vascular spasm** is a mechanism in which the damaged blood vessel constricts to slow the bleeding and to allow clotting to occur. With an injured small vessel, this constriction may be sufficient to stop the bleeding, but with a larger vessel bleeding usually still occurs.
- **Platelets** in the blood then stick to each other and to the walls of the injured vessel to form a **platelet plug,** which may reduce or stop minor bleeding.
- **Clotting** (coagulation) is the process in which **fibrin** produced from blood proteins clumps together with platelets and other blood cells in a fibrin web to seal the leak in the vessel (**Figure 9-1**). These three mechanisms working together may be able to stop or reduce bleeding after an injury. In a more serious injury, however,

these mechanisms may not be sufficient to stop the bleeding, or bleeding may continue long enough that the victim shows the effects of reduced blood volume. Controlling bleeding is therefore an important first aid action.

Bleeding occurs when blood from injured vessels escapes the body through a wound (external bleeding) or gathers in a body space or cavity (internal bleeding). Although the signs and symptoms of each are different, as is the first aid

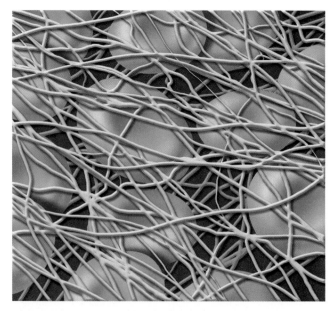

Figure 9-1 View of blood clot showing blood cells in a web of fibrin.

given, both external and internal bleeding can be life threatening when severe and uncontrolled.

EXTERNAL BLEEDING

External bleeding typically occurs when skin and other underlying tissues are damaged by trauma, and blood from cut or torn blood vessels flows out through the wound. The rate at which bleeding occurs depends on the size and type of the vessel(s) damaged. Larger blood vessels are *usually* deeper in the body and more protected, and therefore most superficial wounds damage only smaller blood vessels (**Figure 9-2**). This is not true in all

body areas, however, and a wound where a major vessel is close to the skin surface may result in very heavy bleeding, such as at the wrist or neck.

Types of External Bleeding

There are three types of blood vessels: **arteries,** which carry blood from the heart to body tissues; **veins,** which carry blood back to the heart from body tissues; and **capillaries,** which are tiny vessels between the arteries and veins where oxygen and nutrients in the blood pass into tissues and carbon dioxide and wastes move into the blood for removal. Therefore there are three types of external bleeding (**Figure 9-3**):

- **Bleeding from injured arteries** is more likely with deep injuries and is generally more serious. The blood is bright red and may spurt from the wound, and blood loss can be very rapid. This bleeding needs to be controlled immediately.
- **Bleeding from injured veins** is generally slower and steady but can still be serious. The blood is darker red and flows steadily rather than spurting. This bleeding is usually easier to control.
- **Bleeding from capillaries** occurs with shallow cuts or scrapes and often stops soon by itself. The wound still needs attention to prevent infection.

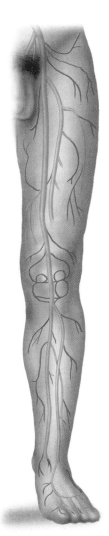

Figure 9-2 Arteries of the leg. Note that the larger arteries are deeper within the leg, and the arteries nearer the skin surface are generally much smaller and will bleed less.

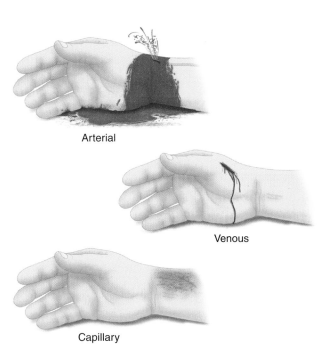

Arterial

Venous

Capillary

Figure 9-3 Arterial, venous, and capillary bleeding.

Controlling External Bleeding

For minor bleeding that stops by itself, clean and dress the wound as described in **Chapter 11**. The bleeding should stop by itself or with light pressure on the dressing, such as the pressure provided by an adhesive bandage around a cut finger.

For more serious bleeding, first aid is needed *immediately* to stop the bleeding. Applying direct pressure on the wound is sufficient to stop the bleeding in most cases (see Skill: "Controlling Bleeding"). Direct pressure on the wound controls bleeding by squeezing shut the bleeding vessel at the point where it is damaged. You apply direct pressure by pressing directly on the wound with a sterile dressing and your gloved hand. If gloves are not available, use any impermeable substance as a barrier to prevent contact between the victim's blood and your skin. Mechanically, this pressure stops the blood from flowing out. When the blood stops flowing, the natural body processes involved in clotting have a chance to function more effectively because platelets and fibrin are not "washed out" of the damaged area by the flow of blood. This is why sometimes pressure is needed only for a short time: the body's natural processes control the bleeding once they have the opportunity to work. With more severe vessel damage, however, pressure may have to be maintained for some time before the clotting is successful. Releasing the pressure on the wound too soon would allow the normal blood pressure to break through the "dam" made of platelets, fibrin, and other cells. This is also the reason why you should add more dressings on top of blood-soaked bandages when bleeding continues, rather than removing the first dressings—because removing them would release pressure and remove blood that is clotting.

Direct pressure should not be put on certain wounds, such as skull fractures or objects impaled in the wound, because the pressure may cause additional damage. In such cases pressure is applied around the wound or object, as described in **Chapter 11.**

Call 9-1-1 for any severe bleeding or bleeding that does not stop quickly. The victim should seek medical attention for any significant wound (see **Chapter**

11). Do not remove the dressing or bandage; the wound will be cleaned later by medical personnel.

Pressure Bandages

To control severe bleeding as quickly as possible, apply direct pressure with your gloved hand on a sterile dressing (or clean cloth) placed on the wound. You can then apply a **pressure bandage** over a wound in an extremity to maintain this pressure so that you can give other first aid as needed. Use a roller bandage wrapped around the limb to completely cover the wound and to maintain sufficient pressure to keep bleeding from starting again (see Skill: "Applying a Pressure Bandage").

Whenever you apply a bandage around an extremity, be sure that it is not so tight that it cuts off circulation to the limb. Periodically check the victim's fingers or toes for signs of good circulation: normal skin color, warmth, and sensation (not a tingling or numbness). If you find signs that circulation is reduced, loosen the bandage and apply it less tightly. Note that injuries often cause swelling that may increase after you apply the bandage, making the bandage tighter and possibly cutting off circulation. Therefore continue to check for signs of circulation until the victim receives medical attention. **Chapter 11** describes bandaging more fully.

Preventing Bloodborne Infection

When giving first aid to control bleeding, remember always to follow standard precautions to prevent disease transmission. If you do not have medical exam gloves with you, put your hand in a plastic bag or use a barrier such as plastic wrap between your hand and the wound. If nothing is available to use as a barrier, you can use the victim's own hand to apply pressure on the wound.

After providing care for bleeding, remember also not to touch your face or other parts of your body until you have thoroughly washed your hands. Since objects or surfaces contaminated with blood can remain infectious for some time afterwards, be sure to dispose of soiled supplies properly and disinfect all contaminated items. **Chapter 2** describes guidelines for preventing bloodborne disease transmission.

Skill | **Controlling Bleeding**

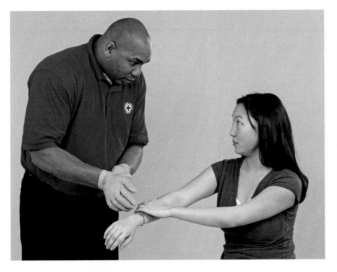

1   Put on gloves.

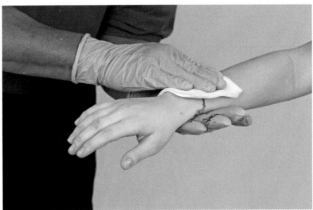

2   Place a sterile dressing on the wound and apply direct pressure with your hand.

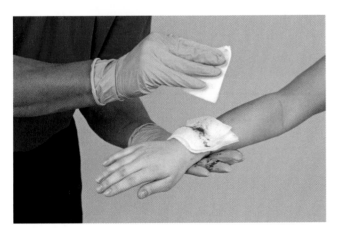

3   If needed, put another dressing or cloth pad on top of the first and keep applying pressure.

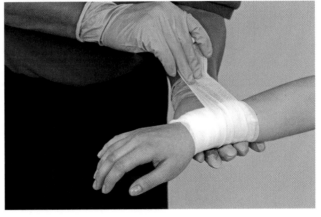

4   Apply a roller bandage to keep pressure on the wound.

5   If appropriate, treat the victim for shock (see **Chapter 10**), and call 9-1-1.

ALERT

- Use your bare hands only if no barrier is available, and then wash immediately.
- Do not put pressure on an object in a wound.
- Do not put pressure on the scalp if the skull may be injured.
- Do not use a tourniquet to stop bleeding except as an extreme last resort because the limb will likely be lost (see **Chapter 24**).

Skill   Applying a Pressure Bandage

Hold end in place for
first turn of bandage

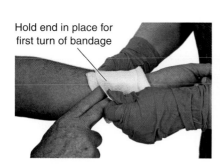

1 Anchor the starting end
   of the bandage below the
   wound dressing.

Overlap turns by about
³/₄ of previous turn

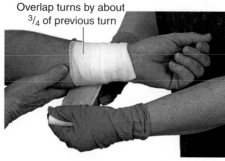

2 Make several circular turns,
   then overlap turns.

Cover the
dressing completely

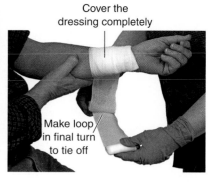

Make loop
in final turn
to tie off

3 Work up the limb.

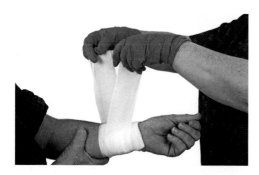

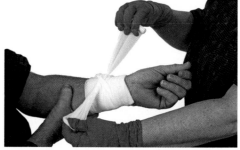

4 Tape or tie the end of the bandage in place.

Learning
Checkpoint ①

1. True or False: Arterial bleeding is the most serious because blood loss can be very rapid.

2. True or False: The first thing to do with any bleeding wound is wash it and apply antibiotic ointment.

3. Describe the skin characteristics of a victim who has been bleeding severely. _____
_____

4. If you do not have medical exam gloves with you, what other materials or objects can be used as a barrier between your hand and the wound when applying direct pressure? _____
_____

INTERNAL BLEEDING

Internal bleeding is any bleeding within the body in which the blood does not escape from an open wound. Internal bleeding is typically caused by a blunt impact on the body. The body may be impacted by a large force, such as being struck by a car, or a smaller force that leaves only a bruise. A serious injury can cause organs deep within the body to bleed severely. This bleeding, although unseen, can be life threatening. A closed wound resulting from a minor injury may involve only minor local bleeding in the skin and other superficial tissue, appearing as a bruise (also called a contusion). Internal bleeding may also occur in the absence of trauma, such as with a bleeding ulcer.

Because you cannot see internal bleeding, it is important to consider the nature of the injury when you assess the victim. With any injury involving a fall or a moving vehicle, even a bicycle, consider the possibility of internal bleeding. The victim may complain of pain. With internal bleeding the victim may experience shock—which may cause cool, clammy skin that is pale or bluish or ashen—thirst, and possible confusion or light-headedness. In some cases the victim may vomit or cough up blood, or blood may be present in urine. With bleeding into the abdominal cavity, the victim's abdomen may be tender, swollen, bruised, or hard.

Minor bleeding just below the skin surface can be reduced to some extent with a cold pack or ice and wrapping an injured extremity (see First Aid: "Simple Bruises"). Deeper internal bleeding cannot be controlled by first aid. Call 9-1-1 immediately if you suspect internal bleeding, and treat for shock (see **Chapter 10**). Be prepared to give basic life support if the victim's condition worsens (see First Aid: "Internal Bleeding").

First Aid   Simple Bruises

When You See
- Bruising
- Signs of pain

Do This First

1 Check for signs and symptoms of a fracture or sprain (see **Chapter 15**) and give appropriate first aid.

2 Put ice or a cold pack on the area to control bleeding, reduce swelling, and reduce pain.

3 With an arm or leg, wrap the area with an elastic bandage. Keep the part raised to help reduce swelling.

Additional Care
- Seek medical attention if you suspect a more serious injury such as a fracture or sprain.

First Aid Internal Bleeding

When You See

- Abdomen is tender, swollen, bruised, or hard
- Blood vomited or coughed up, or present in urine
- Cool, clammy skin, may be pale, bluish, or ashen in color
- Thirst
- Possible confusion, light-headedness

Do This First

1 Have the victim lie on his or her back with legs raised about 12 inches.

2 Call 9-1-1.

3 Be alert for vomiting. Put a victim who vomits or becomes unresponsive in the recovery position.

4 Keep the victim from becoming chilled or overheated.

ALERT

- Do not give the victim anything to drink even if he or she is thirsty.

Additional Care

- Calm and reassure the victim.
- If the victim becomes unresponsive, monitor breathing and give basic life support (BLS) as needed.
- Treat for shock (see **Chapter 10**).

Learning Checkpoint ②

1. True or False: Internal bleeding is seldom life-threatening because there is no loss of blood from the body.

2. Put a check mark next to the signs and symptoms of internal bleeding.

_____ Cool, clammy skin   _____ Confusion or light-headedness

_____ Vomiting or coughing up blood   _____ Blood in urine

_____ Tender, swollen, or hard abdomen   _____ Bruise

3. First aid for serious internal bleeding includes

a. calling 9-1-1.

b. positioning the victim lying down with feet raised.

c. keeping the victim from becoming chilled or overheated.

d. all of the above

Concluding Thoughts

Many people are frightened of or upset by bleeding. Fortunately the body's own mechanisms make it easy to control external bleeding with direct pressure in most cases. Because serious bleeding can be life threatening, however, always call 9-1-1. In **Chapter 10**, you will learn more about caring for a victim who is in shock as a result of serious bleeding.

Learning Outcomes

You should now be able to do the following:

1. Explain the effects of blood loss and the body's mechanisms to control bleeding.

2. Describe the different types of external bleeding.

3. Demonstrate the steps for controlling external bleeding.

4. Demonstrate the steps for applying a pressure bandage.

5. List the steps for caring for a bruise.

6. List the signs and symptoms of internal bleeding and describe the first aid to give.

Review Questions

1. The body attempts to slow or stop bleeding from a damaged blood vessel by
   a. skeletal muscle contraction.
   b. blood clotting.
   c. producing more red blood cells.
   d. stopping the heartbeat.

2. Which type of bleeding is usually most serious?
   a. Arterial bleeding
   b. Venous bleeding
   c. Capillary bleeding
   d. All bleeding is equally serious.

3. To prevent bloodborne disease transmission, apply pressure on a bleeding wound with
   a. your gloved hand.
   b. any impermeable substance.
   c. the victim's hand.
   d. Any of the above

4. What do you do if blood soaks through the pressure bandage?
   a. Ignore the blood but maintain the pressure.
   b. Put a new bandage on top of the first and maintain pressure.
   c. Replace the bloody bandage with a new bandage and maintain pressure.
   d. Apply a tourniquet on top of the bandage.

5. A pressure bandage is applied
   a. around the extremity from the joint above the wound to the joint below the wound, to apply equal pressure to the whole area.
   b. above the wound to cut off the blood flow.
   c. on the wound to control bleeding.
   d. both above and below the wound to control blood flow and bleeding.

6. Which is a sign or symptom that a pressure bandage is too tight on the arm?
   a. Red color under the fingernails
   b. Hot fingers
   c. Cold fingers
   d. Extreme thirst

7. Internal bleeding into the abdomen may result in the abdomen feeling
   a. hard.
   b. hot.
   c. pulsing.
   d. soft and squishy.

8. Severe internal bleeding may cause
   a. the victim to feel thirsty.
   b. the victim's skin to be cool and clammy.
   c. the victim to be confused.
   d. All of the above

References and Resources

American College of Emergency Physicians. *First aid manual: a comprehensive guide to treating emergency victims of all ages in any situation.* DK Publishing; 2001.

American Heart Association. 2005 International consensus on cardiopulmonary resuscitation (CPR) and emergency cardiovascular care (ECC) science with treatment recommendations. *Circulation*, 112(22). November 29, 2005.

American Medical Association. *Handbook of first aid and emergency care.* Revised edition. New York: Random House; 2000.

Barquist ES. Hemorrhagic shock. Emergency Medical Services: The Journal of Emergency Care, Rescue, and Transportation. 1999 October.

Limmer, D., Karren, K., Hafen, B. First responder. 6th ed. Englewood Cliffs, New Jersey: Prentice-Hall; 2003.

National Safety Council. www.nsc.org

Chapter 10
Shock

Chapter Preview

- Shock

- Anaphylaxis

Seated at a nearby table at a local Mexican restaurant are a woman, her two daughters, and her daughter's friend. They are sharing a variety of dishes and having a good time—until abruptly the friend puts down her fork and leans back in her seat, looking ill. You notice her face seems puffy around the mouth, and she is obviously having trouble breathing. The mother and two daughters are asking her if she is okay but don't seem to know what to do. With your first aid training, you recognize the situation as a possible food allergy. What should you do?

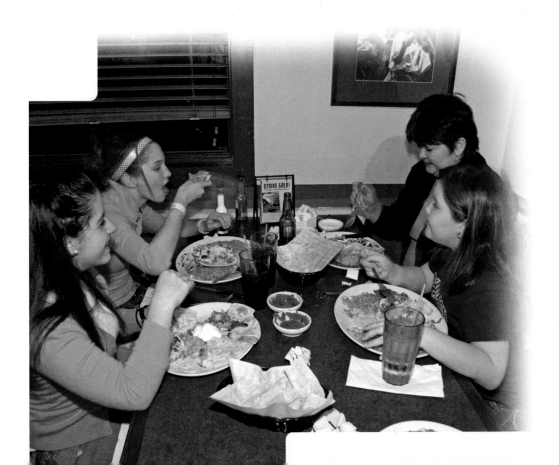

Shock is a dangerous condition in which not enough oxygen-rich blood reaches vital organs in the body. The brain, heart, and other organs need a continual supply of oxygen. Anything that happens to or in the body that significantly reduces blood flow can cause shock. Severe bleeding is a common cause of shock in first aid situations.

Shock is a life-threatening emergency. It may develop quickly or gradually. Always call 9-1-1 for a victim in shock.

SHOCK

For enough blood to reach the body's vital organs and keep them well oxygenated, three general conditions must be met:

1. The heart must be efficiently pumping blood.
2. Blood volume in the body must be sufficient to fill blood vessels, so that the pumping action circulates blood to vital organs.
3. Blood vessels throughout the body must be intact and functioning normally. A loss of blood through injured blood vessels may reduce the blood volume to the point where not enough blood is circulated to vital organs. Certain conditions may also dilate blood vessels to the extent that there is not enough blood volume to fill blood vessels.

Normally the body easily meets these conditions. The heart rate varies as needed to pump more or less blood throughout the body. The body controls blood volume by moving fluid into or out of the blood as needed. Blood ves-sels constrict or dilate in different conditions to ensure that enough blood is circulated to vital organs at all times. In a healthy person these mechanisms work automatically to supply the constant supply of oxygen that the brain, heart, and other vital organs need.

In cases of injury or illness, however, one or more of these necessary conditions may be disrupted. Disruption of the heart, the blood volume, or the blood vessels may reduce the blood flow to vital organs, causing shock (**Figure 10-1**).

Causes of Shock

Shock may develop in a victim in many different situations. Following are descriptions of the primary types of shock. You do not need to know which exact type a victim has, as long as you recognize the problem and give appropriate first aid. **Box 10-1** lists the specific types of injuries and conditions that may lead to shock.

- **Hypovolemic shock** occurs when blood volume drops. Severe bleeding, either external or internal, is a common cause of shock when not enough blood is left circulating in the body to bring required oxygen to vital organs (this is called **hemorrhagic shock**). Other conditions may also lower blood volume. Severe burns result in a loss of fluid from the blood. Severe vomiting or diarrhea, or other causes of dehydration, may also result in the body moving fluid from the blood to meet other body needs, causing shock. Infants and young children are especially vulnerable to hypovolemic shock caused by persistent vomiting or diarrhea.

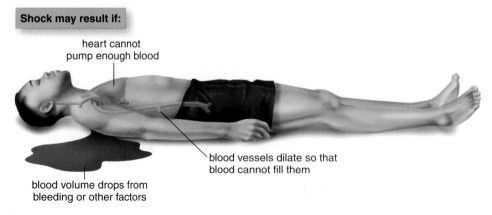

Shock may result if:

heart cannot
pump enough blood

blood vessels dilate so that
blood cannot fill them

blood volume drops from
bleeding or other factors

Figure 10-1 Shock may result from disruption of the heart, blood volume, or blood vessels.

Box 10-1 Injuries and Conditions that May Cause Shock

- Severe bleeding
- Severe burns
- Heart failure
- Heart attack
- Head or spinal injuries
- Allergic reactions

- Dehydration (common with heatstroke or severe vomiting or diarrhea)
- Electrocution
- Serious infections
- Extreme emotional reactions (temporary, less dangerous form of shock)

- **Cardiogenic shock** occurs when any condition causes the heart function to be reduced to the point that blood is not circulating sufficiently. Heart attack is a common cause. An abnormal heartbeat, such as ventricular fibrillation, is another cause of inadequate circulation. As described in the chapters on basic life support, CPR and an AED are used to restore a normal heartbeat and keep blood moving to vital organs and thereby to help prevent the occurrence of shock.
- **Neurogenic shock** occurs when a problem related to the nervous system's control of blood vessels allows vessels to dilate excessively. If blood vessels throughout the body expand too much, the volume of blood is not sufficient to fill blood vessels, and not enough blood can be pumped to vital organs. Certain spinal cord injuries may cause neurogenic shock. A similar condition may result from extreme fear or similar emotions that cause fainting when blood vessels temporarily dilate because of the nervous system reaction.
- **Anaphylactic shock** is an extreme allergic reaction, typically to an insect sting, a particular food, medication, or some other substance. Anaphylaxis produces shock because part of the allergic reaction causes the dilation of blood vessels and the movement of fluid out of the blood through capillary walls. Since anaphylaxis causes other signs and symptoms and requires different first aid treatment, it is discussed separately later in this chapter.

First Aid for Shock

A victim in shock has various signs and symptoms depending on its cause and severity. Note, however, that the victim's signs and symptoms are not always correlated with the severity of the shock; therefore all cases of shock should be treated as severe. A victim with any serious injury should be assumed to be at risk of shock, even if you do not see all the signs and symptoms. Remember that internal bleeding can be life threatening even though you cannot see it or know for certain whether it is occurring.

Shock generally occurs in stages that may progress either gradually or so quickly that the victim is in full shock very soon after the injury. Early signs include feelings of anxiety, restlessness, or fear along with increased breathing and heart rates. Mental status continues to deteriorate, leading to confusion, disorientation, or sleepiness. Breathing becomes rapid and shallow, and the heartbeat rapid (but the pulse weak because of decreased blood volume). The skin becomes pale or ashen and cool as blood is shunted from the extremities to vital organs. Nausea and thirst occur as blood is shunted from the digestive system. As oxygen levels drop in body tissues, the lips and nail beds may look bluish. The victim ultimately becomes unresponsive. Without medical treatment, shock leads to respiratory and cardiac arrest. Once it develops, shock cannot be reversed without professional medical care, so it is important to recognize situations in which shock is likely or is beginning to occur and to give care to minimize it.

Not all victims experience all symptoms of shock or have them in the same order. But a victim who has several of these signs and symptoms after a serious injury is probably beginning to experience shock. It is crucial to call 9-1-1 immediately because, once it begins, shock will continue to develop unless medical treatment begins. EMS professionals often refer to the "golden hour"—the period of time from a shock-producing traumatic injury until the victim is receiving emergency medical treatment in a hospital. A victim reaching medical care later has much lower chances for survival. Calling 9-1-1 immediately is necessary to start the emergency response process so that the victim can receive help before shock leads to death.

After EMS is called, first aid for shock is directed at helping minimize or delay the onset of shock; first aid at the scene cannot reverse shock. If the victim is bleeding, it is essential to control the bleeding immediately to prevent further blood loss. Then position the victim lying on his or her back with legs raised about 8 to 12 inches unless the victim may have a spinal injury, head injury, or stroke; this is often called the *shock position*. Put a victim who is having breathing difficulty in a reclining position partly sitting up.

Ensure that the airway is open. Help the victim to maintain normal body temperature by covering him or her with a blanket or coat, but avoid overheating. Outdoors in cold weather, put a blanket or coat under the victim unless the victim may have a spinal injury (see First Aid: "Shock").

Blood loss in infants or children may quickly lead to shock, and young children and infants are also more susceptible to shock caused by dehydration resulting from repeated vomiting or diarrhea. Call 9-1-1 for any infant or child with persistent vomiting or diarrhea; do not wait for the signs of shock to develop.

Early shock may be less obvious in children because a child's body is generally more efficient in compensating initially for the blood volume decrease. As shock progresses, however, the child's condition rapidly declines. An infant or child in shock may look limp and unresponsive, with eyes partially open or closed, the skin pale, bluish, or ashen. Call 9-1-1 immediately. Treatment is the same as for adults, but because the child's decline is rapid, you should be prepared to give basic life support as needed.

Learning
Checkpoint ①

1. True or False: Because a shock victim is thirsty and may be dehydrated, offer clear fluids to drink.

2. True or False: A spinal injury can cause shock.

3. Which of these actions should you take *first* for a victim in shock because of external bleeding?

   a. Stop the bleeding.

   b. Raise the legs.

   c. Loosen tight clothing.

   d. Cover the victim with a blanket.

4. A shock victim is likely to have which signs and symptoms?

   a. Vomiting; diarrhea; red, blotchy face

   b. Nausea, thirst, clammy skin

   c. Incontinence, hives, swollen legs

   d. Headache, painful abdomen, coughing

5. What is the most important action to take for *all shock victims?*

When You See

- Anxiety, confusion, agitation, or restlessness
- Dizziness, light-headedness
- Cool, clammy or sweating skin, pale, bluish, or ashen in color
- Rapid, shallow breathing
- Thirst
- Nausea, vomiting
- Changing responsiveness

Do This First

1 Check for normal breathing and severe bleeding, and care first for life-threatening injuries.

2 Call 9-1-1.

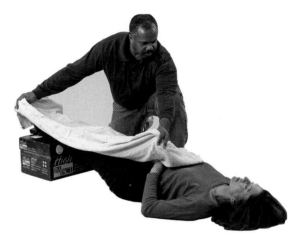

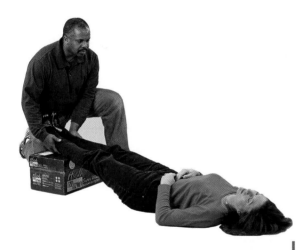

3 Have the victim lie on his or her back and raise the legs about 8 to 12 inches (unless the victim may have a spinal injury). Loosen any tight clothing.

4 Try to maintain the victim's normal body temperature. If lying on the ground, put a coat or blanket under the victim. If in doubt, keep the victim warm with a blanket or coat over the victim.

((•ALERT•))

- Do not let a shock victim eat, drink, or smoke.
- Note that sweating in a shock victim is not necessarily a sign of being too warm. If in doubt, it is better to maintain a shock victim's body temperature by keeping the victim warm.

Additional Care

- Stay with the victim and offer reassurance and comfort.
- Be alert for the possibility of vomiting; turn the victim's head to drain the mouth.
- Put an unresponsive victim (if no suspected spinal injury) in the recovery position.
- Keep bystanders from crowding around the victim.

ANAPHYLAXIS

As described earlier, **anaphylaxis,** also called anaphylactic shock, involves a severe allergic reaction. In addition to the circulatory problems of shock, the victim's airway may swell, making breathing difficult or impossible. The breathing problem is usually the immediate life-threatening emergency. Always call 9-1-1 for an anaphylaxis emergency.

Causes of Anaphylaxis

The immune system has several mechanisms that protect the body from foreign substances that enter the body. When the individual is allergic to the substance (called an **allergen**), such as pollen that is inhaled or a food that is ingested, the normal action of the immune system results in a physiological response that includes various signs and symptoms, depending on the type and strength of the allergy. Typical mild allergic reactions include nasal congestion and watery eyes, or itching, blotchy skin.

Anaphylaxis, or anaphylactic shock, is a more extreme allergic reaction that causes more severe signs and symptoms that can rapidly become life threatening. The most common causes of anaphylaxis are:

- Certain drugs (such as penicillins, sulfa)
- Certain foods (such as peanuts, shellfish, eggs)
- Insect stings and bites (such as bees or wasps)

The signs and symptoms of anaphylactic shock may begin within minutes, even seconds, of the victim's contact with the allergen. As a general rule, the more quickly the reaction occurs, the more serious it is likely to be. Anaphylaxis is frightening and demands immediate action because you cannot know if the reaction will continue to worsen and become fatal without medical care, or whether the victim may recover on his or her own. Even if the victim has had what feels like a similar reaction in the past, he or she cannot know for certain that it will not be worse this time.

Prevention of Anaphylaxis

Prevention of anaphylaxis resulting from allergic reaction depends on avoiding the specific allergen.

Medication allergies are the most common cause of anaphylaxis and death resulting from anaphylaxis. Unfortunately, most reactions occur in people without a history of reaction, so prevention is difficult. Healthcare professionals are trained to watch for the early effects of an ana-phylactic reaction, however, and to provide early treatment. Following are preventive actions for people with known medication allergies:

- Maintain a complete history of medication reactions and share this with all healthcare providers.
- Wear a medical alert ID in case you cannot communicate about an allergy in an emergency.
- For those allergic to nonprescription medications, read product labels carefully because many products include a number of possibly unexpected ingredients.

Food allergies occur in about 4% of adults and 6% to 8% of children under age four. Peanut and nut allergies are the most common. About 150 people die every year in the United States from food-induced anaphylaxis, mostly adolescents and young adults. Prevention of food allergic reactions depends on avoiding foods known to cause a reaction, which can be more difficult than it may seem:

- Check food product labels for alternate names of foods.
- In restaurants and other settings where exact ingredients cannot be known, do not trust what wait staff or other people may say. Avoid foods that may contain hidden ingredients, such as sauces, or that may have been prepared using equipment contaminated by an allergenic food.
- Educate a child's caretakers, teachers, and friends' parents about an allergy and its dangers to prevent the child from eating something shared by another child.

About 3% of adults and 1% of children have an allergic reaction to the venom of stinging insects, including honeybees, hornets, wasps, yellow jackets, and fire ants. There are about 40 to 100 deaths every year in the United States from anaphylactic reactions to such stings. Again, prevention is based on avoiding stinging insects whenever possible. When outdoors, these actions help you to avoid attracting or provoking stinging insects:

- Stay away from insect nesting areas. Check around the home for insect nests to destroy.
- Do not wear bright colors or sweet-smelling perfumes or colognes.
- Wear clothing that covers arms and legs; wear shoes to prevent stings from stepping on insects.
- Do not swat at or try to wave insects away.
- When getting into a car, if the windows were left open, check for insects that may have flown in.

- Be cautious when near areas where insects gather, such as around flowering plants and garbage cans.
- If stung, do not pull the stinger out with your fingers because the attached venom sac may eject more venom when squeezed; instead, scrape it off with something similar in size and rigidity to a credit card (**Figure 10-2**).

Immunotherapy, often called *allergy shots,* is also available to lessen a person's reaction to insect venoms. Injections, usually given over three years, gradually desensitize the body, eventually preventing allergic reactions in most people undergoing therapy. People with severe insect allergies should see their healthcare provider for information about this immunotherapy.

As described in the following section, emergency medication is also available for those at risk for severe allergic reactions. Although this medication cannot prevent the exposure to the allergen, it can stop the progress of an allergic reaction and prevent the victim from experiencing anaphylaxis.

First Aid for Anaphylaxis

If the victim knows he or she has the allergy and knows about the exposure, the victim may be able to tell you about the allergy when the reaction begins. Following the guidelines for the SAMPLE history in **Chapter 4**, ask all victims about allergies and the things they ate or drank most recently. For example, a victim who is severely allergic to bee stings, and who has just been stung, may say he or she needs medication immediately to prevent anaphylaxis. Or someone who is allergic to nuts may feel the start of the reaction and wonder if there were nuts in something he or she just ate. In many cases, however, the person may not know about the allergy and may not have had an allergic reaction before. Therefore you cannot depend on having this information but should suspect an allergic reaction based on the situation and the victim's signs and symptoms.

The early signs and symptoms of anaphylaxis include skin flushing, itching or burning, and rash; sneezing and watery eyes and nose, coughing or a feeling of a tickle or lump in the throat that does not go away; and gastrointestinal upset. As symptoms worsen, the victim becomes anxious and may have the feeling that the throat is closing and the chest is becoming tight. Other signs include fast breathing, coughing, wheezing, or hoarseness and altered mental status. The victim may have severe headache, a feeling of weakness or fainting, and pale or ashen skin or cyanosis (bluish color of lips and nail beds), along with other shock signs and symptoms.

First aid begins with making sure 9-1-1 is called; medical care is urgently needed because first aid usually cannot stop or reverse anaphylactic shock. Help the victim into a position for easiest breathing and offer reassurance. Be prepared to give basic life support if needed. If the victim becomes unresponsive, put him or her in the recovery position and continue to monitor breathing.

Some people who know they have a severe allergy carry an emergency epinephrine kit such as an **EpiPen**®, EpiPen Jr.® (for children), or Anakit® (**Figure 10-3**). This medication usually will stop the anaphylactic reaction. Ask a victim about

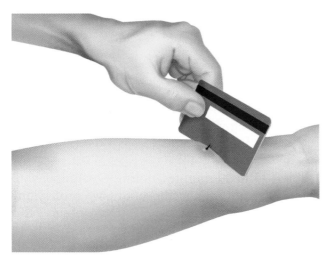

Figure 10-2 Use a rigid piece of plastic to scrape away a stinger.

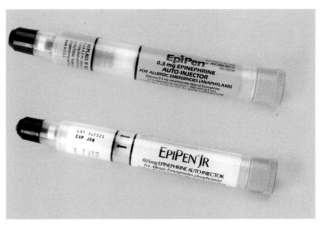

Figure 10-3 Emergency epinephrine kits.

First Aid Anaphylaxis

When You See

- Difficulty breathing, wheezing
- Complaints of tightness in throat or chest
- Swelling of the face and neck, puffy eyes
- Anxiety, agitation
- Nausea, vomiting
- Changing levels of responsiveness

Do This First

1 Call 9-1-1.

2 Give BLS as needed.

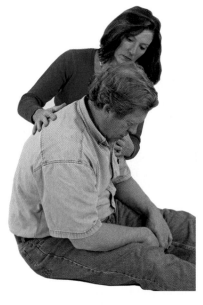

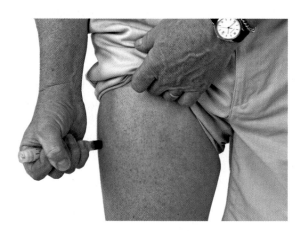

3 Help a responsive victim to use his or her emergency epinephrine kit and sit up in the position of easiest breathing.

4 Put a breathing, unresponsive victim (if no suspected spinal injury) in the recovery position.

Additional Care

- Stay with the victim and offer reassurance and comfort.

this and help him or her to open and use the kit as needed. The EpiPen® is removed from its case and the cap removed. The tip is then jabbed into the outer part of the thigh muscle and held there 5 to 10 seconds while the medication is injected. The injection site is then massaged for a few seconds. The effects of the emergency epinephrine will last 15 to 20 minutes, during which time you should stay with the victim until EMS professionals arrive and take over care. You may observe the victim experiencing the side effects of epinephrine: fast heartbeat, breathing difficulty, nausea and vomiting, dizziness or nervousness, and headache (see First Aid: "Anaphylaxis").

Learning Checkpoint ②

1. True or False: Ask a victim having an anaphylactic reaction about any allergies and medication for allergies.

2. True or False: A bee sting can cause a severe allergic reaction.

3. The major risk for a victim in anaphylaxis is

   a. swelling around the eyes.

   b. heart attack.

   c. internal bleeding.

   d. breathing problems.

4. How should a victim in anaphylaxis be positioned if he or she is having trouble breathing?

_____

Concluding Thoughts

Most commonly, shock is caused by heavy blood loss, so the most important thing to do for a victim who is bleeding is to control the bleeding as quickly as possible. Call 9-1-1 because shock is a serious threat to life. In most cases the first aid for a victim in shock is primarily supportive, but a victim with severe allergies may carry an emergency medication kit that can be used to treat anaphylactic shock caused by an allergic reaction.

Learning Outcomes

You should now be able to do the following:

1. Explain what happens inside the body with severe blood loss.

2. List common causes of shock.

3. Describe first aid steps for a victim in shock.

4. Describe ways to prevent exposure to known allergens.

5. Describe the first aid for anaphylaxis.

Review Questions

1. Which is fundamental to the definition of shock?

   a. Not enough oxygen reaching vital organs

   b. Too much waste building up in the urine

   c. The heartbeat stopping

   d. An abdominal injury

2. When should you call 9-1-1?
   a. Call only if the shock victim becomes unresponsive.
   b. Call only for blood loss over 30% of blood volume.
   c. Call for all victims in shock.
   d. Call for all victims who had any bleeding.

3. Which is a possible cause of shock?
   a. Bleeding
   b. Spinal cord injury
   c. Severe burn
   d. All of the above

4. Which is important in first aid for shock?
   a. Giving the victim water to drink to replace lost fluids
   b. Raising the victim's legs
   c. Keeping the victim moving to prevent his or her becoming unresponsive
   d. Applying ice to the injury

5. Signs and symptoms of shock include
   a. confusion.
   b. rapid, shallow breathing.
   c. pale, bluish, or ashen skin.
   d. All of the above

6. Shock in a child is similar to shock in an adult *except*
   a. a child's condition may decline more rapidly.
   b. early shock is more dramatically obvious in a child.
   c. a greater blood loss is required in a child to produce shock.
   d. a child's skin does not become pale with shock.

7. Anaphylaxis is commonly caused by allergic reactions to
   a. campfire smoke.
   b. insect stings.
   c. poison ivy.
   d. animal fur.

8. How soon may an allergic reaction occur following exposure?
   a. Within seconds or minutes
   b. Within about 30 minutes
   c. Within 1 to 2 hours
   d. Within 6 to 12 hours

9. If a person who has just been stung by a bee says he is allergic to bee stings, you should
   a. call 9-1-1 immediately.
   b. wait for the development of signs and symptoms, then call 9-1-1.
   c. send someone to the nearest drugstore to buy an EpiPen®.
   d. use the shock position and see if that reverses the problem.

10. First aid for a victim experiencing anaphylaxis includes
    a. cooling the victim's body with ice packs.
    b. giving the victim an aspirin as quickly as possible.
    c. positioning the victim for easiest breathing.
    d. using the pressure points on arms and legs.

References and Resources

American College of Emergency Physicians. *First aid manual: a comprehensive guide to treating emergency victims of all ages in any situation.* DK Publishing; 2001.

American Heart Association. 2005 International consensus on cardiopulmonary resuscitation (CPR) and emergency cardiovascular care (ECC) science with treatment recommendations. *Circulation*, 112(22). November 29, 2005.

American Medical Association. *Handbook of first aid and emergency care.* Revised edition. New York: Random House; 2000.

Harvard Medical School Consumer Health Information. Allergy. 2005. www.intelihealth.com

Johns Hopkins Children's Center. *First aid for children fast.* DK Publishing; 1995.

National Institute of Allergy and Infectious Diseases, National Institutes of Health. Allergy statistics. 2005; www.niaid.nih.gov

National Safety Council. www.nsc.org

Chapter 11

Wounds and Soft Tissue Injuries

Chapter Preview

- Types of Open Wounds
- Cleaning Wounds
- Wound Infection

- Dressing and Bandaging Wounds
- When to Seek Medical Attention for a Wound
- Special Wounds

Your co-worker has cut his arm while trying to repair some office equipment. It is not bleeding heavily, but the wound seems dirty. You get the first aid kit and put on gloves, then take him to a nearby sink. How should you wash the wound? What other first aid should you give?

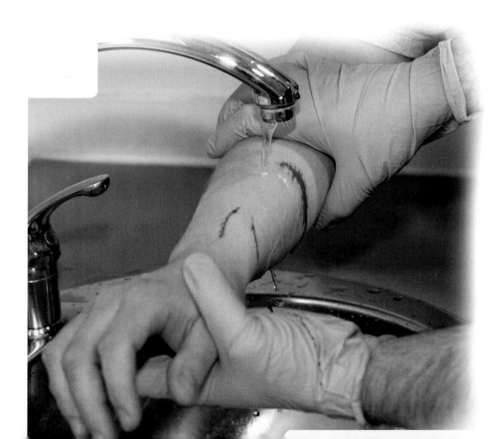

A wound is an injury to the skin and sometimes other deeper soft tissues. In an **open wound** the skin is torn or cut open, often leading to bleeding. Different types of wounds require different specific first aid, but all wounds have a risk for becoming infected by pathogens that may enter the body through the break in the skin. In addition to controlling bleeding (see **Chapter 9**), first aiders should also know how to care for different kinds of wounds and how to apply dressings and bandages.

Wound care involves cleaning and dressing a wound to prevent infection and protecting the wound so that healing can occur. Remember: *Do not waste time cleaning a wound that is severely bleeding. Controlling bleeding is always the priority.* Healthcare personnel will clean the wound as needed.

This chapter describes first aid for open wounds. Care of internal bleeding caused by **closed injuries** is described in **Chapter 9**. The care of musculoskeletal injuries, another type of closed injury, is described in **Chapter 15**.

TYPES OF OPEN WOUNDS

Different mechanisms of injury cause different types of damage to soft tissues. The main types of open wounds are abrasions, lacerations, punctures, avulsions, and amputations. The type and amount of bleeding caused by an injury depend on the type of wound, its location, and its depth. Different types of wounds also have different implications for first aid.

- **Abrasions** occur when the top layers of skin are scraped off (**Figure 11-1**). Skinned elbows or knees, for example, are common in children. Abrasions are often painful but are not

serious injuries because underlying tissues are not usually injured. Bleeding is usually limited to capillary bleeding that typically stops soon by itself. Foreign material may be present in the wound, which can cause infection.

- **Lacerations,** or cuts, frequently penetrate the skin and may also damage underlying tissue (**Figure 11-2**). Lacerations are either smooth cuts with straight edges (called incisions), such as those caused by knives or other sharp objects, or jagged cuts with rough edges. Depending on the depth and location of the cut, lacerations may cause heavier bleeding. A laceration through a major artery may cause life-threatening bleeding.

- **Punctures** occur when sharp objects penetrate the skin and possibly deeper tissues (**Figure 11-3**). The wound may penetrate through the body part, as with a gunshot wound, causing both entrance and exit wounds. Puncture wounds are more likely to trap foreign material in the body, increasing the risk for infection.

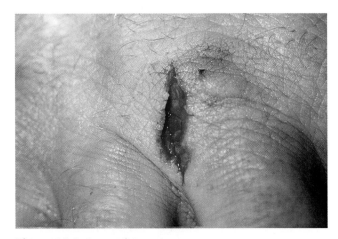

Figure 11-2 Laceration.

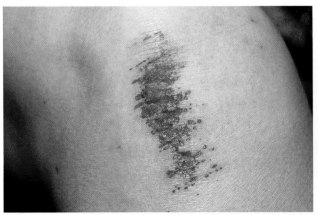

Figure 11-1 Abrasion.

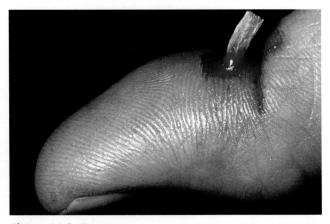

Figure 11-3 Puncture.

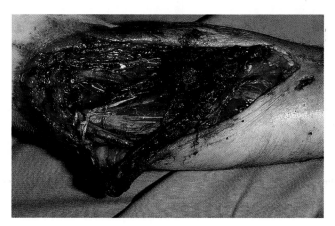

Figure 11-4 Avulsion.

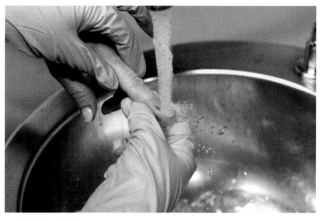

Figure 11-5 Irrigate a shallow wound with running water to help clean it.

- An **avulsion** is an area of skin or other soft tissue torn partially from the body, like a flap (**Figure 11-4**). Any area of skin, or a whole soft tissue structure like the ear, may be avulsed.
- An **amputation** is the complete cutting or tearing off of all or part of an extremity: a finger or toe, hand or foot, arm or leg. This wound is often called a traumatic amputation to distinguish it from an amputation performed surgically. Depending on the nature of the wound and the time that passes before the victim reaches the hospital, the amputated part may be reattached.
- **Burns** are damage caused to skin and other tissue by heat, chemicals, or electricity. Because of the significant differences among first aid approaches for burns, burn care is covered in detail in **Chapter 12**.

First aid care for open wounds varies depending on their location in the body. Wounds to certain body areas require special first aid measures as described later in this chapter.

CLEANING WOUNDS

When a wound is bleeding heavily, the first aid priority is to control the bleeding (see **Chapter 9**). Do not delay or interrupt efforts to stop bleeding in order to clean the wound. Healthcare professionals who treat the victim later will clean the wound. Even after you have stopped the bleeding with direct pressure or other means, do not remove the dressing from the wound in order to clean it. Removing the dressing may disturb clotted blood and start the wound bleeding again.

Unless the wound is very large, deep, or bleeding seriously, or the victim has other injuries needing

attention, the first step in minor wound care is to clean the wound to help prevent infection. Wash your hands first and wear gloves if available. You may need to expose the wound first by removing clothing, taking care to avoid contact with the wound. Then gently wash the wound with soap and water, letting clean tap water run over the wound for at least five minutes or until there appears to be no foreign matter in the wound (**Figure 11-5**). Do not merely soak the wound in water but actively run water over it. Washing out a wound like this under running water is called **irrigation.** If necessary, use sterile gauze or tweezers to remove any dirt or large particles you see in the wound. Then carefully dry the wound and apply a sterile dressing and bandage to protect and keep the dressing in place (see First Aid: "Wound Care").

WOUND INFECTION

Infection is an invasion of the body by a pathogen that may potentially cause disease. Because a wound lacks the protection offered by intact skin and allows pathogens into body tissues and/or the blood, infection may occur with any open wound. Some pathogens cause local tissue damage, while others spread throughout the body and may become life threatening. The bloodborne diseases described in **Chapter 2** may be transmitted from one person to another through an open wound, but many other pathogens are also present in the environment. Pathogens may be transmitted into a wound by the object that caused the wound, by any substance that comes into contact with the wound, or even by pathogens in the air. Because infection is an ever-present threat, wound care includes steps to prevent infection.

First Aid Wound Care

When You See

- A shallow, open wound

Do This First

1 Gently wash the wound with soap and water to remove dirt. Let clean tap water run in and over the wound for at least five minutes to flush it clean.

2 Use sterile gauze or tweezers to remove any dirt or large particles.

3 Pat the area dry. With abrasions and shallow wounds, apply an antibiotic ointment.

4 Cover the wound with a sterile dressing and bandage (or adhesive bandage with nonstick pad).

Additional Care

- If stitches may be needed, or if the victim does not have a current tetanus vaccination, seek medical attention.

- Change the dressing daily or if it becomes wet. (If a dressing sticks to the wound, soak it in water first.) Seek medical attention if the wound later looks infected.

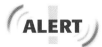

- Do not try to clean a major wound after controlling bleeding—it may start bleeding again. Healthcare personnel will clean the wound as needed.
- Do not put antibiotic ointment on a puncture wound or deep wound; use only on abrasions and shallow wounds.
- Do not use alcohol, hydrogen peroxide, or iodine on the wound. Such substances may not kill pathogens or may damage healthy body tissue along with pathogens.
- Avoid breathing or blowing on the wound, since this may transmit pathogens.
- Do not attempt to remove clothing stuck to a wound; cut around the clothing and leave it in place for healthcare providers to manage.
- Do not scrub a wound, because this can cause further tissue damage.

Box 11-1 Tetanus

Tetanus, also called lockjaw because a stiff neck and jaw is an early symptom, is an infection caused by common bacteria. Tetanus bacteria are found in soil, on skin surfaces, and elsewhere in the environment, including the home and other indoor locations. The bacteria enter the body through a wound, multiply, and produce a powerful toxin that acts on the nervous system, causing death in about 10% of cases.

The number of cases of tetanus in the United States has fallen dramatically since immunization became common in the late 1940s. Tetanus immunization is included in routine childhood vaccinations, but adults need a tetanus booster at least every 10 years. A tetanus booster may be recommended before 10 years in a victim with a significant wound. Tetanus infection is more common following puncture wounds or deep lacerations but can occur also with abrasions or any break in the skin, including burns, dental infections, and animal bites. It is important, therefore, for adults to maintain their immunization status with periodic boosters. In addition, medical attention should be sought for any deep or puncture wound. A tetanus shot must be given within 72 hours of receiving a wound to be effective.

Although infection is a risk with all open wounds, some types of wounds are at greater risk, including wounds resulting from bites (even human bites), puncture wounds, wounds contaminated with dirt or other substances, and wounds with jagged, uneven edges that are not easily cleaned.

As noted earlier, **antibiotic** ointment may be used on abrasions or shallow wounds, after the wound is cleaned, to help healing and prevent infection. Antibiotic ointment should not be used on other types of open wounds because the ointment may seal the wound and block the drainage that is part of the normal healing process. If you see signs of infection occurring in a wound, do not just apply an antibiotic ointment and hope it will kill the pathogen. See a healthcare provider, before the infection becomes worse (**Box 11-1**).

Any wound can become infected (**Figure 11-6**), in which case medical attention is needed. The signs and symptoms of an infection are:

- Wound area is red, swollen, and warm.
- Pain
- Pus
- Fever
- Red streaks or trails on the skin near the wound are a sign the infection is spreading—see a healthcare provider immediately.

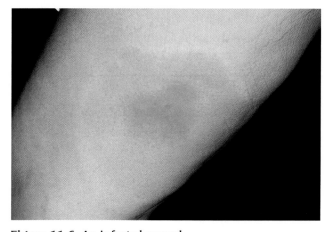

Figure 11-6 An infected wound.

DRESSING AND BANDAGING WOUNDS

Dressings

Dressings are put on wounds to help stop bleeding, prevent infection, and protect the wound while it is healing.

Types of Dressings

First aid kits should include sealed sterile dressings in many sizes (**Figure 11-7**). Common types of dressings include:

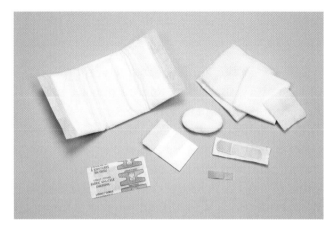

Figure 11-7 A variety of dressings.

- Gauze squares of various sizes
- Roller gauze
- Nonstick pad dressings
- Adhesive strips such as Band-Aids® and other dressings combined with a bandage
- Bulky dressings, also called **trauma dressings** (for large wounds or to stabilize an object impaled in a wound)
- **Occlusive dressings** (which create an airtight seal over certain types of wounds)

In some situations it may be necessary to improvise a dressing. If a sterile dressing is not available, use a clean cloth as a dressing; non-fluffy cloth works best because it is less likely to stick to the wound. Look for a clean towel, handkerchief, or other material. Avoid using cotton balls or cotton cloth if possible because cotton fibers tend to stick to wounds. To improvise bulky dressings, use sanitary pads if available, which although not sterile are generally individually wrapped and very clean. Bulky dressings can also be made of towels, baby diapers, or many layers of gauze. A ring dressing can be used around an area on which direct pressure should not be used (**Box 11-2**).

Guidelines for Using Dressings

After washing and drying the wound, apply the dressing this way:

1. Wash hands and wear gloves.
2. Choose a dressing larger than the wound. Do not touch the part of the dressing that will contact the wound.

3. Carefully lay the dressing on the wound (do not slide it on from the side). Cover the whole wound (**Figure 11-8**).
4. If blood seeps through, do not remove the dressing but add more dressings on top of it.
5. Apply a bandage to hold the dressing in place.

When a dressing is later removed—to clean the wound or change a soiled dressing, for example—do not tug on a dressing that sticks to the wound. Soak it in warm water to release the dressing.

Bandages

Bandages are used for covering a dressing, keeping the dressing on a wound, and maintaining pressure to control bleeding. Because only dressings touch the wound itself, bandages need to be clean but not necessarily sterile. As described in **Chapter 15**, bandages are also used to support or immobilize an injury to bones, joints, or muscles and to reduce swelling.

Types of Bandages

Different types of bandages are available for different uses (**Figure 11-9**). Following are common types of bandages:

- Adhesive compresses or strips for small wounds that combine a dressing with an adhesive bandage
- Adhesive tape rolls (cloth, plastic, paper)
- Tubular bandages for fingers or toes
- Elastic bandages
- Self-adhering roller bandages

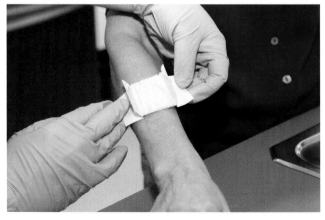

Figure 11-8 Cover the wound with a sterile dressing and apply a bandage.

Box 11-2 Ring Dressing

Direct pressure should not be used over the entire surface of certain types of wounds. For example, pressure should not be put on a skull fracture (see **Chapter 13**), a fractured bone protruding from a wound (see **Chapter 15**), or an object impaled in a wound. In these cases bleeding is controlled by a dressing around the object or fracture. A dressing made into a ring shape is appropriate for controlling bleeding and dressing such wounds.

Make a ring dressing from a long strip of gauze or other material. First make a circular wrap the right size to surround the area. With the remainder of the strip or an additional strip, wrap around the circular wrap to give the ring more bulk. Then position the ring around the wound and apply pressure as needed.

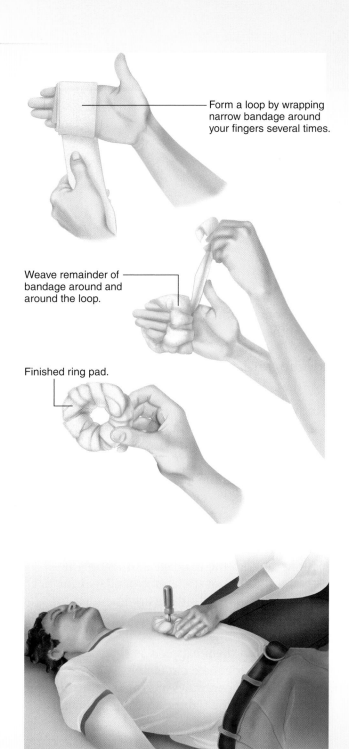

Form a loop by wrapping narrow bandage around your fingers several times.

Weave remainder of bandage around and around the loop.

Finished ring pad.

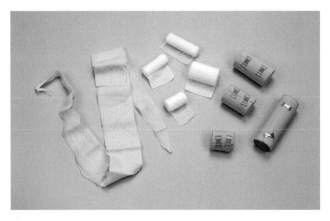

Figure 11-9 Types of bandages.

- Gauze roller bandages
- Triangular bandages (or folded square cloths)
- Any cloth or other material improvised to meet the purposes of bandaging

Guidelines for Bandaging

Follow these guidelines for bandaging:

1. To put pressure on a wound to stop bleeding or to prevent the swelling of an injury, apply the bandage firmly, but not so tightly that it cuts off circulation. Never put a circular bandage around the neck. With a bandage around a limb, check the fingers or toes for color, warmth, and sensation (normal touch, not tingling) to make sure circulation is not cut off. If there are signs of reduced circulation, unwrap the bandage and reapply it less tightly. Do not use elastic bandages for dressings on wounds; these are intended for muscle and joint injuries.

2. Do not cover fingers or toes unless they are injured. Keep them exposed so they can be checked for adequate circulation.

3. Since swelling continues after many injuries, keep checking the tightness of the bandage. Swelling may make a loose bandage tight enough to cut off circulation.

4. With a bandaged wound, be sure the bandage is secure enough that the dressing will not move and expose the wound to possible contamination.

5. With elastic and roller bandages, anchor the first end and tie, tape, pin, or clip the ending section in place. Loose ends could get caught on something and pull the bandage loose

or disrupt the wound (see Skill: "Applying a Roller Bandage").

6. Use a nonelastic roller bandage to make a pressure bandage around a limb to control bleeding and protect the wound (see **Chapter 9**).

7. An elastic roller bandage is used to support a joint and prevent swelling. At the wrist or ankle a figure-eight wrap is used.

8. Wrap a bandage from the bottom of the limb upward to avoid cutting off circulation.

9. Avoid bending a joint once it has been bandaged because movement may loosen the dressing or cut off circulation.

WHEN TO SEEK MEDICAL ATTENTION FOR A WOUND

Remember: call 9-1-1 for severe bleeding. In addition, the victim should see a healthcare provider as soon as possible in the following cases:

- Bleeding that is not easily controlled
- Any deep or large wound (e.g., wounds into muscle or bone)
- Significant wounds on the face
- Signs and symptoms that the wound is infected
- Any bite from an animal or human
- Foreign object or material embedded in the wound
- Puncture wounds
- The victim is unsure about tetanus vaccination
- Any wound you are unsure about
- Wounds that may require stitches (**Figure 11-10**):
  - Cuts on the face or hands when the edges do not close together
  - Gaping wounds
  - Cuts longer than one inch

SPECIAL WOUNDS

In addition to the general guidelines for all wounds, certain types of wounds require special first aid considerations. These include puncture wounds, impaled objects, amputations, and injuries to the genitals, head, or face.

Injury Prevention

Wounds may occur anywhere in the body as a result of any kind of trauma. Prevention focuses on injury prevention in general, as described throughout this text. Following are

Skill **Applying a Roller Bandage**

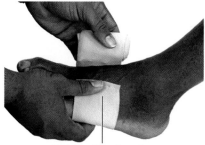

Hold end in place for
first turn of bandage

1 Anchor the starting end of
the bandage.

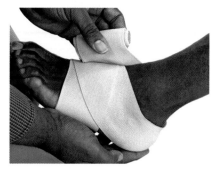

2 Turn bandage diagonally
across top of foot and
around ankle.

Overlap turns by about
³/₄ of previous turn

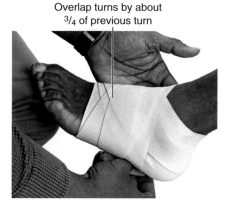

3 Continue with overlapping
figure-eight turns.

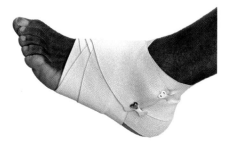

4 Fasten end of bandage with
clips, tape, or safety pins.

guidelines for preventing certain special kinds
of wounds:

- Many traumatic amputations result from
  industrial emergencies and the use of power
  tools in the home. Always follow OSHA
  guidelines in the work setting to prevent
  injury, and when using power tools at home,
  follow the specific guidelines provided by the
  tool's manufacturer. Never disassemble safe-
  guards built into tools or equipment.

- Wearing the appropriate helmet at work or in
  relevant sports and recreational activities can
  prevent skull injuries and injuries to the face
  and ears.

- Eye injuries frequently result from small
  objects or particles being unexpectedly pro-
  pelled into the eye. Eye shields should be
  worn whenever one is working with power
  equipment.

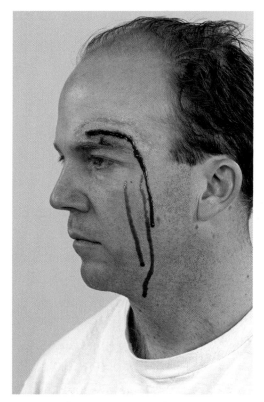

Figure 11-10 A large, open wound may require stitches.

Learning
Checkpoint ①

1. Check off the actions that are included in wound care:

____ Irrigate minor wounds with running water.

____ Pour rubbing alcohol on any wound.

____ Wash major wounds to help stop the bleeding.

____ Use tweezers to remove large dirt particles from a minor wound.

____ Cover any wound with a sterile dressing and bandage.

____ Let a scab form before washing a minor wound.

____ See a healthcare provider for a deep or puncture wound.

____ Blow on a minor wound to cool the area and relieve pain.

2. If you are changing a wound dressing a day after the injury and the dressing sticks to the wound, what should you do?

_____

3. True or False: Puncture wounds have little risk for infection.

4. True or False: You don't need to bother putting on gloves to dress a minor wound if you know the victim well.

5. For what type(s) of wound(s) is an antibiotic ointment appropriate?

_____

6. Check off which signs and symptoms may indicate a wound is infected:

____ Headache   ____ Cool, clammy skin

____ Warmth in the area   ____ A scab forms that looks dark brown

____ Red, swollen area   ____ Nausea and vomiting

____ Fever   ____ Pus drains from the wound

7. Which of these victims need to seek medical attention? (Check all that apply.)

____ Jose has a deep laceration from a piece of equipment, but you managed to stop the bleeding in 15 minutes.

____ Rebecca had lunch in a nearby park and was bitten by a squirrel she was feeding, but the bleeding stopped almost immediately.

____ Carl scraped his knee when he fell off his bicycle on the way to work, but the abrasion washed out clean and you have applied an antibiotic ointment.

____ Kim got a bad gash on her cheek when a bottle broke in the supply room, but she had already stopped the bleeding by the time you saw her.

8. True or False: To control bleeding, make a pressure bandage as tight as you can get it.

Learning
Checkpoint ① *(continued)*

9. You have put a roller bandage around a victim's arm to control bleeding from a laceration. A few minutes later she says her fingers are tingling. You feel her hand, and her fingers are cold. What should you do?

_____

10. When applying a bandage over a dressing, the bandage should

    a. hold down only the corners of the dressing so the wound can breathe.

    b. be soaked first in cold water.

    c. cover the entire dressing.

    d. be loose enough so it can be slid to one side to change the dressing.

- The American Dental Association recommends wearing a mouthguard during any activity that can result in a blow to the face or mouth. Ask your dentist about having a custom mouthguard made to provide a safe, comfortable fit.
- To avoid breaking a tooth, do not chew ice, hard candy, or popcorn kernels.
- To prevent injuries to the genitals, males engaging in contact sports should wear an athletic cup and females a pelvic shield or groin pad or protector.
- To prevent stretching and potentially tearing ligaments and other supportive breast tissues, women should wear a sports bra during exercise or sport activities.

Puncture Wounds

Puncture wounds may involve deeper injuries you cannot see. If the puncturing object may have penetrated the body, check also for an exit wound. In general, puncture wounds carry a greater risk of infection than other types of wounds because often they bleed less and therefore germs may not be flushed out. In addition to routine wound care, follow these steps:

1. Remove any small objects or dirt but not larger impaled objects.
2. Gently press on wound edges to promote bleeding.
3. Do not put any medication inside or over the puncture wound.
4. Wash the wound well in running water directed at the puncture site.
5. Dress the wound and seek medical attention.

Impaled Objects

Removing an object from a wound could cause more injury and bleeding, because often the object is sealing the wound or damaged blood vessels. Leave it in place and dress the wound around it **(Figure 11-11)**. Use bulky dressings (trauma dressings) to stabilize the object and keep it from moving. If there is blood or sweat on the skin, adhesive tape may not stick well enough to hold bulky dressings in place; use a roller bandage or strips of cloth to tie the bandage in place

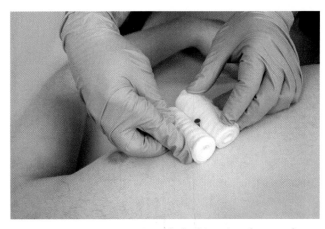

Figure 11-11 Leave an impaled object in place and use bulky dressings to keep it from moving.

around the impaled object. Follow these guidelines:

1. Control bleeding by applying direct pressure at the sides of the object.
2. Dress the wound around the object.
3. Pad the object in place with large dressings or folded cloths.
4. Support the object while bandaging it in place.
5. Keep the victim still and seek medical attention.

An impaled object in the eye or the cheek is a unique circumstance requiring special care, as described in the later sections on eye and cheek injuries.

Avulsions and Amputations

An avulsion is a piece of skin or other soft tissue torn partially from the body, like a flap. Try to move the skin or tissue back into its normal position unless the wound is contaminated, and then control bleeding and provide wound care. If the avulsed tissue is completely separated from the body, care for it the same as you would for an amputated part.

In an amputation, a part has been severed from the body. Control the bleeding and care for the victim's wound first, then recover and care for the amputated part. Bleeding can usually be controlled with the same measures as for other wounds, using bulky dressings. Follow these steps to care for the severed body part, which surgeons may be able to reattach to the victim:

1. Wrap the severed part in a dry, sterile dressing or clean cloth. Do not wash it.
2. Place the part in a plastic bag and seal it.
3. Place the sealed bag in another bag or container with ice. Do not let the part touch water or ice directly, and do not bury it in ice **(Figure 11-12)**.
4. Make sure the severed part is given to the responding EMS crew or taken with the victim to the emergency room.

Genital Injuries

Injuries to the genitals are rare because of their protected location. Injuries may occur from blunt trauma, an impact that creates a wound, or sexual abuse. Provide privacy for a victim when giving first aid for a wound in the genital area. Follow these guidelines:

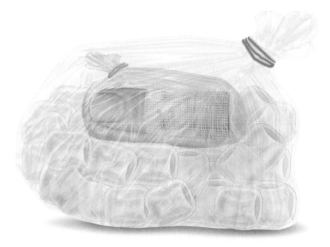

Figure 11-12 Keep amputated part cold but not directly touching ice.

- Use direct pressure with a sterile dressing or sanitary pad to control external bleeding. Then use a large triangular bandage applied like a diaper to secure the dressings in place **(Figure 11-13)**.
- For injured testicles, provide support with a towel between the legs like a diaper. For a closed injury caused by blunt trauma, a cold pack may help reduce pain.
- For vaginal bleeding, have the woman press a sanitary pad or clean folded towel to the area to control the bleeding.
- Call 9-1-1 for severe or continuing bleeding, significant pain or swelling, or the possibility of sexual abuse.
- In the case of rape or sexual abuse, preserve evidence for law enforcement personnel by following the guidelines in **Chapter 22**.

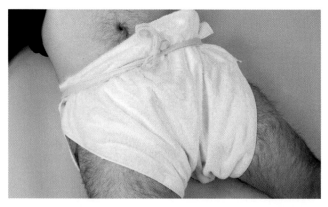

Figure 11-13 Apply a triangular bandage like a diaper to secure dressings in the genital area.

Head and Face Wounds

Wounds to the head or face may require special first aid. The following sections provide guidelines for these special injuries. Skull injuries, such as fractures, are described in **Chapter 13**.

With any significant injury to the head, the victim may also have a neck or spinal injury. If you suspect a spinal injury, be careful not to move the victim's head while giving first aid for head and face wounds.

Scalp Wound Without Suspected Skull Fracture

If signs and symptoms of a skull fracture are not present, and the wound is restricted to the scalp, apply a dressing and use direct pressure as usual to control bleeding. Then apply a roller bandage around the head to secure the dressing. *Never wrap a bandage around the neck because of the risk of impeding breathing if the injury causes swelling* (see First Aid: "Scalp Wound Without Suspected Skull Fracture").

First Aid   **Scalp Wound Without Suspected Skull Fracture**

When You See
- Bleeding from the head
- No sign of skull fracture

Do This First

1 Replace any skin flaps and cover the wound with a sterile dressing.

2 Use direct pressure to control bleeding.

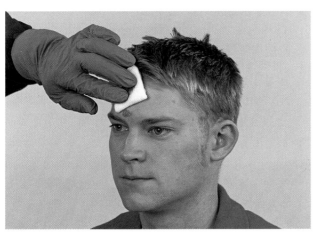

(a) Place dressing against wound.

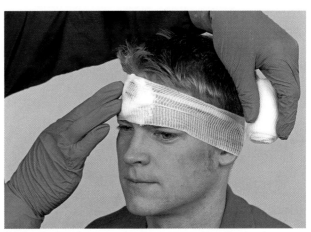

(b) A roller bandage secures the pressure dressing in place.

3 Put a roller or triangle bandage around the victim's head to secure the dressing.

Additional Care
- Position the victim with head and shoulders raised to help control bleeding.
- Seek medical attention if the victim later experiences nausea and vomiting, persistent headache, drowsiness or disorientation, stumbling or lack of coordination, or problems with speech or vision.

Eye Injuries

Eye injuries are serious because vision may be affected. Eye injuries include blows to the eye, impaled objects in the eye, dirt or small particles in the eye, and chemicals or other substances splashed into the eye. When caring for any eye injury, avoid putting pressure directly on the eyeball because this tissue is easily injured.

With most eye injuries, movement of the eye will continue to worsen the injury. Bandaging or otherwise covering an injured eye discourages the victim from moving it. Because the eyes move together, the unaffected eye must also be covered; otherwise the victim, in using the unaffected eye, will also be moving the injured eye. Having both eyes covered or bandaged is often frightening, especially to an injured victim. Explain what you are doing and why before covering the good eye. To minimize the anxiety, keep talking to the victim or have another person offer reassurance with conversation and touch.

For a blow to the eye:

1. If the eye is bleeding or leaking fluid, call 9-1-1 or get the victim to the emergency department immediately.
2. Put a cold pack over the eye for up to 15 minutes to ease pain and reduce swelling, but do not put pressure on the eye. If the victim is wearing a contact lens, do not try to remove it (**Figure 11-14**). Also cover the uninjured eye.
3. Have victim lie still.
4. Seek medical attention if pain persists or vision is affected in any way.

For a large object embedded in the eye:

1. Do not remove the object. Stabilize it in place with dressings or bulky cloth. Be careful not to put any pressure on the eye from the object. With a large impaled object or one that may move, use a paper cup or something similar to stabilize the object and keep it from moving in the eye (**Figure 11-15**).
2. Cover both eyes because movement of the uninjured one causes movement of the injured one.
3. Call 9-1-1 or get the victim to the emergency department immediately.

For dirt or a small particle in the eye:

If the victim complains of something small caught in the eye, do not let the victim rub the eye with his or her hands, which could cause scratching of the eye or other soft tissue. The body's natural way to remove small particles from the eye is to wash it out with tears and blinking. Wait a minute to see if the victim's tears flush out the object. If not, try these methods:

1. Gently pull the upper eyelid out and down over the lower eyelid. This allows the lower lashes to catch a particle caught under the upper eyelid.
2. If the particle remains, gently flush the eye with water from a medicine dropper or water glass. Have the victim tilt the head so that the affected eye is lower than the other; this prevents water from flowing into the unaffected eye. Flush from the corner

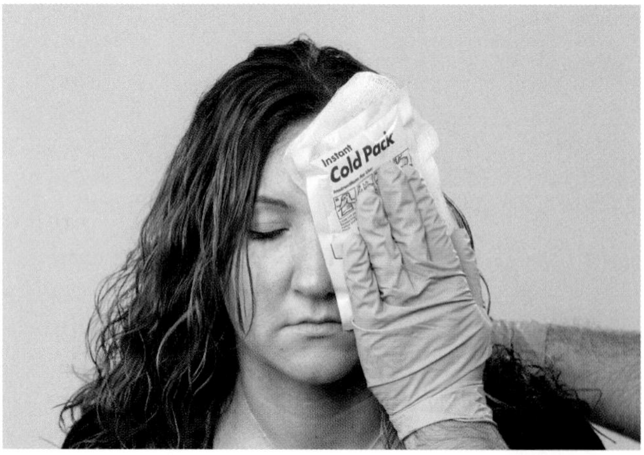

Figure 11-14 For a blow to the eye, hold a cold pack on the eye.

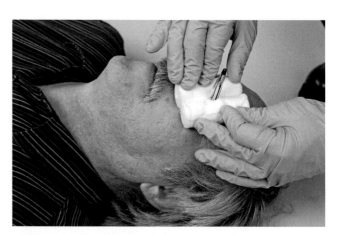

Figure 11-15 Stabilize an object impaled in the eyeball.

nearer the nose. Ask the victim to hold the eyelids open with his or her fingers if needed, and to look in all directions and blink during the flushing.

3. If the particle remains and is visible, carefully try to brush it out gently with a wet, sterile dressing. Lift the upper eyelid and swab its underside if you see the particle (**Figure 11-16**).

4. If the particle remains or the victim has any vision problems or pain, cover the eye with a sterile dressing and seek medical attention. Also cover the uninjured eye to prevent movement of the injured one.

For a chemical or substance splashed in the eye:

1. Rinse the eye with running water for at least 20 minutes.

2. Have the victim hold his or her head with the affected eye lower than the other so that water does not flow into the unaffected eye (see **Chapter 12**).

Ear Injuries

With bleeding from the external ear, control the bleeding with direct pressure and dress the wound.

Remember that bleeding or clear fluid (cerebrospinal fluid) from within the ear can be a sign of a serious head injury. Do not use direct pressure to try to stop fluid from coming out the ear. Give care as described in **Chapter 13**.

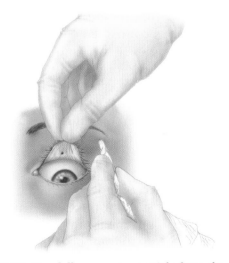

Figure 11-16 Carefully remove a particle from the eyelid.

If the victim complains of a foreign object in the ear, do not try to remove it with any tool or object. Never insert tweezers, a pin, or cotton swab into the ear in an attempt to remove an object. The object may be pushed further into the ear, or the tool may damage the eardrum or other tissues. Leave the object in place and seek medical attention. Only if the foreign object is clearly visible and easily grasped with your fingers is it safe to remove an object, but do not remove an impaled object. Occasionally an insect may crawl into the ear when a person is sleeping. If you see or know that an insect is in the ear, gently pour lukewarm water into the ear to try to float it out. If it does not come out, seek medical attention.

For bleeding from within the ear, follow the guidelines in First Aid: "Ear Injuries."

Nose Injuries

Injury to the nose can cause heavy bleeding. Nosebleeds can also be caused by pressure changes or a child aggressively picking at the nose. Nosebleeds can usually be controlled by positioning the victim leaning slightly forward and pinching the nostrils closed until bleeding stops, usually within a few minutes. With an unresponsive victim or a victim who cannot sit leaning forward, position the victim on one side with the head turned to allow drainage from the nose and mouth while you pinch the nostrils closed. Do not try to pack the nostrils with a dressing in an effort to control the bleeding.

Bleeding that runs from the back of the nose down the throat is more serious and needs immediate medical attention. Do not tilt the victim's head backward but keep the victim positioned to allow blood to drain out the mouth so that the airway is not threatened (see First Aid: "Nosebleed").

Small children often put small objects in their noses. If a foreign object is clearly visible and easily grasped with tweezers, you may safely remove it, but do not remove an impaled object. Do not push tweezers or your finger into the nostril to try to remove an object because of the risk of pushing it in deeper. Do not have a child try to blow an object out, because it may be sucked in deeper instead.

First Aid **Ear Injuries**

When You See
- Bleeding inside the ear
- Signs of pain
- Possible deafness

Do This First

1 If the blood looks watery, this could mean a skull fracture. Call 9-1-1.

2 Help victim to sit up, tilting the affected ear lower to let blood or other fluid drain.

3 Cover the ear with a loose, sterile dressing, but do not apply pressure.

4 Seek medical attention immediately.

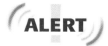

ALERT

- Do not plug the ear closed to try to stop bleeding.

Additional Care
- Keep the ear covered to reduce the risk of infection.

Cheek Injuries

A wound on the outside of the cheek is cared for by following the general guidelines for wounds. If an object is impaled in a wound in the cheek, check inside the mouth to see if the object has penetrated through. If you can see both sides of the object and can remove it safely, do so. *This is the one exception to the rule about not removing an impaled object from a wound.* The object may pose a risk to the airway if it protrudes into the mouth or later falls into the mouth. Gently pull the object out, in the direction from which it penetrated the cheek, taking care with a sharp object not to cut the cheek further. Then place a dressing inside the mouth between the cheek wound and the teeth; watch that this dressing does not come out of position and block the airway. Apply another dressing to the outside of the wound, applying pressure as needed to control bleeding. Position an unresponsive victim with the head turned to the side so that blood and other fluid will run out of the mouth.

Teeth and Mouth Injuries

Injuries to the mouth may cause bleeding anywhere in the mouth and may knock out a tooth. Bleeding is controlled with direct pressure on a dressing over the wound. A tooth that has been knocked out can usually be replanted if the tooth is properly cared for. The priority of first aid for the mouth is always to ensure that the airway is open and that blood can drain from the mouth until bleeding is controlled.

A tooth that has been knocked out requires care if it is to be successfully replanted because delicate tissues attached to the tooth may quickly die. Do not try to put the tooth back in the socket. The tooth should not be allowed to dry out. Immerse the tooth in milk, or use a commercial tooth saver kit.

First Aid   Nosebleed

When You See
- Blood coming from either or both nostrils
- Blood possibly running from back of nose down into the mouth or throat

Do This First

1   Have victim sit and tilt head slightly forward with mouth open. Carefully remove any object you see protruding from the nose.

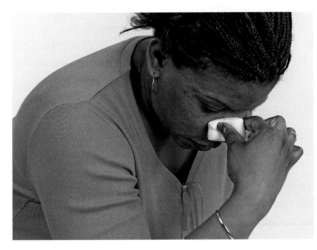

2   Have victim pinch the nostrils together just below the bridge of the nose for 10 minutes. Ask victim to breathe through the mouth and not speak, swallow, cough, or sniff.

3   If victim is gasping or choking on blood in the throat, call 9-1-1.

4   After 10 minutes, release the pressure slowly. Pinch the nostrils again for another 10 minutes if bleeding continues.

ALERT

- Do not tilt the victim's head backward.
- Do not have the victim lie down.
- Do not probe inside the nose to remove an object.

Additional Care
- Place a cold compress on the bridge of the nose.
- Seek medical attention if:
    - Bleeding continues after two attempts to control bleeding.
    - you suspect the nose is broken.
    - there is a foreign object in the nose.
    - the victim has high blood pressure.
- Have the person rest for a few hours and avoid rubbing or blowing the nose.

If a tooth is knocked loose enough that there is a risk it may fall out, make a pad from rolled gauze and have the victim bite down on it to keep the tooth in place until the victim reaches the dentist. If a tooth is broken, rinse the victim's mouth with warm water, and then apply a cold pack to reduce swelling and pain; see a dentist as soon as possible.

For a tooth knocked out:

1. Have the victim sit with head tilted forward to let blood drain out.
2. To control bleeding, fold or roll gauze into a pad and place it over the tooth socket. Have the victim bite down to put pressure on the area for 20 to 30 minutes (**Figure 11-17**).
3. Save the tooth, which may be replanted if the victim sees a dentist very soon. Touching only the tooth's crown, rinse it in water if it is dirty (but do not scrub it or remove attached tissue fragments) and put it in a container of milk or a commercial tooth saver solution.

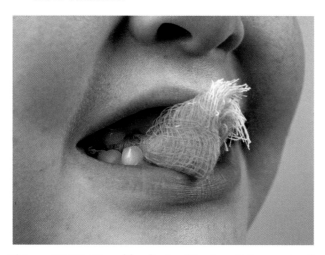

Figure 11-17 Stop bleeding with dressing over tooth socket.

4. Get the victim and the tooth to a dentist as soon as possible. (Most dentists have 24-hour emergency call numbers.)

For other bleeding in the mouth:

1. Have the victim sit with head tilted forward to let blood drain out.
2. **For a wound penetrating the lip:** Put a rolled dressing between the lip and the gum. Hold a second dressing against the outside lip.
3. **For a bleeding tongue:** Put a dressing on the wound and apply pressure.
4. Do not repeatedly rinse the mouth (this may prevent clotting).
5. Do not let victim swallow blood, which may cause vomiting.
6. When the bleeding stops, tell the victim not to drink anything warm for several hours.
7. Seek medical attention if bleeding is severe or does not stop.

Blisters

Blisters usually occur because of friction on the skin, as when a shoe rubs the back of the ankle or heel. They can be painful and may become infected after breaking. Burns may cause a different kind of blister (see **Chapter 12**).

Blisters can usually be prevented by protecting the feet with socks or with tape where socks rub. A small blister can be protected with an adhesive bandage. Try to prevent it from breaking open, which can lead to infection. For a larger blister, cut a hole in several layers of gauze or moleskin and position this dressing over the blister with the blister itself protected within the hole (see First Aid: "Blisters").

If a blister breaks, wash the area and care for it as you would care for a wound (see **Chapter 10**).

First Aid **Blisters**

When You See

- **A raised, fluid-filled blister, often surrounded by red skin**

Do This First

1 Wash the blister and surrounding area with soap and water. Rinse and gently pat dry.

2 Cover the blister with an adhesive bandage big enough that the gauze pad covers the whole blister. Bandages with an adhesive strip on all four sides are best because they keep the area cleaner if the blister breaks. For a larger blister, use a donut-shaped dressing to surround the blister and prevent pressure on it.

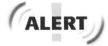 **ALERT**

- **Never deliberately break a blister. This could lead to infection.**

Additional Care

- **Prevent continued friction in the area**

Learning Checkpoint ②

1. Name one circumstance in which you might want to promote bleeding.

2. True or False: The first thing to do when you see an impaled object in a wound is to pull it out so that you can put direct pressure on the wound to stop the bleeding.

3. True or False: An amputated part should be kept cold but not put in direct contact with ice.

4. With an eye injury, why would you cover the *uninjured* eye, too?

5. Describe three ways you can try to remove a small particle from the eye.

6. True or False: For bleeding from within the ear, roll a piece of gauze into a plug and try to seal the ear with it.

Learning
Checkpoint ② *(continued)*

7. A nosebleed victim should first try to stop the bleeding by pinching the nostrils closed for _____ minutes. During this time, list two or three things the victim should *not do.*

_____

8. True or False: A knocked-out tooth can be reimplanted if it is kept in milk and the victim reaches a dentist soon.

9. True or False: Repeatedly rinsing the mouth with cool water is the best way to stop bleeding in the mouth.

Concluding Thoughts

Wounds are among the most common injuries requiring first aid. In most cases the care is simple and straightforward: clean the wound, apply a dressing, and cover and secure the dressing with an appropriate bandage. Particular kinds of wounds, and injuries in certain areas of the body, require additional specific care. Following these guidelines will, in most cases, prevent infection of the wound and lead to effective healing.

Learning Outcomes

You should now be able to do the following:

1. Describe how to clean a wound.
2. Describe the signs and symptoms of an infected wound and what to do about it.
3. List standard guidelines for using dressings and bandages.
4. Explain how to determine when a wound needs medical attention.
5. Describe first aid for punctures, wounds with impaled objects, avulsions and amputations, and for injuries of the genitals, scalp, and specific facial areas.
6. Demonstrate how to apply a roller bandage.

Review Questions

1. What is the first priority for a severely bleeding wound?
   a. Seeking medical attention
   b. Controlling the bleeding
   c. Preventing infection
   d. Irrigating the wound

2. Infection is more likely in which kind of wound?
   a. Puncture
   b. Laceration
   c. Abrasion
   d. Avulsion

3. What is the best way to clean a wound?
   a. Soak in alcohol
   b. Apply iodine
   c. Irrigate with water
   d. Apply a cool, moist compress

4. Antibiotic ointment is best used on what kinds of wounds?
   a. Abrasions
   b. Punctures
   c. Deep burns
   d. Open abdominal wounds

5. A pressure bandage to control bleeding
  a. should be applied directly over the wound.
  b. should be as tight as you can get it to stop the bleeding.
  c. should use an elastic roller bandage.
  d. All of the above

6. Signs of good circulation in a limb below a pressure bandage include
  a. cool skin.
  b. normal skin color.
  c. tingling sensations.
  d. ability to move fingers or toes

7. What wounds should be seen by a health-care provider?
  a. Wounds through the skin into muscle tissue
  b. Human bite wounds
  c. Wounds that may require stitches
  d. All of the above

8. How would you best care for a traumatically amputated finger?
  a. Wash it under running water and put it in a glass or jar of ice water.
  b. Wrap it in a dressing, place it inside a plastic bag, and put the bag on ice.
  c. Keep it dry and at body temperature (held against victim's body).
  d. Put it in a plastic bag and place the bag in the freezer until help arrives.

9. For a painful blow to the eye,
  a. flush constantly with warm, running water for up to 30 minutes.
  b. have victim sit in a dark room with both eyes covered for 30 minutes.
  c. put a cold pack over the eye for up to 15 minutes.
  d. give the victim aspirin or ibuprofen.

10. Care for a nosebleed includes
  a. having the victim "blow" the nose into a handkerchief to clear out blood.
  b. pinching the nostrils closed up to 10 minutes.
  c. packing the nose with sterile gauze.
  d. having the victim tilt head back while sucking on ice chips.

References and Resources

American Academy of Ophthalmology. First aid for the eye. 2004. www.aao.org

American College of Emergency Physicians. *First aid manual: a comprehensive guide to treating emergency victims of all ages in any situation.* New York: DK Publishing; 2001.

American Dental Association. Dental emergencies and injuries. 2005. www.ada.org/public

American Dental Association. Mouthguards. 2005. www.ada.org/public

American Heart Association. 2005 American Heart Association Guidelines for Cardiopulmonary resuscitation and emergency cardiovascular care (ECC) science with treatment recommendations. *Circulation.* 112(22). November 29, 2005.

American Medical Association. *Handbook of first aid and emergency care.* Revised edition. New York: Random House; 2000.

Centers for Disease Control and Prevention. Tetanus. 2005. www.cdc.gov

National Safety Council. www.nsc.org

Chapter 12

Burns

Chapter Preview

- What Happens with a Burn?
- Prevention of Fires and Burns
- Heat Burns
- First Aid for Heat Burns

- Smoke Inhalation
- Chemical Burns
- Electrical Burns and Shocks

While visiting your aunt at her home, you join her in the kitchen as she cooks pasta for dinner. On the stove front burner is a large pot of boiling water. She is telling you about something that happened earlier that day and is not paying close attention to her cooking. Before you can react to stop her, you see her reach across the boiling water for the kettle on the back burner. She yelps as the steam burns her forearm and jerks her arm back. What should you do immediately? What additional care should you give for this burn?

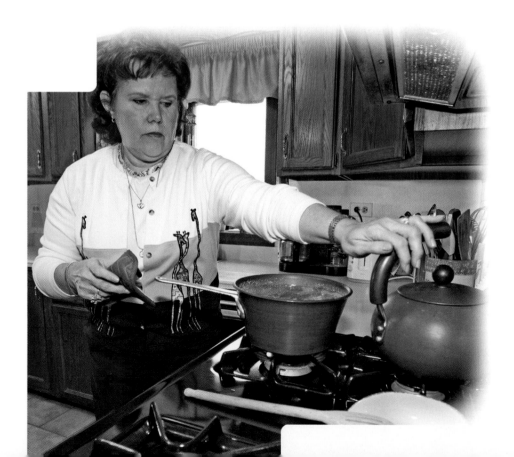

Fires and burns are a major cause of death and injury. In 2004 there were 3900 deaths in the United States caused by fires and burns and about 500,000 burn injuries leading to emergency department visits. Fires and burns may occur in almost any setting, but the great majority occur in the home, and experts believe that 75% to 80% of fires and burns can be prevented. Even with preventive steps, however, it is essential to know what to do when fire occurs and how to treat victims of burns.

Burns of the skin or deeper tissues may be caused by the sun, heat, chemicals, or electricity. Mild heat burns and sunburn may need only simple first aid, but severe burns can be a medical emergency.

What Happens with a Burn?

A burn is an injury to the skin and potentially deeper structures caused by heat, electricity, or chemicals. Burns can cause severe effects in the body because the skin has several important functions:

- *Protection.* The skin protects the body against the entry of **pathogens** that can cause infection as well as other harmful substances. Specialized cells also have an immune function.
- *Fluid retention.* The skin prevents the loss of fluids and other important substances such as electrolytes.

- *Temperature regulation.* The skin has a major role in controlling the body's temperature, preventing heat loss in cold environments and promoting heat loss in hot environments.
- *Sensation.* The skin contains sensory and other nerves and blood vessels.

Although a minor burn like a sunburn may damage only the **epidermis,** the outer layer of skin, more severe burns damage the **dermis,** or middle layer, which contains nerves and blood vessels, or the deepest layer of **subcutaneous** tissue, through which larger blood vessels and nerves pass **(Figure 12-1).**

Burns that extend into the dermis expose tissues to the outside environment and carry a high risk of infection from pathogens present almost everywhere. The more extensive and deeper a burn, the more likely infection becomes because pathogens may enter more easily and medical treatment becomes more difficult.

Burns extending into the dermis or deeper also cause fluid loss. Injured capillaries in the dermis leak fluid; this is the cause of watery blisters in second-degree burns. Deeper burns cause fluid loss from larger blood vessels. Significant fluid loss from severe burns can cause shock, a further threat to the burn victim that can be life threatening (see **Chapter 10**).

To function well, the human body must maintain a fairly consistent internal temperature.

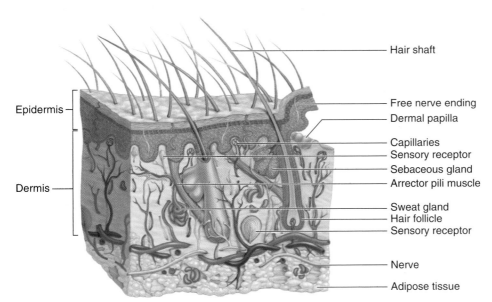

Epidermis

Dermis

Hair shaft

Free nerve ending
Dermal papilla

Capillaries
Sensory receptor
Sebaceous gland
Arrector pili muscle

Sweat gland
Hair follicle
Sensory receptor

Nerve

Adipose tissue

Figure 12-1 Layers of the skin.

Because the skin helps regulate this function, a severe burn can cause a loss of body heat, further stressing vital organs. Therefore a victim with extensive severe burns should not be cooled with water over much of the body, because of the increased risk of **hypothermia,** which would further threaten the victim's condition.

Because the skin is rich in sensory nerves, burns can be very painful due to damage to these nerves. With burns entirely through the skin, however, the victim may not feel pain because the nerve endings are completely destroyed. In such cases there are often less severely burned areas around the pain-free areas that do cause significant pain. Pain is therefore present in most burns but is not an indication of the burn's severity.

Finally, burns may damage body tissues other than just the skin. A full-thickness burn that penetrates all the way through the skin may damage muscle and fat tissue beneath as well as underlying organs, resulting in additional trauma to the body and increasing the urgency for medical treatment. Victims with burns caused by fires may also have respiratory damage caused by inhaling smoke, fumes, or hot air. Respiratory tract tissues may swell, causing breathing difficulty.

PREVENTION OF FIRES AND BURNS
Common Causes of Burns

Of the 3900 deaths by fire and burns in a recent year, 3190 occurred in the home. Following are some sobering facts and statistics about fires in the home: *

- The United States has one of the highest fire death rates among industrialized countries. Fire kills more people than all natural disasters combined.
- Every year, more than 10,000 infants are burned seriously enough to require hospitalization.
- In 2004 about 395,500 residential fires involved responses by fire departments.
- About 15,000 structure fires occur every year from children playing with fire, causing about 220 deaths, 1370 injuries, and $438 million in

*Sources: The Burn Institute, The National Fire Protection Association, The American Burn Association, and The National Safety Council.

property damage. About 85% of these victims were the children themselves.
- Children and the elderly have higher rates of fire and burn injuries and deaths. About 1000 Americans over age 65 die from fire every year.
- 70% of deaths caused by residential fires occurred in the 25% of homes without functioning smoke alarms.

Following are the most common causes of fires leading to injury or death:

- Smoking
- Heating
- Cooking
- Playing with fire
- Electrical wiring
- Open flames
- Appliances or other equipment

Preventing Burns

Preventing burns involves both preventing fires and preventing burns from hot water and other sources of heat such as stoves.

Preventing Fires

Follow these guidelines to prevent a fire in the home and other settings (**Figure 12-2**):

- Make your home and workplace safe:
  ○ Make sure enough smoke detectors are installed and have good batteries (change batteries twice a year when you change your clocks for daylight savings time).
  ○ Do not allow smoking, or ensure that it is done safely and materials are safely extinguished. Never allow smoking in bed.
  ○ Keep curtains and other flammable objects away from fireplaces and stoves; use fireplace screens.
  ○ Have chimneys regularly inspected and cleaned to prevent chimney fires.
  ○ Never store gasoline or other highly flammable liquids indoors.
- Prevent fires in the kitchen:
  ○ Keep a fire extinguisher in the kitchen and know how to use it.
  ○ Tie back long hair or loose clothing when cooking or working around flames.
  ○ If food catches on fire in a microwave or toaster oven, leave the food there and turn

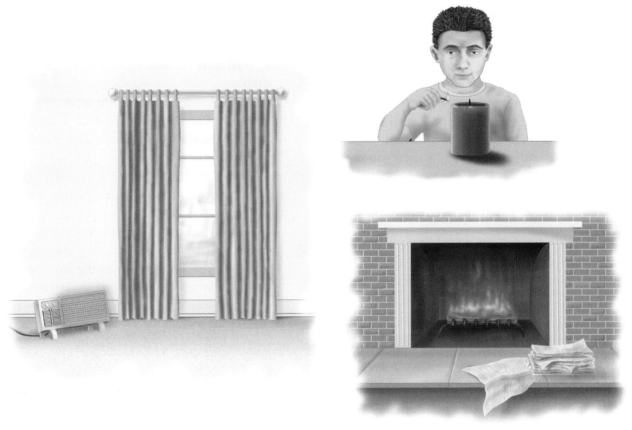

Figure 12-2 Inspect all rooms for fire hazards, and keep children away from flames and sources of heat.

the appliance off; keep other objects away until the flames go out.

- Prevent fires caused by electricity:
  - Keep power cords safely out of the way and away from children.
  - Check appliance cords for damaged areas or fraying.
  - Do not overload electrical outlets or use multiple extension cords.
  - Unplug appliances and extension cords when not in use.
- Keep children from playing with fire:
  - Store matches, lighters, candles, and other ignition sources away from children.
  - Teach young children that matches, candles, and lighters are only for adults to use, and model safe behavior when using them yourself.
  - Accept that "child-resistant" lighters are not childproof but can be used even by toddlers to start fires.
  - Understand that children who know that fire is "bad" are likely to play with matches or lighters in their bedrooms or elsewhere where they think they won't be caught.
  - Any child may play with fire because of peer pressure or simple curiosity. Teach *all* children the dangers, and keep matches and ignition sources away from *all* children. Remember the 80,000 structure fires every year set by children.
- Protect children from burns caused by fire:
  - Use only flame-resistant pajamas and bedding for children.
  - Plan escape routes and teach children where to go if a fire breaks out.
  - Teach children to "stop, drop, and roll" if their clothing catches on fire.

If a Fire Happens

Because a fire may occur even when you try to prevent it, know what to do if one should break out:

- Evacuate everyone first. Do not delay evacuation while you call 9-1-1 or use a fire extinguisher. Follow the rehearsed evacuation route.
- Do not use an elevator.

- Feel doors before opening them, and do not open a door that is hot.
- If the air is smoky, stay near the floor where there is more oxygen.
- Do not throw water on an electrical or grease (cooking) fire.
- If you cannot escape a building on fire, stuff clothing or rags in door cracks and vents; call 9-1-1 and give the dispatcher your exact location.

Preventing Heat Burns

After house fires, the most common cause of serious burns to children and the elderly is scalding from hot gases and liquids. Follow these guidelines to prevent burns from *anything* that may be hot:

- Do not use steam vaporizers, or keep them away from areas children can reach.
- Keep hot irons, curling irons, toasters, and similar appliances away from children. Never leave a child alone in a room with a hot object.
- Do not use space heaters on the floor or anywhere children can reach them. Install heat guards around radiators and heaters. Move a child's bed away from radiators or other heat sources.
- Keep children away from barbecues, which stay hot for a long time after use.
- Keep children away from campfires, which may have hot or burning coals many hours after the fire was "put out." Never use flammable liquids to start a campfire or leave children unsupervised near a fire. Keep tents and other gear well away.
- Never let children use fireworks.
- In the bathroom:
  - Prevent scalding burns by turning down the temperature of the water heater to 120 degrees Fahrenheit or lower. If you cannot do this (as in an apartment building with shared hot water), purchase an anti-scald device from a children's or hardware store.
  - Check the temperature of bath water with your wrist. Stir the water with your hand to prevent hot spots.
  - Supervise children in the bathtub.
- In the kitchen:

  - When cooking, use the back burners on the stove and keep pot handles turned toward the back of the stove.
  - Do not store food near the stove because children may attempt to reach it on their own.
  - Do not hold an infant when cooking or drinking a hot liquid.
  - Do not open the oven door with a child nearby.
  - Check the temperature of microwaved baby food or a baby bottle before feeding it to an infant.
  - Do not let young children use a microwave oven by themselves.
  - Keep high chairs away from the stove and counters where hot foods or electrical cords may be present.

Preventing Heat Burns in the Elderly

The elderly are less likely to hear, see, or feel fire and burn threats and are less able to escape a fire. In addition to the guidelines described previously, take these preventive actions in a home with an elderly family member:

- Ensure that all exits are kept clear.
- Keep eyeglasses, a telephone, and needed walking aids next to the bed.
- Wear short sleeves or tight garments when cooking, and use oven mitts for protection.
- Avoid cooking when sleepy or taking medications.
- Do not let anyone smoke near a device that supplies oxygen.
- Use a timer to remind you to turn off electric heating pads and blankets.
- Be aware of the special risks of hot objects such as cooking materials and utensils.
- Understand the limitations imposed by any physical impairments or cognitive deficits.
- Contact an organization such as the American Burn Association (http://www.ameriburn.org) for additional safety tips to prevent burns to the elderly.

Preventing Sunburn

Sunburns cause pain and damage the skin. Since repeated sunburns can cause skin cancer later in life, steps should always be taken to prevent sunburns.

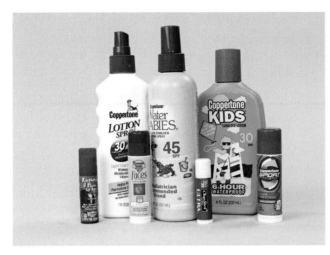

Figure 12-3 Protect against sunburn with frequent use of sunscreen.

- Keep infants under age one out of direct sunlight as much as possible. Sun-blocking clothing and shade are recommended for infants under six months old, although sunscreen can safely be used on small areas of skin. Protect an infant's eyes from sunlight as well.
- For everyday outdoors activities, the American Cancer Society recommends applying sunscreen or sunblock with a **sun protection factor (SPF)** of at least 15 on all exposed areas of skin 20 minutes before sun exposure and at least every two hours while in the sun **(Figure 12-3)**. Use a higher SPF for prolonged sun exposure.
- Wear a wide-brimmed hat and protective clothing, and keep infants and young children covered with light clothing, hats, and sunglasses.
- Limit sun exposure between 10:00 A.M. and 4:00 P.M.
- Be aware that reflective surfaces like water and snow increase the risk of burning.
- Use sunscreen even on cloudy, hazy, or foggy days, when sunburn may still occur.
- Use a lip balm with at least 15 SPF when in direct sun for an extended time.

HEAT BURNS

Heat burns may be caused by flames or contact with steam or any hot object. The severity of a burn depends on the amount of damage to the skin and other tissues under the skin.

Put Out the Fire!

If the victim's clothing is on fire, use a blanket or water to put out any flames, or have the victim roll on the ground. Even when the fire is out, the skin will keep burning if it is still hot, so cool the burn area with water immediately, except with very severe burns. Also remove the victim's clothing and jewelry, if possible without further injuring the victim, because they may still be hot and continue to burn the victim.

Assessing a Burn

Assess burns to determine the appropriate first aid to give and decide whether to call 9-1-1 or transport the victim to medical care. Assessment involves consideration of several factors:

- What type of burn(s) does the victim have? (first-, second-, or third-degree?)
- How extensive is the burn? (how much body area?)
- What specific body areas are burned?
- Are special circumstances present? (the victim's age and health status)

Because these variables can be complex, there is no one simple rule for determining when to call 9-1-1 or seek medical care. Whenever *any* burn may be serious, call 9-1-1 and let medical professionals guide your decision.

Classification of Burns

Burns are classified according to their depth into or through the skin:

- **First-degree burns** (also called **superficial burns**) damage only the skin's outer layer, the epidermis, like a typical sunburn. The skin is red, typically dry, and painful. These minor burns usually heal well by themselves but may require medical attention if they cover an extensive area.
- **Second-degree burns** (also called **partial-thickness burns**) damage the skin's deeper layer, the dermis. The skin is red, may look mottled, and is very painful. Blisters are often present and may be weeping clear fluid. Scarring may be present after healing. Depending on size and other factors, second-degree burns may require medical attention.
- **Third-degree burns** (also called **full-thickness burns**) damage the skin all the way

through the subcutaneous layer and may burn muscle or other tissues. The skin is charred or blackened or may look white and leathery. Pain is not present where the skin has burned through but is likely in adjacent areas. These burns are medical emergencies.

Often a victim with serious burns has a mix of different burn classifications. One area may have a third-degree burn, for example, while nearby areas have first- or second-degree burns. Follow the first aid guidelines for the most severely burned area first.

Assessing Burn Size and Severity

In addition to burn depth, the size of the burned area is an important part of the assessment. This is usually calculated as a percentage of body surface area. A common method used by medical professionals to estimate the body surface area of a burn is the **rule of nines.** In this system the adult body is divided into a number of areas with percentages based on increments of 9%. As shown in **Figure 12-4**, the percentages are different for a small child.

- Each arm is 9% (front or back alone is 4.5%).
- Each leg is 18% (front or back alone is 9%).
- The front of the torso is 18% (9% for abdomen and 9% for chest).
- The back of the torso is 18% (9% for lower back and buttocks, 9% for upper back).
- The head is 9% (face or back of head alone is 4.5%).
- The genital region is 1%.

In some cases the percentage of body surface area burned influences the decision to call EMS and determines some aspects of advanced medical care. Any third-degree burn larger than a 50-cent piece or second-degree burn more than 10% of the body in an adult (5% in a child or older adult) is an emergency. Seek medical attention also for a first-degree burn over more than 50% of the body.

Also important is the location of the burn on the body. Second- or third-degree burns on the face, genitals, or hands or feet are considered emergencies and require immediate medical care. Circumferential burns that wrap around an extremity or a finger or toe should also receive immediate medical attention. Burns around the nose and mouth may affect breathing and are medical emergencies.

Finally, consider the victim's age and health. A burn in a child under age five or an adult over age 55 is more serious than in a younger adult. Many **chronic** health disorders also make burns more serious. When in doubt whether a victim needs immediate emergency treatment, call 9-1-1 (**Box 12-1**).

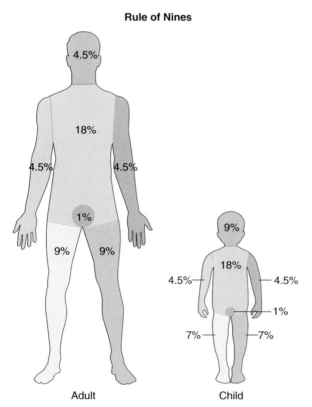

Rule of Nines

Adult

Child

Figure 12-4 The rule of nines for calculating body surface area burned. These numbers represent one half of the body.

BOX 12-1 CALL 9-1-1 FOR A BURN IF:

- The victim has a third-degree burn.
- The victim has a second-degree burn that is large (over 10% of body area in adult, or 5% of body area in a child, older adult, or someone with chronic illness) or that affects the head, genitals, or hands or feet.
- The victim is having trouble breathing.
- The victim may have inhaled smoke or fumes.

Learning Checkpoint (1)

1. List at least three of the most common activities during which fires occur.

2. Describe at least three things you can do to help prevent fires from occurring in the kitchen.

3. True or False: If a fire breaks out in a building where you and others are present, the first thing you should do is call 9-1-1.

4. Name four factors that affect how serious a burn may be.

FIRST AID FOR HEAT BURNS

First aid for heat burns is based on four general principles of burn care:

1. Stop the burning and cool the area.
2. Protect the burned area from additional trauma and pathogens.
3. Provide supportive care.
4. Ensure medical attention.

The specific first aid varies somewhat depending on the severity of the burn.

Care for First-Degree Burns

First-degree burns include most cases of sunburn and minor burns caused by heat or scalding. The skin is pink or red and remains unbroken, but some swelling may occur. Although first-degree burns may seem minor, they still cause pain and damage the skin. The first goal, as in all burns, is to stop the burning by removing the heat source and cooling the area with cold water; do not use ice, which can cause further damage. Be sure the water stays cold—a wet cloth on a burn, for example, may absorb the burn's heat and no longer be cold. Since swelling may occur, jewelry and constrictive clothing should be removed from the area. Thereafter, protect the burned skin from contact with objects that may rub or put pressure on it. Do not apply ointment or other oily or greasy substances on the burn, although **aloe vera** gel may provide some comfort (see First Aid: "First-Degree Burns").

Care for Second-Degree Burns

A second-degree burn is deeper than a first-degree burn, involving the dermis and causing more dam-

age to capillaries and nerve endings. The skin is red and swollen, often blotchy in appearance, and has blisters that may leak a clear fluid. If blisters break, pathogens may enter the skin and cause infection; first aid therefore includes protecting the skin. Pain is more severe than with a first-degree burn.

A small second-degree burn (smaller than your palm) may be treated at home, but a larger burn requires immediate medical attention. If larger than 10% of the body surface area (or 5% in a child, older adult, or person with chronic illness), the burn should be treated as an emergency and 9-1-1 called. Stop the burning immediately and cool the area with water. Be sure the water stays cool by continually adding fresh water. Remove jewelry and constricting clothing from the area. While waiting for medical care, keep the burn covered with a dry, loose, nonstick dressing. As with all burns, do not apply ointment or other substances to the burn (see First Aid: "Second-Degree Burns").

Care for Third-Degree Burns

Third-degree burns are usually emergencies and when large may be life threatening. Third-degree burns penetrate all the way through the skin and may damage underlying tissues. Infection is likely. It is important to act immediately to stop the burning and cool the burn, although a very large burn area (over 20% of body surface area) should not be immersed in water because of the risk of causing hypothermia. The victim may rapidly develop the signs of shock, a life-threatening condition requiring treatment in addition to the burn first aid. Call 9-1-1.

First Aid   First-Degree Burns

When You See
- Skin is red, dry, and painful
- May be some swelling
- Skin not broken

Do This First

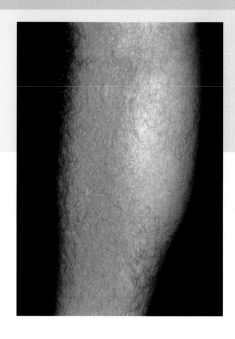

1 Stop the burning by removing the heat source.

2 Cool the burned area with cold water. Immerse a small area in a sink or bucket, or cover a larger area with a wet cloth for at least 10 minutes—but not most of the body.

3 Remove clothing and jewelry or any other constricting item before the area swells.

4 Protect the burn from friction or pressure.

ALERT
- Do not put butter on a burn.
- Do not use ice on a burn because even though it may relieve pain, the cold may cause additional damage to the skin. Ice-cold water should not be used longer than 10 minutes.

Additional Care
- Aloe vera gel can be used on the skin for comfort.

Stop the burning immediately and cool the area. Be sure the water stays cool by continually adding fresh water. Remove jewelry and constricting clothing from the area. Cover the burn with a dry, loose, nonstick dressing. As with all burns, do not apply ointment or other substances to the burn. While waiting for emergency personnel, treat the victim for shock by having the victim lie down, elevating the legs, and maintaining normal body temperature. Monitor the victim's breathing and give basic life support (BLS) if needed (see First Aid: "Third-Degree Burns").

When You See

- Skin is swollen and red, may be blotchy or streaked
- Blisters that may be weeping clear fluid
- Signs of significant pain

Do This First

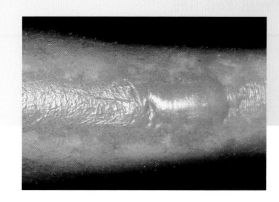

1 Stop the burning by removing the heat source.

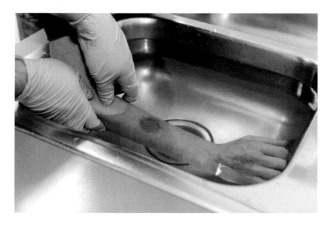

2 Cool the burned area with cold water. Immerse a small area in a sink or bucket, or cover a larger area (but not most of the body) with wet cloths for at least 10 minutes or until the area is free of pain even after removal from the water.

3 For large burns, call 9-1-1.

4 Remove clothing and jewelry from the area before the area swells.

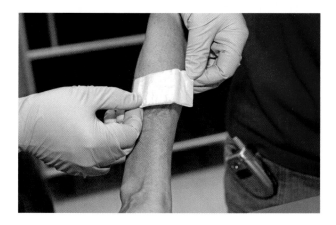

5 Put a nonstick dressing over the burn to protect the area, but keep it loose and do not tape it to the skin.

ALERT

- Do not break skin blisters; this could cause an infection.
- Be gentle when covering the area.

Additional Care

- For burns on the face, genitals, hands, or feet, seek medical attention.

First Aid Third-Degree Burns

When You See

- Skin damage, charred skin, or white, leathery skin
- May have signs and symptoms of shock (clammy, pale, or ashen skin; nausea and vomiting; fast breathing)

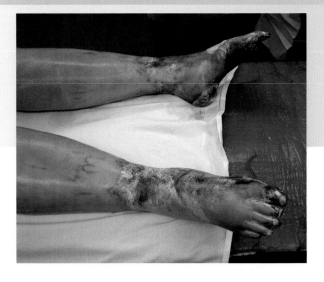

Do This First

1 Stop the burning by removing the heat source.

2 Cool surrounding first- and second-degree burns only.

3 Remove clothing and jewelry before the area swells.

4 Call 9-1-1.

5 Prevent shock: have the victim lie down, elevate the legs, and maintain normal body temperature.

6 Carefully cover the burn with a nonstick dressing. Do not apply a cream or ointment.

ALERT

- With third-degree burns do not cool more than 20% of the body with water (10% for a child) because of the risk of hypothermia and shock.
- Do not touch the burn or put anything on it.

- Do not give the victim anything to drink.

Additional Care

- Watch the victim's breathing and be ready to give basic life support (BLS) if needed.

Learning Checkpoint 2

1. True or False: For a victim with a second-degree burn, you should break skin blisters and cover the area with a burn ointment to promote faster healing.

2. For a victim with a third-degree burn, you should cool only a _____ area with water because of the risk of shock or hypothermia.

3. As you are leaving work, you see a man working on his car in the parking lot. He suddenly screams and backs away, his clothing on fire. What do you do? List in correct order the first four actions you should take.

SMOKE INHALATION

Any victim who was in the vicinity of a fire could have airway or lung injuries from inhaling smoke or other fumes resulting from fires. Even hot air can cause such injuries. This can be a medical emergency. The lining of the airway may swell and make breathing difficult. The small sacs in the lungs where oxygen enters the lungs, the alveoli, may be damaged and affect the ability of the body to receive enough oxygen through normal breathing. A victim of smoke inhalation may also have carbon monoxide poisoning (see **Chapter 18**).

The signs and symptoms of smoke inhalation include coughing, wheezing, or hoarseness; burns or blackening around the mouth or nose; coughing up a sooty substance; and difficulty breathing. Note that symptoms from smoke inhalation may not become obvious for up to 48 hours after exposure.

Care for Smoke Inhalation

First, get the victim to fresh air or fresh air to the victim. A victim who can safely be moved should be assisted outdoors or to an area of fresh air. If the victim cannot be moved, ventilate the area by any means available to remove smoke and fumes. Call 9-1-1 immediately, even if the victim is not experiencing signs and symptoms, because injury may have occurred even though the effects are not yet showing. While waiting for medical care, help the victim into a position for easiest breathing (often semireclining) and keep him or her calm. If the victim becomes unresponsive, position him or her in the recovery position and monitor breathing. Be prepared to give basic life support if needed (see First Aid: "Smoke Inhalation").

First Aid   Smoke Inhalation

When You See

- Smoke visible in area
- Coughing, wheezing, hoarse voice
- Possible burned area on face or chest
- Difficulty breathing

Do This First

1 Get the victim to fresh air, or fresh air to the victim.

2 Call 9-1-1.

3 Help the victim into a position for easy breathing.

Additional Care

- Put an unresponsive victim in the recovery position.
- Be ready to give BLS if needed.

CHEMICAL BURNS

Many strong chemicals found in workplaces and the home can burn the skin on contact. Sometimes the burn develops slowly and in some cases the victim may not be aware of the burn for up to 24 hours. Acids and alkalis, liquids and solids can all cause serious chemical burns (**Figure 12-5**).

Preventing Chemical Burns

- Read directions before using any household products. Heed warnings on products, and keep all products in their original containers. Do not mix different products.
- Protect hands with heavy rubber gloves, and cover other exposed areas of the body.
- Ensure adequate ventilation when using products with dangerous fumes.

Care for Chemical Burns

In most cases you can see the substance on the victim's skin, and the victim feels a burning or stinging sensation. Since the chemical reaction can continue as long as the substance is on the skin, you must remove it immediately. With a dry chemical, brush it off with a cloth, piece of cardboard or paper, spare article of clothing, or any other item available. Be careful not to get the chemical on your own skin or to spread it to other areas of the victim's skin. Wear gloves if available. Then flush the area with water as soon as possible.

Remove any clothing and jewelry from the burned area. With a liquid spilled on the victim's skin, start flushing with water immediately.

Call 9-1-1 for any chemical burn, and keep flushing the area with water until medical care arrives, or for at least 30 minutes. Remember that a chemical may give off fumes, even if you cannot smell it, and therefore the victim should be moved (if safe) to fresh air. Even a dry chemical may give off fumes once it is in contact with water. Note: Do not try to neutralize an acid by applying an alkaline substance, or vice versa, because of the risk of further damage caused by the chemical reaction.

After flushing the burn with water, if the victim is still waiting for medical care to arrive or is being transported for medical care, cover the burn with a loose, dry, nonstick dressing and protect the area (see First Aid: "Chemical Burns").

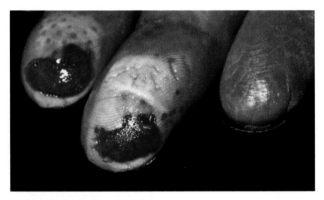

Figure 12-5 A chemical burn.

Learning
Checkpoint ③

1. A co-worker has splashed an unknown liquid in her eye and is holding her hand over the eye. What should you do first?

   a. Have her keep holding the eye closed so that her tears will wash out the chemical.

   b. Call 9-1-1 and wait for healthcare personnel to take care of her eye.

   c. Immediately flush the eye with running water.

   d. Mix baking soda with water and pour it into her eye.

2. Describe the first action to take if a victim has a dry chemical on the skin.

   _____

3. True or False: If a person who was in a smoky area near a fire does not have any signs and symptoms within an hour, that person does not need medical care.

First Aid   Chemical Burns

When You See

- A chemical on the victim's skin or clothing
- Complaints of pain or a burning sensation
- A spilled substance on or around an unresponsive victim
- A smell of fumes in the air

Do This First

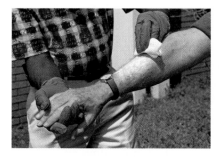

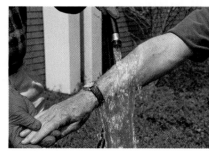

4 Remove clothing and jewelry from the burn area while flushing with water.

5 Call 9-1-1 for any chemical burn.

1 With a dry chemical, first brush it off the victim's skin, but do not contaminate skin that has not been in contact with the chemical. (Wear medical exam gloves to avoid contact with the substance yourself.)

2 Because of the risk of fumes, move the victim or ventilate the area.

3 Wash off the area as quickly as possible with running water for at least 30 minutes. Use a sink, hose, or even a shower to flush the whole area of contact.

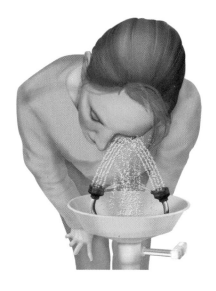

((ALERT))

Chemical in the Eyes

- With a chemical splashed into the eye, flush immediately with running water and continue for at least 20 minutes. Have the victim remove a contact lens.
- Tilt the victim's head so that the water runs away from the face and not into the other eye.
- After flushing, have the victim hold a dressing over the eye until he or she receives medical care.

Additional Care

- If chemicals were spilled in a confined area, leave the area with the victim because of the risk of fumes.
- Put a dry, nonstick dressing over the burn.

ELECTRICAL BURNS AND SHOCKS

An electrical burn or shock occurs whenever any part of the body comes in contact with electricity. Typical injuries occur with electricity from faulty appliances or power cords or when an appliance comes into contact with water. Water easily conducts electricity to anyone who touches the water. Many deaths caused by electricity occur when an appliance such as a hair dryer or radio falls into bathwater.

Preventing Electrical Shocks and Burns

Electricity may cause life-threatening shocks as well as electrical burns. Follow these guidelines to stay safe (**Figure 12-6**):

- Use outlet caps to block unused electrical outlets.
- Do not use a nightlight in a young child's bedroom that looks like a toy; it can cause an electrical burn if the child tries to play with it.
- Never use electrical appliances near water or when your hands are wet.
- Inspect electrical cords for broken or frayed insulation.
- Be careful not to touch the wire prongs when inserting or removing electrical plugs from a receptacle. Pull the plug itself out, not the cord.
- Install a **ground fault circuit interrupter (GFCI)** in outlets in bathrooms and kitchens; this device automatically turns off electricity when appliances become wet.
- Outdoors, keep everyone away from downed power lines, and do not let children play near electrical poles or fly kites near electrical wires.

Preventing Lightning Strikes

Each year, about 1200 people in the United States are struck by lightning, causing significant injuries and more than 100 deaths. If you are caught outdoors in a thunderstorm, follow these guidelines:

- Realize the lightning risk even if the storm seems far off. Seek shelter if you hear thunder within 30 seconds of seeing a lightning strike. Lightning has been known to "jump" miles away from a storm cloud.
- Get out of water immediately, or off a boat.
- Try not to be the tallest object around. Crouch near the ground or get beneath a group of trees—but not a tall, isolated tree. Avoid high ground and open spaces.
- Stay away from metal fences and power lines. Do not take shelter near metal objects.
- A closed motor vehicle is safer than being caught in the open. Keep the doors and windows completely shut.
- If you are caught in the open, crouch or squat down (but do not lie down) with your feet together. A group of people should stay about 15 feet away from each other.
- Indoors, stay away from doors and windows, and do not use electrical appliances or devices. Also keep away from telephone lines and plumbing fixtures.

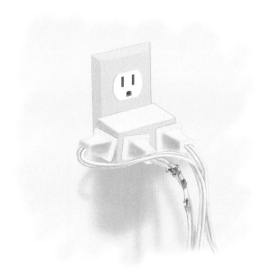

Figure 12-6 Overloaded outlets or extension cords pose a risk of fire or electrical shocks.

Box 12-2 High-Voltage Shocks

High Power Lines

If a power line is down, do not approach a victim in contact with the line. Call 9-1-1 immediately. Do not try to move the wire away using any object. Wait for emergency workers to arrive, and keep others away from the scene.

Lightning Strikes

Lightning strikes often cause serious injury. In addition to burns, the electrical shock may affect the heart and brain and cause temporary blindness or deafness, unresponsiveness or seizures, bleeding, bone fractures, or cardiac arrest. Call 9-1-1 immediately and give basic life support, treating the most serious injuries first.

Care for Electrical Burns

Two possible injuries may occur from electricity:

- External burns caused by the heat of electricity
- Electrical injuries caused by electricity flowing through the body

High-voltage electricity flowing through the body can cause significant injuries to many different tissues. Heart damage may cause heart rhythm irregularities that threaten the victim's circulation or cause the heart to stop (**Box 12-2**).

As with all types of burns, the urgent first step is to stop the burning. If the victim is still in contact with a source of electricity, ensure that the power is disconnected or turned off immediately. Do not touch a victim still in contact with electricity because of the risk of receiving a shock or burn yourself.

External burns resulting from heat or flames caused by electricity are cared for in the same manner as heat burns. Electrical injuries may cause only minor external burns where the electricity entered and left the body; these are called **entrance** and **exit wounds** (**Figure 12-7**).

Internal damage caused by an electrical shock is seldom as obvious as an external burn. Signs and symptoms may include unresponsiveness, seizures, or changing levels of responsiveness. Call 9-1-1 and monitor the victim's breathing while waiting for medical assistance. Be prepared to give basic life support if needed (see First Aid: "Electrical Burns").

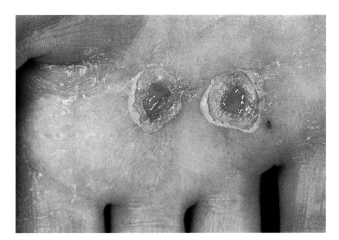

Figure 12-7 An electrical burn.

First Aid · Electrical Burns

When You See

- A source of electricity near the victim: bare wires, power cords, an electrical device
- Burned area of skin, possibly both entrance and exit wounds
- Changing levels of responsiveness

Do This First

1 Do not touch the victim until you know the area is safe. Unplug or turn off the power.

2 With an unresponsive victim, give BLS.

3 Call 9-1-1.

4 Care for the burn (stop the burning, cool the area, remove clothing and jewelry, cover the burn).

5 Prevent shock by having the victim lie down, elevating the legs, and maintaining normal body temperature.

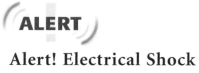

Alert! Electrical Shock

- Do not touch a victim you think is receiving an electrical shock! First make sure the power is turned off or the person is well away from the power source. Turn off the circuit breaker and call 9-1-1.
- Note that electrical burns can cause massive internal injuries even when the external burn may look minor.

Additional Care

- Keep an unresponsive victim in the recovery position and monitor breathing until help arrives.

Learning
Checkpoint ④

1. True or False: The first thing to do for an unresponsive victim in contact with an electrical wire is pour water over the area of contact.

2. What is the safest way to stop the electricity when someone is shocked by an electrical appliance? How should you *not* try to stop it?

_____

3. Driving home from work, you are stopped behind a car that has struck a telephone pole. You get out to help the driver and see a power line dangling from the pole in contact with the roof of the car. Your first action should be to

   a. use your cell phone to call 9-1-1.

   b. look for a stick or piece of wood to push the wire away from the car.

   c. try to pull the victim out the car window.

   d. give any needed first aid by leaning in the car window.

Concluding Thoughts

First aid for burns may seem complex because of the variations in care depending on the type of burn, its size and location on the body, and its depth. Most importantly, remember the general first aid principles for all burns:
- Act fast to stop the burning.
- Cool or flush the area.
- Seek help.
- Protect the victim.

Learning Outcomes

You should now be able to do the following:

1. Explain common causes of fires and burns and how to prevent them.

2. Describe what happens to the body when it receives a burn.

3. List the differences between first-, second-, and third-degree burns.

4. Describe first aid for first-, second-, and third-degree heat burns.

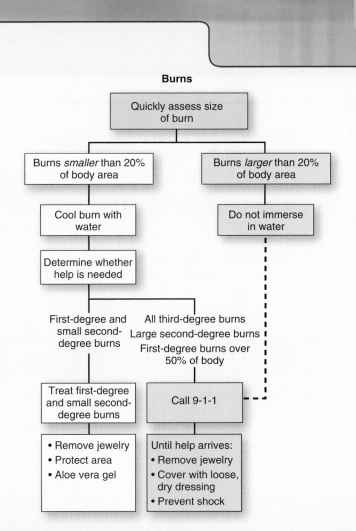

Burns

Quickly assess size of burn

Burns *smaller* than 20% of body area | Burns *larger* than 20% of body area

Cool burn with water | Do not immerse in water

Determine whether help is needed

First-degree and small second-degree burns | All third-degree burns / Large second-degree burns / First-degree burns over 50% of body

Treat first-degree and small second-degree burns | Call 9-1-1

• Remove jewelry
• Protect area
• Aloe vera gel

Until help arrives:
• Remove jewelry
• Cover with loose, dry dressing
• Prevent shock

5. Describe first aid for smoke inhalation.

6. Describe first aid for chemical burns.

7. Describe first aid for electrical burns and shocks.

Review Questions

1. Most fires occur
   a. in the home.
   b. in the workplace.
   c. in schools.
   d. in public gathering places.

2. A first-degree burn is characterized by
   a. the presence of white, fluid-filled blisters.
   b. pink or red skin.
   c. white, leathery areas of skin.
   d. bleeding.

3. Factors that influence the severity of a burn include
   a. the depth of the burn.
   b. the percentage of body area burned.
   c. the location of the burn.
   d. All of the above

4. Which of the following is true about burns?
   a. The deeper the burn, the more painful it is.
   b. Third-degree burns are more painful than others.
   c. The level of pain is not an indicator of burn severity.
   d. Blisters are more painful than charred or red skin.

5. Which of the following is the best substance to put on a burn immediately after it has occurred?
   a. Antibiotic ointment
   b. Aloe vera
   c. Butter
   d. Water

6. The purpose of putting a dressing over a burn is to
   a. protect the area.
   b. absorb the fluid from blisters.
   c. keep the area moist for 24 hours.
   d. prevent swelling.

7. Using icy water to cool a burn that covers 25% of the body may result in
   a. hypothermia and shock.
   b. shock and cardiac arrest.
   c. hypothermia and severe bleeding.
   d. electrolyte imbalances and infection.

8. A ring should be removed from a burned finger because
   a. gold and silver are toxic metals on exposed skin.
   b. swelling may cut off circulation.
   c. the ring is a likely source of infection.
   d. the ring makes it difficult to cool the burn.

9. First aid for a dry chemical burn includes
   a. neutralizing an acid with an alkaline substance.
   b. neutralizing an alkaline burn with an acidic substance.
   c. brushing off the chemical and then flushing the skin with water.
   d. tightly taping a dressing over the burn.

10. Call 9-1-1 for
   a. a second-degree burn larger than 10% of body surface area in an adult victim.
   b. a second-degree burn larger than 5% of body surface area in an elderly victim.
   c. a third-degree burn.
   d. All of the above

References and Resources

American Academy of Pediatrics. AAP makes new recommendations on infant use of sunscreen. 1999. www.aap.org

American Burn Association. Burn incidence and treatment in the US: 2000 fact sheet. 2004. www.ameriburn.org

American Burn Association. National Burn Awareness Week campaign kit: educator's guide. 2003.

American Cancer Society. Cancer reference information. 2005. www.cancer.org

American College of Emergency Physicians. *First aid manual: a comprehensive guide to treating emergency victims of all ages in any situation.* New York: DK Publishing; 2001.

American Heart Association. 2005 International consensus on cardiopulmonary resuscitation (CPR) and emergency cardiovascular care (ECC) science with treatment recommendations. *Circulation,* 112(22). November 29, 2005.

Burn Institute. www.burninstitute.org

National Fire Protection Association. www.nfpa.org

National Safety Council. www.nsc.org

Occupational Safety and Health Administration. OSHA fact sheet: fire safety in the workplace. 2004. www.osha.gov

Chapter 13

Head and Spinal Injuries

Chapter Preview

- Prevention of Head and Spinal Injuries
- Assessing Head and Spinal Injuries
- Skull Fractures

- Brain Injuries
- Spinal Injuries

You have stopped by a neighborhood school on your way home to see a friend who helps coach the girls' gymnastic team. While talking in a corner of the gym, you are horrified to see a young girl on the uneven bars attempt a release move and miss the bar. You run to her and find that she is unresponsive. What should you do?

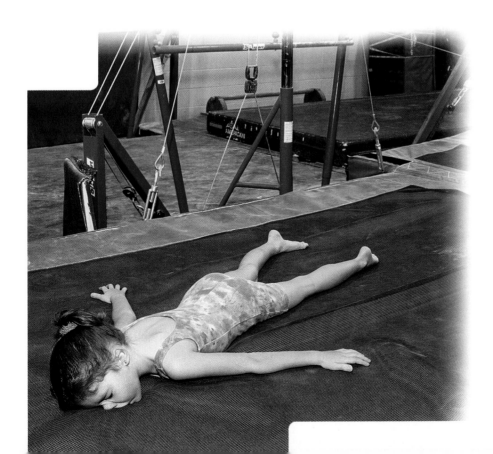

Head and spinal injuries may be life threatening or may cause permanent damage to the brain or spinal cord, producing nervous system deficits such as paralysis. Any trauma to the head, neck, or back may result in a serious injury. Injuries that cause unresponsiveness or loss of sensation in a body part are especially likely to be serious, but even injuries without immediate, obvious signs and symptoms may create a potentially life-threatening problem.

Because of the forces involved, any injury to the head may also injure the spine. Whenever you find a serious head injury, suspect a neck or back injury.

This chapter considers head and spinal injuries that involve deeper injuries to the skull or spine, including bone and nerves. **Chapter 11** describes the first aid for more superficial wounds to the head and face.

PREVENTION OF HEAD AND SPINAL INJURIES

Motor vehicle crashes are the leading cause of head and spinal injuries in people under age 65, and falls are the leading cause of these injuries over age 65. Sports and recreation activities cause about 18% of spinal cord injuries. About 11,000 people in the United States have a spinal injury each year, and nearly 200,000 live with a disability resulting from a spinal cord injury.

Many head and spinal injuries can be prevented by following accepted guidelines for safety in vehicles, recreation, and work.*

- Always wear seatbelts and shoulder restraints in vehicles.
- Use approved car seats for infants and small children, and make sure they are installed correctly (incorrect installation is a frequent cause of injury).
- Wear appropriate helmets, headgear, or hard hats for bicycling, skating and skateboarding, sports, and work activities.
- At work, follow appropriate OSHA guidelines for equipment and safety practices.

*Source: The Centers for Disease Control and Prevention and the Brain Injury Association of America.

- Avoid risky activities, including driving, when you are under the influence of drugs, alcohol, or medications that produce drowsiness.
- Ensure that children's playground surfaces are made of a shock-absorbing material.
- Store firearms in a locked cabinet with ammunition in a separate secure location.
- Do not dive into murky or shallow water (shallow means less than nine feet deep).
- To prevent falls, keep yourself and your house safe for children and older adults:
  - To reach high shelves, use a step stool with a grab bar.
  - Make sure all stairways have handrails.
  - Use safety gates at the top and bottom of stairs when young children are present.
  - Remove tripping hazards such as small area rugs and loose electrical cords.
  - Use nonslip mats in the tub and shower.
  - Install grab bars by the toilet and in the tub or shower.
  - Get regular exercise to improve strength, balance, and coordination.
  - See an eye doctor regularly for vision checks.
  - Since falls often result from dizziness caused by medications, have your healthcare provider review your medications.

ASSESSING HEAD AND SPINAL INJURIES

Assessing a victim with a potential head and spinal injury begins with considering the cause of the injury and the forces involved. An understanding of the general signs and symptoms of head and spinal injuries helps you to focus the physical examination. It is essential to recognize the possibility of a head or spinal injury immediately because the possibility of a spinal injury determines how and when a victim is positioned and moved.

Causes of Head and Spinal Injuries

Any trauma to the head may cause a head or spinal injury. In addition, spinal injuries may be caused by forces to the back, chest, or even the pelvis or legs by indirect force. Common causes of head and spinal injuries include the following:

- Motor vehicle crashes (including whiplash injuries without direct impact to the head)
- Falls from a height of more than a few feet
- Diving emergencies involving impact to the head (even blows that do not cause bruises or wounds)
- Skiing emergencies and other sports injuries
- Any forceful blow to the head, neck, or back

Suspect a head or spinal injury in any of these situations or when wounds or other injuries in the body suggest large forces were involved. If so, observe the victim carefully and thoroughly for the signs and symptoms of a head or spinal injury even as you are carrying out the initial assessment.

General Signs and Symptoms of Head and Spinal Injuries

Head and spinal injuries are closely related because a traumatic injury to one may injure the other as well. For example, a blow to the head that fractures the skull may also put enough force on vertebrae in the neck that a spinal injury occurs. Although a head injury may occur in a victim without a spinal injury, and a spinal injury may occur in a victim without a head injury, the assessment of a victim with such injuries should look for both head and spinal injuries.

The general signs and symptoms of head and spinal injuries may overlap in victims with an injury of the head, neck, or back. Suspect a head or spinal injury in a victim if any of these signs and symptoms is present:

- Lump or deformity in the head, neck, or back
- Changing levels of responsiveness, drowsiness, confusion, dizziness (see AVPU scale in **Chapter 4**)
- Unequal pupils
- Headache
- Clear fluid from the nose or ears
- Stiff neck
- Inability to move any body part
- Tingling, numbness, or lack of feeling in feet or hands

Noting any of these signs and symptoms in the initial assessment or physical examination of a victim should lead to a more specific assessment looking for a head or spinal injury. These specific injuries are described in following sections in this chapter.

Physical Examination of Head and Spinal Injuries

Chapter 4, "Assessing the Victim," describes general procedures for assessing all victims, including a physical examination of a victim not being treated for a life-threatening injury. In the initial assessment of an unresponsive victim, consider whether the victim may have a spinal injury based on these factors:

- The cause of the victim's injuries (e.g., blow to the head, a fall, strong forces)
- Observations of bystanders at the scene who saw the injury occur
- Immediately apparent injuries and wounds (e.g., a serious head wound, or the neck twisted at an unusual angle)—but do not take the time to do a physical examination if the victim is not breathing
- Any observed sign of a head or spinal injury

During the initial assessment of the victim, you may have to position the victim to open the airway, to check breathing, to give CPR, to control bleeding, or to allow blood, vomit, or other fluid to drain from the mouth. If you have determined that the victim may have a spinal injury, take great care when moving or repositioning the victim, as described later in this chapter. Unless it is necessary, do not move the victim.

If the victim is unresponsive and the initial assessment does not reveal a life-threatening condition for which you must care, do not perform a physical examination but observe the victim for other injuries. If an unresponsive victim may have a spinal injury, do not move the victim unless it is necessary. Check only for serious injuries such as bleeding that must be controlled. Otherwise, maintain the victim's head position to prevent movement and wait for EMS professionals.

If the victim is responsive and the nature of injuries suggests the possibility of a spinal injury, carefully assess for the signs and symptoms of spinal injury during the physical examination. Ask the victim to stay in position and not move more than you ask during the examination, to prevent further damage to the spine.

Perform the physical examination in the same manner as described in **Chapter 4**, paying particular attention to signs and symptoms of a head or spinal injury. Gently feel the skull for bumps or depressions. Check the ears and nose for blood or a clear fluid. Check the pupils of both eyes, which should be of equal size and should respond to light when you cover and uncover the eyes with your hand. Check the neck for deformity or swelling, bleeding, or pain. When checking the torso, observe for impaired breathing and loss of bladder or bowel control, a sign of nerve damage. When assessing the extremities, check for sensation and the ability to move the hand or foot, comparing strength from one side of the body to the other.

If your examination reveals any problem suggesting a head or spinal injury, call 9-1-1 and keep the victim still until EMS professionals arrive. Note that it can be very difficult for first aiders without advanced training to recognize a spinal injury with certainty. ***Do not depend on any specific assessment of a victim to decide whether or not the victim may have a spinal injury. Do not assume a victim without specific symptoms does not have a possible spinal injury.*** Consider the forces involved in the injury, and when in doubt, keep the victim's head immobile while waiting for help to arrive. With a responsive victim, encourage the victim not to move, and with an unresponsive victim, hold the head in place to prevent movement.

In addition, the results of the examination are not always clear-cut. For example, even though the spinal cord may be intact, an injury may put pressure on the cord that results in limited sensation, pain, or partial inability to move. If the victim can move a hand or foot only weakly, for example, assume a spinal injury has occurred.

Follow this assessment approach for all suspected cases of head or spinal injuries (see Skill: "Assessing Head and Spinal Injuries").

Skull Fractures

If the victim had a blow to the head, consider the possibility of a skull fracture or a brain injury. The skull is generally strong and is fractured only with severe trauma. When you find bleeding from the scalp, check carefully for a possible skull fracture before applying direct pressure to the wound. If the skull is fractured, direct pressure on the wound could push bone fragments into the brain, causing serious injury.

Feel the scalp gently for signs of a skull fracture: a depressed or spongy area or the presence of bone fragments. Blood or a clear fluid leaking from the nose or eyes may also be a sign of a skull injury. In such a case, to control bleeding, apply pressure around the wound rather than directly on it. Note that a skull fracture may occur even without an open wound.

A skull fracture is life threatening. Call 9-1-1 immediately. Note that a skull fracture often also causes injuries to the brain (see First Aid: "Skull Injury").

Skill **Assessing Head and Spinal Injuries**

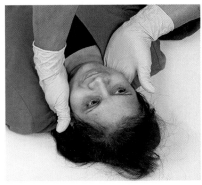

1 Check the victim's head.

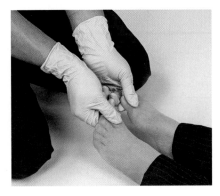

2 Check neck for deformity, swelling, and pain.

3 Touch toes of both feet and ask victim if the sensation feels normal.

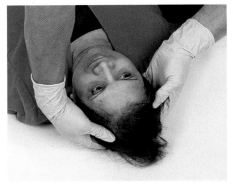

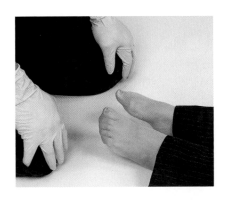

4 Ask victim to point toes.

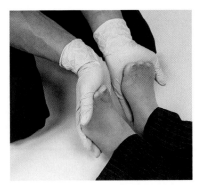

5 Ask victim to push against your hands with the feet.

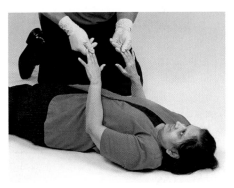

6 Touch fingers of both hands and ask victim if the sensation feels normal.

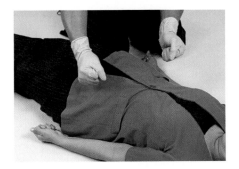

7 Ask victim to make a fist and curl (flex) it in.

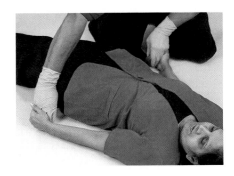

8 Ask victim to squeeze your hands.

First Aid Skull Injury

When You See

- A deformed area of the skull
- A depressed area in the bone felt during the physical examination
- Blood or fluid coming from the ears or nose
- Eyelids swollen shut or becoming discolored (bruising)
- Bruising behind the ears
- Unequal pupils
- Impaled object in the skull

Do This First

1 Call 9-1-1.

2 If the victim is unresponsive, check for normal breathing.

3 *Do not* clean the wound, press on it, or remove an impaled object.

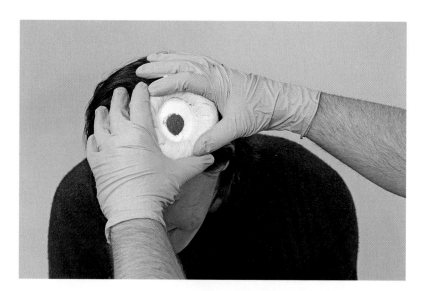

4 Cover the wound with a sterile dressing.

5 If there is significant bleeding, apply pressure only around the edges of the wound, not on the wound itself. You may use a ring dressing to apply pressure around the wound (see **Chapter 11**).

6 Do not move the victim unnecessarily, since there may also be a spinal injury. Stay with the victim until help arrives.

Additional Care

- Put an unresponsive victim in the recovery position (unless there may be a spinal injury).
- Do not raise the victim's legs.

BRAIN INJURIES

Brain injuries may occur with a blow to the head with or without an open wound. A brain injury is likely with a skull fracture. Injury results when the traumatic force is transmitted to brain tissue, causing bleeding or swelling of the brain and concussion. Brain injuries may cause a range of signs or symptoms, including headache, altered mental status, confusion, or unresponsiveness; weakness, numbness, loss of sensation, or **paralysis** of body areas; nausea and vomiting; seizures; and unequal pupils **(Figure 13-1)**. If breathing is impaired, the victim may need basic life support.

Call 9-1-1 for any victim with a suspected brain injury. Even if the signs and symptoms seem mild at first, swelling and/or bleeding in the brain may continue, and the victim's condition may rapidly deteriorate and become life threatening. Stay with the victim and be prepared to give basic life support if needed. With any force strong enough to injure the brain, suspect a possible spinal injury as well and support the victim's head to prevent movement while waiting for help to arrive. Since vomiting commonly occurs with brain injuries, be prepared to move the victim into the recovery position to allow fluid to drain from the mouth. Enlist the help of bystanders to keep the victim's head in line with the body whenever you move the victim (see First Aid: "Brain Injuries").

In some cases after a blow to the head the victim does not immediately have the signs and symptoms of brain injury and does not seek medical care. Signs and symptoms may appear within the next 48 hours that indicate a more serious injury. Seek medical attention immediately if any of the following late signs and symptoms occurs following a head injury:

- Nausea and vomiting
- Severe or persistent headache
- Changing levels of responsiveness
- Lack of coordination, movement problems
- Problems with vision or speech
- Seizures

Concussion

A **concussion** is a type of brain injury that involves a temporary impairment of brain function but usually not permanent damage. Usually there is no head wound, and the victim may not have many of the signs and symptoms of a more serious brain injury. The victim may have been "knocked out" by a blow to the head but regained consciousness quickly. A concussion typically causes these signs and symptoms:

- Temporary confusion
- Memory loss about the traumatic event
- Brief loss of responsiveness
- Mildly or moderately altered mental status
- Unusual behavior
- Headache

Although a victim with a concussion may seem to recover quickly and to experience no signs or symptoms, it is generally difficult to determine the seriousness of the injury. More

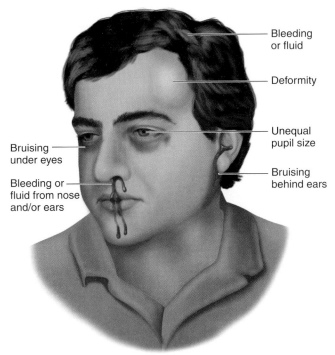

Bleeding or fluid

Deformity

Unequal pupil size

Bruising behind ears

Bruising under eyes

Bleeding or fluid from nose and/or ears

Figure 13-1 The signs of a brain injury.

First Aid   Brain Injuries

When You See

- Head wound suggesting there was a blow to the head
- Changing levels of responsiveness, drowsiness
- Confusion, disorientation, memory loss about the injury
- Headache
- Dizziness
- Seizures
- Nausea, vomiting
- Breathing problems or irregularities
- Unequal pupils

Do This First

For a responsive victim:

1 Have the victim lie down.

2 Keep the victim still and protect him or her from becoming chilled or overheated.

3 Call 9-1-1 and monitor the victim's condition until help arrives.

4 Support the head and neck, even in a responsive victim, if you suspect a spinal injury.

For an unresponsive victim:

1 Call 9-1-1.

2 Check the victim's breathing without moving the victim unless necessary. Suspect there may be a spinal injury.

3 Control serious bleeding and cover any wounds with a dressing.

(ALERT))

- Do not let the victim eat or drink anything.

serious signs and symptoms may occur over time. Therefore it is important to seek medical care for all suspected brain injuries. If a brain injury may be possible, call 9-1-1 and keep the victim still and give supportive care while waiting for help to arrive. In no situation should a victim with a suspected head injury, no matter how mild, continue an activity, such as a sport, in which a second injury may occur (see **Box 13-1**).

Box 13-1 Second Impact Syndrome

The CDC reports that an estimated 300,000 concussions occur each year during sports activities. Such brain injuries are more likely to occur in contact sports such as football. In the last two decades, sports physicians have become increasingly aware of the fact that a second head impact after even a mild concussion can cause severe brain swelling that may lead to death. In the 1990s, for example, a high school and a college football player both died of brain swelling after a second impact. In both cases the first injury was so mild that the player reported only a headache to friends or family members—and did not tell the coach at all—before returning to play. Even mild injuries can have this cumulative fatal effect. Since an athlete with only a mild concussion may not tell anyone at all, statistics are lacking for how often second impact syndrome occurs, although over 20 cases have been described in the medical literature.

The problem occurs in part because it is difficult to diagnose a concussion quickly and to know whether it is safe for the player to get back into the game. Pressure from coaches and other players to stay in the game may contribute to an athlete's not admitting to a mild injury.

There is hope, however, that the situation may improve with a new device that may be able to determine on the athletic field within minutes whether a player has a mild head injury. The device, called DETECT (for "display enhanced testing for concussions and mild traumatic brain injury system"), began testing in 2005. The device conducts several neuropsychological tests such as showing the person series of shapes and words to test for short-term memory, response time, and other cognitive abilities. The device is worn like a helmet and screens out sounds and visual stimuli that often make it difficult to assess an athlete's mental status on the often noisy, congested, distracting athletic field.

Learning
Checkpoint ①

1. List two or three signs of a possible skull fracture. What is one thing you should *not* do to stop bleeding from the head if you suspect a skull fracture?

_____

2. True or False: You can easily distinguish a mild concussion from a serious brain injury by the signs and symptoms.

3. Check off the possible signs and symptoms of a brain injury:

____ Headache   ____ Fingernail beds look blue

____ Rapid blinking   ____ Dizziness or confusion

____ Memory loss   ____ Nausea and vomiting

4. The one sure way to know whether the victim has a spinal injury is

    a. pain in the neck.

    b. headache.

    c. unresponsiveness.

    d. None of the above

5. How long after a blow to the head might signs and symptoms of a more serious injury appear?

_____

SPINAL INJURIES

A fracture of the neck or back is a spinal injury. These injuries are always serious because of possible damage to the **spinal cord,** the bundle of nerves that runs down from the base of the skull and through the neck to branch off to all parts of the body. As **Figure 13-2** shows, these nerves pass through openings in the **vertebrae,** the bones of the neck and back. Even a small displacement or fracture of these bones can damage the soft tissue of the spinal cord or the nerves that lead from the cord to the body. Spinal injuries are so serious because the spinal cord, unlike bones and some soft tissues, cannot grow back to heal the injury. Although medical care can improve the condition of a victim with partially damaged nerves, if the spinal cord is severed by the injury, the victim will have permanent paralysis and loss of function.

The effects of nerve damage caused by a spinal injury depend on the nature and location of the injury. In general, body functions con-

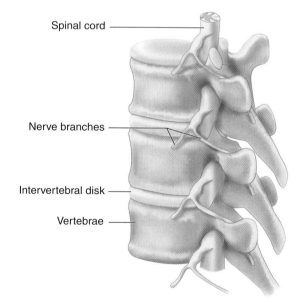

Figure 13-2 The spinal cord passes through openings in the vertebrae. Nerve branches exit the spinal cord to reach all body areas.

trolled by nerves exiting the spinal cord below the level of injury may be affected. An injury to the lower spine may result in paralysis of the legs, for example, while an injury to the spinal cord at a higher level may paralyze the arms as well as the legs. If the nerves controlling the muscles involved in breathing are damaged, the victim may have a life-threatening breathing problem. Any spinal cord damage can cause permanent paralysis.

Although an injury to the spine may cause immediate nerve damage with immediate signs and symptoms, in some cases nerve damage may not yet have occurred. For example, a fractured vertebra in the neck could put the nerves of the spinal cord at risk for damage if the neck vertebrae were to move. The victim may not have signs and symptoms of a spinal injury, but if the neck were moved carelessly, fractured bone could damage nerve tissue and cause permanent paralysis or a life-threatening condition. Similarly, when signs and symptoms of spinal nerve damage are present, movement of the head or neck could make the injury worse. Therefore it is critical to prevent head and neck movement in all victims suspected of having a spinal injury.

The primary care for a suspected spinal cord injury is to prevent movement of the spine by preventing movement of the head, neck, and body. Unless you must move the victim, support the victim's head in the position in which you find the victim **(Figure 13-3)**. Although it is generally better for the head to be in line with the body, *do not move the victim's head to put it in line with the body.* Damage to the spinal cord and nerves could be worsened by any unnecessary movement of the head. When the victim's head is already in line with the body when you reach the scene, support it in that position in line; this can be done with the victim lying down or sitting up. This technique is called **inline stabilization,** which simply means to prevent movement of the head by supporting it manually in line with the body (see Skill: "Inline Stabilization"). A responsive victim is likely to be in this position, and you should encourage the victim not to move while you provide support. If the victim is unresponsive and must be moved in order to give CPR, keep the head in line with the body while you move the victim with assistance from others.

While supporting the victim's head manually until help arrives, continue to maintain the victim's open airway if needed, and monitor the victim's breathing (see First Aid: "Spinal Injuries").

Positioning the Victim

Generally you support the victim's head and neck in the position found. Move the victim only if absolutely necessary. If the victim is lying on his or her back and vomits, you must roll the victim onto his or her side to let the mouth drain and allow breathing. If the victim is lying on his or her side or face down and

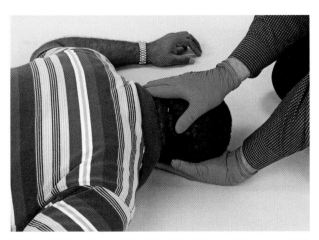
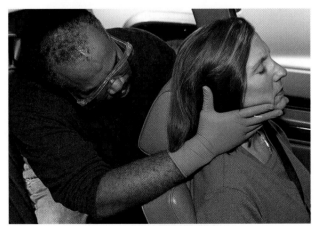

Figure 13-3 Support the head in the position in which you find the victim.

Skill | **Inline Stabilization**

1 Assess a responsive victim for spinal injury.

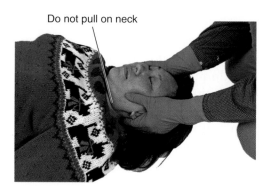

Do not pull on neck

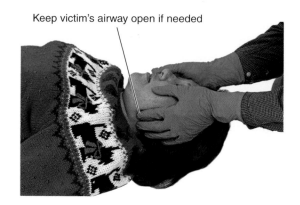

Keep victim's airway open if needed

2 Hold the victim's head with both hands to prevent movement of neck or spine.

3 Monitor the victim's breathing.

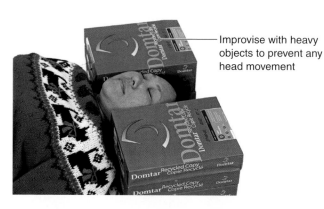

Improvise with heavy objects to prevent any head movement

4 If needed, use objects to maintain head support.

---

requires CPR, you must move the victim onto his or her back.

The help of two or three others is necessary to keep the back and neck aligned during the move. The technique called a log roll is used by mul-tiple rescuers to turn the victim while keeping the head supported in line with the body (see Skill: "Rolling a Victim with Spinal Injury [Log Roll]"). Continue to monitor the victim's breathing until help arrives.

When You See

For a responsive victim:

- Inability to move any body part
- Tingling or a lack of sensation in hands or feet
- Deformed neck or back
- Breathing problems
- Headache

For an unresponsive victim:

- Deformed neck or back
- Signs of blow to head or back
- Nature of the emergency suggests possible spinal injury

Do This First

1 Assess a responsive victim:
- Can the victim move his or her fingers and toes?
- Can the victim feel you touch his or her hands and feet?

2 Stabilize the victim's head and neck manually in the position found.

3 Monitor the victim's breathing. Keep the airway open if necessary in an unresponsive victim.

4 Send someone to call 9-1-1.

5 For a long wait, or if you must leave the victim to call 9-1-1, use padding or heavy objects on both sides of the head to prevent movement.

Additional Care

- Reassure a responsive victim and tell him or her not to move.
- Continue to monitor the victim's breathing until help arrives.

If you are alone and the victim vomits, move him or her into the HAINES recovery position, supporting the head and neck at all times.

Injuries to Lower Back

Spinal injuries include lower back injuries that may not damage the spinal cord or be as serious as other spinal injuries. Such injuries generally occur as a result of a stressful activity rather than a traumatic injury such as a fall or blow to the head or neck. For example, the victim may have been lifting or moving a heavy object or working in an unusual position. A strained muscle or ligament may

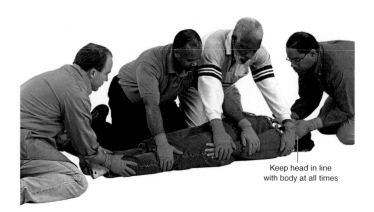

Keep head in line
with body at all times

1   Hold the victim's head with hands on both sides
over ears.

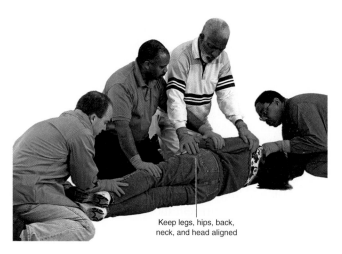

Keep legs, hips, back,
neck, and head aligned

2   The first aider at the victim's head directs others
to roll the body as a unit.

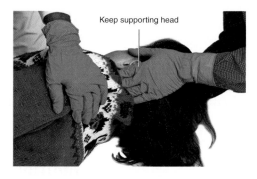

Keep supporting head

3   Continue to support head in new
position on side.

result, or a disk (soft tissue between vertebrae) may be damaged. Such injuries may not
be emergencies, although often they require
medical attention.

Signs and symptoms of a less serious lower
back injury may include sharp pain in the
lower back, stiffness and reduced movement
in the back, and possible sharp pain in one
leg. If any of the signs and symptoms of a
spinal injury are present, call 9-1-1 and keep
the victim from moving. Otherwise, the victim
should see a healthcare provider.

Learning
Checkpoint ②

1. True or False: Suspect a spinal injury in any victim with a serious head injury.

2. For an unresponsive victim you suspect may have a spinal injury,

    a. immediately place the victim on his or her back in case you have to give CPR.

    b. check the victim's breathing in the position in which you found the victim.

    c. turn the head to one side in case the victim vomits.

    d. move all body parts to see if anything feels broken.

3. A spinal injury should be suspected in which of these situations? (Check all that apply.)

    _____ The victim fell from a roof 20 feet high.

    _____ A victim with diabetes passes out at lunch.

    _____ The victim was in a car that hit a telephone pole.

    _____ A piece of heavy equipment fell from a shelf on the victim's head.

    _____ You find a victim slumped over in a desk chair.

4. Which of these are signs and symptoms of a spinal injury? (Check all that apply.)

    _____ Victim cannot stop coughing.   _____ Victim's face is bright red.

    _____ Victim's hands are tingling.   _____ Unresponsive victim has a fever.

    _____ Victim has breathing problem.   _____ Victim's neck seems oddly turned.

5. When do you call 9-1-1 for a victim with a potential spinal injury?

    a. Call for all victims with potential spinal injury.

    b. Call only if the victim is unresponsive.

    c. Call for a responsive victim only if feeling is lost on one side of the victim's body.

    d. Call after waiting 10 minutes to see if an unresponsive victim awakes.

6. In what position do you stabilize the head of a victim with a suspected spinal injury?

_____

7. Roll a victim with a spinal injury onto his or her side only if the victim _____ .

8. In the company parking lot you see a car skid on an icy patch and smash into another car. The driver is still behind the wheel and looks dazed. Her forehead is bleeding. You ask her how she feels and she does not answer but just stares ahead. What should you do?

_____

_____

Concluding Thoughts

Because of the risk of brain damage or paralysis, head and spinal injuries can be frightening experiences. Most important, remember that you do not have to assess the injury with certainty before acting. Any time you suspect a victim has a head or spinal injury, call 9-1-1 and keep the victim still until help arrives.

Learning Outcomes

You should now be able to do the following:

1. List the signs and symptoms of head and spinal injuries.

2. Perform a physical examination of a victim with head or spinal injury.

3. Describe the first aid for a victim with a possible brain injury.

4. Explain why a victim with a possible spinal injury should not be moved unnecessarily.

5. Perform manual inline stabilization.

6. With other rescuers, perform a log roll of a victim with a spinal injury.

Review Questions

1. Assessing a victim with a potential head or spinal injury includes
   a. considering the cause of the injury.
   b. asking the victim to turn his or her head to the side.
   c. assessing how the victim holds his or her head when sitting.
   d. comparing skin color in different parts of the body.

2. Which of the following is *not* a sign or symptom of a possible head or spinal injury?
   a. Unequal pupils
   b. Sudden red rash around neck
   c. Tingling in hands
   d. Headache

3. What is the best way to stop bleeding from the scalp at the site of a skull fracture?
   a. Apply direct pressure on the wound.
   b. Apply indirect pressure on the pulse point in the neck.
   c. Apply pressure only around the edges of the wound.
   d. Tightly bandage the wound but do not apply pressure at all.

4. What is the one sure way to know whether a head injury victim has a serious brain injury?
   a. The victim feels temporarily confused.
   b. The victim is acting unusually.
   c. The victim was briefly unconscious.
   d. There is no certain way.

5. A spinal cord injury can cause
   a. paralysis.
   b. a breathing problem.
   c. numbness in feet.
   d. All of the above

6. You find an unresponsive victim at the base of a ladder with his head turned to one side. He is breathing. You should
   a. support the head in the position found.
   b. gently move the head in line with the body.
   c. roll the victim onto his side.
   d. try to move his body in line with his head.

7. In your physical examination of a victim with a suspected spinal injury, the victim squeezes your hand only very softly with her left hand. To further assess this victim you can
   a. squeeze her hand hard and ask what she feels.
   b. ask her to squeeze with both hands at the same time and compare them.
   c. ask her to snap her fingers with her left hand.
   d. have her clasp her hands together and pull with each, to see which arm pulls the other.

8. When might you have to move a victim with a suspected spinal injury?
   a. To position the victim for CPR
   b. To drain vomit from the victim's mouth
   c. To escape an encroaching fire
   d. All of the above

9. When should you call 9-1-1 for a suspected spinal injury?
   a. Call only if the victim is unresponsive.
   b. Call only if the victim is unresponsive, or if a responsive victim is experiencing a severe headache.
   c. Call for any suspected spinal injury.
   d. Call if no one else is present to help you transport the victim to the emergency department.

References and Resources

American College of Emergency Physicians. *First aid manual: a comprehensive guide to treating emergency victims of all ages in any situation.* New York: DK Publishing; 2001.

American Heart Association. 2005 International consensus on cardiopulmonary resuscitation (CPR) and emergency cardiovascular care (ECC) science with treatment recommendations. *Circulation,* 112(22). November 29, 2005.

American Medical Association. *Handbook of first aid and emergency care.* Revised edition. New York: Random House; 2000.

Basic Trauma Life Support International. www.btls.org

Campbell JE. *Basic trauma life support.* Upper Saddle River, New Jersey: Pearson Prentice Hall; 2004.

Centers for Disease Control and Prevention. Sports-related recurrent brain injuries—United States. 2005. www.cdc.gov

JAMA Patient Page: Head injury—protecting against head injuries. *Journal of the American Medical Association* 1999; 282. www.medem.com

National Association of Emergency Medical Technicians. *Basic and advanced prehospital trauma life support.* Revised 5th edition. St. Louis: Mosby; 2003.

National Center for Injury Prevention and Control. Spinal cord injury: fact sheet, 2005. www.cdc.gov/ncipc/factsheets

National Safety Council. www.nsc.org

Portable device to check for concussions. www.news-medical.net

Prehospital trauma life support. www.phtls.org

Chapter 14

Chest, Abdominal, and Pelvic Injuries

Chapter Preview

- Chest Injuries

- Abdominal Injuries

- Pelvic Injuries

The car in front of you suddenly swerves to the right and runs into the back of a parked car. Fortunately, it was not moving very fast at the time. You pull over and get out to see if you can help. The driver is slumped forward against the steering wheel, apparently not wearing a seat belt and shoulder harness. As you approach, he at first seems unresponsive, but then he leans back and opens the car door. He gets out, holding his chest on one side, and staggers a few feet before you reach him. He does not seem to be bleeding, but obviously he is in pain. What do you do?

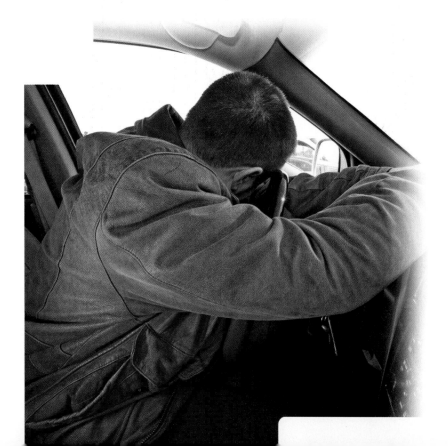

Injuries to the chest, abdomen, or pelvis can result from either blunt or penetrating forces. Blunt trauma typically occurs from motor vehicle crashes, falls, industrial emergencies, fights, and similar events. Open injuries can result from any object that breaks the skin, including gunshots and stab wounds. Both closed and open injuries to the chest, abdomen, and pelvis can be life threatening when bleeding is severe or internal organs are injured. Shock often occurs. Always call 9-1-1 for these injuries.

CHEST INJURIES

The chest contains many important structures that may be damaged with a chest injury, including the heart, lungs, and large blood vessels. Trauma may injure the chest wall, including the ribs and soft tissues or structures within the chest, or both. Serious chest injuries include broken ribs, objects impaled in the chest, and sucking chest wounds in which air passes in and out of the chest cavity. These wounds can be life threatening if breathing is affected. Chest injuries may result from such things as:

- Striking the steering wheel in a motor vehicle crash
- A blow to the chest
- A fall from a height
- Sports injuries
- Physical assault
- A penetrating injury or impaled object

The general signs and symptoms of a serious chest injury include:

- Breathing problems
- Severe pain
- Bruising, swelling
- Deformity of the chest
- Coughing blood

Because the condition of a victim with a chest injury may be life threatening and may worsen over time, it is essential to continue checking the victim's breathing and provide basic life support as needed. The forces involved may also suggest the possibility of a spinal injury. In addition, specific first aid is given for the particular injury.

Closed Chest Injuries

Common chest injuries involving the lungs include pneumothorax and hemothorax, which may occur with either open or closed injuries. In a pneumothorax, air escapes from an injured lung into the thoracic cavity—the space inside the chest around the lungs—causing collapse of some or all of the lung and resulting in respiratory distress. In a hemothorax, blood from an injury accumulates in the thoracic cavity, compressing the lung and causing respiratory distress and possibly shock.

The fact that the skin is not broken in a closed chest injury does not mean that there is not serious underlying damage. Because organ damage or internal bleeding could be serious, call 9-1-1 and monitor the victim's breathing while waiting for help to arrive. In an unresponsive victim, maintain an open airway and keep checking breathing. Let a responsive victim find the position that is most comfortable and allows for easiest breathing.

Broken Ribs

Rib fractures typically result from blunt trauma to the chest. Rib fractures are more common in the lower ribs and along the side. Rib fractures usually cause severe pain, discoloration, and swelling at the site of the fracture. The pain is often sharper upon breathing in, and the victim may be breathing shallowly. Another sign of a rib fracture is the victim holding or supporting the area. Many rib fractures involve only the fracture, but with severe trauma there may also be injuries to the lungs or other underlying organs (**Figure 14-1**). Because of the possibility of serious injury and the risk that the injury may become worse with movement, always call 9-1-1 for a rib fracture.

The first aid for rib fractures is primarily supportive. Let a responsive victim assume a

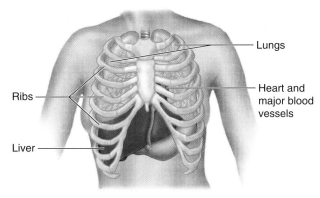

Figure 14-1 The rib cage protects underlying organs in the chest.

Labels: Lungs; Heart and major blood vessels; Ribs; Liver

First Aid **Broken Ribs**

When You See

- Signs of pain with deep breathing or movement
- Victim holding ribs
- Shallow breathing

Do This First

1 Have person sit or stand in position of easiest breathing.

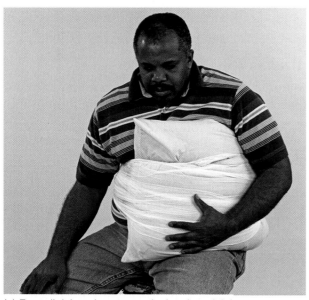

(a) For a rib injury do not wrap the bandage tightly.

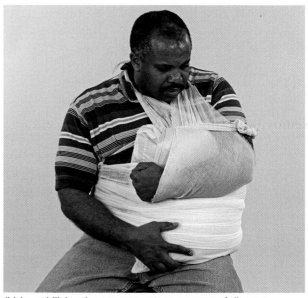

(b) Immobilizing the arm prevents movement of rib area.

2 Support the ribs with a pillow or soft padding loosely bandaged over the area and under the arm.

3 Call 9-1-1.

Additional Care

- Monitor the victim's breathing while waiting for help
- If helpful, immobilize the arm with a sling and binder (**see Chapter 16**) to prevent movement and ease pain

comfortable position. The victim may sit or stand and often leans toward the side of the injury with an arm compressed against the rib. Use a pillow or blanket to help immobilize the area and reduce pain. Do not tightly wrap a bandage or padding around the chest, because this could restrict breathing (see First Aid: "Broken Ribs").

Flail Chest

A **flail chest** is the fracture of two or more ribs in two or more places **(Figure 14-2)**. Flail chest usually results from a severe blow to the chest. The injury actually separates a segment of the chest wall from the remainder of the chest.

With breathing, the flail segment moves in the opposite direction from the rest of the chest wall in what is called **paradoxical movement.** This part of the chest wall moves outward during exhalation because of the increased pressure within the chest. During inhalation the segment moves inward. The larger the flail segment, the greater the threat to the victim's respiratory function.

First aid for flail chest includes monitoring the victim's breathing and supporting the affected chest area with a bulky dressing, towel, or pillow secured with tape or bandages (see First Aid: "Flail Chest").

Impaled Object

Removing an impaled object from the chest could cause additional bleeding, injury, and breathing problems. Leave the object in place and use bulky dressings bandaged around the object, as described in **Chapter 9**. Call 9-1-1 and treat the victim for shock (see **Chapter 10**). Monitor the victim's breathing while waiting for help to arrive (see First Aid: "Impaled Object").

Sucking Chest Wound

A **sucking chest wound** is an open wound in the chest caused by a penetrating injury that lets air move in and out of the chest during breathing. When the chest expands during inhalation, the pressure inside the chest decreases, and air is sucked in through the wound. When the chest contracts during exhalation, air is forced out through the wound. You may hear a gurgling or sucking sound and may see air bubbles in the blood around the wound.

A sucking chest wound can be life threatening because breathing can be affected. First aid includes sealing the wound to help the victim to maintain adequate respiratory function. The dressed wound should be covered with an **occlusive** dressing such as plastic food wrap, a plastic bag, or a piece of aluminum foil. This occlusive dressing should be taped on three sides, with the fourth left open **(Figure 14-3)**. This kind of dressing prevents air from being sucked into the chest, allowing more normal breathing, while allowing allow air to escape from the wound, to prevent a buildup of pressure in the chest (see First Aid: "Sucking Chest Wound").

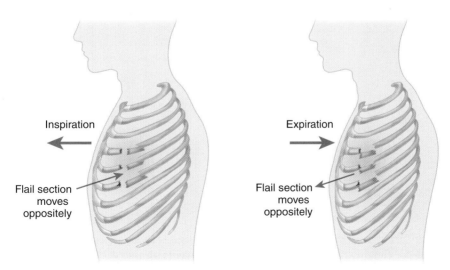

Figure 14-2 In flail chest, a section of the chest wall moves in and out opposite to the normal motion of breathing.

First Aid   **Flail Chest**

When You See
- Victim holding ribs
- Shallow breathing
- Paradoxical movement of chest segment
- Severe pain
- Swelling or chest deformity

Do This First

1 Have person lie down or sit in position of easiest breathing.

2 Splint the flail area with a small pillow or thick padding loosely bandaged in place (but not completely around the chest).

3 Position the victim lying on the injured side to give more support to the area.

4 Call 9-1-1.

Additional Care
- If padding is not available to splint the flail area, support it with pressure from your hand.
- Monitor the victim until help arrives.

On inspiration, dressing seals wound, preventing air entry.

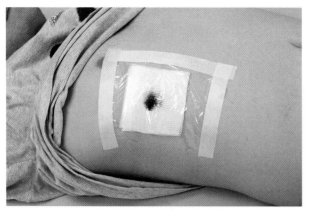
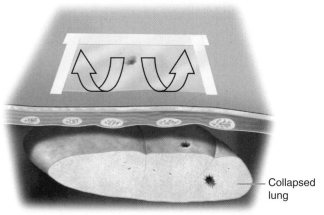

Collapsed lung

Figure 14-3 First aid for sucking chest wound. (a) Tape only three sides to let air escape from a sucking chest wound. (b) When victim breathes in, the dressing seals the wound and prevents air entry.

First Aid   **Impaled Object**

When You See

- An object impaled in a chest wound

Do This First

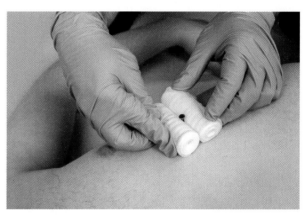

1 Keep victim still. Victim may be seated or lying down.

2 Use bulky dressings or cloth to stabilize the object.

3 Bandage the area around the object.

4 Call 9-1-1.

((ALERT))

- Do not give the victim anything to eat or drink.

Additional Care

- Reassure the victim.
- Monitor the victim's breathing until help arrives.

First Aid   Sucking Chest Wound

When You See

- Air moving in or out of a penetrating chest wound
- Sucking sounds on inhalation

Do This First

1 Put a thin, sterile dressing over the wound.

2 Cover the dressing with a plastic wrap or bag to make an airtight seal. As the victim exhales, tape it in place on three sides, leaving one side untaped to let exhaled air escape.

3 Position victim lying down inclined toward the injured side, or in a position for easiest breathing.

4 Call 9-1-1.

Additional Care

- If the victim's breathing becomes more difficult, remove the plastic bandage to let air escape; then reapply it.
- If an occlusive dressing is not available, cover the wound with your gloved hand during inhalation to prevent air from entering the chest.
- Monitor the victim's breathing until help arrives.
- Treat the victim for shock.

Learning Checkpoint ①

1. True or False: Broken ribs are treated by taping the entire rib cage tightly.

2. Immobilize the arm of a victim with a rib fracture to

   a. prevent movement.

   b. ease pain.

   c. help immobilize that side of the chest.

   d. All of the above

Learning
Checkpoint 1 *(continued)*

3. What should you do with a screwdriver you see embedded in the chest of an unresponsive friend after an explosion in his garage?

_____

4. A gunshot victim has a small, bleeding hole in the right side of his chest. You open his shirt to treat the bleeding and see air bubbles forming in the hole as air escapes. How do you dress this wound?

_____

ABDOMINAL INJURIES

Abdominal injuries include closed and open wounds that result from a blow to the abdomen or a fall. Because large blood vessels are present within the abdomen along with many organs, injury may cause internal and/or external bleeding. The abdominal cavity is not protected from injury as the chest is by the ribs. The posterior abdomen is afforded some protection by the spine and lower part of the rib cage, but the anterior abdomen is relatively unprotected **(Figure 14-4)**. Internal organs may be damaged, and organs may protrude from an open wound.

The external appearance of an injured abdomen can sometimes be deceptive, even when serious or life-threatening injuries to organs are present. Often the only indication of abdominal injury is a small bruise or wound. Because of the potential for serious injury, all abdominal wounds should be regarded as potentially life threatening and treated accordingly.

Closed Abdominal Injury

A closed abdominal injury can threaten life because internal organs may have ruptured and there may be serious internal bleeding. Blunt abdominal trauma commonly occurs in motor vehicle crashes but may also result from sports injuries, falls, physical assault, or industrial emergencies.

The signs and symptoms of abdominal trauma can vary. Often, the only symptom is pain. The physical examination may reveal bruising or an obvious abdominal wound. If

bleeding is severe, shock may also be present and the abdomen may appear very firm, almost rigid. Abdominal muscles may also contract to minimize movement or agitation of the affected site, a condition called guarding.

First aid for a victim with an abdominal injury includes monitoring the victim's breathing and giving supportive care as well as first aid for an open wound. Do not move the victim, who should try to avoid coughing or straining. The victim may feel more comfortable with the knees slightly bent because this position lessens tension in abdominal

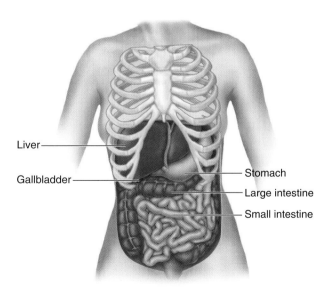

Figure 14-4 Abdominal organs have little protection from injury.

Liver

Gallbladder

Stomach

Large intestine

Small intestine

First Aid   Closed Abdominal Injury

When You See

- Signs of severe pain, tenderness in area, victim protecting the abdomen
- Bruising
- Swollen or rigid abdomen
- Rapid, shallow breathing
- Nausea, vomiting

Do This First

1 Carefully position the victim on his or her back and loosen any tight clothing.

2 Allow the victim to bend knees slightly if this eases the pain; put support under the knees.

3 Call 9-1-1.

4 Treat the victim for shock and monitor the victim's breathing.

ALERT

- Do not let the victim eat or drink.

Additional Care

- Continue to monitor the victim's breathing until help arrives.

---

muscles. Unless you suspect a spinal injury, slightly elevate the patient's feet. Keep the victim warm. Do not give the victim anything to eat or drink because emergency surgery may be needed (see First Aid: "Closed Abdominal Injury").

Open Abdominal Wound

An open abdominal injury usually injures internal organs such as the intestines, liver, kidneys, or stomach. A large wound in the abdominal wall may allow abdominal organs to protrude through the wound (**Figure 14-5**);

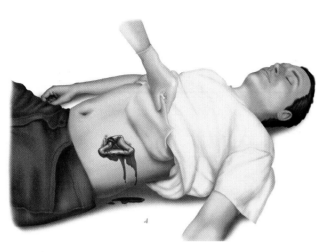

Figure 14-5 Open abdominal wound.

this is called **evisceration.** This is a serious emergency because organs can be further damaged by drying out, bleeding from associated blood vessels, or infection.

First aid includes positioning the victim as with a closed abdominal injury and providing wound care and treatment for shock. If abdominal organs are protruding through an open wound, do not touch them or try to push them back into the abdomen. Do not pack the wound with dressings. Instead, cover the wound with a dry, nonadherent dressing or a moist, sterile dressing, and cover with an occlusive dressing or plastic wrap loosely taped in place to keep the organs from drying (see First Aid: "Open Abdominal Wound").

Learning
Checkpoint ②

1. After a sports injury you find an unresponsive victim on the ground. Which of the following are signs and symptoms he may have a closed abdominal injury? (Check all that apply.)

_____ Bruises below the rib cage   _____ Blotchy skin around the eyes

_____ Abrasions on the chest   _____ Swollen abdomen

_____ Skin feels hot all over   _____ Tight skin around the neck

2. Describe the best position in which to put a victim with either an open or closed abdominal wound.

_____

3. True or False: To treat a victim for shock, help maintain normal body temperature.

4. If the victim has an organ protruding from an open abdominal wound, what should you do?

   a. Push the organ back into the abdomen.

   b. Spray clean water over the organ to keep it moist.

   c. Leave the wound exposed to the air.

   d. Cover the wound with a nonadherent dressing and plastic wrap.

5. In what circumstances do you call 9-1-1 for a victim with an open or closed abdominal wound?

_____

First Aid | Open Abdominal Wound

When You See

- Open abdominal wound
- Bleeding
- Severe pain
- Organs possibly protruding from wound
- Signs of shock

Do This First

1 Lay the victim on his or her back and loosen any tight clothing. Allow the victim to bend knees slightly if this eases the pain.

2 Cover the wound with a dry, nonadherent dressing or a moist, sterile dressing.

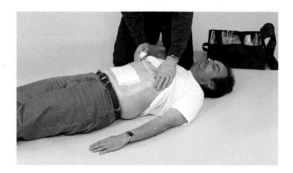

3 Cover the dressing with a large, occlusive dressing or plastic wrap, taped loosely in place. Then cover the area with a blanket or towel to help maintain warmth.

4 Call 9-1-1.

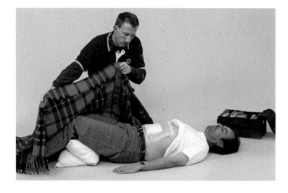

5 Treat the victim for shock and monitor the victim's breathing.

 ALERT

- Do not push protruding organs back inside the abdomen, but keep them from drying out with an occlusive dressing or plastic covering.
- Do not apply direct pressure on the wound.

Additional Care

- Monitor the victim until help arrives.

PELVIC INJURIES

The most common pelvic injury is fracture of the pelvis. Such fractures in healthy adults are usually caused only by large forces, which are likely to cause other injuries as well. Pelvic fractures are more common in the elderly and may be caused by lesser forces, such as falls. Pelvic fractures are generally very serious. A broken pelvis may cause severe internal bleeding and organ damage. A broken pelvis can be life threatening. With severe bleeding the victim may be in shock.

A victim with a pelvic fracture cannot move and often has severe pain. In the physical examination you may note instability in the pelvic area. The victim may be bleeding from the genitalia or rectum or leaking urine.

Because of the large forces that typically cause the injury, consider that the victim may also have a spinal injury, and support the head and neck accordingly. The care for a suspected pelvic fracture is primarily supportive. Do not move the victim or let the victim move. Take steps to minimize shock, including maintaining the victim's body temperature, but do not elevate the legs (see First Aid: "Pelvic Injuries").

First Aid   **Pelvic Injuries**

When You See

- Signs of pain and tenderness around the hips
- Inability to walk or stand
- Signs and symptoms of shock

Do This First

1 Help the victim lie quietly on the back and bend knees slightly if this eases the pain.

2 Call 9-1-1.

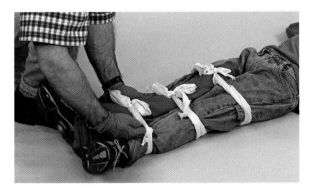

3 If help may be delayed, immobilize the victim's legs by padding between the legs and then bandaging them together, unless this causes more pain.

4 Treat the victim for shock.

Additional Care

- Monitor the victim until help arrives.
- Care for any open wounds, such as wounds to the genitals.

Learning
Checkpoint ③

1. First aid for a pelvic fracture prevents _____ of the area.

2. True or False: Internal bleeding can be severe with a broken pelvis.

3. True or False: Bending the victim's knees slightly may ease the pain of a broken pelvis.

Concluding Thoughts

Victims with serious injuries to the chest, abdomen, or pelvis usually have experienced significant trauma, and often there are injuries to internal organs you cannot observe. The victim may have other wounds or injuries as well, complicating the situation. Most important, ensure that 9-1-1 is called immediately to get help on the way. Then care for any life-threatening conditions first and provide specific first aid for the injuries.

Learning Outcomes

You should now be able to do the following:

1. Explain why chest injuries may be life threatening, and list the general signs and symptoms of chest injuries.

2. Describe the specific first aid steps for broken ribs, flail chest, an impaled object in the chest, and a sucking chest wound.

3. Describe the signs and symptoms of a closed abdominal injury and the first aid to give.

4. Explain how to care for an open abdominal wound.

5. Describe the signs and symptoms of a pelvic fracture and the first aid to give.

Review Questions

1. Chest injuries may be life threatening because
   a. breathing may be affected.
   b. rib fractures usually involve nerve damage.
   c. chest abrasions can bleed heavily.
   d. All of the above

2. First aid for a rib fracture includes
   a. tightly bandaging around the chest to prevent movement.
   b. using a pillow or blanket to help support the area.
   c. taping the arm against the side down to the waist.
   d. applying rigid splints on both sides of the thorax.

3. When should an impaled object be removed from the chest wall?
   a. Always
   b. Only when there is no heavy bleeding around it
   c. Only when air bubbles from the lungs are escaping around it
   d. Never

4. The dressing and bandage over a sucking chest wound should
   a. allow air to escape but prevent air from being sucked in.
   b. allow air to be sucked in but prevent air from escaping.

c. allow air to flow in and out of the wound.

d. prevent air from flowing in or out of the wound.

5. Which of the following is a sign of a closed abdominal injury with severe internal bleeding?

   a. Breathing is slow and very deep.

   b. The area of skin below the umbilicus looks red.

   c. The abdomen feels hard.

   d. The victim always has a fever.

6. The position that is usually most comfortable for a victim with an abdominal injury is

   a. curled up on side in fetal position.

   b. lying on back with knees slightly bent.

   c. lying on back with knees straight.

   d. lying face down.

7. Internal organs protruding from an abdominal wound should be protected by

   a. covering them with a clean, dry cloth.

   b. covering them with a sterile, moist dressing.

   c. pushing them back into the body.

   d. placing the victim's hand over them.

8. What should you do if you suspect the victim has a pelvic fracture?

   a. See if the victim can stand up.

   b. Carefully roll the victim into a face-down position.

   c. Elevate the legs to prevent shock.

   d. Keep the victim still and call 9-1-1.

References and Resources

American College of Emergency Physicians. *First aid manual: a comprehensive guide to treating emergency victims of all ages in any situation.* New York: DK Publishing; 2001.

American Heart Association. 2005 International consensus on cardiopulmonary resuscitation (CPR) and emergency cardiovascular care (ECC) science with treatment recommendations. *Circulation,* 112(22). November 29, 2005.

American Medical Association. *Handbook of first aid and emergency care.* Revised edition. New York: Random House; 2000.

Basic Trauma Life Support International. www.btls.org

Campbell JE. *Basic trauma life support.* Upper Saddle River, New Jersey Pearson Prentice Hall; 2004.

National Association of Emergency Medical Technicians. *Basic and advanced prehospital trauma life support.* Revised 5th ed. St. Louis: Mosby; 2003.

National Center for Injury Prevention and Control (NCIPC). www.cdc.gov/ncipc

National Safety Council. www.nsc.org

Prehospital Trauma Life Support. www.phtls.org

Chapter 15

Bone, Joint, and Muscle Injuries

Chapter Preview

- Prevention of Sports and Recreation Injuries
- Assessing Musculoskeletal Injuries
- General First Aid

- Fractures
- Joint Injuries
- Muscle Injuries

On a Saturday morning you are jogging the trail through a local park when you see a woman jogging some distance in front of you suddenly tumble to the ground. When you reach her, she is holding her ankle, which she says really hurts. She says she came down on the side of her foot and felt her ankle twist. She thinks it is sprained, but she doesn't know what to do. How can you help?

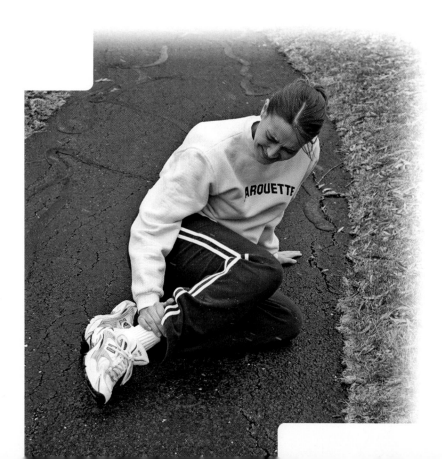

Injuries of the bones, joints, and muscles are among the most common injuries in the home, at work, and in sports and recreation (**Figure 15-1**). Injuries may result from a blow, the impact of a body part against an object or surface (as in a fall), or other forces acting on the body's bones, joints, or muscles. Most sports injuries are musculoskeletal injuries. Although this chapter focuses on first aid for more serious injuries, the most common musculoskeletal injuries are less serious, such as muscle strains resulting from overexertion, and they are seldom an emergency.

This chapter covers musculoskeletal injuries to the extremities. Injuries to the skull or spine are discussed in **Chapter 13**, and injuries to the rib cage and pelvis are discussed in **Chapter 14**.

Musculoskeletal injuries are generally classified as injuries of bones (**fractures**), **joints** (dislocations and sprains), or muscles (strains, contusions, cramps). A **dislocation** is movement of a bone out of its usual position in a joint. A **sprain** is a tearing of **ligaments** in a joint. A **strain** is the tearing of a muscle or **tendon,** and a **contusion** is a bruised muscle. It is not necessary to know the exact nature of the injury, however, to provide effective first aid. Remember always to assess the victim's breathing first and look for any threats to life before looking for musculoskeletal injuries.

PREVENTION OF SPORTS AND RECREATION INJURIES

Injuries from almost all sports and recreational activities are very common. Death from such injuries is very rare, usually caused by head injuries in victims not wearing helmets, but emergency department visits are very common (**Table 15-1**). In addition to causing pain and temporary disability, sports injuries may cause long-term or even permanent disabilities.

Preventing sports and recreational injuries begins with the correct use of sports equipment such as helmets and other protective wear and following established safety guidelines for the particular sport. No sport can be made 100% safe, however, and specific sports have certain risks for injury—a factor that should be considered by those involved and the parents of children. Sports medicine is increasingly investigating the long-term effects of some kinds of sports injuries, such as the potential for disabling conditions such as arthritis or pain from hairline fractures that appear years or decades after the injury.

To reduce the risk of injury, before beginning a strenuous new activity, check with a healthcare provider. In addition, to prevent common sprains and strains in sports and recreational activities, the Orthopedic Surgery Department of Massachusetts General Hospital recommends:

- Maintain a healthy, well-balanced diet to keep muscles strong.
- Maintain a healthy weight.
- Practice safety measures to help prevent falls (for example, keep stairways, walkways, yards, and driveways free of clutter, and salt or sand icy patches in the winter).
- Wear shoes that fit properly. Replace athletic shoes as soon as the tread wears out or the heel wears down on one side.
- Do stretching exercises daily.
- Be in proper physical condition to play a sport.

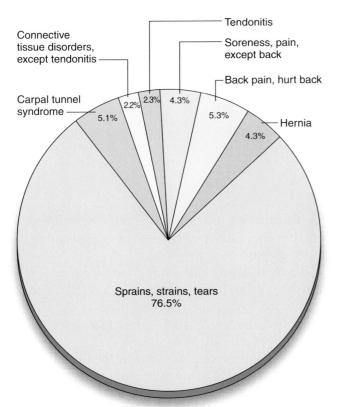

Figure 15-1 Musculoskeletal disorders causing days away from work by nature of injury or illness.

Table 15-1

Sports and Recreation Injuries Resulting in U.S. Emergency Department Visits per Year

Activity	Children 5 to 14[*]	All People Ages 5 to 24[**]
Group Sports		
Basketball	193,000	447,000
Football	186,000	271,000
Baseball/softball	116,000	245,000
Soccer	85,000	95,000
Other group sports	—	112,000
Individual Sports/Activities		
Bicycling	373,000	421,000
Ice/roller skating/boarding	99,000	150,000
Gymnastics/cheerleading	—	146,000
Playground injuries	—	137,000
Trampoline	68,000	—
Sledding/skiing/snowboarding	42,000	111,000
Water sports	—	100,000
Other individual sports/activities	—	381,000
All Sports/Recreation	—	2,616,000

Sources: [*]National Youth Sports Safety Foundation. Available from: http://www.nyssf.org
[**]National Center for Health Statistics, 2005. Available from: http://www.cdc.gov/nchs

- Warm up and stretch before participating in any sports or exercise.
- Wear protective equipment when playing.
- Avoid exercising or playing sports when tired or in pain.
- Run on even surfaces.

ASSESSING MUSCULOSKELETAL INJURIES

Remember to first perform the initial assessment of any victim and to care for any life-threatening conditions before performing a physical examination. Musculoskeletal injuries are usually not life threatening, except in cases of severe bleeding, but they may nonetheless be serious and result in pain and disability.

When assessing the injury, consider the type and size of the forces involved. Ask a responsive victim what happened and what he or she felt when the injury occurred. **Figure 15-2** describes common mechanisms of injury.

If large forces were involved in the injury, consider the potential also for a spinal injury, and assess the victim accordingly (see **Chapter 13**). Particularly if the victim is unresponsive, do not move him or her unnecessarily to assess a musculoskeletal injury.

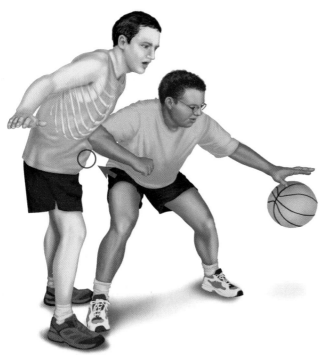

Direct forces, such as a blow to a bone, joint, or muscle, often injure that impacted area of the body; the larger the force, the more likely is a serious injury like a fracture.

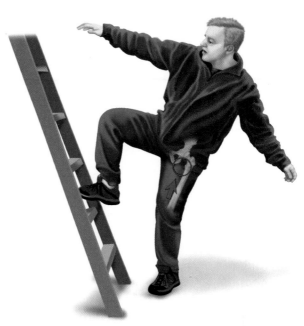

An indirect force may also be transferred up or down an extremity, as when falling on one leg. Similarly falling on an outstretched arm may cause dislocation of shoulder bones.

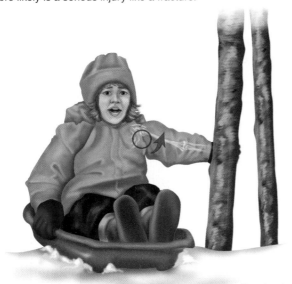

Twisting forces occur when the body moves in one direction but a force keeps some part of an extremity from moving with the rest of the body. Twisting forces may cause fractures or dislocations of bones at joints.

Figure 15-2 Common mechanisms of injury.

When you perform a physical examination on an injured extremity, remember to look for the following signs and symptoms (**Figure 15-3**). Compare the injured arm or leg to the opposite one.

- Pain when an area is touched
- Bleeding or other wounds
- Swelling
- An area that is deformed from its usual appearance (compare to other extremity)
- Skin discoloration
- Abnormal sensation (numbness, tingling)
- Inability to move the area
- Difference in temperature

In addition, with a fracture, you may hear the broken bone ends grating together, or the victim may feel them grinding together. This is called **crepitus.**

Remove the victim's clothing as needed to examine an injured area and check for an open wound that may require care. Pain occurs with most musculoskeletal injuries and may be more severe with serious injuries, although less painful injuries should not be assumed to be minor. When checking for the ability to move the extremities, do not ask the victim to move an injured area that causes pain. A lack of sensation in the injured area or below it (for example, the finger or toes) may be a symptom of a serious injury involving nerve damage. Swelling occurs in most musculoskeletal injuries because of

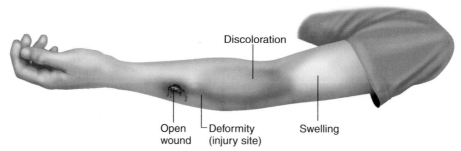

Figure 15-3 Signs of a musculoskeletal injury.

bleeding in injured tissues, but the amount of swelling is not a good indication of the severity of the injury. An obvious deformity or difference between the injured extremity and its uninjured opposite is usually a sign of a fracture or dislocation, both of which are serious injuries. Skin discoloration may include the "black and blue" color of bruising or a pale or light blue skin color (ashen in dark-skinned individuals) that, along with cool skin, may indicate a lack of blood flow below the injured area, a sign of a serious injury.

GENERAL FIRST AID

Later sections in this chapter describe the specific care for fractures, dislocations, sprains, strains, and other injuries. The general first aid for all musculoskeletal injuries is similar, however, based on the same principles of care. You do not have to know the specific type of injury before caring for the victim. The general first aid for most bone, joint, and muscle injuries involves four steps that are summarized in the acronym **RICE (Box 15-1):**

R = Rest

I = Ice

C = Compression

E = Elevation

Rest

Any movement of a musculoskeletal injury can cause further injury, pain, and swelling. With a fracture or dislocation, for example, any movement of the extremity could cause movement of the bone, further injuring soft tissues such as blood vessels and nerves around the bone. In addition, movement generally increases blood flow, which may increase internal bleeding and swelling. With serious injuries call 9-1-1 and have the victim rest until help arrives. Usually the victim can assume whatever position is the least painful. With less serious injuries, when the victim will be transported to a healthcare provider or home, minimize movement of the injured extremity as much as possible. With a fracture or dislocation, if medical care may be delayed or the victim must be moved, use a **splint** to immobilize the injured area, as described in **Chapter 16.**

Rest is also important for healing. The victim should follow the healthcare provider's advice to continue to rest the injured area after treatment.

Ice

Cold applied to a musculoskeletal injury reduces swelling, lessens pain, and minimizes bruising. Broken blood vessels constrict, reducing the bleeding into tissues. Nerves are numbed by cold, thereby reducing pain. Cold also helps relieve muscle spasms.

With any musculoskeletal injury other than an open fracture, put ice or a cold pack on the injury as soon as possible. Cubed or crushed ice in a plastic bag, a commercial cold pack, or an improvised cold pack such as a bag of frozen peas or a cloth pad soaked in cold water can be used. A cold pack that undergoes a phase change (melts) is preferred to refreez-

Box 15-1 RICE and Other Acronyms

RICE is a widely used acronym to help first aiders remember the treatment for most musculoskeletal injuries, but other acronyms also have been devised for the care of these injuries.

One that is becoming more commonly used now is PRICE, in which the P stands for protection. This is intended to remind the first aider also to protect the injured area by immobilizing it either with a splint (when appropriate) or by protecting the area from movement until the victim is seen by emergency personnel. (Some would argue that this protection is already implied by the R in RICE—resting the injured area.)

Other old standards are PIE (pressure, ice, elevation) and PIES (pressure, ice, elevation, splinting). The P for pressure is equivalent to the C for compression—both referring to wrapping the injury. Proponents of these acronyms suggest the R in RICE for rest is not necessary because the pain and discomfort of the injury will force the victim to rest the area, anyway. Still other acronyms that have been used as memory aids include ICE, ICES, and PRICES. Occasionally the same acronym has been defined in different ways, such as having I stand for ice in one definition but immobilization in another, and C for cold in one definition but compression in another.

What matters, of course, is remembering the first aid steps behind the acronym.

able gel packs. The ice or cold pack should be wrapped in cloth to prevent injury caused by cold in direct contact with the skin.

Cold works best if applied to the injury as soon as possible, preferably within 10 minutes. Apply it for 20 minutes each hour for the first few hours, then for 20 minutes at a time every 2 or 3 hours for the first 24 to 48 hours, or for 72 hours for severe injuries. For any injury for which the victim sees a healthcare provider, follow the provider's instructions for the use of cold (and later heat) after the injury and during the healing period **(Box 15-2)**.

Compression

Compression provides comfort and support and may prevent swelling. Compression of an injured extremity is done with an elastic roller bandage. Wrap the bandage over the injured area, starting at least two inches below the injury and using overlapping turns for at least two inches above the injury. The bandage should be firm but not so tight that it cuts off circulation. Compare the fingers or toes before the injury to those on the other extremity to ensure that circulation is not impeded by the bandage. If the fingers or toes look pale and feel cold compared to the other side, or feel numb or tingling, loosen the bandage (see Skill: "Applying a Spiral Bandage" and Skill: "Applying a Figure-Eight Bandage").

A compression bandage can also be applied around a cold pack. Remove the bandage just long enough to remove the cold pack after 20 minutes, and then rewrap it until it is time to apply cold again. Because in some cases swelling may increase after bandaging, causing the bandage to become tighter, it is necessary to continue checking the fingers or toes for circulation.

A compression bandage can be used for 24 to 48 hours as long as it is not too tight and the person can assess the injury to ensure that the bandage is not too tight.

Box 15-2 Cold First, Heat Later

People sometimes become confused about applying cold to an injury because they know heat is also used to treat musculoskeletal injuries. It is true that heat is beneficial for healing—just not soon after the injury.

Heat is beneficial for the healing of sprains and strains in part because it causes blood vessels to dilate, or enlarge, which allows more blood to reach the injured area. This increased circulation helps speed up the body's healing processes.

But heat should not be used for about three days, or until the initial swelling of the injury is diminished. Heat applied too early would have the opposite of the desired effect of cold: heat would encourage more internal bleeding because of the increased circulation, would increase swelling, and would make nerve endings more sensitive to pain. Follow your healthcare provider's guidelines and wait at least 72 hours after the injury, or until the swelling goes down, before soaking the injured area in warm water or applying a heat pad.

Elevation

Elevating an injured arm or leg uses gravity to help slow the blood flow to the injury, thereby helping minimize swelling and bleeding. First apply cold and a compression bandage, and then elevate the injured area above the level of the heart if possible (Figure 15-4). Do not try to elevate an extremity with a suspected fracture or dislocation—or move it at all—without first splinting it as described in **Chapter 16**. In all cases, elevate the injured extremity only if moving the limb does not cause pain (see Skill: "RICE: Wrist Injury").

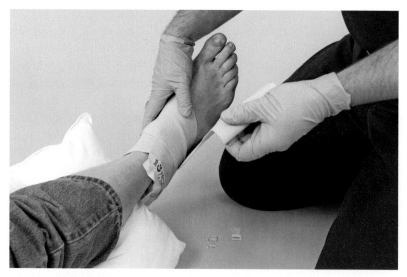

Figure 15-4 Remember the acronym RICE for treatment of musculoskeletal injuries.

Skill Applying a Spiral Bandage

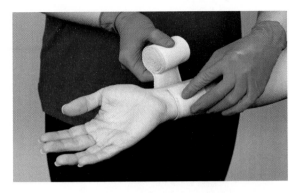

1 Anchor the starting end of the elastic roller bandage below the injured area, farther from the trunk.

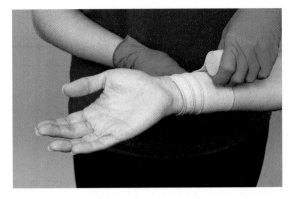

2 Wrap the bandage in spirals up the limb.

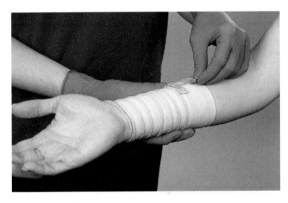

3 Fasten the end of the bandage with clips, tape, or safety pins.

Controversy in First Aid

Compression for Musculoskeletal Injuries

Compression provided by an elastic bandage wrapped around an extremity injury has long been believed to help reduce swelling and internal bleeding. In 2005, the National First Aid Science Advisory Board studied this issue and concluded that that there is insufficient evidence to recommend for or against using a compression bandage for such injuries. The scientific studies this group examined did not show a clear benefit for compression bandages, but they also did not show that harm might result from their use. It may be that sufficient scientific studies have not yet been performed to demonstrate a benefit.

Skill   **Applying a Figure-Eight Bandage**

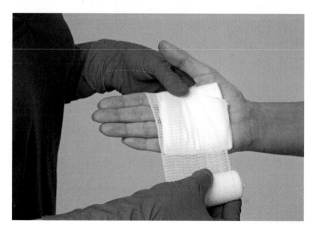

1   Anchor the starting end of the roller bandage.

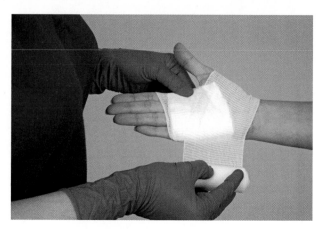

2   Turn the bandage diagonally across the wrist and back around the hand.

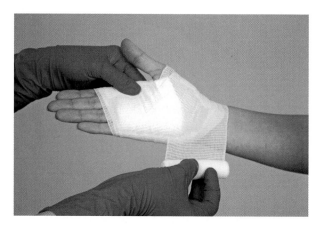

3   Continue with overlapping figure-eight turns.

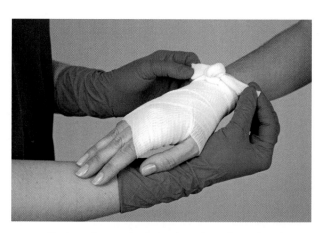

4   Fasten the end of the bandage by tying it or using clips, tape, or safety pins.

Skill   **RICE: Wrist Injury**

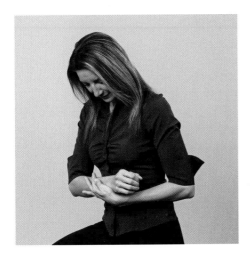

1 Rest the injured wrist.

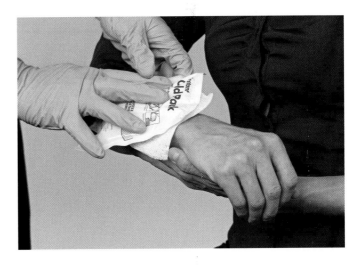

2 Put ice or cold pack on the injured area.

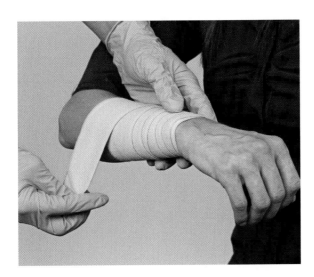

3 Compress the injured area with an elastic roller bandage.

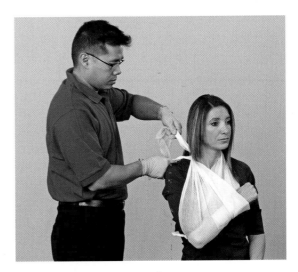

4 Elevate the injured area. Use a sling to hold the wrist in place.

Learning
Checkpoint ①

1. Use RICE for:

   a. most musculoskeletal injuries.   **c.** muscle injuries only.

   b. fractures only.   **d.** muscle and joint injuries only.

2. True or False: Putting a commercial cold pack directly on the skin is the best way to relieve pain and reduce swelling.

3. What is important about how you apply a compression bandage?

   a. Using an elastic roller bandage

   b. Putting the cold pack under the bandage if needed

   c. Checking that circulation is not cut off

   d. All of the above

4. Describe the steps you would follow to use RICE for an injured ankle.

FRACTURES

A fracture is a broken bone. The bone may be completely broken with the pieces separated or still together, or it may only be cracked.

With a closed fracture the skin is not broken. Internal bleeding may occur. With an open fracture there is an open wound at the fracture site, and the bone end may protrude through the wound (**Figure 15-5**). An open fracture can be more serious because there is a greater chance of infection and more serious bleeding. **Figure 15-6** describes common types of fractures.

Although most fractures are not life threatening, external or internal bleeding can be severe with fractures of large bones such as the femur (thigh bone). Nerves and organs nearby may also be injured. A fracture can also result in extended or permanent disability. Fractures are more likely in elderly adults whose bones are often weaker due to osteoporosis, a gradual thinning of bone with aging. In more severe cases of osteoporosis, a bone may fracture with relatively little force.

A fracture causes pain, swelling, bruising, deformity, and an inability to use the affected

body part. You may hear, or the victim may feel, the broken bone ends grating together. With severe bleeding the victim may also experience shock. Check the victim first for any life-threatening conditions, and then care for

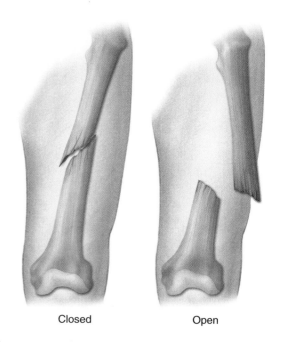

Closed   Open

Figure 15-5 Closed and open fractures.

When You See

- A deformed body part (compare to other side of body)
- Signs of pain
- Swelling, discoloration of skin
- Inability to use the body part
- Bone exposed in a wound
- Victim heard or felt a bone snap
- Possible signs and symptoms of shock

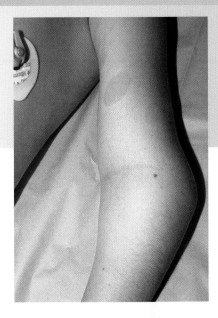

Do This First

1 Immobilize the area. With an extremity, also immobilize the joints above and below the fracture.

2 Call 9-1-1 for a large bone fracture. A victim with a fracture in the hand or foot may be transported to the emergency department.

3 With an open fracture, cover the wound with a dressing and apply gentle pressure around the fracture area only if needed to control bleeding.

4 Apply RICE.

5 If help may be delayed or if the victim is to be transported, use a splint to keep the area immobilized (see **Chapter 16**). Elevate a splinted arm.

ALERT

- Do not try to align the ends of a broken bone.
- Do not put pressure on bone ends when controlling bleeding,
- Do not give the victim anything to eat or drink.

Additional Care

- Treat the victim for shock.
- Monitor the victim's breathing.
- Remove clothing and jewelry if they may cut off circulation as swelling occurs.

---

the fracture. Assess the victim's fingers or toes below the injury to determine if circulation has been disrupted; if so, call 9-1-1 immediately. Also call 9-1-1 for fractures of large bones or bones of the spine, head, or trunk. The first aid for fractures includes resting and immobilizing the area, the use of ice or a cold pack, the use of a compression bandage (except for open fractures), and, when practical, elevating a splinted arm (never elevate a leg with a leg fracture). The victim needs to see a healthcare provider as soon as possible (see First Aid: "Fractures"). The splinting of specific injuries is described in **Chapter 16**.

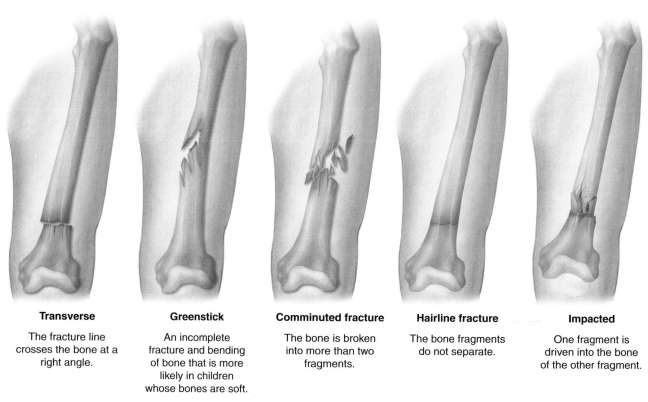

Transverse	**Greenstick**	**Comminuted fracture**	**Hairline fracture**	**Impacted**
The fracture line crosses the bone at a right angle.	An incomplete fracture and bending of bone that is more likely in children whose bones are soft.	The bone is broken into more than two fragments.	The bone fragments do not separate.	One fragment is driven into the bone of the other fragment.

Figure 15-6 Common types of fractures.

JOINT INJURIES

In joints, bones are held in place by ligaments and other structures that allow for movement. Every joint allows a certain normal range of motion. Forcing a body part beyond the normal range of a joint, or in a direction in which the joint normally cannot move, causes a joint injury.

Injuries to joints include dislocations and sprains. In a dislocation, one or more bones have been moved out of their normal position in a joint; this usually involves the tearing of ligaments and other joint structures. In a sprain, the bones remain in place in the joint, but ligaments and other structures are injured. Both kinds of joint injuries often look similar to a fracture and may be just as serious. When in doubt about the seriousness of any injury, assume the worst: treat the injury as severe and call 9-1-1.

Dislocations

In a dislocation, one or more of the bones at the joint are displaced from their normal position when the ligaments that normally hold the bone in place are torn (**Figure 15-7**). Dislocations typically result from strong forces and are sometimes accompanied by bone fractures or other serious injuries.

Pain, swelling, and bruising usually occur. The victim is unable to use the joint because of both pain and structural damage in the joint. Because major blood vessels and nerves are located near joints in many parts of the body, a significant displacement of the bones can damage nearby nerves and cause serious bleeding. If the dislocation is severe, the joint or limb will look deformed. Dislocations can be serious because of the potential for nerve and blood

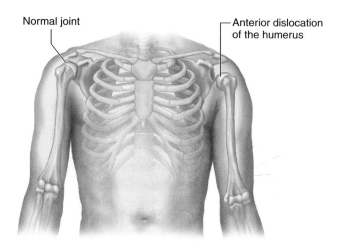

Normal joint

Anterior dislocation of the humerus

Figure 15-7 In a dislocation, the bones at the joint are not in normal position.

First Aid **Dislocations**

When You See

- The joint is deformed (compare to other side of body)
- Signs of pain
- Swelling
- Inability to use the body part

Do This First

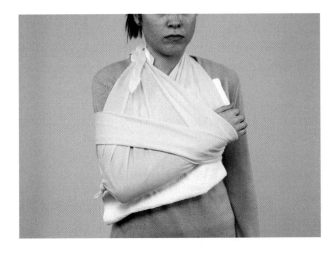

1 Immobilize the area in the position in which you find it.

2 Call 9-1-1. A victim with a dislocated bone in the hand or foot may instead be transported to the emergency department.

3 Apply RICE, but do not use a compression bandage if moving the joint causes pain.

4 If help may be delayed or if the victim is to be transported, use a splint to keep the area immobilized in the position in which you find it (see **Chapter 16**).

ALERT

- Do not try to put the displaced bone back in place.
- Do not let the victim eat or drink.

Additional Care

- Treat the victim for shock if needed.
- Monitor the victim's breathing.
- Remove clothing and jewelry if they may cut off circulation as swelling occurs.

vessel injury, which may be indicated by a loss of sensation or cool, pale skin in the extremity below the injury.

It is not always possible to tell a dislocation from a closed fracture, but the first aid is very similar for both. With severe bleeding, the victim may experience shock. Check the victim first for any life-threatening conditions, and then care for the dislocation. Assess the victim's fingers or toes below the injury to determine if circulation

has been disrupted; if so, call 9-1-1 immediately. Except for a dislocation in the hand or foot, which can be immobilized so that the victim can be transported to a hospital, call 9-1-1 for suspected dislocations. The first aid includes resting and immobilizing the area, the use of ice or a cold pack, use of a compression bandage, and, when practical, elevating a splinted hand or foot (see First Aid: "Dislocations"). The splinting of specific injuries is described in **Chapter 16**.

When to See a Healthcare Provider for a Musculoskeletal Injury

Since you cannot always judge the type or severity of an injury by the signs and symptoms, you may be unsure whether you need medical attention. You should see a healthcare provider if any of the following is true:

- You have the signs and symptoms of a fracture or dislocation.
- The injury causes severe pain.
- You cannot put any weight on an injured leg or walk more than a few steps without significant pain, or the leg buckles when you try to walk.

- An injured joint or the area around it is very tender to touch or feels numb.
- The injured area looks different from the same area on the other extremity (other than swelling).
- The injured joint cannot move.
- Redness or red streaks spread out from the injured area.
- An area that has been injured several times before is reinjured.
- You are unsure how serious an injury is or what treatment to give.

Sprains

A sprain is a joint injury involving the stretching or tearing of ligaments. Sprains typically occur when the joint is overextended or forced beyond the range of normal movement, as when the ankle is twisted by a sideways force on the foot. Sprains can range from mild to severe. The ankles, knees, wrists, and fingers are the body parts most often sprained.

Sprains cause swelling, pain, bruising, and an inability to use the joint because of the pain. The swelling may be considerable and often occurs rapidly. It can be difficult to tell a severe sprain from a fracture, but the first aid is similar for both. Check the victim first for any life-threatening conditions, and then care for the sprain. Assess the victim's fingers or toes below the injury to determine if circulation has been disrupted; if so, call 9-1-1. Use RICE, immobilize the joint with a splint if the victim is to be moved, and seek medical attention (see First Aid: "Sprains"). The splinting of specific sprains is described in **Chapter 16**.

Removing a Ring

When an injury to the hand or fingers causes swelling, the victim's watch or rings can cut off circulation. Try to remove a watch and rings before swelling occurs. Removal of a ring is easier if you first soak the finger in cold water or wrap it in a cold pack and then put oil or butter on the finger.

First Aid **Sprains**

When You See

- Signs of pain
- Swollen joint
- Bruising of joint area
- Inability to use joint

Do This First

1 Immobilize the area in the position in which you find it.

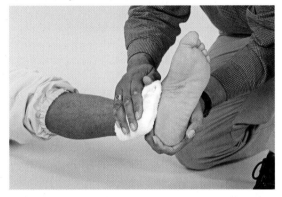

2 Apply RICE.

4 Seek medical attention.

3 Use a soft splint (bandage, pillow, blanket) to immobilize and support the joint.

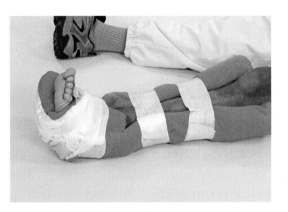

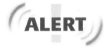 **ALERT**

Additional Care

- Remove clothing or jewelry if they may cut off circulation as swelling occurs.

Learning Checkpoint ②

1. True or False: Call 9-1-1 for a fracture of a large bone such as the thigh bone.

2. When you are immobilizing a fracture injury, what body area should be immobilized?

   a. The immediate fracture area

   b. The fracture area and the joint above it

   c. The fracture area and the joints both above and below it

   d. The entire victim

Learning
Checkpoint ② *(continued)*

3. True or False: With a fracture, you may also need to treat the victim for shock.

4. The signs and symptoms of a bone or joint injury include which of the following? (Check all that apply.)

_____ Deformed area   _____ Pain

_____ Small or unequal pupils   _____ Inability to use part

_____ Skin is hot and red   _____ Fever

_____ Swelling   _____ Spasms and jerking of nearby muscles

5. True or False: A victim with a sprained ankle should "walk it off."

MUSCLE INJURIES

Common muscle injuries include strains, contusions, and cramps. These injuries are usually less serious than fractures and joint injuries. Muscle injuries are often easy to identify because, unlike sprains and dislocations, they do not usually involve the joint. Muscle injuries are typically caused by overexertion, careless or sudden uncoordinated movements, or poor body mechanics, such as lifting a weight with back bent or twisted. Repetitive forces, as frequently occur in some sports, may also inflame or injure tendons. Repeated injury can lead to chronic problems.

Strains

A strain is a tearing of a muscle or a tendon, which connects the muscle to bone. Usually the tear is partial, but in extreme cases the muscle or tendon may tear completely. A strain occurs when the muscle is stretched too far by overexerting the body area. The victim experiences pain, swelling, and sometimes an inability to use the muscle. Back strains are common occupational injuries, and strains in extremities are common in sports. In most cases strains can be prevented by avoiding overexertion, using good body mechanics, and following accepted guidelines for sports safety.

Use RICE to treat strains (see First Aid: "Strains"). Follow-up light exercise may help with healing and later muscle strengthening. With a very serious muscle or tendon tear, surgical repair may be required.

Contusions

A contusion is a bruised muscle as may result from a blow. The blow causes blood vessels within the muscle to rupture, leaking blood into the muscle tissue. This injury often occurs when the muscle is compressed between the object causing the blow and an underlying bone. Contusions cause pain, swelling, and discoloration (**Figure 15-8**) and are treated with

First Aid   **Strains**

When You See

- Signs of dull or sharp pain when muscle is used
- Stiffness in the area of the injury
- Weakness or inability to use the muscle normally

Do This First

1 Apply RICE.

2 Keep the cold pack on the area for 20 minutes on, then at least 30 minutes off.

Additional Care

- Seek medical attention if pain is severe or persists, or if there is a significant or prolonged (three days or more) impairment of function.

RICE (see First Aid: "Contusion"). The discoloration may persist up to a month.

Cramps

A muscle **cramp** is a tightening of a muscle that usually results from prolonged use but may occur with no apparent cause. Cramps are most common in the thigh and calf muscles, but they may also occur in abdominal or back muscles, in any muscle that is overused, or with dehydration. These cramps are different from heat cramps, which result from fluid loss in hot environments (see **Chapter 21**). A cramp may last only a few seconds or up to 15 minutes. You may see the muscle bunching up or twitching under the skin. Cramps are treated with gentle stretching and massage after the cramping stops (see First Aid: "Muscle

Cramp"). Cramps may be prevented with flexibility exercises and stretching before engaging in physical activity.

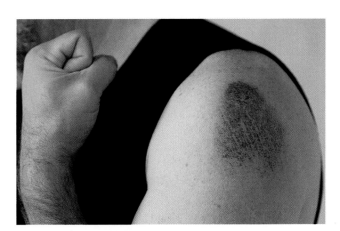

Figure 15-8 Contusion.

First Aid **Contusion**

When You See
- Signs of pain
- Swollen, tender area
- Skin discoloration (black and blue)

Do This First

1 Apply RICE. Do not massage the muscle.

2 Keep the cold pack on the area for 20 minutes, then at least 30 minutes off.

Additional Care
- Seek medical attention if pain is severe or impaired function persists.

First Aid **Muscle Cramp**

When You See
- Signs of muscle pain and tightness

Do This First

1 Stop the activity.

2 Gently stretch out the muscle if possible.

3 Massage the muscle after active cramping stops.

Additional Care
- Drink plenty of fluids.

Learning
Checkpoint ③

1. True or False: For a muscle strain, keep an ice pack on the injury for at least two hours.

2. True or False: Vigorous massage is the best treatment for a muscle contusion.

3. True or False: You can distinguish a contusion from a fracture because only a contusion causes an area of skin discoloration.

4. Name two things you can do to ease a muscle cramp.

Concluding Thoughts

Millions of people every year go to the emergency department with musculoskeletal injuries. Countless others sustain less serious injuries that do not require a healthcare provider's attention. Most people will experience at least a sprain or a strain in their lifetime and will also care for another person with such an injury. Fortunately, most of these injuries are not life threatening or very severe, and the victim recovers well. Giving the appropriate first aid, however, is important for making a good recovery without future disability. Remember that you do not have to know the exact nature of the injury before helping: use RICE (Rest, Ice, Compression, Elevation) for most injuries, and call 9-1-1 or seek medical attention for more serious injuries.

Learning Outcomes

You should now be able to do the following:

1. Describe ways to prevent common sports and recreation injuries.

2. Explain what to look for when assessing musculoskeletal injuries.

3. Demonstrate how to use RICE to care for a musculoskeletal injury.

4. Describe the first aid for fractures, dislocations, and sprains.

5. Explain the differences among strains, contusions, and cramps and describe the first aid for each.

Review Questions

1. Steps to help prevent sports and recreational injuries include
   a. maintaining a healthy weight.
   b. wearing shoes that fit properly.
   c. wearing protective equipment.
   d. All of the above

2. What is true about swelling in most musculoskeletal injuries?
   a. Swelling occurs because of internal bleeding in tissues.
   b. Swelling occurs with all injuries except fractures.
   c. The amount of swelling indicates the seriousness of the injury.
   d. Swelling is promoted because it aids healing.

3. Cold that can be applied to a musculoskeletal injury may include
   a. ice.
   b. a commercial cold pack.
   c. a bag of frozen peas.
   d. All of the above

4. Which statement is generally true of treatment for a musculoskeletal injury?
   a. Apply heat for up to three days, then apply cold.
   b. Apply cold for up to three days, then apply heat.
   c. Apply cold for the first 12 hours, then apply heat.
   d. Apply cold and heat alternating every six hours.

5. The purpose of using a compression bandage on a musculoskeletal injury is to
   a. dress the injured area.
   b. cut off circulation to the area.
   c. help support injury and prevent swelling.
   d. prevent infection.

6. The most important aspect of fracture care is to
   a. apply antibiotic ointment to an open fracture.
   b. put the bone ends together in their normal position.
   c. apply traction to prevent shortening of the limb.
   d. immobilize the area.

7. What should *not* be done with a dislocation?
   a. Apply ice or a cold pack on the joint.
   b. Try to move the bone ends back into their normal position in the joint.
   c. Apply a compression bandage over the joint if it is in an extremity.
   d. Prevent the victim from moving the joint.

8. To assess for circulation in the foot when the victim has an ankle sprain,
   a. check the toes for color, temperature, and sensation.
   b. ask the victim to push against your hand with the foot.
   c. determine whether the victim can stand without feeling pain.
   d. have the victim take a few steps and report whether the toes tingle.

9. A strain occurs when a muscle
   a. is bruised by a blunt blow.
   b. is separated from ligaments in a joint.
   c. is stretched too far with overexertion.
   d. becomes dehydrated.

10. First aid for a muscle cramp may include
   a. returning to activity as soon as possible.
   b. massaging the muscle.
   c. applying a heat pad.
   d. soaking the extremity in icy cold water.

References and Resources

American Academy of Orthopedic Surgeons. Sprains and strains. 2005. orthoinfo.aaos.org

American College of Emergency Physicians. *First aid manual: a comprehensive guide to treating emergency victims of all ages in any situation.* New York: DK Publishing; 2001.

American Heart Association. 2005 International consensus on cardiopulmonary resuscitation (CPR) and emergency cardiovascular care (ECC) science with treatment recommendations. *Circulation*, 112(22). November 29, 2005.

American Medical Association. *Handbook of first aid and emergency care.* Revised ed. New York: Random House; 2000.

Basic Trauma Life Support International. www.btls.org

Campbell, JE. *Basic trauma life support.* Upper Saddle River, New Jersey: Pearson Prentice Hall; 2004.

Massachusetts General Hospital Orthopedic Surgery Department. Pediatric orthopaedic ailments. 2005. www.massgeneral.org/ortho

National Association of Emergency Medical Technicians. *Basic and advanced prehospital trauma life support.* Revised 5th ed. St. Louis: Mosby; 2003.

National Center for Health Statistics. www.cdc.gov/nchs

National Safe Kids Campaign. Sports injury fact sheet. 2004. www.safekids.org

National Safety Council. www.nsc.org

National Youth Sports Safety Foundation. www.nyssf.org

Prehospital Trauma Life Support. www.phtls.org

Chapter 16

Extremity Injuries and Splinting

Chapter Preview

- Types of Splints
- Guidelines for Splinting
- Applying Slings
- Splinting Extremity Injuries

Your young daughter is playing with two friends in the playground while you watch from a nearby bench. While climbing up a climbing structure, she loses her grip and tumbles to the ground. Although she falls only a couple feet, she lands hard on her arm. When you reach her a few seconds later, she is crying and clutching her arm tightly. What do you do?

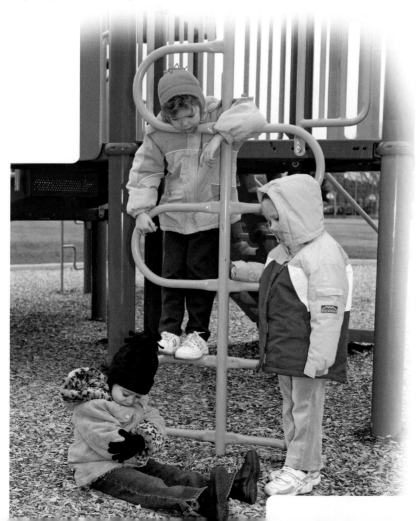

As described in **Chapter 15**, with most musculoskeletal injuries there is a risk of movement worsening the injury and causing more pain. All such injuries should be stabilized to prevent movement. When a victim has a fracture, dislocation, or sprain in an arm or leg, the arm or leg may be splinted if there is a risk for moving the injured area unless help is expected within a few minutes. Always splint an extremity before transporting the victim to a healthcare provider or the emergency department. Splinting helps prevent further injury, reduces pain, and minimizes bleeding and swelling. Splints can be improvised when needed and tied in place with bandages, belts, neckties, or strips of cloth torn from clothing.

This chapter describes splinting and other first aid for specific musculoskeletal injuries of the arms and legs. Remember always to first check the victim's breathing and provide care for life-threatening conditions. Consider the forces involved in the injury and whether a spinal injury may be present. If you suspect a spinal injury, the priority is to support the head and neck and prevent spinal movement. Since splinting a fracture may involve moving some part of the victim or may distract from care given for the spinal injury, unless multiple rescuers are present, leave an extremity injury unsplinted while waiting for help to arrive.

TYPES OF SPLINTS

A splint is any object you can use to help keep an injured body area from moving. Various kinds of commercial splints are available and are used by professional rescuers, but splints can also be made from many different materials at hand. There are three general types of splints (**Figure 16-1**):

- **Rigid splints** may be made from a board, a cane or walking stick, a broom handle, a piece of plastic or metal, a rolled newspaper or magazine, or thick cardboard.

- **Soft splints** may be made from a pillow, a folded blanket or towel, or a triangular bandage folded into a sling.

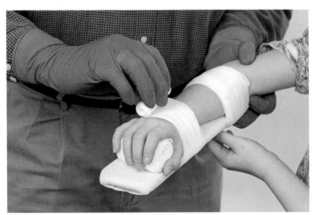

(a) Rigid splint.

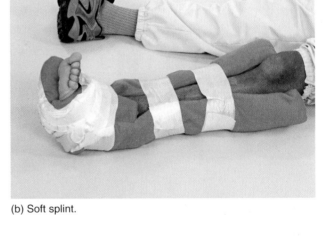

(b) Soft splint.

(c) Anatomic splint.

Figure 16-1 Examples of general types of splints.

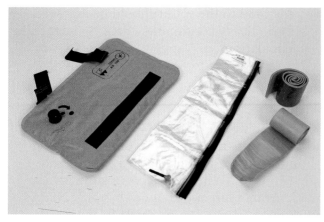

Figure 16-2 Commercial splints.

- **Anatomic splints** involve splinting one part of the body with another part, such as an injured leg to the uninjured leg or splinting fingers together, or splinting the arm to the chest to immobilize the shoulder.

The splint is the object to which the injured extremity is secured to prevent movement. The splint is usually secured by wrapping bandages, strips of cloth (often called **cravats**), Velcro® straps, or other materials around the splint and extremity. Because you may have to loosen or remove a splint if it interferes with circulation to the limb, use knots that can be untied if needed. Do not secure a splint with tape, which can be difficult to remove, unless no other materials are available; if tape is used, do not tape to the skin directly but put a dressing or other material over the skin first.

In addition to common rigid and soft splints, commercial splints are available that are typically used by rescuers with more training. **Figure 16-2** shows some examples of commercial splints.

GUIDELINES FOR SPLINTING

Regardless of the specific type of injury and its location, always apply the following general guidelines for splinting. Later sections in this chapter show how to use these guidelines when splinting specific extremity injuries.

- *Put a dressing on any open wound before splinting the area.* This helps protect the wound, control bleeding, and prevent infection.
- *Splint an injury only if it does not cause more pain for the victim.* Splinting usually involves touching and perhaps manipulating the injured

area, which may cause pain and may worsen the injury. If the victim complains, stop the splinting and have the victim immobilize the area as well as possible until help arrives.

- *Splint the injury in the position in which you find it* (**Figure 16-3**). Trying to straighten out a limb or joint will likely cause pain and could worsen the injury. Blood vessels or nerves near a fracture or dislocation, for example, could be damaged by moving the bone ends. Almost always the injured extremity can be splinted in the position in which you find it, as shown later in this chapter. Only if the victim is in a remote location and will not receive medical attention for a long time, and if circulation has been cut off in the extremity by the injury, should the limb be straightened (see **Chapter 24**).
- *Splint to immobilize the entire injured area.* For example, the splint should extend to the joints above and below the injured area. With a bone fracture near a joint, assume that the joint, too, is injured, and extend the splint well beyond the joint to keep it immobilized as well as the fracture site.
- *Put padding such as cloth between the splint and the victim's skin.* This is especially important with rigid splints, which otherwise may press into soft tissues and cause pain and further injury. Use whatever materials are at hand that will conform to the space between the splint and the body part. Pad body hollows, and ensure that the area of the splint close to the injury is well padded.

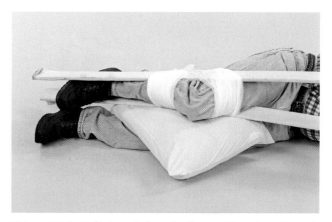

Figure 16-3 Splint an injury in the position found, such as this knee injury. Do not try to straighten the limb to splint it.

- *Put splints on both sides of a fractured bone if possible.* If the injury makes this difficult or splinting materials are limited, splint one side.
- *Do not secure the splint on an open wound because the securing bandage or strap could cut into or irritate the wound.* Tie the bandages or other materials used to hold the splint in place on both sides of the wound.
- *Elevate the splinted extremity if possible.* Do not move the injured area to elevate it if it causes the victim pain or may worsen the injury.
- *Apply a cold pack to the injury around the splint.* Since the ice or cold pack must be removed after 20 minutes, it should not be positioned inside the splint. Placing it inside would require removal and repositioning of the splint. This may cause pain and movement in the injured area. Splint the injury first, and then position the cold pack as close to the injury as possible around the splint **(Figure 16-4)**.
- *With a splinted extremity, do not completely bandage over the fingers or toes, and check them frequently to make sure circulation is not cut off.* To be effective, the splint must be tied firmly enough to the extremity to prevent movement but not so tight that circulation is cut off. Swelling, pale or bluish discoloration, tingling or numbness, and cold skin are signs and symptoms of reduced circulation. If any of these occurs, the splint should be removed or the bandages holding

the limb to the splint should be loosened. Periodically continue to check for adequate circulation.

APPLYING SLINGS

A **sling** is a device used to support and immobilize the upper extremity. A sling may be used for most upper extremity injuries, including shoulder, upper and lower arm, elbow, and wrist injuries. When available, a sling is best made from a large, triangular bandage, but improvised slings can be made of many other materials, such as strips of cloth torn from clothing, neckties, and so on. Cloth or soft, flexible material is generally best.

A sling is used to prevent movement of the arm and shoulder, thereby preventing a worsening of the injury, helping to limit pain, and elevating the extremity to help control bleeding and swelling. In some instances a binder is used along with the sling. A binder (or swathe) is an additional supportive bandage or cloth tied over the sling and around the chest to provide additional support (see Skill: "Applying an Arm Sling and Binder").

Follow these guidelines when using a sling:

- *Splint the injury first, when appropriate.* A fracture of the upper or lower arm or a dislocation of the elbow or wrist should be splinted to prevent movement of the area. Then a sling is applied to provide additional support and to keep the injury elevated.
- *If you splint the injury in the position found and this position makes the use of a sling impossible or difficult, do not try to use a sling.*
- *Do not move the arm into position for a sling if this causes the victim more pain.* If so, splint the arm in the position found, not using a sling, and have the victim immobilize it until help arrives.
- *A cold pack can be used inside the sling.* Follow the standard guidelines for removing the cold pack after 20 minutes and reapplying later (see **Chapter 15**).
- *Do not cover the fingers inside the sling.* Ensure circulation in the extremity periodically by checking the fingers for color, temperature, and normal sensation.

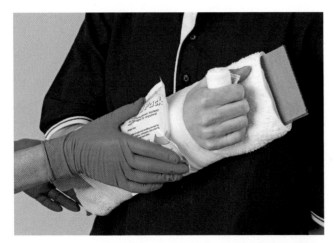

Figure 16-4 Apply a cold pack to the injured area around the splint.

Skill **Applying an Arm Sling and Binder**

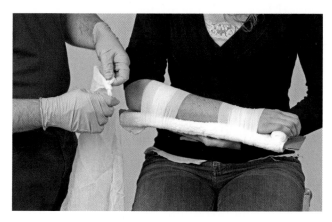

1 Secure the point of the bandage at the elbow.

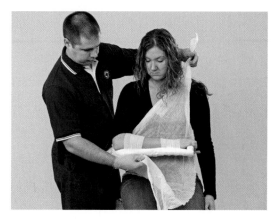

2 Position the triangular bandage.

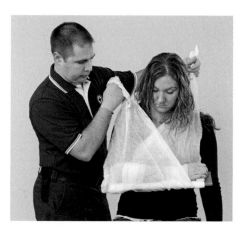

3 Bring up the lower end of the bandage to the opposite side of the neck.

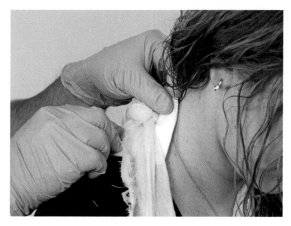

4 Tie the ends.

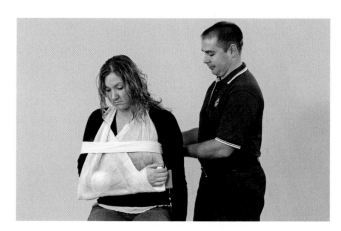

5 Tie a binder bandage over the sling and around the chest.

Learning
Checkpoint ①

1. You encounter a victim with an obviously fractured forearm. What materials might you be able to find around the home that you can use to make a rigid splint?

_____

2. When using a splint, which of the following are actions you should take? (Check all that apply.)

___ Put a heating pad on the area.   ___ Pad the splint.

___ Straighten out a limb before splinting it.   ___ Put a cold pack around the splint.

___ Dress an open wound before splinting.   ___ Splint in the position found.

3. List signs that circulation has been cut off in an extremity below the splint:

_____

4. Name two things you should *not* do when contemplating putting a victim's arm in a sling:

_____

SPLINTING EXTREMITY INJURIES

The following sections describe first aid and splinting techniques for specific bone and joint injuries of the extremities. Remember to follow the RICE acronym described in **Chapter 15** and the splinting guidelines listed earlier.

Upper Extremity Injuries

Upper extremity injuries include fractures, dislocations, and sprains of the shoulder, upper arm, elbow, lower elbow, wrist, and hand.

Shoulder Injuries

Shoulder injuries can fracture the clavicle (collar bone), the scapula (shoulder blade), or joint structures. The clavicle is the most frequently fractured bone in the body. Victims have pain and cannot use the shoulder, which often is lower than the opposite shoulder. Swelling and tenderness are present. Fractures of the scapula are very rare. Dislocations of the shoulder are common and cause pain, deformity of the shoulder, and an inability to move the shoulder.

The goal of splinting the shoulder is to stabilize the area from the trunk to the upper arm with a soft splint. First check for signs of circulation and sensation in the hand. Have the victim wiggle the fingers and ask whether he or she can feel your light touch on the palm. Then apply a sling and binder.

1. Use a soft, not rigid splint for shoulder injuries. Do not move the extremity.
2. Check for signs of circulation and sensation in the hand and fingers. If they are absent, call 9-1-1 for immediate care.
3. Pad the hollow between the body and the arm with a small pillow or towels, and apply a sling and binder to support the arm and immobilize it against the chest (**Figure 16-5**). If moving the arm closer to the chest causes pain, use a larger pillow between the arm and the trunk.
4. Follow the general guidelines for safe splinting. Check the fingers periodically for circulation.

Upper Arm Injuries

Fractures of the **humerus,** the bone of the upper arm, cause pain, swelling, and deformity of the arm. Fractures near the shoulder should be treated in a manner identical to shoulder injuries with soft splinting.

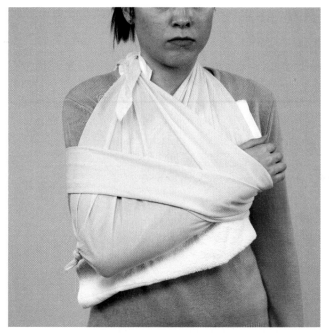

Figure 16-5 Immobilize a shoulder injury with a sling and binder.

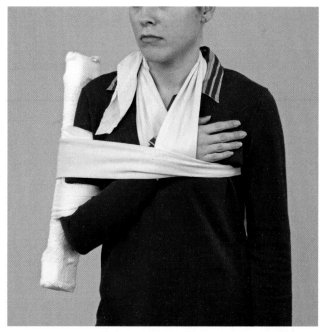

Figure 16-6 Immobilize an upper arm injury with a splint, sling, and binder.

The goal of splinting is to stabilize the bone between the shoulder and the elbow by using a rigid splint on the outside of the arm and placing the wrist in a sling. The fracture site can then be further secured by applying a wide binder around the arm and chest. Be careful not to apply the binder directly over the fracture site.

1. Check for signs of circulation and sensation in the hand and fingers. If they are absent, call 9-1-1 for immediate care.
2. Apply a rigid splint along the outside of the upper arm, tied above the injury and at the elbow.
3. Support the wrist with a sling, and then apply a wide binder to support the arm and immobilize it against the chest (**Figure 16-6**). If it causes pain to raise the wrist for a sling, a long, rigid splint may be used that supports the arm in a straighter position.
4. Follow the general guidelines for safe splinting. Check the fingers periodically for circulation.

Elbow Injuries

The elbow can be injured by a blow or force that moves the joint beyond its normal limits. Sprains and dislocations are the most common injuries to the joint itself. Fractures of the bones above or below the elbow are also common. Nerves and arteries pass close to the bones of the elbow and may also be injured. Usually the victim is unable to move the joint and may say the joint is "locked."

The goal of splinting the elbow is to stabilize the joint from the arm to the forearm in the position in which you find it. If the elbow is bent, a soft splint with sling and binder may be sufficient, but a rigid splint provides greater stability. If the elbow is straight, then a rigid splint should be applied.

1. Check for signs of circulation and sensation in the hand and fingers. If they are absent, call 9-1-1 for immediate care.
2. If the elbow is bent, apply a rigid splint from the upper arm to the wrist as shown in **Figure 16-7a**. If more support is needed, use a sling at the wrist and a binder around the chest at the upper arm.
3. If the elbow is straight, apply a rigid splint from the upper arm to the hand as shown in **Figure 16-7b**. If more support is needed, binders may be used around the chest and upper arm and around the lower arm and waist.
4. Follow the general guidelines for safe splinting. Check the fingers periodically for circulation.

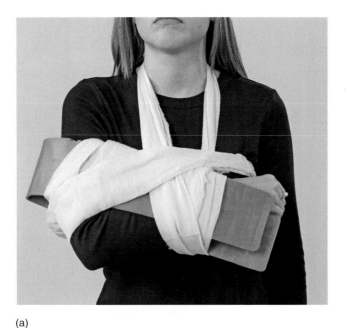

(a)

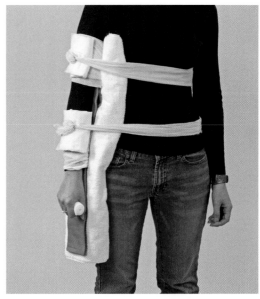

(b)

Figure 16-7 Immobilize an elbow injury with a rigid splint in the position found. (a) Splinting a bent elbow. (b) Splinting a straight elbow.

Forearm Injuries

The forearm is frequently injured by direct blows that may fracture either or both bones. Pain, swelling, and deformity typically result.

The goal of forearm splinting is to stabilize and support the area from the elbow to the hand. You may use a splint on the palm side of the forearm or on both sides. After splinting the arm, secure it with a sling and binder (see Skill: "Splinting the Forearm").

Wrist Injuries

Common wrist injuries include sprains and fractures. Movement of the wrist produces pain. Swelling, discoloration, and deformity may be present.

Wrist injuries should be stabilized from the forearm to the hand. In some cases a soft splint is sufficient, with the area then elevated and supported with a sling. A rigid splint provides more support, and the joint is stabilized in a manner similar to a forearm injury.

1. Check for signs of circulation and sensation in the hand and fingers. If they are absent, call 9-1-1 for immediate care.

2. Apply a rigid splint on the palm side of the arm from the forearm past the fingertips, tied above and below the wrist. Leave the fingers uncovered.

3. Support the forearm and wrist with a sling, and then apply a binder around the upper arm and chest (**Figure 16-8**).

4. Follow the general guidelines for safe splinting. Check the fingers periodically for circulation.

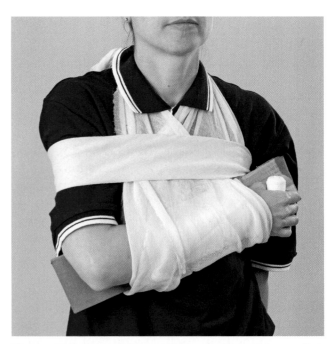

Figure 16-8 Immobilize an injured wrist with a splint, sling, and binder.

Skill **Splinting the Forearm**

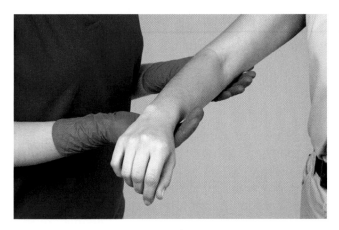

1 Support the arm. Check circulation.

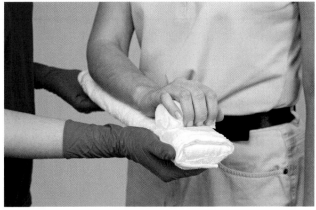

2 Position the arm on a rigid splint.

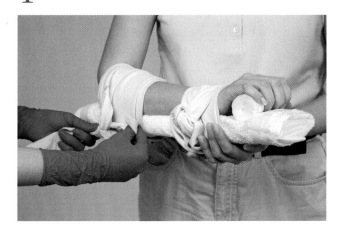

3 Secure the splint.

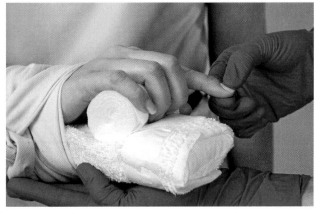

4 Check circulation.

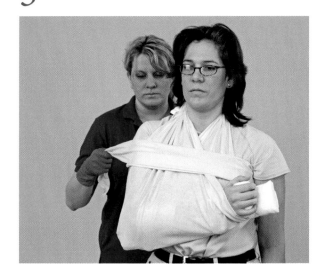

5 Put the arm in a sling, and tie a binder over the sling and around the chest.

Hand and Finger Injuries

The hand may be injured by a direct blow. Fractures often occur, for example, when the victim punches something with a closed fist. Pain and swelling of the hand typically result.

An injured hand may be immobilized with a soft or rigid splint. First place a roll of gauze or similar padding in the palm, allowing the fingers to take a naturally curled position. The entire hand is then bandaged. Place a rigid splint on the palm side of the hand extending from above the wrist to the fingers, the same as with a wrist injury. Pad the area well between the hand and the splint. Then support the injury further with a sling and binder.

Finger injuries include fractures and dislocations. Both are common in both sports and industrial injuries. Often a splint is not required, but a victim with a painful injury will benefit from splinting. Use a soft splint if the finger cannot be straightened without pain. Do not try to manipulate the finger to move a bone into its normal position. Use a rigid splint such as a tongue depressor or ice cream stick secured in place with tape, or make an anatomic splint by taping the finger to an adjoining finger with gauze in between (**Figure 16-9**).

Lower Extremity Injuries

Lower extremity injuries include fractures, dislocations, and sprains of the hip, upper leg, knee, lower leg, ankle, and foot. Because the bones of the thigh and lower leg are larger than those of the arm,

larger forces are typically involved in these injuries. This means that there is a greater risk that a spinal injury may have occurred. Assess the victim carefully, being careful not to move the extremity. A fracture of the femur, the large bone of the thigh, can also damage the large femoral artery and cause life-threatening bleeding.

Hip Injuries

The hip is the joint where the top of the femur meets the pelvis. Hip injuries include fractures, and, less commonly, dislocations. A hip fracture is actually a fracture of the top part of the **femur.** Hip fractures are more common in the elderly, whose bones are often more brittle because **osteoporosis,** a loss of calcium from bones, is common in old age, and because some older people are less stable and more likely to experience a fall. Bleeding and pain may be severe.

Hip dislocations can occur at any age. The victim feels pain and cannot move the joint. Hip dislocations result from falls, vehicular crashes, and blows to the body.

First aid is similar to that for a pelvic injury, from which it is often difficult to differentiate a hip injury. Do not move the victim, and immobilize the leg and hip in the position in which you find it. Call 9-1-1 immediately. Immobilize the victim's legs by padding between the legs with a soft pillow or blanket and gently bandaging them together, unless this causes more pain. Treat the victim for shock but do not elevate the legs.

Learning Checkpoint (2)

1. For an injured shoulder, use a _____ splint.

2. A splint for a fracture of the forearm should extend from the _____ to the _____ .

3. Why is a binder used over a sling?

    a. To prevent movement and give additional support

    b. To pull the fractured bone ends back into position

    c. To promote good circulation

    d. All of the above

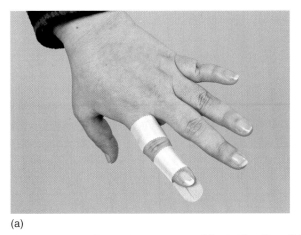
(a)

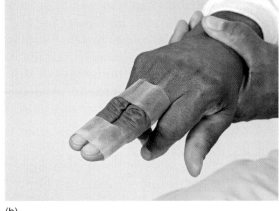
(b)

Figure 16-9 Splint a finger injury. (a) Rigid splint. (b) Anatomic splint.

Upper Leg Injuries

Fractures of the femur are serious because bleeding even with a closed injury can be profuse. The victim experiences severe pain and may be in shock. Swelling and deformity are common.

Call 9-1-1 immediately for a fracture of the femur, and keep the victim from moving. If the victim is lying down with the leg supported by the ground, a rigid splint may be unnecessary. Provide additional support with folded blankets or coats to immobilize the leg in the position found. If help may be delayed, splinting can be used to stabilize the injury. To use an anatomic splint, pad between the legs, move the uninjured leg beside the injured one, and carefully tie the legs together. A rigid splint provides better support if needed:

1. Check for signs of circulation and sensation in the foot and toes.
2. If possible, put a rigid splint on each side of the leg. Pad bony areas and voids between the leg and the splints. The inside splint should extend from the groin past the foot, and the outside from the armpit past the foot.
3. Tie the splints with cravats or bandages (**Figure 16-10**).
4. Follow the general guidelines for safe splinting. Check the toes periodically for circulation.

Knee Injuries

The most common knee injuries are sprains, but dislocations also occur. These injuries commonly result from sports injuries, motor vehicle crashes,

and falls. With large forces the knee can actually be dislocated, which is a serious emergency because nearby nerves and blood vessels are often injured as well. In addition, fractures of the end of the femur or the tibia or fibula (the bones of the lower leg) can be indistinguishable from other knee injuries. Dislocations of the patella (kneecap) may be mistaken for knee dislocations because they too cause the knee to appear deformed.

Knee injuries cause pain and an inability to move the knee. The knee joint may appear to be "locked." Swelling is usually present with or without bruising. With a dislocation the knee may be deformed or angulated.

Do not try to transport a victim with a knee injury but call 9-1-1. With any knee injury, the knee should be splinted in the position found. A soft splint can be applied by rolling a blanket or placing a pillow around the knee. If

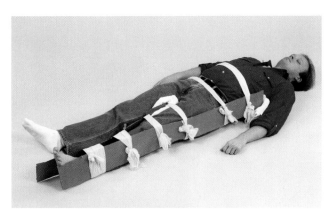

Figure 16-10 Splinting a fractured femur.

the knee is straight, you can make an anatomical splint by tying the upper and lower leg to the unaffected leg. Rigid splints provide additional support. If the knee is straight, ideally two splints are applied along both sides of the knee. If the knee is bent, splint the joint in the position found.

1. Check for signs of circulation and sensation in the foot and toes.
2. If possible, put a rigid splint on each side of the leg in the position found. Pad bony areas and voids between the leg and the splints.
3. Tie the splints with cravats or bandages.
4. Follow the general guidelines for safe splinting. Check the toes periodically for circulation.

Lower Leg Injuries

Injuries to the lower leg commonly result from sports, motor vehicle crashes, and falls. Either or both of the bones of the lower leg can be fractured.

Do not move or transport a victim with a lower leg injury. Call 9-1-1 and immobilize the leg from the knee to the ankle. Either a soft splint or a rigid splint may be used. A rigid splint is applied the same as for a knee injury; a three-sided cardboard splint can also be used (**Figure 16-11**). Be sure not to tie the splint over the fracture site.

A leg fracture can be splinted using either a rigid splint or an anatomic splint (see Skill: "Anatomic Splinting of Leg"). A similar anatomic splint can be used for an upper leg fracture, with the bandages tied higher (including the hips).

Ankle Injuries

The most common ankle injury is a sprain, which typically occurs when the foot is forcefully twisted to one side. The victim experiences pain and swelling of the ankle. The swelling can be significant, and the victim is unable to put weight on the ankle due to pain. Fracture or dislocation may also occur, often involving torn ligaments and possibly also nerve and blood vessel damage.

Usually a soft splint is best for ankle injuries, along with having the victim avoid the use of the foot and leg:

1. Check for circulation.
2. Position the foot in the middle of a soft pillow and fold the pillow around the ankle.
3. Using cravats or bandages, tie the pillow around the foot and lower leg (**Figure 16-12**).
4. Check for signs of circulation and sensation in the foot and toes. If they are absent, call 9-1-1 for immediate care.
5. Follow the general guidelines for safe splinting. Check the toes periodically for circulation.

Foot Injuries

Foot injuries most commonly result from direct blows to the foot or from falls. Foot injuries may involve almost any bone or ligament of the foot. Foot injuries should be treated identically to ankle injuries.

Fractures of the toes can be quite painful. The toe often is swollen, tender, and discolored. Usually no splinting is required. If the toe is significantly bent, more than one toe is involved, or the foot is very painful, a pillow splint can be used as for an ankle injury.

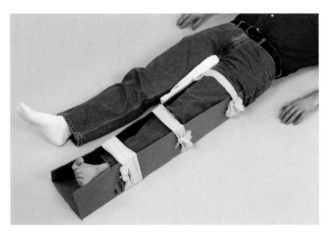

Figure 16-11 Rigid splinting of a lower leg fracture using cardboard.

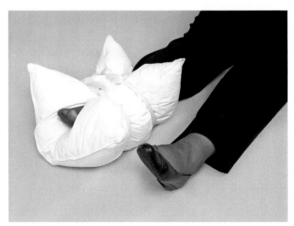

Figure 16-12 Soft splint for an ankle injury.

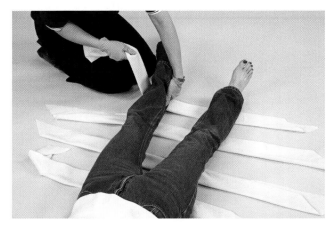

1   Check circulation. Gently slide four or five bandages or strips of cloth under both legs.

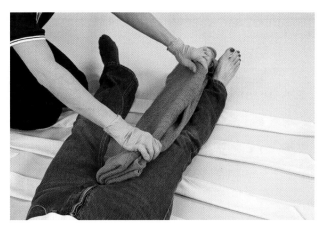

2   Put padding between the legs.

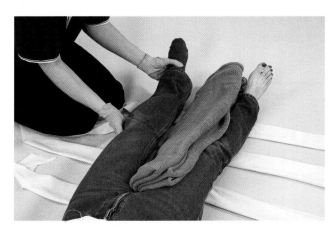

3   Gently slide the uninjured leg next to the injured leg.

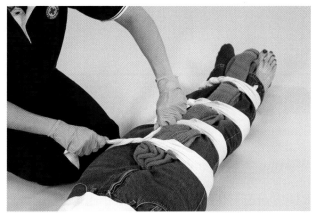

4   Tie the bandages. Check circulation.

Learning
Checkpoint ③

1. You come upon a scene where a woman on a bicycle apparently ran into a light post. She is lying on the ground and says she has severe pain in her lower leg below the knee. You cannot tell whether the bone is broken, but there is no open wound and she says she cannot move her leg. What should you do?

_____

2. A victim with a fracture of the femur may also experience what other condition?

   a. Severe bleeding   **c.** Shock

   b. Open or closed wound   **d.** All of the above

3. Explain when you may use two rigid splints.

_____

Concluding Thoughts

Although this chapter details how to splint all the different areas of the extremities, it is most important to remember the key principles of splinting for any body area:

- Do not splint if it causes more pain.
- Splint an injury in the position found.
- Splint to immobilize the entire area.
- Check the circulation below the injury and splint.
- Call 9-1-1 or seek medical attention.

Learning Outcomes

You should now be able to do the following:

1. Describe the three general types of splints and how to improvise splints with common materials.

2. List the general guidelines for splinting and the use of arm slings.

3. Describe how to splint the different areas of the upper and lower extremities.

4. Demonstrate how to apply an arm sling.

5. Demonstrate how to apply a rigid splint to an injured forearm.

6. Demonstrate how to use an anatomic splint for a leg injury.

Review Questions

1. Which of the following could make an effective rigid splint?
   a. A board
   b. A rolled magazine
   c. A walking stick
   d. All of the above

2. Which statement is true about how splints should be applied?
   a. Tape the splint tightly in place.
   b. For greatest support, tie a cravat directly over the wound.
   c. Straighten the limb as much as possible before splinting.
   d. Dress an open wound before splinting the area.

3. Which is a sign of reduced circulation below an injury?
   a. Cold skin
   b. Hot skin
   c. Red skin
   d. Itching skin

4. Where is a cold pack applied to a splinted open injury?
   a. Outside the dressing but under the bandage and splint
   b. Outside the dressing and bandage but under the splint
   c. Around the splint
   d. Cold packs are not used with splints.

5. How is an injured elbow splinted when you find it in a bent position?
   a. Gently straighten the arm and use a long, rigid splint from shoulder to hand.
   b. Gently bend the elbow to 90 degrees and put it in a sling.
   c. Keep the elbow in its original bent position and use a rigid splint from the upper arm to the hand.
   d. Do not splint the arm, but bind it directly to the chest with bandages.

6. How is an injured hand positioned for splinting?
   a. Let the fingers curl naturally around a soft padding in the palm.
   b. Ask the victim to make a fist before bandaging the hand.
   c. Straighten out the fingers on the surface of a rigid splint.
   d. Keep the fingers spread wide apart with bandaging and padding between them.

7. How can you tell the difference between a hip displacement and a hip fracture?
   a. A fracture is more painful than a displacement.
   b. With a fracture, you can still move the leg, but not with a displacement.
   c. With a displacement the leg is in an unusual position, but not with a fracture.
   d. You cannot easily tell the difference between a displacement and a fracture.

8. With which of these injuries is it safe for the victim to attempt to walk?
   a. Ankle sprain
   b. Ankle displacement
   c. Ankle fracture
   d. None of the above

References and Resources

American College of Emergency Physicians. *First aid manual: a comprehensive guide to treating emergency victims of all ages in any situation.* New York: DK Publishing; 2001.

American Heart Association. 2005 International consensus on cardiopulmonary resuscitation (CPR) and emergency cardiovascular care (ECC) science with treatment recommendations. *Circulation,* 112(22). November 29, 2005.

American Medical Association. *Handbook of first aid and emergency care.* Revised ed. New York: Random House; 2000.

Basic Trauma Life Support International. www.btls.org

Campbell JE. *Basic trauma life support.* Upper Saddle River, New Jersey: Pearson Prentice Hall; 2004.

National Association of Emergency Medical Technicians. *Basic and advanced prehospital trauma life support.* Revised 5th ed. St. Louis: Mosby; 2003.

National Safety Council. www.nsc.org

Prehospital Trauma Life Support. www.phtls.org

Chapter 17

Sudden Illness

Chapter Preview

- General Care for Sudden Illness
- Heart Attack
- Angina
- Stroke
- Respiratory Distress

- Fainting
- Seizures
- Altered Mental Status
- Diabetic Emergencies
- Severe Abdominal Pain

Returning to your office after lunch, you find a co-worker leaning over her desk looking ill. Her breathing is labored and noisy. You ask her what is wrong and she says she doesn't know but she feels like she can't breathe. She pauses, gasping, between words. Her skin is pale. What do you do?

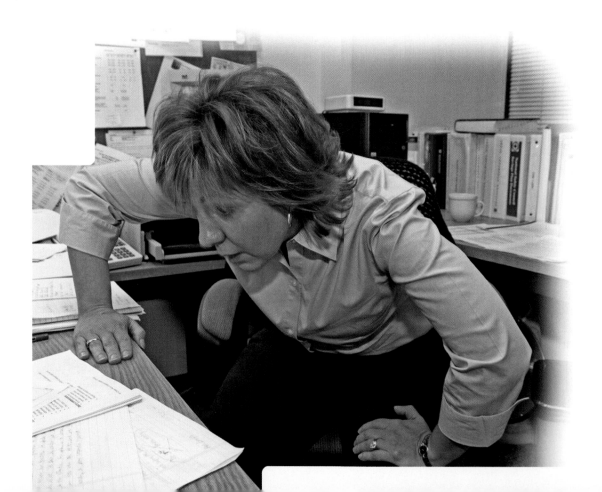

Most chapters in this text involve first aid for injuries. Illness too can cause an emergency, especially if the person becomes ill suddenly. With most illnesses, a person has time to see a healthcare provider long before the illness becomes an emergency, but with the specific health problems described in this chapter, the emergency may develop very quickly. Life-saving action by first aiders and others at the scene is often needed. Because some sudden illnesses, such as a heart attack, may occur with little or no warning and can result in death within minutes if no action is taken, it is important to be aware of the common signs and symptoms and to be prepared to act any time in any place.

GENERAL CARE FOR SUDDEN ILLNESS

Many different illnesses can occur suddenly and become medical emergencies. In some cases you may know or suspect the cause of the problem, such as when a heart attack victim clutches his or her chest and complains of a crushing pressure before collapsing. In other cases neither you nor the victim may know the cause of the problem. The general first aid principles are the same for all sudden illness emergencies, however, so you do not have to know what the victim's illness is before you give first aid.

Following are common general signs and symptoms of sudden illness:

- Person feels ill, dizzy, confused, or weak
- Skin color changes (flushed or pale), sweating
- Breathing changes
- Nausea, vomiting

Following are the general steps to follow for any sudden illness:

1. Call 9-1-1 for unexplained sudden illness.
2. Help the victim rest and avoid getting chilled or overheated.
3. Reassure the victim.
4. Do not give the victim anything to eat or drink.
5. Watch for changes, and be prepared to give basic life support (BLS).

In some cases of sudden illness the most difficult decision is whether to call 9-1-1. How can you tell if the illness is an emergency? Two key factors can help you decide. First, if the illness is *sudden,* it is more likely to be an emergency. Many common illnesses come on gradually. For example, with the flu a person gradually develops a headache or achy joints, fever may begin mildly and slowly rise, respiratory symptoms gradually increase, and so on. The illness seldom becomes an emergency before the person seeks healthcare. Problems that come on suddenly and unexpectedly often do become emergencies, however, such as a sudden heart attack or asthma attack.

Second, is the illness *unexplained?* A person suddenly has an excruciating, pounding headache—but this person has never had bad headaches before and nothing special has happened today that might cause a headache. This headache is likely to be a symptom of an emergency developing. In contrast, a child who develops a "tummy ache" after gobbling down a whole carton of ice cream is unlikely to be having an emergency—unlike some victims with sudden, unexplained severe abdominal pain.

In rare instances, if you cannot decide whether someone's sudden illness might be an emergency, call 9-1-1. Tell the dispatcher exactly what you know and have observed, and let the dispatcher help decide the best course of action.

In addition to these general care principles, when you can identify the specific illness, give first aid as described in the following sections.

HEART ATTACK

Heart attack, or **acute myocardial infarction (AMI),** involves a sudden reduced blood flow to the heart muscle. It is a medical emergency and often leads to cardiac arrest. Heart attack can occur at any age **(Box 17-1)**. Heart attack is caused by a reduced blood flow or blockage in the coronary arteries, which supply the heart muscle with blood, usually as a result of atherosclerosis (see **Chapter 6**).

Prevention of Heart Attack

Heart attack, angina, and stroke are all cardiovascular diseases. **Chapter 6** describes how one can minimize the risk factors for cardiovascular disease by not smoking, eating a healthy diet low in cholesterol and salt, controlling blood pressure, maintaining a normal weight, getting exercise, and controlling stress.

Box 17-1 Facts About Heart Attack

- 180,000 people a year in the United States die from heart attacks. Many of them could have been saved by prompt first aid and medical treatment.
- Heart attack is more likely in those with a family history of heart attacks.

- One-fifth of heart attack victims do not have chest pain, but they often have other symptoms.
- Heart attack victims typically deny that they are having a heart attack. Do not let them talk you out of getting help!

First Aid for Heart Attack

The signs and symptoms of heart attack vary considerably, from vague chest discomfort (which the victim may confuse with heartburn) to crushing pain, with or without other symptoms (**Figure 17-1**).

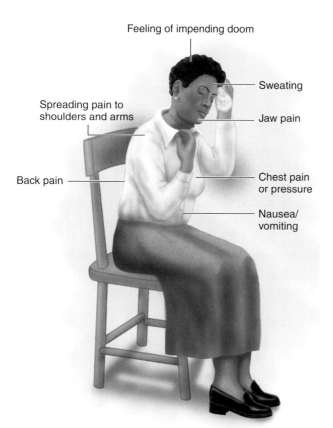

Feeling of impending doom

Sweating

Spreading pain to shoulders and arms

Jaw pain

Back pain

Chest pain or pressure

Nausea/ vomiting

Figure 17-1 Signs and symptoms of a heart attack.

The victim may have no signs and symptoms at all before collapsing suddenly. Sometimes the victim has milder symptoms that come and go for two or three days before the heart attack occurs. It is important to consider the possibility of heart attack when a wide range of symptoms occurs rather than expecting only a clearly defined situation. Note that some heart attack symptoms are more common in women. Chest pain or discomfort is still the most common symptom, but women are somewhat more likely to have shortness of breath, jaw or back pain, and nausea and vomiting.

It is important to act quickly when the victim may be having a heart attack, because deaths from heart attack usually occur within an hour or two after symptoms begin. Healthcare professionals can administer medications to reduce the effects of heart attack and save the victim's life—but only if EMS is involved quickly.

First aid for heart attack begins with calling 9-1-1 to get help on the way immediately. Then help the victim to rest in the most comfortable position. A sitting position is often easiest for breathing. Loosen any constricting clothing. Try to calm the victim and reassure him or her that help is on the way. Since heart attack frequently leads to cardiac arrest, be prepared to give BLS if needed (see First Aid: "Heart Attack").

In recent years the value of aspirin as a clot-preventing medication has become well known, and many healthcare providers advise

When You See

- Complaints of persistent pressure, tightness, ache, or pain in the chest
- Complaints of pain spreading to neck, shoulders, or arms
- Complaints of shortness of breath
- Complaints of dizziness, lightheadedness, feeling of impending doom
- Pale, moist skin or heavy sweating
- Nausea

Do This First

1 Call 9-1-1 immediately, even if the victim says it is not serious.

2 Help the victim to rest in a comfortable position (often sitting). Loosen any tight clothing. Keep the victim from moving.

3 Ask the victim if he or she is taking heart medication, and help obtain the medication for the victim.

4 Allow the victim to take one aspirin (unless allergic).

5 Stay with the victim, and be reassuring and calming, and be prepared to give care if the victim becomes unresponsive and breathing stops.

Additional Care

- **Do not let the victim eat or drink anything.**

---

their patients who are at risk for cardiovascular disease to take one low-dose aspirin daily unless they are allergic or experience side effects such as gastrointestinal bleeding. Some benefit has been demonstrated for taking aspirin during a heart attack, and for victims who do not need to avoid aspirin, taking one aspirin is often recommended when they experience heart attack symptoms. First aiders should never on their own give aspirin or any medication to a victim, but they may allow the victim to take an aspirin.

Nitroglycerin is another medication of benefit for a heart attack victim who has been prescribed this drug. Nitroglycerin increases blood flow through partially restricted arteries by dilating them. Nitroglycerin is generally prescribed for angina, a condition of pain in the chest caused by narrowed coronary arteries. If the victim has nitroglycerin, you can help the person to use it. Nitroglycerin comes in small tablets that are dissolved under the tongue, tablets that dissolve in the cheek, extended-release capsules, oral sprays, and extended-release patches that are applied to the chest, usually daily (**Figure 17-2**). Follow the victim's instructions to help with the drug. The victim should be seated because dizziness or fainting may occur. Do not try to give the drug yourself if the victim is unresponsive.

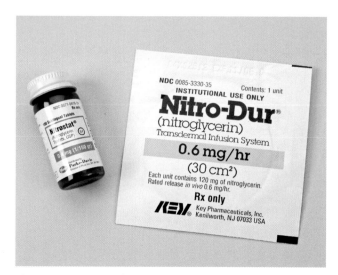

Figure 17-2 Nitroglycerin tablets and patch.

ANGINA

Angina pectoris, usually just called angina, is chest pain caused by heart disease that usually happens after intense activity or exertion. Other factors may trigger the pain of angina, such as stress or exposure to extreme heat or cold. The pain is a sign that the heart muscle is not getting as much oxygen as needed, usually because of narrowed or constricted coronary arteries. The pain usually goes away after a few minutes of rest. The pain may also radiate to the jaw, neck, or left arm or shoulder. People usually know when they have angina and may carry medication for it, usually nitroglycerin.

Help a person with angina to take his or her own medication and then to rest. If the pain persists more than 10 minutes or stops and then returns, or if the victim has other heart attack symptoms, give first aid as for a heart attack.

STROKE

A **stroke,** also called a cerebrovascular accident (CVA) or a brain attack, is an interruption of blood flow to a part of the brain, which kills nerve cells and affects the victim's functioning. Stroke, like heart attack, may be caused by atherosclerosis. A blood clot may form in a brain artery or may be carried there in the blood and lodge in the artery, obstructing flow to that part of the brain. Stroke may also result when an artery in

the brain ruptures or other factors impede flow. As noted in **Chapter 6**, some 700,000 people in the United States have a stroke each year, resulting in over 162,000 deaths. Strokes are more common in older adults.

Because a stroke victim needs medical help immediately to decrease the chance of permanent damage, it is important to be able to identify the signs and symptoms of stroke. Stroke generally causes a sudden weakness or numbness in the face, arm, or leg on one side; dizziness, confusion, and difficulty understanding speech; and difficulty speaking or swallowing, possibly with vision problems. The exact signs and symptoms vary somewhat depending on the exact site in the brain where an artery is blocked. First aiders who are not thinking about the possibility of a stroke might attribute the victim's signs and symptoms to some other condition. Because it is so important that medical care begin as soon as possible, screening assessments have been devised to accurately identify strokes (**Box 17-2**).

The most important thing to do for a stroke victim is to call 9-1-1 immediately to access advanced medical care. Drugs can often minimize the effects of a stroke—but only if administered very soon after the stroke. Tell the dispatcher you believe the victim has had a stroke and describe his or her signs and symptoms. With the victim, be calming and reassuring, because often a stroke victim does not understand what has happened and is confused or fearful. Have the victim lie down on the back with head and shoulders slightly raised; this is often called the "stroke position." Monitor the victim and be prepared for vomiting and to give BLS if needed. Move an unresponsive victim into the recovery position (see First Aid: "Stroke").

Transient Ischemic Attack

A **transient ischemic attack (TIA),** sometimes called a ministroke, is a temporary interruption to blood flow in an artery in the brain. A TIA produces signs and symptoms similar to those of a stroke, except they usually disappear within a few minutes. Since a person who experiences a TIA is at a high risk for a stroke, you should always call 9-1-1 for a victim who exhibits the signs and symptoms of stroke, even if they seem milder or soon disappear.

Box 17-2 The Cincinnati Prehospital Stroke Scale

Among EMS professionals, the need to accurately identify a potential stroke victim is well recognized. The more quickly stroke is recognized, the more quickly the victim can be given appropriate prehospital care and rushed to a stroke center or other appropriate treatment center. Several screening processes have proved accurate in the rapid identification of stroke, and most professional rescuers now use a screening process.

A screening process can also be used effectively by lay first aiders. Emergency dispatchers who answer 9-1-1 calls in many areas are guiding callers to use such assessments. The **Cincinnati Prehospital Stroke Scale (CPSS)** is used widely and is similar to other methods. The CPSS uses three simple assessments:

1. Ask the victim to smile.
2. Ask the victim, with eyes closed, to raise both arms out in front of the body.
3. Ask the victim to repeat this sentence: "You can't teach an old dog new tricks."

A stroke victim typically manifests these signs:

1. Only one side of the face makes a smile; the other side seems to droop.
2. One arm drifts down lower than the other in front of the body.
3. The victim slurs words, uses the wrong words, or cannot speak at all.

A first aider who identifies these signs of stroke in a victim and relays that information to EMS speeds the process of quickly getting the most appropriate care to the victim. The arriving EMS crew can quickly begin medical care at the scene and plan to transport the victim to the best setting for immediate care. Calling ahead helps ensure that resources are mobilized to provide advanced care on arrival.

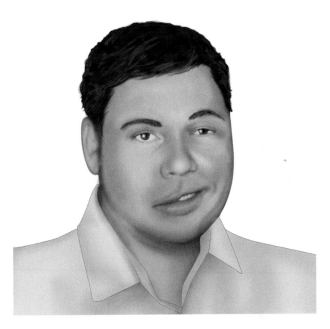

When gathering SAMPLE history information from a potential stroke victim, as explained in **Chapter 4**, try to learn when the signs and symptoms first occurred. Ask family members or others present at the scene as well as the victim. This information is important for the EMS treatment of the victim.

First Aid | Stroke

When You See

- Complaints of sudden, severe headache
- Complaints of sudden weakness or numbness of face, arm, or leg on one side
- Dizziness, confusion, difficulty understanding speech
- Difficulty speaking or swallowing, vision problems
- Changing levels of responsiveness or unresponsiveness

Do This First

1 Call 9-1-1.

2 Monitor the victim and be prepared to give BLS.

3 Have the victim lie on his or her back with head and shoulders slightly raised. Loosen a constrictive collar.

4 If necessary, turn the victim's head to the side to allow drool or vomit to drain.

ALERT

Alert!

- Do not let a stroke victim eat or drink anything.

Additional Care

- Keep the victim warm and quiet until help arrives.
- Put an unresponsive victim in the recovery position.

Learning
Checkpoint ①

1. True or False: With an unknown sudden illness, do not give the victim anything to eat or drink.

2. Check off the common signs and symptoms of heart attack:

___ Skin red and flushed	___ Nausea
___ Tingling in fingers and toes	___ Headache
___ Shortness of breath	___ Pale skin
___ Chest pain or pressure	___ Unusual cheerfulness
___ Sweating	___ Dizziness

3. How do you decide if a victim's chest pain may be a heart attack or angina?

_____

4. The immediate first action to take for a heart attack victim is _____

5. It may be important to position a stroke victim such that

   a. fluids drain from the mouth.

   b. the victim's head is protected from injury during convulsions.

   c. the victim can sit up even if partially paralyzed.

   d. the victim's head is lower than rest of the body.

RESPIRATORY DISTRESS

Respiratory distress, or difficulty breathing, can be caused by many different illnesses and injuries.

Prevention of Respiratory Distress

People with asthma generally have learned what factors may trigger an asthma attack so that they can try to avoid them when possible, and many carry medication with them that can stop an attack when one occurs. People with other chronic respiratory problems, such as chronic obstructive pulmonary disease (COPD), should also learn to avoid situations in which respiratory difficulty may occur and should learn what actions to take if a problem does occur.

First Aid for Respiratory Distress

A victim in respiratory distress may be gasping for air, panting, breathing faster or slower than normal, or making wheezing or other sounds with breathing. Typically the victim cannot speak a full sentence without pausing to breathe. The victim's skin may look pale or ashen and may be cool and moist; the lips and nail beds may be bluish. Lowered oxygen levels in the blood may make the victim feel dizzy or disoriented (**Figure 17-3**). The victim may be sitting and leaning forward, hands on knees, in what is called the **tripod position (Figure 17-4).**

Because respiratory distress in an infant or child may rapidly progress to respiratory arrest, it is crucial to act quickly when an infant or child is having a problem breathing. In addition to the signs and symptoms just described, an infant or child may have obviously flaring nostrils and more obvious movements of chest muscles with the effort to breathe.

If the cause of a victim's breathing problem is not obvious, look for other signs and symptoms

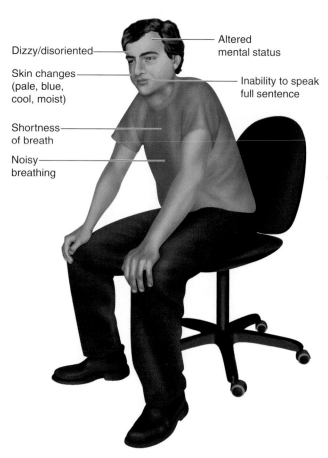

Altered
mental status

Dizzy/disoriented

Skin changes
(pale, blue,
cool, moist)

Inability to speak
full sentence

Shortness
of breath

Noisy
breathing

Figure 17-3 Signs and symptoms of respiratory distress.

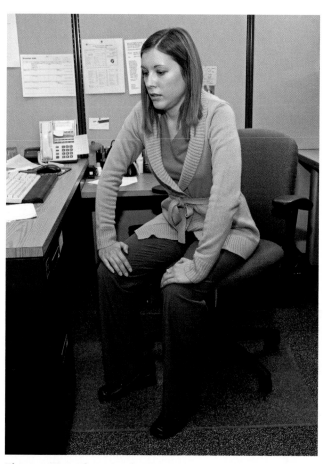

Figure 17-4 The tripod position, commonly assumed by victims in respiratory distress.

that may reveal the problem. Respiratory distress can be a sign of many of the injuries described in other chapters throughout this text. If you can determine the cause of a victim's breathing difficulty, give first aid for that problem. For example, a victim of a heart attack may have shortness of breath; while it is important to care for this breathing difficulty also, it is most crucial to call 9-1-1 immediately for the heart attack and give the first aid described earlier.

Respiratory distress may also result from sudden illness. Asthma and chronic obstructive pulmonary disease (COPD) are two common diseases that may cause episodes of breathing difficulty. These are described in more detail in the following sections along with specific first aid steps.

In some cases you will not be able to identify the cause of a victim's respiratory distress. In this situation give the general breathing care described in First Aid: "Respiratory Distress." Call 9-1-1 for

a victim of respiratory distress because this condition may progress to respiratory arrest, a life-threatening condition.

Asthma

Asthma is a common problem affecting 1 in 20 adults and 1 in 7 children. Asthma attacks in the United States result in over 1.5 million emergency department visits a year and over 5500 deaths. The prevalence of asthma has been increasing gradually in the United States for over two decades. Asthma is a chronic disease—it cannot be cured, although attacks often become less common as a child becomes older and moves through adulthood. In an asthma attack, the airway becomes narrow and the person has difficulty breathing. Many asthma victims know they have the condition and carry medication for emergency situations, typically an inhaler. They may also have learned what situations and factors can trigger an asthma attack and thus they try

When You See

- Victim is gasping or unable to catch his or her breath.
- Breathing is faster or slower, or deeper or shallower, than normal.
- Breathing involves sounds such as wheezing or gurgling.
- Victim feels dizzy or lightheaded.

Do This First

1 Call 9-1-1 for sudden, unexplained breathing problems.

2 Help the victim to rest in the position of easiest breathing (often sitting up).

3 Ask the victim about any prescribed medicine he or she may have, and help the victim to take it if needed.

4 Stay with the victim and be prepared to give BLS.

Additional Care

- Calm and reassure the victim (anxiety increases breathing distress).
- Administer supplemental oxygen to the victim if available and if you are trained in its use.

---

to avoid these (**Box 17-3**). When left untreated, a severe asthma attack can be fatal. If a young child who is away from usual caretakers has trouble breathing, always ask if he or she has medication (see First Aid: "Asthma").

When an asthma attack occurs and the victim has an inhaler, you may assist the victim in using the inhaler under these conditions:

- The victim confirms that it is an asthma attack occurring.
- The victim identifies the inhaler as his or her asthma medication.
- The victim cannot self-administer the medication.

Helping a Child with an Inhaler

Parents and child care providers may need to help a small child with asthma to use an inhaler during an asthma attack. An inhaler is a device that contains and delivers the asthma medication in automatically measured doses (**Figure 17-5**). The medication is usually a **bronchodilator,** a drug that relaxes the muscles of the airway, allowing airway passages to open wider (dilate) to make breathing easier. Always follow the healthcare provider's specific instructions for the inhaler. Use only the child's own prescribed inhaler. Never use an inhaler belonging to another child.

Box 17-3 Asthma Triggers

Asthma attacks are usually triggered by some factor in the person's internal or external environment. Understanding these factors helps prevent or minimize attacks. Common triggers include:

- Respiratory infection, including the common cold (the most common cause of asthma attacks in children under age 5)
- Allergic reaction to pollen, mold, dust mites, animal fur, or dander
- Exercise (especially in cold, dry air)
- Certain foods (nuts, eggs, milk)
- Emotional stress
- Medications
- Air pollution caused by such things as cigarette smoke, vehicle exhaust, or fumes of cleaning products
- Temperature extremes

Knowing the specific triggers that provoke asthma can help prevent attacks. A person with asthma may have had a skin test to detect specific allergens that trigger his or her asthma. In addition to avoiding the factors just listed, follow these guidelines:

- Use a damp cloth to dust furniture and surfaces.
- Vacuum rugs frequently and when the person with asthma is not present.
- Avoid fluffy blankets and pillows that collect dust and that contain feathers.
- Enclose mattresses and pillows in plastic covers.
- Do not use air fresheners or products with strong odors.
- Use an air purifier and stay indoors when pollen counts are high.

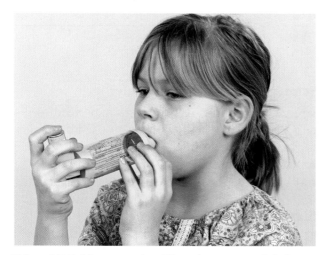

Figure 17-5 Many people with asthma use an inhaler.

Following are general instructions that may need modification for the specific medication device or for a particular child.

1. Shake the inhaler.
2. If a spacer is used, position it on the inhaler. (A spacer is a tube or chamber that fits between the inhaler and the child's mouth.)
3. Have the child breathe out fully through the mouth.
4. With the child's lips around the inhaler mouthpiece or the spacer, have the child inhale slowly and deeply; press the inhaler down to release one spray of medication as the child inhales. (A face mask is generally used for an infant instead of a mouthpiece.)
5. Have the child hold his or her breath for up to 10 seconds if possible and then exhale slowly. Follow the directions for the inhaler or follow the child's treatment plan to repeat doses if needed.

Asthma

When You See

- Wheezing and difficulty breathing and speaking
- Dry, persistent cough
- Fear, anxiety
- Gray-blue skin
- Changing levels of responsiveness

Do This First

1 If the victim does not know he or she has asthma (first attack), call 9-1-1 immediately.

2 Help the victim to use his or her medication (usually in an inhaler).

3 Help the victim to rest and sit in a position for easiest breathing.

Additional Care

- The victim may use the inhaler again in 5 to 10 minutes if needed.
- If the breathing difficulty persists after using the inhaler, call 9-1-1.
- If the difficulty persists, give supplemental oxygen if available and if you are trained in its use (see Appendix A).
- Never unnecessarily separate a child from a parent or loved one when providing care.

Chronic Obstructive Pulmonary Disease

Chronic obstructive pulmonary disease (COPD) includes emphysema, chronic bronchitis, and other conditions. Over 12 million people in the United States have chronic bronchitis or emphysema, leading to over 124,000 deaths a year. It is the number four cause of death in the United States. Both of these diseases may cause respiratory distress and breathing emergencies.

Emphysema is a disease that affects the alveoli of the lungs, the tiny sacs where oxygen enters the blood. The alveoli lose elasticity and decrease in number, which reduces oxygen absorption. Chronic bronchitis affects the bronchial tubes into the lungs, causing inflammation and a buildup of mucus. Both diseases are mainly caused by smoking, air pollution, and other factors. Both often become worse over time. People with these diseases often get colds and respiratory infections, and they are likely to become short of breath even with mild exertion such as walking. In advanced cases the person may need a home oxygen system.

Victims with breathing difficulty related to COPD generally have the same signs and symptoms as described earlier for respiratory distress, and the first aid care is the same. Ask the victim whether he or she has a chronic disease, and give this information to the dispatcher when you call 9-1-1. If the victim has a prescribed medication to help with breathing, you may help the person to take the medication.

Hyperventilation

Hyperventilation is fast, deep breathing usually caused by anxiety or stress, although it may also be caused by some injuries or illnesses. The rapid breathing causes an imbalance in the body's levels of oxygen and carbon dioxide, which may add to the person's anxiety and cause confusion or dizziness. Numbness or tingling of the fingers, toes, and lips may occur.

Hyperventilation caused by emotional stress usually does not last long or become an emergency. Help the person to calm down and relax and breathe more slowly. Do not have the person breathe into and out of a bag, which could lower the person's oxygen level too far. Breathing slowly along with the victim often helps the victim to slow his or her breathing rate.

Since rapid breathing may also be caused by injury or sudden illness, do not assume that the victim is simply hyperventilating. Look for other signs of injury or illness, and ask the victim what happened to start the problem. If there are other signs or symptoms that suggest injury or illness, or if the victim's breathing does not return to normal in a few minutes, call 9-1-1 (see First Aid: "Hyperventilation").

Learning Checkpoint ②

1. True or False: You cannot give first aid for a person with difficulty breathing unless you know the specific cause of the problem.

2. To help someone to breathe more easily,

   a. position the victim flat on his or her back.

   b. have the victim stand, and clap him or her on the back with each breath.

   c. have the victim sit and put his or her head between the knees.

   d. let the victim find the position in which he or she can breathe most easily.

3. What is the best thing a victim with asthma can do when having an asthma attack?

_____

4. True or False: Have a hyperventilation victim breathe into a bag in order to start breathing normally again.

5. When should you call 9-1-1 for a victim who seems to be hyperventilating?

_____

Hyperventilation

When You See
- Very fast breathing rate
- Dizziness, faintness
- Tingling or numbness in hands, feet, and lips
- Muscle twitching or cramping

Do This First

1 Make sure there is no other cause for the breathing difficulty that requires care.

2 Reassure the victim and ask him or her to try to breathe slowly.

3 Call 9-1-1 if the victim's breathing does not return to normal within a few minutes.

ALERT
- Do not ask the victim to breathe into a bag or other container. A victim who repeatedly rebreathes his or her exhaled air will not be getting enough oxygen.

Additional Care
- A victim who often has this problem should seek medical care, because some medical conditions can cause rapid breathing.

FAINTING

Fainting is caused by a temporary reduced blood flow to the brain. This commonly occurs in hot weather or after a prolonged period of inactivity, or from other causes such as fright, emotional shock, or lack of food. A temporary drop in blood pressure caused by suddenly standing after prolonged sitting or lying down may cause dizziness or fainting, especially in the elderly. In a young, healthy, nonpregnant adult, fainting is usually not a sign of a more serious problem, unless the person faints often or does not recover quickly. In someone who has heart disease, is pregnant, or is over age 65, fainting may be a sign of a serious problem requiring immediate medical attention.

Injury may result if the fainting person falls—try to catch the person and gently lower him or her to the floor. Sometimes a person has signs or symptoms before fainting, including dizziness, sweating, nausea, blurring or dimming of vision, and generalized weakness. If fainting is anticipated, have the person sit or lie down (see First Aid: "Fainting").

SEIZURES

Seizures, or convulsions, result from a brain disturbance caused by many different conditions, including epilepsy, high fever in infants and young children, head injuries, low blood sugar in a person with diabetes, poisoning, and

First Aid Fainting

When You See
- Sudden, brief loss of responsiveness and collapse
- Pale, cool skin, sweating

Do This First

1 Check the victim and provide BLS if needed.

2 Lay the victim down and raise the legs about 12 inches. Loosen constricting clothing.

3 Check for possible injuries caused by falling.

4 Reassure the victim as he or she recovers.

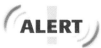

ALERT
- Do not pour or splash water on the victim's face; it could be aspirated into the lungs.

Additional Care
- Call 9-1-1 if the victim does not regain responsiveness soon or faints repeatedly. Always call 9-1-1 for all older adults, people with heart disease, and pregnant women.
- Place a victim who remains unresponsive in the recovery position.

---

electric shock. The brain's normal electrical activity becomes out of balance, resulting in a sudden altered mental status and uncontrolled muscular contractions that cause jerking or shaking of the body. Most seizures are caused by epilepsy (**Box 17-4**).

Prevention of Seizures
First-time seizures can seldom be prevented, but someone with a diagnosed seizure disorder usually has prescribed medication that will prevent most seizures. Sometimes specific factors may increase the risk of a seizure occurring (such as inadequate sleep, or flashing lights), and the individual can learn to control these factors. Seizures caused by head injuries can be prevented by preventing inju-

ries (**see Chapter 13**)—for example, by wearing a helmet in appropriate sports and other activities.

First Aid for Seizures
Seizures generally occur suddenly and without warning. Some victims have an unusual feeling in advance of the seizure called an **aura.** An aura may be a generalized sensation or a hallucinated sensation involving any of the senses.

Seizures follow a wide variety of different patterns, depending in part on the cause. Several different patterns occur in people with epilepsy; some may have only one type of seizure, while others experience different types at different times. Following are some of the more common types of seizures:

Box 17-4 Facts About Epilepsy

- Epilepsy and seizures affect 2.5 million people of all ages in the United States.
- Approximately 181,000 new cases of seizures and epilepsy occur each year.
- 10% of the U.S. population will experience a seizure in their lifetime.
- 45,000 children under the age of 15 develop epilepsy each year.
- Males are slightly more likely to develop epilepsy than females.
- The incidence is greater in African American and socially disadvantaged populations.

- In 70% of new cases, no cause is apparent.
- 70% of people with epilepsy can be expected to enter remission, defined as five or more years seizure-free using medication.
- 75% of people who are seizure-free on medication after two to five years can be successfully withdrawn from medication.
- 10% of new patients may still have seizures despite optimal medical management.

Source: Epilepsy Foundation. 2005. Available from: www.epilepsyfoundation.org

- **Complex partial seizures.** These occur in some people with epilepsy. The person is conscious but does not interact normally with others and is not in control of movements or speech. These seizures are called "partial" because only part of the brain is involved. The person seems dazed and may mumble or wander. This type of seizure is often mistaken for a behavioral problem.
- **Absence seizures.** These occur in some people with epilepsy. The person seems to stare blankly into space and does not respond to others; the seizure begins and ends abruptly, often lasting only a few seconds.
- **Generalized tonic clonic seizures.** These occur in some people with epilepsy. This type is also called convulsions or grand mal seizures. The person loses consciousness and falls; the person is at first stiff (tonic), then experiences jerking of muscles (clonic) throughout the body. Breathing may stop momentarily but restarts spontaneously. After the seizure the person may be confused or agitated.
- **Febrile seizures.** These seizures are not related to epilepsy. Febrile seizures are caused by high fever (usually over 102° F) in infants or young children. The convulsions are similar to those of tonic clonic seizures, and the first aid is the same, followed by measures to bring down the victim's body temperature.

The first aid for all kinds of seizures is primarily directed toward protecting the person until the seizure ends, almost always within seconds to minutes. If the person seems conscious, stay with him or her until it passes. Someone having a complex partial seizure may wander about; if the person is moving into a hazardous situation, gently guide the person away from danger. Look for a medical identification bracelet or necklace if you are unsure why the person is suddenly acting oddly. Reassure the person as the seizure ends. If the person seems agitated or angry, stay back but close enough to protect the person from danger. Never try to restrain a person who is having any kind of a seizure.

For a person who is having a convulsive seizure, gently turn the person on one side to prevent choking. Do not put anything in the person's mouth because objects may damage teeth or other tissues during the seizure or break and obstruct the airway. Protect the head from injury with a pillow or folded jacket. Keep track of how long the seizure lasts because 9-1-1 should be called for any seizure lasting over five minutes. There is nothing you can do to stop or shorten the seizure, but try to keep the person as comfortable as possible during the seizure. Afterwards the person is likely to be confused or disoriented and drowsy or agitated; be reassuring and help the person to rest as needed (see First Aid: "Seizures"). Commonly the victim is unresponsive

First Aid | Seizures

When You See

- Minor seizures: staring blankly ahead; slight twitching of lips, head, or arms and legs; other movements such as lip-smacking or chewing
- Major seizures: crying out and then becoming unresponsive; body becomes rigid and then shakes in convulsions; jaw may clench
- Fever convulsions in young children: hot, flushed skin; violent muscle twitching; arched back; clenched fists

Do This First

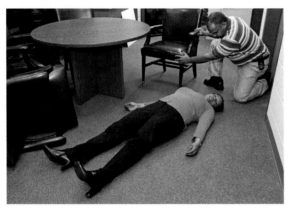

1 Prevent injury during the seizure by moving away dangerous objects and putting something flat and soft under the head. Remove eyeglasses.

2 Loosen clothing around the neck to ease breathing. Check for a medical identification.

3 Gently turn the person onto one side to help keep the airway clear if vomiting occurs.

4 Be reassuring as the person regains responsiveness.

ALERT

- Do not try to stop the person's movements or restrain the person.
- Do not place any objects in the person's mouth.

Additional Care

- Call 9-1-1 if the seizure lasts more than five minutes, if the person is not known to have epilepsy, if the person recovers very slowly or has trouble breathing or has another seizure, if the person is pregnant or is wearing a medical ID for a condition other than epilepsy, or if the person is injured.
- Place an unresponsive victim in the recovery position and monitor breathing.
- For an infant or child with fever convulsions, sponge the body with lukewarm water to help cool the victim, and call 9-1-1.

for a time after a seizure; place the victim in the recovery position and monitor breathing.

Seizures in Special Circumstances

A person who has a seizure while in the water is at risk of aspirating water into the lungs or even drowning. Since a seizure lasts only a few minutes at most, do not try to move the person from the water but support him or her with the head tilted to keep water out of the mouth. After the seizure, help the person out of the water. If the person is not responsive, check for breathing and give CPR if needed.

Another special circumstance is a seizure that occurs in an airplane, motor vehicle, or other confined area. If there are empty seats around the person, fold back the armrests so the person can lie on his or her side across the seats with his or her head on a cushion. If there is no room to lie down, use pillows to protect the person's head from striking hard objects around the seat. Try to lean the person to one side to keep the airway open.

ALTERED MENTAL STATUS

Altered mental status is a phrase used to refer to a change from a person's normal responsiveness and awareness. The person may be confused, disoriented, combative, drowsy, or partially or wholly unresponsive. Altered mental status is not a condition itself but is a sign or symptom that may result from many different injuries and illnesses. Following are just a few of the many causes of altered mental status:

- Seizures
- Stroke
- Head injury
- Poisoning, drug use or overdose
- High fever
- Diabetic emergencies
- Any condition causing lowered blood oxygen levels

When you encounter someone with altered mental status, determine the nature of the problem if possible. If the victim is responsive, perform a physical examination and gather a SAMPLE history. Then give first aid for any problems found.

If the person's altered mental status is due to drug or alcohol use, and the person is acting erratically or in a potentially violent manner, the situation may involve a behavioral emergency. In such cases it is important to ensure your own safety and that of other bystanders. **Chapter 22** describes how

to manage behavioral emergencies. Never assume, however, that a person with altered mental status is intoxicated or is using drugs, or that someone on the street acting strangely has a mental illness. Certain injuries and sudden illnesses such as a diabetic emergency can produce behavior that is easily mistaken for intoxication. Even if the person is intoxicated, he or she may still have an injury or illness that could become an emergency if not cared for.

Altered mental status is often a sign of deteriorating condition. If you cannot determine a cause for the person's condition or behavior, or if you are unsure what to do, call 9-1-1. Describe the situation and the person's signs and symptoms to the dispatcher, who will determine the correct course of action.

DIABETIC EMERGENCIES

Diabetes is actually a group of related diseases in which blood sugar (glucose) levels are not well regulated by the body. The hormone insulin, normally produced in the pancreas, is needed for body cells to be able to use glucose. When insulin levels are too low, glucose levels rise too high. The problem results if the body is not producing enough insulin or if the body does not use the insulin well, a condition called insulin resistance. Currently over 18 million people in the United States have diabetes, five million of whom have not been diagnosed. The disease is chronic and incurable.

There are two primary types of diabetes. In type 1, formerly called insulin-dependent diabetes or juvenile-onset diabetes, the body does not produce enough or any insulin. The person must receive insulin by injection or a pump. In type 2 diabetes, formerly called non-insulin-dependent or adult-onset diabetes, body cells do not use insulin well. Eventually the pancreas may not produce as much insulin. Either way, blood glucose levels may be too high. Over 90% of all diabetics have type 2 diabetes, which becomes more common as one grows older or becomes more overweight. Most people with type 2 diabetes can control the problem with diet, exercise, weight control, and oral medication when needed.

Blood glucose levels vary moment by moment in the body as a result of many factors including what one has eaten, when it was eaten, one's level of activity, and other factors. In a person who is not diabetic, insulin maintains a dynamic balance with blood glucose to prevent levels from becoming too high or too low. People with diabetes, however, sometimes have problems maintaining this balance even with careful attention to diet, activity levels, and blood glucose monitoring.

Prevention of Diabetes and Diabetic Emergencies

Diabetes is a serious and growing problem in the United States. It kills almost 70,000 people yearly, making it the sixth leading cause of death. Diabetes contributes to another 210,000 deaths annually from related causes. In addition, diabetes causes complications throughout the body. Diabetes contributes to heart disease and stroke, is the most common cause of blindness in people 20 to 74 years old, causes severe kidney disease, and damages the nervous system. Because of resulting circulation problems, foot infections in diabetics often lead to amputation. An alarming current trend is the increasing numbers of children and adolescents who are developing type 2 diabetes related to overweight and lack of exercise.

Type 2 diabetes often can be prevented or delayed in people at a high risk for developing the problem. Diet, exercise, and weight control are critical for prevention—the same lifestyle factors that can reduce one's risk for cardiovascular disease (see **Chapter 7**). For those with diabetes, careful control of their glucose levels, blood pressure, and cholesterol levels along with preventive care for the eyes, kidneys, and feet can help prevent complications from developing.

Diabetic emergencies can usually be prevented by careful monitoring of blood glucose levels and by controlling diet, medication use, and activity levels (**Figure 17-6**).

First Aid for Diabetic Emergencies

In a person with diabetes, the blood sugar level may become either too low or too high as a result of many interacting factors. Low blood sugar, called **hypoglycemia,** may result if a person takes too much insulin, does not eat enough or the right foods, or uses blood sugar too quickly through exercise or emotional stress. High blood sugar, called **hyperglycemia,** may result if a person takes too little insulin, eats too much or the wrong foods, or does not use blood sugar with activity (**Figure 17-7**). Other factors, too, can affect blood sugar levels.

Either hypoglycemia or hyperglycemia can quickly progress to a medical emergency if the person is not treated. In many cases you may know if a victim experiencing this emergency has diabetes. Both hypoglycemia and hyperglycemia cause altered mental status (drowsiness, disorientation) and a generalized

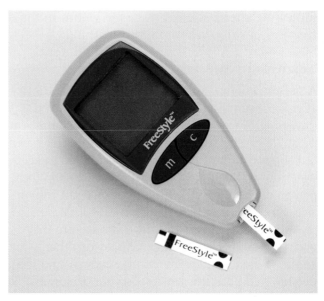

Figure 17-6 People with diabetes often use a blood glucose monitoring system like this one to check their glucose levels using a tiny drop of blood.

feeling of sickness. When taking the SAMPLE history of any victim who suddenly feels ill, ask about diabetes or other medical conditions, and look for a medical alert ID. If the victim is responsive and alert, he or she may know from experience whether the problem is hypoglycemia or hyperglycemia.

Hypoglycemia

The signs and symptoms of hypoglycemia include sudden dizziness, shakiness, or mood change (even combativeness); headache, confusion, and difficulty paying attention; pale skin, sweating; hunger; and

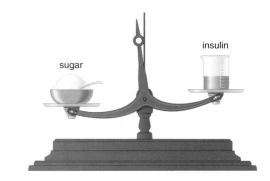

Hypoglycemia
• Sudden dizziness
• Shakiness
• Mood change
• Headache
• Confusion
• Pale skin
• Sweating
• Hunger

Hyperglycemia
• Frequent urination
• Drowsiness
• Dry mouth
• Thirst
• Shortness of breath
• Deep, rapid breathing
• Nausea/vomiting
• Fruity-smelling breath

Figure 17-7 A diabetic emergency may result if the body's balance of insulin and blood sugar is disrupted.

clumsy, jerky movements. A seizure may occur. Although the victim may appear to be intoxicated (slurring words, staggering gait, confusion, etc.), it is important never to dismiss these symptoms without considering the possibility of a diabetic emergency.

First aid for hypoglycemia involves raising the victim's blood sugar level by giving the person food or drink that is high in glucose. Diabetics often carry glucose tablets in case of episodes of low blood sugar **(Figure 17-8)**. Glucose is quickly absorbed into the blood, quickly relieving the problem (see First Aid: "Low Blood Sugar").

Hyperglycemia

The signs and symptoms of hyperglycemia include frequent urination, drowsiness, dry mouth and thirst, shortness of breath and deep, rapid breathing, fruity-smelling breath, and nausea or vomiting. Unresponsiveness eventually occurs.

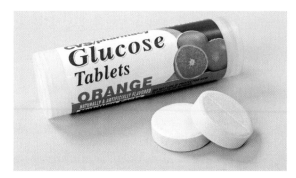

Figure 17-8 Diabetics often carry glucose tablets in case of low blood sugar.

Hyperglycemia generally requires medical treatment. Hyperglycemia usually develops gradually over time, allowing the diabetic person to correct the problem. In a mild case, the victim may follow the instructions from his or her healthcare provider. With more significant symptoms, the victim needs

---

First Aid **Low Blood Sugar**

When You See

- Sudden dizziness, shakiness, or mood change (even combativeness)
- Headache, confusion, difficulty paying attention
- Pale skin, sweating
- Hunger
- Clumsy, jerky movements
- Possible seizure

Do This First

1 Talk to the victim and confirm that he or she has diabetes; look for a medical alert ID.

2 Give the victim sugar: 3 glucose tablets, ½ cup fruit juice, 1 or 2 sugar packets (but not non-sugar sweetener packets), or 5 to 6 pieces of hard candy (unless choking is a risk).

3 If the victim still feels ill or has signs and symptoms after 15 minutes, give more sugar.

ALERT

- If a diabetic victim becomes unresponsive, do not try to inject insulin or put food or fluids in the mouth.

Additional Care

- If the victim becomes unresponsive or continues to have significant signs and symptoms, call 9-1-1 and monitor breathing.

First Aid | High Blood Sugar

When You See

- Frequent urination
- Drowsiness
- Dry mouth, thirst
- Shortness of breath, deep, rapid breathing
- Breath smells fruity
- Nausea, vomiting
- Eventual unresponsiveness

Do This First

1 Talk to the victim and confirm that he or she has diabetes; look for a medical alert ID.

2 Have the victim follow his or her healthcare provider's instructions for hyperglycemia.

3 If you cannot judge whether the victim has low or high blood sugar, give sugar as for low blood sugar. If the victim does not improve in 15 minutes, seek medical care.

4 Call 9-1-1 if the victim becomes unresponsive or continues to have significant signs and symptoms.

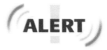

Additional Care

- **Put an unresponsive victim in the recovery position and monitor breathing.**

---

help. The victim may be taken to an emergency department, or if the victim becomes unresponsive, call 9-1-1 (see First Aid: "High Blood Sugar").

In some situations you may know or discover the person has diabetes but not know whether the problem is high or low blood sugar. In this case, give sugar as for low blood sugar. If it happens that the victim has high blood sugar, this additional sugar will not worsen the victim's condition, but it could solve the problem if the victim has low blood sugar. If the victim does not improve in 15 minutes, seek medical care.

SEVERE ABDOMINAL PAIN

Abdominal injuries were described in **Chapter 14**; always call 9-1-1 for an abdominal injury. Abdominal pain may also result from illness ranging from minor conditions to serious medical

emergencies. Urgent medical care is needed for severe abdominal pain in these situations:

In Adults:

- Sudden, severe, intolerable pain, or pain that causes awakening from sleep
- Pain that begins in the general area of the central abdomen and later moves to the lower right
- Pain accompanied by fever, sweating, black or bloody stool, or blood in urine
- Pain in pregnancy or accompanying abnormal vaginal bleeding
- Pain accompanied by dry mouth, dizziness on standing, or decreased urination
- Pain accompanied by difficulty breathing
- Pain accompanied by vomiting blood or greenish-brown fluid

In Young Children:

- Pain that occurs suddenly, stops, and then returns without warning
- Pain accompanied by red or purple, jelly-like stool; or with blood or mucus in stool
- Pain accompanied by greenish-brown vomit
- Pain with swollen abdomen that feels hard
- Pain with a hard lump in lower abdomen or groin area

Many different factors and illnesses can result in gastrointestinal distress with or without abdominal pain. Vomiting or diarrhea may also occur from many different causes. Again, seek urgent medical care for the signs and symptoms listed here, and talk with a healthcare provider for other unexplained or persistent gastrointestinal distress. Following are additional key points:

- Persistent diarrhea or vomiting in an infant or small child or in an elderly or debilitated person can rapidly cause dehydration, which can become an emergency. Seek medical care immediately.
- While awaiting medical help, do not give a person with abdominal pain anything to eat or drink, which may cause vomiting—except in the case of clear fluids for dehydration.

Learning Checkpoint ③

1. When should you call 9-1-1 for a victim who faints?

_____

2. True or False: When a person has fainted, lay him or her down and raise the head and shoulders about 12 inches.

3. For a victim having seizures,

   a. lay the victim face down on the floor.

   b. ask others to help you hold the victim's head, arms, and legs still.

   c. put something flat and soft under the victim's head.

   d. put something wood, like a pencil, between the victim's teeth.

4. Name at least three situations in which you should call 9-1-1 for a seizure victim.

_____

5. What should you do for a young child whose abdomen is swollen and feels hard?

_____

6. Check off common signs and symptoms of a low blood sugar diabetic emergency.

  ___ Dizziness   ___ Red, blotchy skin

  ___ Hunger   ___ Sweating

  ___ Rapid deep breathing   ___ Confusion

  ___ Clumsiness   ___ Swollen legs

7. In the late afternoon you see a friend at the library who is acting oddly. She is sitting at a table staring into space, and when you ask her if she is okay, she does not seem to understand what you are saying. She looks ill, her skin is pale, and she is sweating even though the room is not warm. You know this woman is diabetic and you suspect that she might have skipped lunch today. You cannot be sure whether she has low or high blood sugar. What should you do?

_____

Concluding Thoughts

It can be a frightening experience to be with someone who is suddenly ill, especially if you do not know the cause. Remember the first steps for all first aid situations: assess the victim and try to find out what happened. If you know the cause of the problem, give appropriate first aid; if you do not know, call 9-1-1 and give supportive care until help arrives. Reassure the victim. Help the victim to rest and to avoid getting chilled or overheated, and do not give anything to eat or drink. Stay with the person, watch for changes, and be prepared to give basic life support if needed.

Learning Outcomes

You should now be able to do the following:

1. Explain why first aid is needed when someone suddenly becomes ill.

2. List the general care steps for any sudden illness.

3. Describe the signs and symptoms of and the first aid for each of the following sudden illnesses:
   - Heart attack
   - Angina
   - Stroke
   - Respiratory distress
   - Fainting
   - Seizures
   - Altered mental status
   - Diabetic emergencies
   - Severe abdominal pain

Review Questions

1. Common general signs and symptoms of sudden illness include
   a. feeling ill, dizzy, confused, or weak.
   b. skin color changes (flushed or pale), sweating.
   c. breathing changes.
   d. All of the above

2. Always call 9-1-1 for a victim whose illness
   a. occurs suddenly and without explanation.
   b. includes a fever.
   c. is chronic.
   d. involves feeling fatigued.

3. The signs and symptoms of heart attack include
   a. chest pain, fever, and flushed skin.
   b. chest pain, headache, and an inability to raise both arms.
   c. chest pain, sweating, and shortness of breath.
   d. chest pain, difficulty speaking or swallowing, and vision problems.

4. The most crucial aspect of first aid for a stroke victim is
   a. calling 9-1-1 immediately.
   b. explaining the situation to family members.
   c. elevating the victim's legs.
   d. performing a complete physical examination before calling 9-1-1.

5. Low oxygen blood levels caused by breathing difficulty may cause
   a. heavy sweating.
   b. dizziness or disorientation.
   c. a reddish coloration of the skin.
   d. hyperactivity.

6. First aid for an asthma attack may include
   a. calling 9-1-1 if the victim is not better in 30 minutes.
   b. asking the victim to try to breathe slowly.
   c. helping the victim to lie down with feet raised.
   d. helping the victim to use an inhaler.

7. To help a person who is hyperventilating
   a. have the victim breathe into a paper bag.
   b. splash cold water on the victim's face.
   c. ask the victim to try to breathe slowly.
   d. ask the victim to hold his or her breath as long as possible.

8. Help to prevent injury to a person having a seizure by
   a. putting something flat and soft under the head.
   b. putting a wooden stick between the teeth.
   c. restraining the person by holding the shoulders.
   d. having bystanders help hold the arms and legs still.

9. Altered mental status may result from
   a. stroke.
   b. poisoning.
   c. head injury.
   d. All of the above

10. If you are unsure whether a diabetic is experiencing hypoglycemia or hyperglycemia,
    a. wait an hour to observe signs and symptoms.
    b. give a sugar substance.
    c. call a family member of the victim to inquire.
    d. give the victim an emergency epinephrine shot in the thigh muscle.

References and Resources

American Academy of Pediatrics. *Caring for your school-age child.* New York: Bantam; 1999.

American Academy of Pediatrics. www.aap.org

American College of Emergency Physicians. *First aid manual: a comprehensive guide to treating emergency victims of all ages in any situation.* New York: DK Publishing; 2001.

American Diabetes Association. National diabetes fact sheet. 2005. www.diabetes.org

American Heart Association. Heart attack, stroke & cardiac arrest warning signs. 2005. www.americanheart.org

American Heart Association. 2005 International consensus on cardiopulmonary resuscitation (CPR) and emergency cardiovascular care (ECC) science with treatment recommendations. *Circulation*, 112(22). November 29, 2005.

American Lung Association. www.lungusa.org

American Medical Association. *Handbook of first aid and emergency care.* Revised ed. New York: Random House; 2000.

Epilepsy Foundation. www.epilepsyfoundation.org

Liferidge AT, et al. Ability of laypersons to use the Cincinnati Prehospital Stroke Scale. *Prehospital Emergency Care 2004;* 8(4), October-December.

National Heart, Lung, and Blood Institute. Angina. 2005. www.nhlbi.nih.gov

National Safety Council. www.nsc.org

Persse D, et al. Improving the chain of recovery for acute stroke in your community. Task force report. 2002 Dec 12-13. National Institute of Neurological Disorders and Stroke. http://accessible.ninds.nih.gov

Chapter 18

Poisoning

Chapter Preview

- Overview of Poisoning
- Preventing Poisoning
- Swallowed Poisons
- Inhaled Poisons
- Poison Ivy, Oak, and Sumac

With your young son, Danny, you are visiting a friend at home. Danny has been playing with his toy truck on the floor, which he now pushes down the hallway into the bathroom. You start to get up to bring him back but your friend says, "That's okay, there's nothing in there he can get into." With the normal curiosity of a child, however, Danny starts looking in the bathroom drawers and soon finds a bottle of what looks to him like little candy mints. He puts a handful in his mouth—they don't taste much like mint but he chews and swallows them anyway. You see pills spilled on the floor when you walk into the bathroom. He admits he ate "some" of the pills. What do you do?

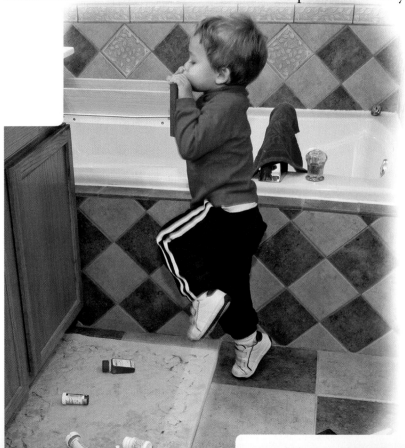

With over two million incidents occurring in the United States every year, resulting in almost 20,000 deaths, poisoning is a huge problem in a world where so many products containing toxins are present in the home and workplace. Most poisonings are accidental, but some victims take a poison intentionally either in a suicide attempt or to experience the effects produced by the substance. This chapter focuses primarily on accidental poisonings. Poisoning caused by the misuse or overdose of alcohol and other drugs, including over-the-counter and prescription medications, is discussed in **Chapter 19**. Behavioral emergencies such as suicide are described in **Chapter 22**.

Virtually all poisonings can be prevented. Parents and other caretakers can protect children from poisoning by keeping them safely away from common products that are poisonous. Most adult poisonings involve the careless use or misuse of medications and cleaning products, which can be prevented by following safety guidelines.

OVERVIEW OF POISONING

A **poison** is any substance that enters or touches the body with effects that are injurious to health or are life threatening. Poisons can enter the body by being swallowed, by being injected (by hypodermic needle or an insect stinger), by being inhaled, or by being absorbed through the skin or mucous membranes. All too often, people think of the risk of poisoning only in terms of ingesting the substance, but inhaling fumes from a product or spilling a chemical on unprotected skin can be just as dangerous. **Chapter 12**, Burns, describes the first aid for poisons (chemicals) that contact the skin or eyes. Injected poisons are described in **Chapters 19** (substance abuse) and **20** (insect stings). This chapter primarily discusses swallowed and inhaled poisons, along with the contact poisons of certain plants, but the prevention guidelines detailed in the next section apply to all forms of poison.

A huge percentage of poisonings occur in the home, most involving common products (**Box 18-1**).

Box 18-1 Facts About Poisonings

- In 2000, Poison Control Centers reported approximately 2.2 million poison exposures. U.S. Poison Control Centers handle an average of one poison exposure every 15 seconds. In 1999, 19,741 poisoning deaths were reported.
- More than 100,000 poisonings resulted in hospitalization.
- More than 90% of poison exposures occur in the home.
- Of the more than two million poison exposures, 52.7% occurred among children younger than age six.
- The most common poison exposures for children were ingestion of household products such as cosmetics and personal care products, cleaning substances, pain relievers, foreign bodies, and plants.

- Adolescents are also at risk for poisonings, both intentional and unintentional. About half of all poisonings among teens are classified as suicide attempts.
- For adults, the most common poison exposures were pain relievers, sedatives, cleaning substances, antidepressants, and bites/stings.
- Childhood lead poisoning is considered one of the most preventable environmental diseases of young children, yet approximately one million children have elevated blood lead levels.
- Carbon monoxide (CO) results in more fatal unintentional poisonings in the United States than any other agent, with the highest number occurring during the winter months.

Source: National Center for Injury Prevention and Control. 2005. Available from: www.cdc.gov/ncipc

The American Association of Poison Control Centers analyzes cases of poisoning in 26 classes of products other than pharmaceuticals. The 12 classes of poisons that cause the greatest number of poisonings are listed in **Table 18-1**. The classes of poisons that cause the most deaths are listed in **Table 18-2**. These are just the most common types of products that contain poisons—a complete list of every product or substance that is poisonous would be many, many pages long. Since there are so many poisons present in so many different products, **the safest thing is to assume that *all* substances that can be swallowed, injected, breathed in, or put in contact with skin are poisonous unless known to be otherwise.** Note that almost any substance can be poisonous in doses larger than intended, including aspirin, vitamins, herbal supplements and natural remedies, and prescribed or over-the-counter medication.

Comparing **Tables 18-1 and 18-2** leads to some insights about common poisonings. Alcohol poisoning, which usually results from beverage alcohol, causes the most poisoning deaths, even though the number of cases is much lower than for other causes of poisoning, such as cosmetics and personal care products, which cause more than three times as many poisonings but less than one-tenth as many deaths. Similarly, poisonings with chemicals and fumes carry a much higher risk of death than many household products. On the other hand, such statistics can be misleading. Even one death that occurs when a child eats the leaves of a houseplant is significant. It is essential, therefore, to pay attention to all possible sources of poisons.

Poison Control Centers

A system of **Poison Control Centers (PCC)** has been developed throughout the United States to provide information and treatment advice for all kinds of poisonings. Presently there are 62 Poison Control Centers throughout the states and U.S. territories. All can be reached by dialing the same telephone number: 1-800-222-1222, 24 hours a day. Your call will be routed to the regional PCC in your area. This telephone number should be

Table 18-1

Top 12 Nonpharmaceutical Product Classes Causing Poisoning (Ranked by Number of Cases)

Rank	Product Class	Cases of Poisoning	Deaths
1	Cosmetics/personal care products	223,187	8
2	Household cleaning substances	211,077	24
3	Foreign bodies/toys/miscellaneous	124,177	4
4	Pesticides	97,677	41
5	Bites and envenomations	92,247	6
6	Plants	77,169	3
7	Alcohols (beverage, rubbing, etc.)	69,524	121
8	Food products (excluding foodborne disease)	69,122	0
9	Hydrocarbons (gasoline, etc.)	55,310	17
10	Chemicals	49,882	43
11	Arts/crafts/office supplies	45,382	0
12	Fumes/gases/vapors	38,462	61

Source of data: AAPCC 2003 annual report. 2005. Available from: www.aapcc.org

Table 18-2

Top 12 Nonpharmaceutical Product Classes Causing Poisoning (Ranked by Number of Deaths)

Rank	Product Class	Cases of Poisoning	Deaths
1	Alcohols (beverage, rubbing, etc.)	69,524	121
2	Fumes/gases/vapors	38,462	61
3	Chemicals	49,882	43
4	Pesticides	97,677	41
5	Household cleaning substances	211,077	24
6	Automotive/aircraft/boat products	14,181	19
7	Hydrocarbons (gasoline, etc.)	55,310	17
8	Cosmetics/personal care products	223,187	8
9	Heavy metals	17,894	7
10	Bites and envenomations	92,247	6
11	Foreign bodies/toys/miscellaneous	124,177	4
12	Mushrooms	8,252	4

Source: AAPCC 2003 annual report. 2005. Available from: www.aapcc.org

posted by your telephone at home and in your workplace. When you are away from this number, call 9-1-1 and if necessary the dispatcher will contact the Poison Control Center. In almost all cases it is better to call the PCC in cases of poisoning than a healthcare provider because the PCC has the most accurate and up-to-date information. Personnel staffing each PCC have information about all known poisons and will advise you what first aid to give in each poisoning case.

The American Association of Poison Control Centers (AAPCC) also provides much valuable information about how to prevent poisonings and information about specific poisons. On request, the AAPCC will provide a list of poisonous plants in your area to help you identify threats in your yard or in places you may visit (http://www.aapcc.org).

PREVENTING POISONING

Most poisonings occur accidentally and can be prevented by following simple guidelines. The safety principles for preventing poisonings in children are based on keeping children away from products and substances that contain poisons and educating children in safe behaviors. Prevention principles for adults, who often use products and medications that can be poisonous, focus on safe and appropriate use and on minimizing or eliminating the risk of accidental exposure.

Preventing Poisoning in Children

Children under age six are at the highest risk for poisoning. Children are often curious about what things taste like and will put many different substances into their mouths. Colorful product packages may attract a young child, who cannot easily distinguish between food products and other products found in the home. Even if they are told to leave certain things alone, young children do not yet have the cognitive skills needed to understand why they should not eat or drink substances they find. Prevention emphasizes keeping all potentially harmful substances where children cannot get to them.

Follow these guidelines provided by the American Association of Poison Control Centers:

Household and Chemical Products

- Use safety locks on all cabinets. Store potential poisons out of reach of small children.
- Store all poisonous household and chemical products out of sight of children.
- If you are using a product and need to answer the telephone or doorbell, take the child with you. Most poisonings occur when the product is in use.
- Store all products in their original containers. *Do not* use food containers such as milk jugs or soda bottles to store household and chemical products.
- Store food and household and chemical products in separate areas. Mistaken identity could cause a serious poisoning. Many poisonous products look like and come in containers very similar to those that contain drinks or food—for example, apple juice and pine cleaner.
- Return household and chemical products to safe storage immediately after use.
- Use extra caution during mealtimes or when the family routine is disrupted. Many poisonings take place at these times.
- Pesticides can be absorbed through the skin and can be extremely toxic. Keep children away from areas that have recently been sprayed. Store these products in a safe place where children cannot reach them.
- Discard old or outdated household and chemical products.
- Take time to teach children about poisonous substances.
- Keep the Poison Control Center telephone number on or near your telephone.

Medicine

- Keep medicines out of sight, locked up, and out of reach of children.
- Make sure that all medicines are in child-resistant containers and are labeled properly. Remember that child-resistant does not mean childproof.
- Never leave pills on the counter or in plastic bags. Always store medicines in their original container with a child-resistant cap.

- Keep purses and diaper bags out of reach of children.
- Do not take medicines in front of children. Young children often imitate adult behaviors.
- Do not call medicine candy. Medicines and candy look alike, and children cannot tell the difference.
- Vitamins are medicine. Vitamins with iron can be especially poisonous. Keep them locked up and out of reach of children.
- Be aware of medicines that visitors may bring into your home. Children are curious and may investigate visitors' purses and suitcases.

Plants

- Contact your local Poison Control Center for more information about toxic plants in your area. **Figure 18-1** shows three common plants that are poisonous when eaten.
- Know the name of the plants in your home and in your yard. Label all of your plants. If you are having difficulty identifying a plant, take a sample to a nursery for identification.
- Keep poisonous plants out of reach of children and pets.
- Teach your children not to eat mushrooms growing in the yard. Some of these mush-

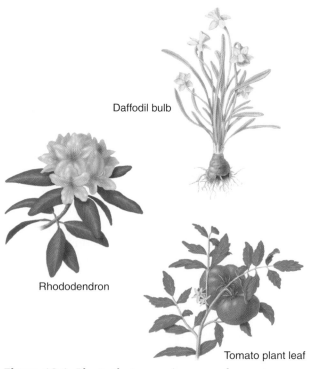

Daffodil bulb

Rhododendron

Tomato plant leaf

Figure 18-1 Plants that are poisonous when eaten.

rooms can be poisonous. Be aware that mushrooms are often abundant after rain.

- Teach your children not to eat leaves and berries that grow in the yard. Do not assume a plant is safe to eat if you see wild animals eating it.
- Keep children and pets away from plants that have recently been sprayed with weed killer, bug killer, or fertilizer.

Preventing Poisoning in Adults

Follow these guidelines provided by the American Association of Poison Control Centers:

- Keep potential poisons in their original containers. Do not use food containers such as cups or bottles to store household and chemical products.
- Store food and household and chemical products in separate areas. Mistaken identity could cause a serious poisoning.
- Read and follow the directions and caution labels on household and chemical products before using them.
- Never mix household and chemical products together. A poisonous gas may be created when mixing chemicals.
- Turn on fans and open windows when using household and chemical products.
- When spraying household and chemical products, make sure the spray nozzle is directed away from your face and other people. Wear protective clothing—long-sleeve shirts, long pants, socks, shoes, and gloves—when spraying pesticides and other chemicals.
- Pesticides can be absorbed through the skin and can be extremely poisonous. Stay away from areas that have recently been sprayed.
- Never sniff containers to discover what is inside.
- Discard old or outdated household and chemical products.
- First aid instructions on product containers may be incorrect or outdated. Call the Poison Control Center instead for guidelines to follow if an exposure occurs.
- Keep the Poison Control Center telephone number on or near your telephone.
- Follow the prevention guidelines in **Chapter 19** to prevent accidental poisoning by the misuse of over-the-counter and prescription medications.

SWALLOWED POISONS

Most cases of poisoning involve substances that are swallowed. Depending on the poison, effects may begin almost immediately or may be delayed. First aid is most effective if given as soon as possible after the poison is swallowed, and in some cases the effects can be prevented or minimized by acting quickly. Poisoning is like sudden illness in that often there is no visible injury and you may not know immediately what happened. The victim may be unresponsive or, even if responsive, may be confused and disoriented and unable to tell you what happened. The most important aspect of first aid for a poisoning often is recognizing that a poisoning has occurred.

As you check the scene and perform your initial assessment of the victim, look around for any sign that the victim may be poisoned. Look for containers nearby or any clue that the person was using a substance or product. Ask others at the scene if anyone saw anything or knows what the person was doing when the problem occurred. If the victim is responsive and identifies a substance to which he or she was exposed, try to learn how much the person may have swallowed and how long ago.

The specific signs and symptoms of poisons depend on the substance and many other factors, although many poisons cause similar general effects:

- The victim may look and feel ill.
- The victim may have abdominal pain, feel nauseous, and may vomit or have diarrhea.
- The victim may have altered mental status or may become unresponsive.
- There may be burns, stains, or odors around the victim's mouth.
- The pupils of the eyes may be dilated or constricted.
- The victim may be breathing abnormally.

Be aware that the condition of a poisoning victim may change rapidly.

First aid for a poisoning depends on the victim's condition. For an unresponsive victim, call 9-1-1 immediately. Check for normal breathing and provide CPR if needed. Because of the risk for vomiting, put a breathing, unresponsive victim in the recovery position, and continue to monitor breathing.

If the victim is responsive, call the Poison Control Center and follow the instructions

Box 18-2 Calling the Poison Control Center

If possible, have the following information with you if you call a PCC for help with a suspected poisoning with any product or substance. This information will help the Center to determine the best care to provide. But do not delay a call to the PCC to look for this information if it is not readily available.

- The victim's present condition
- Name of the product and ingredients
- How much of the product was taken
- The time poisoning happened
- Your name and phone number
- The victim's approximate age and weight

provided (**Box 18-2**). Depending on the poison, the PCC may direct you to take any of various actions. Some poisons may be diluted by having the victim drink water or milk. With some poisons the victim may benefit from drinking a solution of activated charcoal, if available, which absorbs some kinds of poison. Activated charcoal is available in a powder or liquid form without prescription and may be kept in the home medicine cabinet for use if the PCC advises it (**Figure 18-2**). Because none of these actions is used for all kinds of poisons, *never take any of these actions unless told to do so by the Poison Control Center.* The PCC will also tell you whether to call 9-1-1 or seek other urgent medical care for a poisoning incident (see First Aid: "Swallowed Poisons").

Note that syrup of ipecac was in the past used in some situations to induce vomiting in a victim of swallowed poison. Because of problems caused by this and its lack of effectiveness in most cases, PCCs no longer recommend the use of ipecac.

Food Poisoning

Food poisoning occurs after one eats food that is contaminated with microorganisms, usually bacteria, or their toxins. Most cases of food poisoning are acute infections, although some bacteria make toxins that can poison a food even if the bacteria are later killed. The CDC estimates that 76 million people in the United States become sick every year from pathogens in food, and about 5000 die. Botulism is a life-threatening type of food poisoning produced by a certain bacterium present in improperly canned or preserved food.

Contamination can occur at any stage, from growing the food through processing to food

preparation and delivery. Food contamination usually results from improper cooking or leaving a cooked food out for more than two hours at room temperature. Most bacteria grow rapidly and are undetected because they do not change the odor or taste of the food. Freezing a food will slow or stop bacteria growth but will not kill the bacteria.

Food poisoning symptoms may begin soon after eating or within a day. The most common signs and symptoms are nausea, vomiting, abdominal pain, and diarrhea. Talk to your healthcare provider to see if treatment is needed (see First Aid: "Food Poisoning"). Seek urgent medical care if any of the following signs and symptoms occurs:

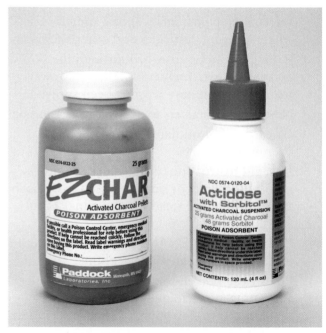

Figure 18-2 The Poison Control Center may advise taking activated charcoal in some cases of poisoning.

When You See

- Open container of poisonous substance
- Nausea and vomiting, signs of abdominal pain or cramps
- Drowsiness, dizziness, disorientation, or other altered mental status
- Changing levels of responsiveness

Do This First

1 Determine what was swallowed, when, and how much.

2 For a responsive victim, call the Poison Control Center (800-222-1222) immediately and follow their instructions.

3 For an unresponsive victim, call 9-1-1 and provide basic life support (BLS) as needed.

(((ALERT)))

- Do not give any substance to eat or drink unless instructed by the PCC or healthcare provider.
- Do not follow first aid instructions present on some household product labels; instead, call the PCC.

Additional Care

- Put an unresponsive victim in the recovery position and be prepared for vomiting.
- If a responsive victim's mouth or lips are burned by a corrosive chemical, rinse the mouth with cold water (without swallowing).

- Signs of shock: shallow breathing; cold, clammy, pale or ashen skin; shaking or chills; or chest pain
- Signs of severe dehydration: dry mouth, decreased urine output, dizziness, fatigue, increased breathing rate
- Confusion or difficulty reasoning

Preventing Food Poisoning

The National Digestive Diseases Information Clearinghouse recommends the following guidelines to prevent food poisoning:

- Refrigerate foods promptly. If you let pre-pared food stand at room temperature for more than two hours, it may not be safe to eat. Set your refrigerator at 40° F or lower and your freezer at 0° F.
- Cook food to the appropriate temperature (145° F for roasts, steaks, and chops of beef, veal, and lamb; 160° F for pork, ground veal, and ground beef; 165° F for ground poultry; and 180° F for whole poultry). Use a thermometer to be sure. Foods are properly cooked only when they are heated long enough and at a high enough temperature to

When You See

- Nausea and vomiting, signs of abdominal pain or cramps
- Diarrhea, possibly with blood
- Headache, fever

Do This First

1 Have the victim rest lying down.

2 Give the victim lots of clear liquids.

3 Seek medical attention.

((ALERT))

Botulism

- Botulism is more likely to occur from the consumption of home-canned foods. If the victim experiences dizziness, muscle weakness, and difficulty talking or breathing, call 9-1-1.

Additional Care

- Check with others with whom the victim has eaten recently.

---

kill the harmful bacteria that cause illness.

- Prevent cross-contamination. Bacteria can spread from one food product to another throughout the kitchen and can get onto cutting boards, knives, sponges, and countertops. Keep raw meat, poultry, seafood, and their juices away from other foods that are ready to eat.
- Handle food properly. Always wash your hands before touching food and after using the bathroom, changing diapers, or handling pets, as well as after handling raw meat, poultry, fish, shellfish, or eggs. Clean surfaces well before preparing food on them.
- Keep cold food cold and hot food hot.
- Maintain hot cooked food at 140° F or higher.
- Reheat cooked food to at least 165° F.
- Refrigerate or freeze perishables, prepared food, and leftovers within two hours.
- Never defrost food on the kitchen counter. Use the refrigerator, cold running water, or the microwave oven.

- Never let food marinate at room temperature; refrigerate it.
- Divide large amounts of leftovers into small, shallow containers for quick cooling in the refrigerator.
- Remove the stuffing from poultry and other meats immediately and refrigerate it in a separate container.
- Do not overfill the refrigerator. Cool air must circulate to keep food safe.

INHALED POISONS

In both home and work settings, various gases and fumes may be present. Products such as paints, thinners, and many chemicals give off fumes that can result in a poisoning if there is not enough fresh air or other protection. Some products' fumes are so toxic that a respirator must be worn when working with them, even outdoors where fresh air is plentiful. Always check product labels for health risks and safety precautions.

Inhaled poisons also include gases that may escape from pipelines or tanks being transported. Whenever you smell gas or have other evidence of a leak, stay away from the scene. Remember that not all hazardous gases or fumes can be smelled. Call 9-1-1 and let a specially trained hazardous materials team manage the situation. In such a situation do not risk your own safety in an attempt to get to a victim. **Chapter 2** describes typical hazardous scenes and the warning placards that may indicate the presence of a poisonous gas.

Smoke and fumes resulting from fires are also poisonous. Fires produce carbon monoxide and, depending on the substances being burned, may produce other highly toxic gases. **Chapter 25** describes actions to take in or near a fire.

The signs and symptoms of inhaled poisons may be similar to those of other poisons. Breathing difficulty with or without chest pain may be present. Altered mental status may include dizziness, disorientation, headache, unresponsiveness, or other symptoms.

In most cases you will not know the specific treatment for an inhaled poison. First try to ensure that the victim is breathing fresh air, if it is safe for you to go to the victim. Move the victim outdoors or to a well-ventilated area, if possible. If the victim should not be moved because of injuries or other factors, ventilate the area. If the victim is responsive, call the PCC and follow its instructions. If the victim is unresponsive, call 9-1-1.

The general first aid for an inhaled poison is the same as for carbon monoxide poisoning, described in the next section. Carbon monoxide is the most common gas involved in poisonings.

Carbon Monoxide

Carbon monoxide is especially dangerous because it is invisible, odorless, and tasteless—and very lethal. This gas results in more fatal unintentional poisonings in the United States than any other poison. Carbon monoxide may be present from motor vehicle or boat exhaust, a faulty furnace, a kerosene heater, industrial equipment, a poorly vented fireplace or wood stove, or fire. Exposure to large amounts causes an immediate poisoning reaction; a small leak may cause gradual poisoning with less dramatic symptoms. To prevent poisoning, carbon monoxide detectors should be used along with smoke detectors in appropriate locations. If your carbon monoxide detector goes off, do not investigate the problem yourself but leave the premises and call your furnace company or appropriate other professional.

Preventing Carbon Monoxide Poisoning

Over 15,000 cases of carbon monoxide poisoning and about 500 deaths occur each year in the United States from carbon monoxide poisoning unrelated to fires. The CDC recommends the following strategies to prevent carbon monoxide exposure in the home:

- Have your heating system, water heater, and any other gas-, oil-, or coal-burning appliances serviced by a qualified technician every year.
- Install a battery-operated carbon monoxide detector in your home, and check or replace the battery when you change the time on your clocks each spring and fall.
- If your CO detector sounds, evacuate your home immediately and telephone 9-1-1.
- Seek prompt medical attention if you suspect CO poisoning and are feeling dizzy, light-headed, or nauseated.
- Do not use a generator, charcoal grill, camp stove, or other gasoline- or charcoal-burning device inside your home, basement, or garage or near a window.
- Do not run a car or truck inside a garage attached to your house, even if you leave the door open.
- Do not burn anything in a stove or fireplace that is not vented.
- Do not heat your house with a gas oven.

First Aid for Carbon Monoxide Poisoning

Carbon monoxide poisoning usually causes altered mental status. Prolonged periods of exposure to CO may cause headaches, dizziness, confusion, poor judgment, and sleepiness. Continued exposure brings on breathing difficulty, nausea, vomiting, and heart palpitations. Exposure to high levels of CO for prolonged periods can result in seizures, unresponsiveness, and death.

The most important first aid for a victim of carbon monoxide poisoning is to get the victim to fresh air, but do not risk your own health if the scene is dangerous. Call 9-1-1. If it is safe to move the victim, do so quickly. Note that even a victim who seems to recover needs medical care for the poisoning (see First Aid: "Carbon Monoxide and Inhaled Poisons").

First Aid   Carbon Monoxide and Inhaled Poisons

When You See

- Headache
- Dizziness, light-headedness, confusion, weakness
- Nausea, vomiting
- Signs of chest pain
- Convulsions
- Changing levels of responsiveness

Do This First

1 Immediately move the victim into fresh air.

2 Call 9-1-1 even if the victim starts to recover.

Additional Care

3 Monitor the victim and give care as needed.

- Put an unresponsive victim in the recovery position.
- Loosen tight clothing around neck or chest.

Learning Checkpoint ①

1. Check off the common signs and symptoms of a swallowed poison.

___ Nausea	___ Red lips
___ Uncontrolled shaking	___ Vomiting
___ Dizziness	___ Unresponsiveness
___ Drowsiness	___ Hyperactivity

2. Name one action you would take for a victim of food poisoning that you would not do for a victim of swallowed poison.

_____

3. The first thing to do for a victim of carbon monoxide poisoning is

   a. loosen tight clothing around the neck.

   b. call 9-1-1.

   c. move the victim to fresh air.

   d. place the victim in the recovery position.

4. You are in a friend's house when you enter the kitchen and find the friend's child unresponsive on the floor. The cabinet under the sink is open, and the cap is off a bottle of a cleaning product. Describe what actions you need to take.

_____

POISON IVY, OAK, AND SUMAC

Contact with poison ivy, oak, and sumac causes an allergic skin reaction, called **allergic contact dermatitis,** in about half the population. A resin in the leaves of these plants causes the reaction. These plants grow in many areas of the country but can be identified by their distinctive leaves **(Figure 18-3).** The resin can rub off on a person's clothing and shoes and then be transferred to the skin. If someone touches the leaves and gets the resin on the fingers, touching other body areas before washing may transfer the irritating resin to other skin areas, including the face and eyes and even the genitals.

If you know you have made contact with one of these plants, wash the area as soon as possible with soap and water. Also wash clothing and wipe off shoes, since the resin on these can still cause the reaction.

The rash may appear within a few hours or up to two days after exposure **(Figure 18-4).** The skin is red and often very itchy, and young children must be kept from scratching it because the skin easily breaks and may become infected with bacteria. Once the rash appears on the skin and has been washed, however, it cannot spread to other people; it is not a contagious condition. First aid is usually to control the itching, which can be intense

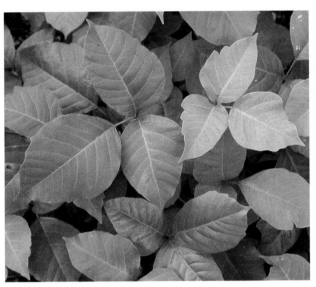

(a) Poison ivy

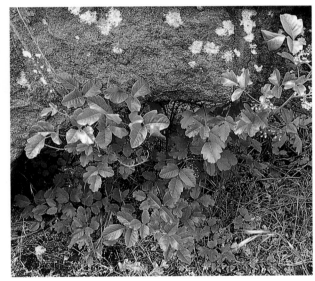

(b) Poison oak

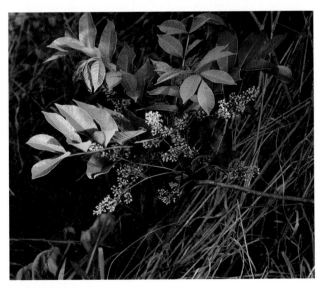

(c) Poison sumac

Figure 18-3 Common poisonous plants causing rashes.

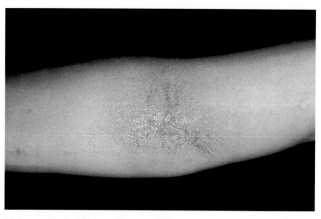

Figure 18-4 Skin rash caused by poison ivy.

and lasts as long as the rash persists, usually less than two weeks. Cool, wet compresses applied four times a day generally help, along with calamine lotion or a paste of baking soda and water between compresses. Make the baking soda paste just thick enough to cling to the skin without running off. Topical hydrocortisone cream or an oral antihistamine may help in more serious cases. See a health-care provider if the reaction is very severe or the rash occurs around the eyes or genitals. Fever or pus oozing from the rash may indicate an infection that should also receive medical treatment (see First Aid: "Poison Ivy, Oak, and Sumac").

First Aid   Poison Ivy, Oak, and Sumac

When You See
- Redness and itching occur first
- Rash, blisters (may weep)
- Possible headache and fever

Do This First

1 Wash the area thoroughly with soap and water as soon as possible after contact.

2 For severe reactions or swelling on the face or genitals, seek medical attention.

3 Treat itching with colloid oatmeal baths; a paste made of baking soda and water, calamine lotion, or topical hydrocortisone cream; and an oral antihistamine (e.g., Benadryl).

ALERT
- Do not burn these poisonous plants to get rid of them, as smoke also spreads the poisonous resin.

Additional Care
- Wash clothing and shoes (and pets) that contacted the plants to prevent further spread.

Learning Checkpoint ②

1. True or False: Never put water on a site of contact with poison ivy because of the risk of spreading the rash further.

2. When should a person with a poison ivy or oak rash see a healthcare provider?

_____

3. Which of the following can help reduce the itching of poison ivy?

   a. Hydrocortisone cream

   b. Rubbing alcohol

   c. A paste made with dishwasher detergent

   d. All of the above

Concluding Thoughts

Remember that a poison is any substance that is injurious to health after it enters the body. In addition to those substances we all think of as obvious poisons, alcohol and drugs, too, can be toxic when misused or abused—prescription and over-the-counter drugs as well as illicit drugs. In fact, poisonings from medications, even everyday aspirin, are more common than poisonings caused by household products. In the next chapter you will learn about the problems of substance abuse and misuse.

Learning Outcomes

You should now be able to do the following:

1. Explain different ways that poisons can enter the body.

2. List things you can do in your own home to prevent the poisoning of both children and adults.

3. Describe the role of Poison Control Centers in the treatment of poisoning.

4. Describe the first aid for swallowed and inhaled poisons.

5. List actions to take when exposed to poison ivy, oak, or sumac.

Review Questions

1. Where do most poisonings occur?
   a. Industrial settings
   b. Homes
   c. Farms
   d. Day care centers

2. What group experiences the largest percentage of poisonings?
   a. Children under age 6
   b. Children 4 to 14
   c. The elderly
   d. Construction workers

3. Which of the following types of products may be poisonous?
   a. Cosmetics
   b. Vitamins with iron
   c. Arts and crafts supplies
   d. All of the above

4. The common signs and symptoms of swallowed poisonings often include
   a. dizziness and aching in the joints.
   b. unresponsiveness and high fever.
   c. nausea and altered mental status.
   d. localized redness and swelling around the joints.

5. For a responsive child who swallowed a substance that might be poisonous, it is best to call
   a. the Poison Control Center.
   b. the child's pediatrician.
   c. the local hospital emergency department.
   d. the child's school nurse.

6. The usual first aid for most swallowed poisons includes
   a. giving the victim milk to drink.
   b. inducing vomiting by any means.
   c. having the victim drink as much water as possible.
   d. calling 9-1-1 or the Poison Control Center for help.

7. When should you seek medical care for a victim who feels ill a few hours after eating food that may have been contaminated?
   a. When the victim is experiencing shaking or chills
   b. When the victim feels dizzy
   c. When the victim's skin is cold and clammy
   d. All of the above

8. What should you do for a breathing, unresponsive victim suspected of having swallowed a poison?
   a. Put the victim in the shock position with the feet raised.
   b. Put the victim on his or her back with the head raised.
   c. Put the victim in the recovery position.
   d. Put the victim in the prone position with his or her head lower than the body.

9. Exposure to carbon monoxide may cause
   a. bleeding at mucous membranes.
   b. dizziness.
   c. dark stains around the mouth.
   d. hyperexcitability.

10. To treat the itching caused by poison ivy, what can be put on the rash?
    a. An oral antihistamine tablet crushed and mixed with water
    b. A paste of baking soda and water
    c. Lemon juice mixed with powdered sugar
    d. Antibiotic cream

References and Resources

Poison Control Center—National Hotline: 1-800-222-1222

American Association of Poison Control Centers (AAPCC). www.aapcc.org

American College of Emergency Physicians. *First aid manual: a comprehensive guide to treating emergency victims of all ages in any situation.* New York: DK Publishing; 2001.

American Heart Association. 2005 International consensus on cardiopulmonary resuscitation (CPR) and emergency cardiovascular care (ECC) science with treatment recommendations. *Circulation,* 112(22). November 29, 2005.

American Medical Association. *Handbook of first aid and emergency care.* Revised ed., New York: Random House; 2000.

National Center for Injury Prevention and Control. Poisonings: fact sheet. 2005. www.cdc.gov/ncipc

National Digestive Diseases Information Clearinghouse (NDDIC). Bacteria and foodborne illness. 2005. http://digestive.niddk.nih.gov/diseases/pubs/bacteria/index.htm

National Safety Council. www.nsc.org

Chapter 19

Substance Misuse and Abuse

Chapter Preview

- Substance Abuse

- Prevention of Substance Abuse

- Prevention of Drug Misuse and Overdose

- Intoxication

- Drug Abuse

- Medication Overdose

You are at a friend's holiday party where some of the guests are drinking rather heavily. At the end of the evening, when most have left, you notice a young woman alone on the sofa, apparently either sleeping or passed out. She seems to be by herself, and others are saying to just leave her alone and let her "sleep it off." You are wondering if you should do something—if it could be a more serious problem—but what can you do?

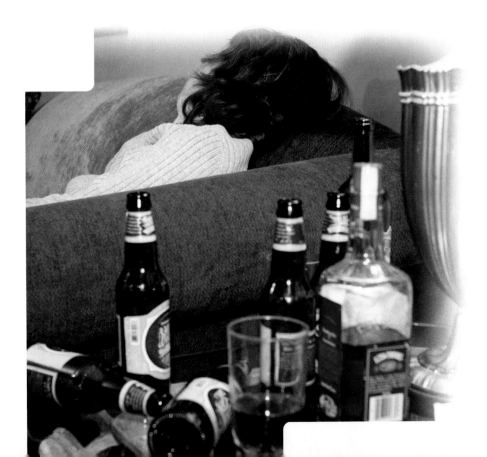

The misuse and abuse of alcohol, illicit drugs, and medication is a huge problem in our society. The effects of alcohol and other drugs may themselves cause a medical or behavioral emergency or may complicate a sudden illness or injury. In either case, first aiders need to understand the effects of alcohol and other drugs and special considerations when giving first aid to victims under their influence.

SUBSTANCE ABUSE

Substance abuse is an inescapable problem virtually everywhere in our society. Consider these U.S. statistics:

- About half of those age 12 or older, or 119 million people, regularly consume alcohol.
- More that one-fifth of those age 12 or older, or 54 million people, participate in binge drinking at least once a month.
- Almost 7% of those age 12 or older, or 16 million people, routinely drink heavily.
- Over 8% of those age 12 or older, or 19 million people, use illicit drugs.

Both heavy drinking and binge drinking are most common in the late teen and early adult years and gradually taper off with age, although they remain a common behavior (**Figure 19-1**). Although some variations in drinking habits are correlated with ethnic group, socioeconomic status, and education levels, studies show alcohol use is a problem at all ages and in all groups. One common problem behavior, driving under the influence of alcohol, is practiced by almost 30% of young adults and by high percentages of other age groups also.

The popularity of alcohol may be due in part to several common myths that suggest that it creates fewer risks than other drugs. Here are some facts about consumption:

- Alcohol and tobacco are "gateway" drugs: someone who smokes or drinks is 65 times more likely to move on to marijuana, and someone who has smoked marijuana is 104 times more likely to move on to cocaine.
- Someone drinking beer is just as likely to become impaired as someone drinking hard liquor. The amount of alcohol in a 12-ounce beer is the same as in a 5-ounce glass of wine or 1.5 ounces of 80-proof spirits.
- Heavier people are no less likely to become impaired by consuming alcohol than lighter people. Many complex factors influence a person's reaction to alcohol, and these cannot easily be predicted. It is therefore unsafe to drink and drive at any time.
- From the first drink, alcohol impairs motor skills, judgment, reaction time, and other abilities needed for safe driving.

The toll of alcohol abuse in society includes automobile death rates, other injuries, and huge medical costs spent on alcohol-related health problems such as liver disease and cardiovascular conditions. Over seven million victims of alcohol-related injuries and illnesses are brought to hospital emergency departments every year. Over 12,000 people die each year in the United States as the result of alcohol-related driving crashes. This represents more than 30% of all traffic deaths. The costs of alcohol-related motor vehicle crashes is estimated at $34 billion annually.

Illicit drugs include marijuana, cocaine, heroin, hallucinogens, inhalants, and the nonmedical use of prescription pain relievers, tranquilizers, stimulants, and sedatives. Like alcohol abuse, illicit drug abuse typically begins in the preteen years, peaks in the late teen and early adult years, and gradually becomes less common thereafter. Marijuana is the most commonly used illicit drug (**Figure 19-2** and **Table 19-1**).

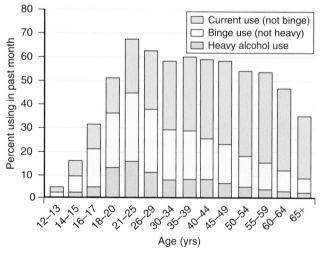

Figure 19-1 Alcohol use and abuse in different age groups. (From the National Survey on Drug Use and Health, 2003.)

Table 19-1

Illicit Drug Use in the U.S.

Drug	Number of Users
Illicit Drugs	
Marijuana	14.6 million
Cocaine	2.3 million
Hallucinogens	1 million
Heroin	119,000
Prescription Drugs Used Illicitly	
Pain relievers	4.7 million
Tranquilizers	1.8 million
Stimulants	1.2 million
Sedatives	300,000

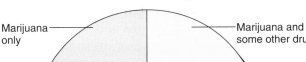

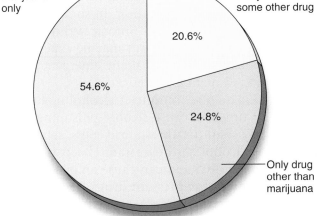

Figure 19-2 Types of illicit drugs abused. (From the National Survey on Drug Use and Health, 2003.)

PREVENTION OF SUBSTANCE ABUSE

Because alcohol and other drug abuse typically begin at young ages, most prevention efforts focus on children and adolescents. For adults who have begun abusing alcohol and other drugs, many treatment centers and organizations have programs available. The National Survey on Drug

Use and Health has identified key risk factors for developing an abuse problem, and a wide range of prevention measures have been developed to address these:

- *Substance abuse is more likely in those who perceive less risk in using the substance.* Education programs in elementary and middle schools teach students the risks of alcohol and drugs, and many public information campaigns strive to make the risks known.

- *Substance abuse is more prevalent among those with easier access to drugs and alcohol.* Law enforcement and other programs strive to reduce the availability of drugs and alcohol to young people, although most youths still report that it is easy to obtain alcohol, marijuana, and other drugs.

- *Substance abuse is about five times as prevalent among youths who perceive that their parents would not strongly disapprove of their substance use as it is among those who feel their parents would strongly disapprove.* Public education campaigns increasingly focus on the role of parents' attitudes and the need for communication with their children.

- *Substance abuse is about twice as prevalent among youths who dislike school.* Many schools have adopted programs aimed at increasing student satisfaction levels and building the self-esteem of students related to their schooling.

- *Substance abuse is more prevalent among youths who engage in delinquent behaviors such as fighting, stealing, or carrying weapons.*

- *Substance abuse is about twice as prevalent among youths who do not attend religious services or youth activities such as sports, band, and other after-school activities.* Recognizing this, many schools and communities have increased the availability of programs for youth.

The 2003 National Survey on Drug Use and Health showed that such prevention programs are having a positive effect. Youths exposed to substance abuse prevention messages in or outside of school, who have talked with their parents about the dangers of drug and alcohol use, and who have participated in various special programs are all less likely to use or abuse alcohol and other drugs. But as the earlier statistics show, abuse remains a huge problem, and clearly more efforts are needed both to understand the many complex factors involved in substance abuse behavior and to develop prevention strategies to successfully counter those factors.

PREVENTION OF DRUG MISUSE AND OVERDOSE

Substance abuse is the intentional and often frequent nonmedical use of a substance for its effects, typically without regard for potential negative health effects. **Substance misuse,** in contrast, may involve using a drug for an unintended purpose or using it in larger amounts than prescribed, including unintentional misuse. Misuse may occur, for example, if a person takes more of a medication than prescribed either by accident or from a false belief that more of the medication is better. Because misuse, like abuse, can lead to a drug **overdose,** it is important to take steps to prevent it:

- Use medications only as prescribed and read product information.
- Keep all medications in their original, clearly labeled containers. Check the label before taking the medication. (Never take a medication in the dark.) Organize medications used by the elderly to prevent accidental overdose.
- If a person's judgment may be diminished by a medical or other condition, make sure that the person cannot accidentally use too much of any prescribed or over-the-counter medication.
- Read and follow the directions and warnings on the label before taking any medicine.
- If you have any questions about the intended use of your medicine, contact your doctor.
- Some medicines are dangerous when mixed with alcohol. Consult your doctor or pharmacist.
- Be aware of potential drug interactions. Some medicines interact dangerously with food or other medicines. Your doctor should be made aware of all medicines, prescription or over-the-counter, you are currently taking. Talk to your doctor before taking any natural or herbal supplements.
- Dispose of old and outdated medicines. Some medications can become dangerous or ineffective over time.
- Never share prescription medicines. Medicines should be taken by the person to whom they are prescribed and for the reason prescribed.
- Remember that *any* over-the-counter drug, including herbal supplements, vitamins, and natural remedies, can be toxic in doses larger than recommended in the product information.

INTOXICATION

Excessive alcohol consumption causes problems that may lead to a medical emergency. In addition to the problems caused by intoxication, the person may have an injury or sudden illness requiring care. Remember not to assume that a victim is experiencing signs and symptoms only as a result of intoxication. In some cases, someone who behaves as if intoxicated may not have drunk alcohol at all but may be experiencing a problem such as a diabetic emergency that causes altered mental status.

Drinking a large amount of alcohol in a short period of time can cause alcohol poisoning, which may result in unresponsiveness, seizures, or death. Alcohol has depressant effects on the respiratory system and can cause an overdose similar to that of depressant drugs. First aid focuses on ensuring that the person receives medical care if needed and protecting the person from injury due to the intoxication (see First Aid: "Intoxication").

Alcohol Withdrawal

Someone who drinks heavily for a long time may develop a physical **dependence** on alcohol. **Withdrawal** from alcohol dependence may then cause delirium tremens (sometimes called "the DTs"), an altered mental status characterized by confusion, disorientation, agitation, and altered perception such as hallucinations or illusions (see First Aid: "Alcohol Withdrawal").

First Aid   **Intoxication**

When You See

- Smell of alcohol about the person
- Flushed, moist face
- Vomiting
- Slurred speech, staggering
- Fast heart rate
- Impaired judgment and motor skills
- Agitated or combative behavior
- Changing levels of responsiveness, coma

Do This First

1 Check for injuries or illness. Do not assume alcohol is the factor, or the only factor, involved.

3 For an unresponsive intoxicated person:
   a. Position the victim in the recovery position (preferably on left side to reduce the risk of vomiting); be prepared for vomiting.
   b. Monitor the victim's breathing and provide BLS if necessary.
   c. Call 9-1-1 if the victim's breathing is irregular, if seizures occur, or if the victim cannot be roused (coma).

4 For an injured intoxicated person:
   a. Because alcohol may keep the person from feeling pain, do not rely on the victim's perception of an injury to guide your care.
   b. Give first aid as you would if the victim were unresponsive, based on your assessment of the signs of injury or illness rather than reported symptoms.
   c. If the mechanism of injury suggests the victim could have a spinal injury, do not move the victim but keep the head aligned with the body.

2 For a responsive intoxicated person:
   a. Stay with the person and protect him or her from injury (take away car keys).
   b. Do not let the person lie down on his or her back.
   c. Care for any injuries.
   d. Calm and reassure the person.
   e. If you have any doubt about whether the person may be injured or ill, may have consumed a dangerous amount of alcohol, or may injure self or others, call 9-1-1 and let the dispatcher decide what help is needed.

((ALERT))

- Intoxication makes some people hostile and violent. Stay a distance away and call law enforcement if the person threatens violence.

Additional Care

- In a cold environment an intoxicated person is likely to experience hypothermia because dilated peripheral blood vessels allow the body's heat to escape more easily. Take steps to keep the victim warm (see **Chapter 21**).

First Aid   Alcohol Withdrawal

When You See

- Hand trembling, head shaking
- Nausea, vomiting
- Seizures
- Hallucination, irrational fears, extreme confusion
- Unusual behavior

Do This First

1 Call 9-1-1.

2 Give first aid as for an intoxicated victim, including the use of the recovery position for an unresponsive victim and monitoring breathing.

Additional Care

- Stay with the victim and protect him or her from injury until help arrives.

Learning Checkpoint ①

1. The most commonly abused drugs in the United States are

- **a.** alcohol and marijuana.
- **b.** marijuana and cocaine.
- **c.** cocaine and pain relievers.
- **d.** heroin and hallucinogens.

2. Substance abuse efforts should focus on people in what age group(s)?

_____

3. Put a check mark next to all actions that are appropriate for helping to prevent the misuse of prescribed drugs.

_____ Take medications only when you feel the symptoms for which the medication is prescribed.

_____ Read product information that comes with prescription medications.

_____ Keep medications in their original labeled containers.

_____ Use medications prescribed for someone else only when you are certain you have the same condition as the person with the medication.

_____ Ensure that a person with diminished judgment cannot accidentally take too much medication.

DRUG ABUSE

Illicit drugs, and prescription drugs used for non-medical purposes, cause a wide variety of effects, depending on the type of drug and the amount used (**Figure 19-3**). The primary effects of drugs commonly abused are described in **Table 19-2**. You do not need to know the type of drug taken in order to care for the victim. Consider the possibility of drug abuse or overdose whenever a victim's behavior or signs and symptoms cannot otherwise be explained. Observe the scene for drug **paraphernalia,** such as needles and syringes, eyedroppers, burnt spoons, straws or rolled-up dollar bill used for snorting, pipes, glass bulbs, razor blades, paper or plastic bags reeking of inhalants, or bottles of pills, powder, or liquid (**Figure 19-4**).

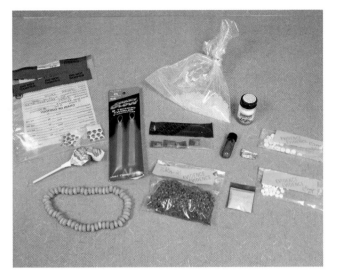

Figure 19-3 Illicit drugs.

Methamphetamine Use on the Rise

The last decade has seen a huge increase in the abuse of methamphetamine. According to the 2004 National Survey on Drug Use and Health, 1.4 million people in the United States used methamphetamine, and about 12 million have used this illicit drug at least once in their lifetime.

Methamphetamine is also known as meth, speed, crank, crystal, and other street names. Methamphetamine is a powerful central nervous system stimulant with no medical uses. The many long-term health effects of methamphetamine include cancer, brain damage, heart problems, birth defects, and miscarriage. The drug can also cause aggression and violence.

Methamphetamine is easily produced in illegal labs that have become increasingly common throughout the United States and now number in the thousands. Methamphetamine can be made from common household and over-the-counter drugs such as decongestants. In addition to the dangers of the drug, the labs themselves raise many public health concerns because of the toxic wastes and poisonous fumes they produce. Fires and explosions are common. Meth labs may be set up in rental units, motel rooms, abandoned buildings, and even campgrounds and rest areas. Warning signs may include blacked-out windows, a strong odor of solvents, unusual nighttime activity, and excessive or unusual trash. Lab supplies often include pill bottles, jars, plastic tubing, metal cylinders, and camp stoves. Meth labs are frequently abandoned, leaving behind potentially explosive and toxic chemicals. Never approach a suspected meth lab site, but report your suspicions to local law enforcement. Because of the chemicals involved, a hazmat team response is required.

Table 19-2

Effects of Commonly Abused Drugs

Drug Class or Type	Specific Drugs	Examples of Street Names	Common Effects
Marijuana	Marijuana, hashish	Grass, pot, dope, weed, bamba, ganja, joint	Elation, relaxation, dizziness, distorted perceptions, hunger, fast pulse
Narcotics	Heroin, morphine, codeine, oxycodone (OxyContin, Percocet, Percodan)	H, horse, junk, stuff, smack, scag, poppy, ox, OCs, perc	Euphoria or stupor, depressant effects, dizziness, pain relief, muscle relaxation, impaired judgment, slowed respiration, coughing and sniffing, contracted pupils, slurred speech
Hallucinogens	LSD, PCP, mescaline, psilocybin	Acid, purple hearts, angel dust, peyote, mushrooms	Stimulant effects, hallucinations, disorientation, anxiety, paranoia, trancelike state, euphoria, dilated pupils, fast pulse
Inhalants	Amyl nitrite, butyl nitrite, nitrous oxide, many solvents and common household products	Sniffing, huffing, snorting, bagging	Mood alterations, depressant or stimulant effects, nausea, excitability, slurred speech, impaired coordination
Stimulants	Amphetamine, methamphetamine, dextroamphetamine, cocaine and crack cocaine, designer drugs such as "ecstasy"	Speed, bennies, uppers, pep pills, white crosses, dex, ice, crank, rock, coke, snow, flake	Increased mental alertness, physical energy, talkativeness, restlessness, irritability or aggressive behavior, dilated pupils, increased respiration and blood pressure
Sedatives, depressants, tranquilizers	Barbiturates, benzodiazepines, muscle relaxants	Downers, goofballs, reds, ludes	Decreased mental alertness, relaxation, dizziness, slurred speech, dilated pupils, nausea and vomiting, delusions, slowed respiration and pulse

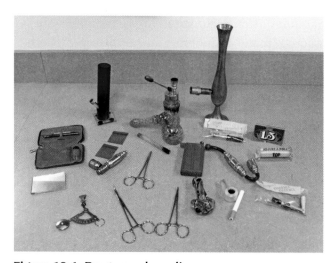

Figure 19-4 Drug paraphernalia.

First Aid for Drug Abuse or Overdose

The signs and symptoms of drug abuse and overdose vary widely, depending on the type and amount of the substance taken, but first aid should always follow the same general principles (see **Table 19-2**). Remember that a drug overdose is a type of poisoning. If you know the drug or other substance taken, call the Poison Control Center (PCC) and follow its instructions (see **Chapter 18**). Otherwise, call 9-1-1 and provide supportive care and give first aid for any injuries until help arrives (see First Aid: "Drug Abuse or Overdose").

In some cases the victim may become violent, suicidal, or act bizarrely under the influence of the drug. Remember the general rule never to enter a

First Aid   ## Drug Abuse or Overdose

When You See

- Unusual or erratic behavior
- The signs and symptoms of drug abuse
- Drug paraphernalia

Do This First

1 Call 9-1-1 for serious signs and symptoms, or the Poison Control Center for instructions if you know the substance taken.

2 Some drugs cause violent behavior. If the victim demonstrates a potential for violent behavior, withdraw and wait for help to arrive.

3 Put an unresponsive victim in the recovery position (preferably on left side to reduce the risk of vomiting), monitor breathing, and give BLS as needed.

4 Check the victim for any injuries requiring care, and provide care for any condition that occurs (seizures, shock, cardiac arrest).

5 Try to keep the victim awake and talking.

6 Keep the victim from harming himself or herself or others.

7 Question the victim and others present at the scene about the drug or substance used, the amount used, and when it was used. Give this information to arriving EMS personnel.

))ALERT))

- Do not try to induce vomiting, which may cause further harm and is unlikely to help the victim.
- Some drugs make people hostile and violent. Stay a distance away and call law enforcement if violence threatens.

Additional Care

- Try to keep the victim calm.

---

scene that is dangerous; withdraw from the scene if a victim's behavior becomes threatening. Note that when illegal drugs are involved, this is also a crime scene: be very careful to avoid potential dangers. **Chapter 22,** "Behavioral Emergencies," provides more information about dealing with victims who act in unusual or unpredictable ways.

MEDICATION OVERDOSE

While many drug overdoses occur in people intentionally abusing drugs, overdose may also result from drug misuse, including accidental drug poisoning caused by taking too much of a prescription or over-the-counter medication. A person having an overdose of a prescription medication may experience a wide range of behaviors and symptoms, depending on the drug. Drug withdrawal can also be an emergency. In some cases it is impossible to know whether behaviors or symptoms are caused by drugs or by an injury or sudden illness. While caring for the victim, try to determine what drug the person may have taken: ask family members or others present at the scene, and look for pill bottles or other evidence of medications taken (see First Aid: "Medication Overdose").

First Aid   Medication Overdose

When You See

- Very small or large pupils of the eye
- Stumbling, clumsiness, drowsiness, incoherent speech
- Difficulty breathing (very slow or fast)
- Irrational or violent behavior
- Changing levels of responsiveness

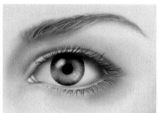
Normal

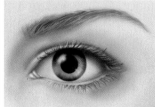
Dilated

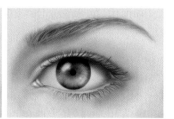
Constricted

Do This First

1 Put an unresponsive victim in the recovery position, monitor breathing, and give BLS as needed. Call 9-1-1.

2 For a responsive victim, first be sure that it is safe to approach the person. If the victim's behavior is erratic or violent, call 9-1-1 and stay a safe distance away.

3 Try to find out what drug the victim took. If there is evidence of an overdose, call 9-1-1.

4 If symptoms are minor and you know the substance taken, call the Poison Control Center and follow their instructions.

5 If the victim vomits, save a sample for arriving medical personnel.

Additional Care

- Monitor the victim's condition while waiting for help.
- Provide care for any condition that occurs (seizures, shock, cardiac arrest).

Learning
Checkpoint ②

1. Describe what to do for an intoxicated person who "passes out."

_____

2. How is alcohol similar to narcotic drugs in high doses?

   a. Both stimulate the user to increased mental alertness.

   b. Both are depressants and can lead to impaired respiration or coma.

   c. Both can cause dangerously high blood pressure and internal bleeding.

   d. All of the above

3. Check off appropriate actions to take for a person with a drug or medication overdose.

   ____ Position an unresponsive victim on the back with feet raised (shock position).

   ____ Call 9-1-1 or the Poison Control Center.

   ____ Restrain a potentially violent person to prevent self-injury.

   ____ Check for injuries that may require first aid.

   ____ Induce vomiting if the person is responsive.

   ____ Try to keep the person awake and talking.

   ____ Try to find out what the person took.

Concluding Thoughts

Although substance abuse is a huge problem in our society, do not jump to the conclusion that someone who is behaving oddly must be on drugs. Remember that many illnesses and injuries also cause altered mental status that may lead to unusual behaviors. Take the time to assess the victim and situation and to call for help and give first aid when needed. Whenever giving first aid it is important not to be judgmental—a state of mind that could lead to not providing the best care for a person in need.

Learning Outcomes

You should now be able to do the following:

1. Explain actions that can be taken to help prevent youth from abusing drugs and other substances.

2. Describe specific steps for preventing someone from accidentally misusing or overdosing on a medication.

3. List the steps of first aid for alcohol intoxication and alcohol withdrawal.

4. Describe the effects of commonly abused drugs.

5. List the steps of first aid for drug abuse or overdose.

6. List the steps of first aid for medication overdose.

Review Questions

1. To help prevent drug misuse or overdose in an elderly person who is taking prescription medications,
   a. consult with the healthcare provider or pharmacist before allowing the person to drink alcohol while using the drug.
   b. always have the person take all medications at the same time.
   c. have the person drink lots of water while taking the medications.
   d. monitor the person continually for two hours after each dose.

2. Substance abuse prevention programs involve
   a. youths at risk.
   b. parents and families.
   c. schools and communities.
   d. All of the above

3. Alcohol poisoning may cause
   a. diabetes.
   b. seizures.
   c. heart attack.
   d. anaphylaxis.

4. Assessment of an intoxicated victim's injuries depends mostly on
   a. the visible signs of injury.
   b. the victim's mental status when first encountered.
   c. the victim's reported symptoms.
   d. how much alcohol the victim drank.

5. Alcohol withdrawal in a dependent person may cause
   a. anaphylaxis.
   b. permanent psychosis.
   c. hallucinations.
   d. circulation problems.

6. You are giving first aid to a man who seems mildly "high." He tells you he took two "percs." To determine how best to treat him, whom should you call for more information?
   a. Law enforcement personnel
   b. A family member
   c. The Poison Control Center
   d. The federal drug information website

7. First aid for a drug overdose is generally the same as first aid for
   a. poisoning.
   b. stroke.
   c. diabetic coma.
   d. hypothermia.

8. A drug overdose may occur with
   a. illicit drugs.
   b. nonprescription medication.
   c. small amounts of some substances.
   d. All of the above

References and Resources

National Treatment Referral 24-Hour Hotline (Alcohol and Drugs): 1-800-662-HELP (1-800-662-4357)

American College of Emergency Physicians. *First aid manual: a comprehensive guide to treating emergency victims of all ages in any situation.* New York: DK Publishing; 2001.

American Heart Association. 2005 International consensus on cardiopulmonary resuscitation (CPR) and emergency cardiovascular care (ECC) science with treatment recommendations. *Circulation,* 112(22). November 29, 2005.

American Medical Association. *Handbook of first aid and emergency care.* Revised ed. New York: Random House; 2000.

Koch Crime Institute. National trends of methamphetamine. 2005. www.kci.org/metho_info

National Alcohol and Drug Abuse Information Call Center 24-hour hotline. 1-800-784-6776. Internet information and live chat. www.addictioncareoptions.com

National Clearinghouse for Alcohol and Drug Information. 1-800-729-6686. www.health.org

National Institute on Drug Abuse. www.nida.nih.gov

National Safety Council. www.nsc.org

Substance Abuse and Mental Health Services Administration. National survey on drug use and health. 2003. www.drugabuse statistics.samhsa.gov/NHSDA

Substance Abuse and Mental Health Services Administration, U.S. Department of Health and Human Services. www.samhsa.gov

Chapter 20

Bites and Stings

Chapter Preview

- Animal Bites
- Human Bites
- Snakebites
- Spider Bites
- Tick Bites

- Mosquito Bites
- Bee and Wasp Stings
- Scorpion Stings
- Marine Bites and Stings

Y ou are at the beach boardwalk with your family on a bright summer day. The girls are thirsty, so Mom opens a carton of juice and pours it into cups, trying to ignore a wasp that has appeared and is buzzing around the juice. As the toddler takes her first sip, she slaps at the wasp, which stings her lip. Her juice spills everywhere, she is screaming with pain, and the wasp now is nowhere to be seen. What, if anything, should you do?

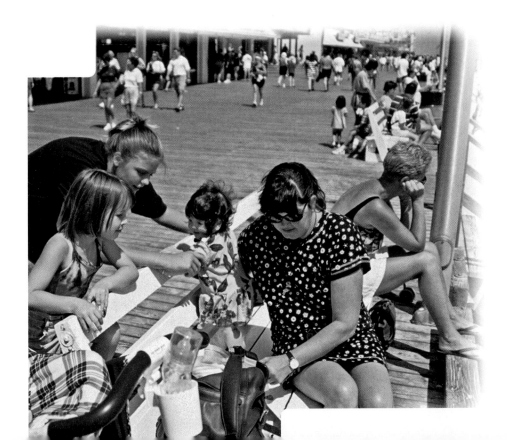

Literally millions of people every year are bitten or stung by animals, snakes, spiders and insects, and marine life, making this a significant first aid issue. Fortunately the majority of cases are not medical emergencies, but often medical treatment is needed for bleeding, wound care, or to treat infection or a reaction to an injected poison. In some cases, particularly when the victim is allergic, a medical emergency does occur, and appropriate, timely first aid is needed.

ANIMAL BITES

About four million people are bitten by dogs in the United States every year, followed by a large number of cat bites and a much lower number of bites from other domestic or wild animals. Over 300,000 bites are serious enough to require emergency department treatment, and on the average about 25 people a year die from dog bites. Most victims are young children who often have not learned how to act around dogs and other animals. With an estimated 68 million pet dogs in the United States, it is crucial that children as well as adults learn how to safely interact with dogs as well as other animals kept as pets (**Box 20-1**). In general, most bites occur to the arm or hand, followed by the leg or foot, but in children under age four about 65% sustain injury to the head or neck—an often dangerous injury (**Figure 20-1**).

Animal bites can be serious for three reasons. Depending on the location and depth of the bite injury, bleeding can be serious. Control bleeding from an animal bite as you would bleeding caused by other injuries (see **Chapter 9**). Second, because bacteria are present in animals' mouths, there is a risk that the wound will become infected. Even a small wound from a dog bite can become infected; the bites of cats have an even higher risk. Give wound care to prevent infection (see **Chapter 11**), and consult with your healthcare provider to see if additional measures may be needed. Finally, the bite of any animal, even a house pet, carries the risk of **rabies.** This risk is much higher with wild animals, since most pets are vaccinated against rabies, but the risk is present with all animals.

In many other countries, dog bites are the most common source of rabies, and any dog bite should immediately be seen by a healthcare provider.

Caused by a virus that can be transmitted by saliva into the blood of a bite victim, rabies remains a major threat in all areas of the United States even though with vaccinations and other precautions, it has become very rare in humans. Because rabies is fatal unless vaccination injections are given early, every bite from a mammal, domestic or wild, must be considered serious. Unless the bite occurs from your own pet and you are certain the animal's rabies vaccination is current, all dog and other animal bites should be reported to your local public health department or animal control office. Because the threat of rabies is so serious, many states have laws that require quarantining or observing any biting animal—even one with a current vaccination—to ensure that there is no risk for the bite victim. In most locations, any wild animal that bites

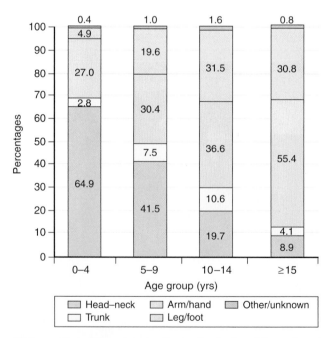

Figure 20-1 Percentage of nonfatal dog bite–related injuries treated in U.S. hospital emergency departments, by primary body part affected and age group. (National Electronic Injury Surveillance System—All Injury Program, United States, 2001.)

Box 20-1 Preventing Dog Bites

The CDC recommends the following to prevent dog bites and rabies:

- Consult with a professional (e.g., veterinarian, animal behaviorist, or responsible breeder) before choosing a dog to determine suitable breeds on the basis of your lifestyle and physical environment.
- Exclude dogs with histories of aggression from households with children.
- Be sensitive to cues that a child is fearful or apprehensive about a dog and, if so, delay acquiring a dog.
- Spend time with a dog before buying or adopting it.
- Use caution when bringing a dog or puppy into the home of an infant or toddler.
- Spay/neuter virtually all dogs (this frequently reduces aggressive tendencies).
- Never leave infants or young children alone with any dog.
- Properly socialize and train any dog entering the household. Teach the dog submissive behaviors (e.g., rolling over to expose abdomen and relinquishing food without growling).
- Seek professional advice (e.g., from veterinarians, animal behaviorists, or responsible breeders) immediately if the dog develops aggressive or undesirable behaviors.
- Do not play aggressive games (e.g., wrestling) with a dog.
- Teach children basic safety around dogs and review regularly:
  - Never approach an unfamiliar dog.
  - Never run from a dog or scream.
  - Remain motionless when approached by an unfamiliar dog (e.g., "be still like a tree").
  - If knocked over by a dog, roll into a ball and lie still (e.g., "be still like a log").
  - Never play with a dog unless supervised by an adult.
  - Report stray dogs or dogs displaying unusual behavior to an adult immediately.
  - Do not disturb a dog that is sleeping, eating, or caring for puppies.
  - Do not pet a dog without allowing it to see and sniff you first.
  - If bitten, report the bite to an adult immediately.

a person is assumed to have rabies, unless the animal can be caught or killed and its brain examined for the virus.

First aid for the bite of any animal focuses on controlling bleeding and wound care to prevent infection. Wash the wound well and apply a sterile dressing (see **Chapter 11**). Seek medical attention immediately for a puncture wound, a wound to the head or neck, and any bite wound from an animal that is not your own pet. Even with a superficial wound caused by the bite of your own pet, it is a good idea to contact your healthcare provider to see whether medical treatment may be needed. In all cases observe the wound carefully over the next few days for any signs of infection (see First Aid: "Animal Bites").

First Aid **Animal Bites**

When You See
- Any animal bite

Do This First

1 Clean the wound with soap and water. Run water over the wound for at least 5 minutes (except when bleeding is severe).

2 Control bleeding.

3 Cover the wound with a sterile dressing and bandage (see **Chapter 11**).

4 The victim should see a healthcare provider or go to the emergency department right away.

((ALERT))

- Do not try to catch any animal that may have rabies.

Additional Care

- Report all animal bites to local animal control officers or police. The law requires certain procedures to be followed when rabies is a risk.
- An antibiotic ointment may be applied to a shallow wound before dressing it.

HUMAN BITES

Small children often bite others when angry or acting out. Human bites are rarer among adults, but the same result may occur in a fight if someone's knuckles striking another person's teeth breaks the skin. Because our mouths harbor many bacteria, a bite from a human can cause an infection the same as an animal bite. Because many of the pathogens that are harmless in the mouth can cause serious infection if they enter the blood, all human bites should be seen by a healthcare provider (see First Aid: "Human Bites").

First Aid Human Bites

When You See

- **A human bite**
- **Open puncture wound**
- **Bleeding**

Do This First

1 Clean the wound with soap and water. Run water over the wound for 5 minutes (except when bleeding is severe).

2 Control bleeding.

3 Cover the wound with a sterile dressing and bandage (see **Chapter 11**).

4 The victim should see a healthcare provider or go to the emergency department right away.

Additional Care

- **An antibiotic ointment may be applied to a shallow wound before dressing it.**
- **If any tissue has been bitten off, bring it with the victim to the emergency department.**

Learning Checkpoint ①

1. To minimize the risk of rabies from an animal bite, you should take which action?

   a. See a healthcare provider immediately.

   b. See a healthcare provider if you experience heavy salivation five to seven days after the bite.

   c. Capture the animal and take it to a veterinarian for examination.

   d. Soak the wound area with rubbing alcohol.

2. Why can a human bite lead to a serious medical condition?

_____

_____

Snakebites

Poisonous snakes in North America include rattlesnakes, copperheads, water moccasins (cottonmouths), coral snakes, and exotic species kept in captivity (**Figure 20-2**). An estimated 7000 to 10,000 snakebites occur every year in the United States, causing an average of about 10 deaths annually. World travelers should be aware, however, that snakebites in many other countries are more common and more lethal, causing about 30,000 deaths annually worldwide.

Snakebite statistics in the United States reveal an interesting pattern. Most venomous snakebites occur in males aged 15 to 30, and most of these occur in the hands and arms. Alcohol is often involved, and experts say many of

these victims were trying to handle the snake to impress their friends. The CDC classifies about 3000 snakebites each year as "illegitimate," meaning they occurred while the victim was handling or molesting the snake. Clearly the first step in preventing snakebite is to avoid a snake when one is seen (**Box 20-2**). The great majority of "legitimate" accidental snakebites occur below the knee.

Even with venomous snakes, in about half of bite cases the snake does not inject venom. In all, the risk of a lethal snakebite is very low. Nonetheless, those who live or work in areas where venomous snakes are common should take preventive steps and know what first aid to give in case a bite occurs. Venomous snakes are

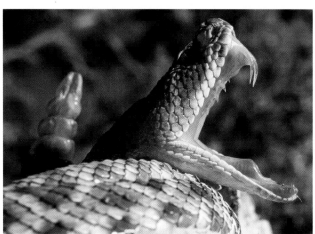

(a) Rattlesnake.

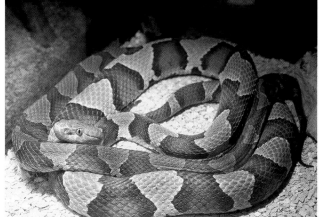

(b) Copperhead.

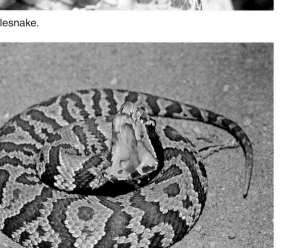

(c) Water moccasin.

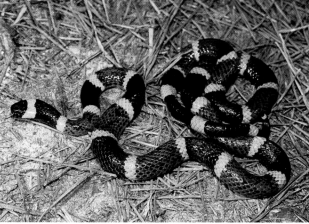

(d) Coral snake.

Figure 20-2 The four poisonous snakes of North America.

Box 20-2 Preventing Snakebites

- Stay away from areas known to have snakes.
- If you see a snake, reverse your direction and retrace your steps, watching for other snakes.
- Stay away from underbrush areas, fallen trees, and other areas where snakes may live.

The Arizona Poison and Drug Information Center (APDIC) makes these additional recommendations for preventing snakebites in areas where venomous snakes are common:

- Leave wild animals alone. Fifty to seventy percent of reptile bites managed by the APDIC were provoked by the person who was bitten—that is, by someone trying to kill, capture, or harass the animal.
- Be aware of peak movement times. Reptiles are most active in the warmer months of April through October. During the hottest months, they will be most active at night. They may be encountered during the day in spring and fall.
- Try to keep your hands and feet out of crevices in rocks, woodpiles and deep grass. Always carry a flashlight and wear shoes or boots when walking after dark.
- Never handle a venomous reptile, even when it is dead. Reflex strikes with envenomation can occur for several hours after death.
- Install outdoor lighting for yards, porches, and sidewalks. If you see a venomous reptile in your yard, it is probably just "passing through." However, if you are concerned about a dangerous animal in your yard, seek professional assistance in removing it.

---

most common in the Southeast and the Southwest. Rattlesnake bites cause most snakebite deaths.

Unless you are absolutely certain that a victim's snakebite was from a nonpoisonous snake, treat all snakebites as potentially dangerous. First, calm the victim and have the victim remain still. Anything that increases the heart rate, including strong emotions and physical movement, will speed the spread of the venom. Try to identify the snake species or be able to describe it to responding EMS personnel, because **antivenin** (antidote to the poison) is available in many areas where snakebites are common. Call 9-1-1. Wash the bite area and remove any constrictive jewelry or clothing from the limb, which will likely swell (see First Aid: "Snakebites").

Many of the traditional myths and techniques for managing snakebites do not in fact improve the victim's condition or minimize the risk. Do not try to suck out the venom, do not cut across the fang holes in an attempt to remove the venom, and do not put a tourniquet on the limb. In addition, do not put ice on the bite because of the potential for injuring tissues further with the cold.

For snakebites from coral snakes only, it is now recommended that a bitten extremity be wrapped snugly but not tightly with an elastic bandage; you should be able to insert one finger under the bandage. Wrap the entire length of the extremity to reduce the spread of the venom by slowing lymph flow. The extremity should also be immobilized and the victim should receive medical attention as soon as possible.

First Aid **Snakebites**

When You See

- Puncture marks in skin
- Complaint of pain or burning at bite site
- Redness and swelling
- Depending on species: difficulty breathing, numbness or muscle paralysis, nausea and vomiting, blurred vision, drowsiness or confusion, weakness

Do This First

1 Have the victim lie down and stay calm. (Do not move the victim unless absolutely necessary.) Keep the bitten area immobile and below the level of the heart.

2 Call 9-1-1.

3 Wash the bite wound with soap and water.

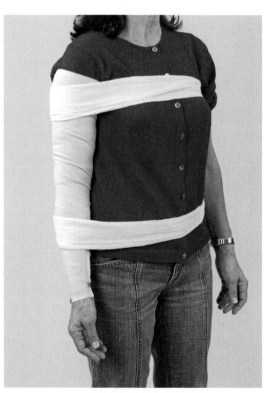

4 For coral snakes only, wrap the extremity with a snug but not tight bandage and immobilize.

5 Remove jewelry or tight clothing before swelling begins.

((ALERT))

- Do not put a tourniquet on the victim.
- Do not cut the wound open to try to drain the venom out or try to suck out the venom.
- Do not put ice on the bite.

Additional Care

- Do not try to catch the snake, but note its appearance and describe it to the healthcare provider.
- Stay with the victim and give BLS if needed.

SPIDER BITES

Many types of spiders bite, but in the United States only the venom of the black widow and brown recluse spiders is serious and sometimes fatal. The black widow often has a red hourglass-shaped marking on the underside of the abdomen. The brown recluse has a violin-shaped marking on its back (**Figure 20-3**). Reliable statistics are not available for how many spider bites occur every year, but annually only about five deaths result, mostly from black widow spiders.

The venom of the brown recluse spider can cause severe tissue damage but rarely causes death.

Both species are more common in warm climates and generally live in areas that are dry and undisturbed. Outside the home, they are often found in woodpiles, sheds, or debris. Inside the home they may live in closets, rarely used cabinets, attics, crawl spaces, and similar areas. Since these spiders are small and usually not seen before the bite occurs, preventive steps are important in areas where these spiders are known to live (**Box 20-3**).

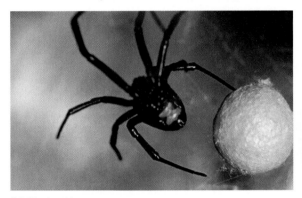

(a) Black widow.

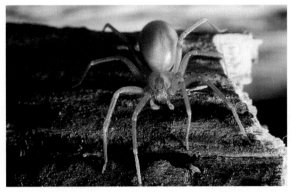

(b) Brown recluse.

Figure 20-3 Poisonous spiders.

Box 20-3 Preventing Spider Bites

Neither black widow nor brown recluse spiders attack humans: they bite defensively when someone comes too close. Preventing these and other spider bites involves two types of actions: avoiding bites in places where spiders are likely, and controlling spider populations.

Avoiding Spider Bites

• Wear gloves and a long-sleeve shirt when cleaning basement or attic areas, seldom used closets, sheds or garages, and similar areas where spiders may live. Wear gloves when gathering wood from a woodpile.

• Before putting on clothing or shoes that have been unused for a time, shake them out. Better, store clothing and shoes in sealed plastic bags or boxes.

• Check inside tents, sleeping bags, and other

seldom-used equipment before using.

• Before sleeping in a bed that has not been used in a while, carefully check between the covers.

Controlling Spider Populations

• Use appropriate pesticides or spider traps (glue traps) in areas where spiders or their nests have been identified.

• Thorough, routine housecleaning helps control spider populations. Vacuum up webs and egg sacs when they are seen, and dispose of the vacuum bag.

• Reduce clutter in storage areas.

• Repair or seal off openings in screens, windows, chimneys, and other openings through which spiders may enter the home.

• Clean up any debris around the home where spiders may breed.

Although the signs and symptoms of the bites of these two spiders vary, the first aid is the same. A black widow bite causes immediate pain, swelling and redness at the site, followed later by sweating, nausea, stomach and muscle cramps, headache, dizziness or weakness, and possible difficulty breathing. A brown recluse bite causes more slowly developing pain or stinging at the site, followed later by blistering at the site, fever, chills, nausea or vomiting, and joint pain; an open sore at the site will continue to grow without medical treatment.

With either bite, the victim needs emergency medical care. An antivenin is available for black widow spider bites. Wash the wound with soap and water to help prevent infection, and apply an ice or cold pack. Keep the bite area below the level of the heart (see First Aid: "Spider Bites").

Tick Bites

Tick bites are not poisonous but can transmit serious diseases like Rocky Mountain spotted fever or **Lyme disease (Figure 20-4)**. Ticks

---

First Aid   **Spider Bites**

When You See

For black widow bite:

- **Complaint of pain or burning at bite site**
- **Red skin at site**
- **After 15 minutes to hours: sweating, nausea, stomach and muscle cramps, increased pain at site, dizziness or weakness, difficulty breathing**

For brown recluse bite:

- **Stinging sensation at site**
- **Over 8 to 48 hours: increasing pain, blistering at site, fever, chills, nausea or vomiting, joint pain, open sore at site**

Do This First

1 If the victim has difficulty breathing, call 9-1-1 and be prepared to give BLS. Call 9-1-1 immediately for a brown recluse spider bite.

2 Keep the bite area below the level of the heart.

3 Wash the area with soap and water.

4 Put ice or a cold pack on the bite area.

Additional Care

- **Try to safely identify the spider for the healthcare provider.**
- **If 9-1-1 was not called, the victim should go to the emergency department.**

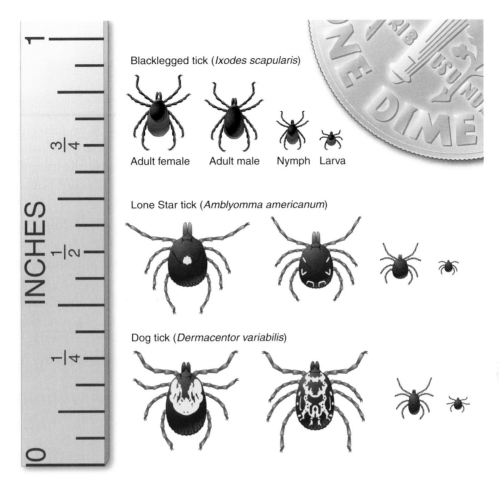

Figure 20-4 Common types of ticks found in the United States. Only the blacklegged tick carries Lyme disease in the United States.

cannot fly but will crawl up clothing or body areas that touch the ground or will fall off vegetation that one brushes against. Ticks may also be brought into the home in the fur of a dog or other pet that has picked up a tick outside. For guidelines to prevent tick bites see **Box 20-4.**

The tick usually crawls to an unexposed part of the body and bites into the skin, embedding its mouthparts in the skin to avoid being brushed off **(Figure 20-5)**. Because ticks are very small and often seek unexposed areas to bite, such as the scalp, an embedded tick may not be found unless you search diligently. If not detected and removed, the tick may remain in the skin for days. A careless attempt

to remove a tick may result in breaking off its body and leaving the head or mouthparts embedded in the skin, which could lead to infection. Remove a tick correctly by pulling gently but steadily with fine-tipped tweezers until the tick lets go. Then wash the area well and apply an antibiotic cream.

Medical treatment is not usually needed with tick bites. In areas where Lyme disease occurs frequently, talk with your healthcare provider about whether treatment may have benefit. Most important, following a tick bite you should watch for the development of the signs and symptoms of Lyme disease. Lyme disease often produces a characteristic "bull's-eye" rash **(Figure 20-6)** typically 7 to 14 days

Box 20-4 Lyme Disease

Lyme disease, spread by ticks, is a potentially serious bacterial infection that has become a serious problem in many parts of the United States. Of the 23,763 reported cases in 2002, most were in the Northeast or Upper Midwest, although as the figure shows, people living in many other areas are at some risk. Lyme disease is a bacterial infectious disease that first causes fever, chills, and other flulike symptoms and often much later causes heart and neurological problems. The longer the tick remains on the body, the greater the chance of transmitting the disease. Look for a bull's-eye rash that appears around the bite site 3 to 30 days later. Get medical attention if you have this rash or flulike symptoms or joint pain after a tick bite.

To prevent tick bites:
- Keep lawns mowed, brush cleaned up, and woodpiles stacked off the ground.
- Wear socks with shoes or boots. Tuck long pants into socks.
- Wear light-colored clothing, which makes it easier to see ticks before they reach your skin. Tuck your shirt into your pants.
- Do not lay clothing or towels on the ground.
- Walk in the middle of paths, away from tall grass and underbrush.
- Comb or brush your hair after being in an infested area.
- Check your body everywhere when bathing or showering, including neck and scalp.

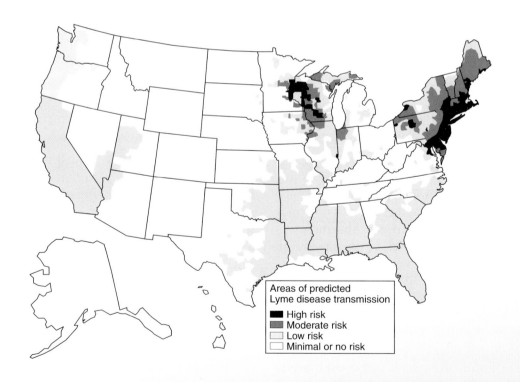

Areas of predicted
Lyme disease transmission

■ High risk
▨ Moderate risk
□ Low risk
□ Minimal or no risk

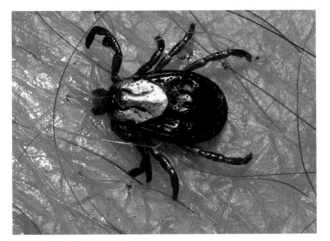

(a) Tick embedded in skin

Figure 20-5 Tick bite.

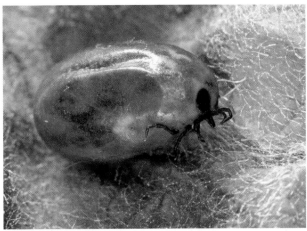

(b) Tick engorged

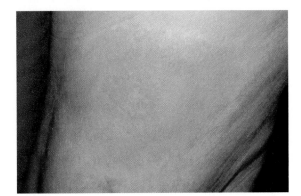

Figure 20-6 Bull's-eye rash characteristic of Lyme disease.

after the bite, but sometimes as soon as 3 or as long as 30 days later. Other nonspecific symptoms include fever, headache, fatigue, muscle and joint pain, or other flulike symptoms (see First Aid: "Tick Bites").

Learning
Checkpoint ②

1. List three key actions to take for a victim of snakebite.

_____

2. Check off situations in which you should call 9-1-1 for a spider bite.

___ All spider bites   ___ If there is any pain at the bite site

___ Any spider bite in a diabetic victim   ___ If the victim has trouble breathing

___ Any brown recluse spider bite   ___ If you have no ice to put on the bite

3. A tick is best removed from the skin using _____ .

4. A prominent initial sign of Lyme disease following a tick bite is

    a. pain and burning at the site.

    b. a bull's-eye rash.

    c. high fever within 24 hours.

    d. All of the above

When You See

- Tick embedded in skin

Do This First

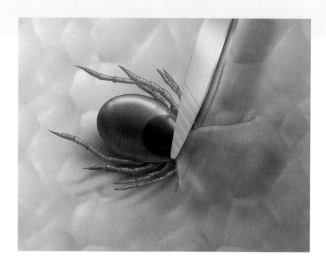

1 Remove the tick by grasping it close to the skin with fine-tipped tweezers and pulling very gently until the tick finally lets go. Avoid pulling too hard or jerking, which may leave part of the tick in the skin.

2 Wash the area with soap and water.

3 Put an antiseptic such as rubbing alcohol on the site. Apply an antibiotic cream.

ALERT

- Do not try to remove an embedded tick by covering it with petroleum jelly, soaking it with bleach, burning it away with a hot pin or other object, or similar methods. These methods may result in part of the tick remaining embedded in the skin.

Additional Care

- Seek medical attention if a rash appears around the site or the victim later experiences fever, headache, chills, muscle and joint pain, or other flulike symptoms.

MOSQUITO BITES

With the spread of **West Nile virus (WNV)** throughout the United States, mosquitoes are now a greater public health issue. WNV is a bloodborne disease that is a seasonal epidemic in many parts of North America **(Figure 20-7)**. According to the CDC, 2448 human cases were reported nationwide in 2004, causing 88 deaths. A low percentage of people infected with WNV develop severe illness, however, and more than half have no signs and symptoms at all. WNV is spread mostly by the bite of infected mosquitoes, which often transmit the virus from infected birds.

In the eastern United States, eastern equine encephalitis (EEE) is another serious mosquito-borne infection that is fatal in 35% of those infected. Fortunately, there have been only 200 confirmed cases in the last 40 years. EEE trans-mission is prevented the same as WNV: by preventing mosquito bites.

Many affected states and communities have expanded mosquito control programs, but in many areas people still need to take precautions to prevent mosquito bites. The best way to avoid WNV is to prevent mosquito bites in these ways:

- Wear long-sleeve shirts and pants.
- Use an insect repellent when outside in areas where mosquitoes are common **(Box 20-5)**.
- Be aware of peak mosquito hours from dusk to dawn.
- Mosquito-proof your home by draining standing water around your home and installing or repairing screens.
- Report dead birds to local authorities.
- Support local mosquito control programs.

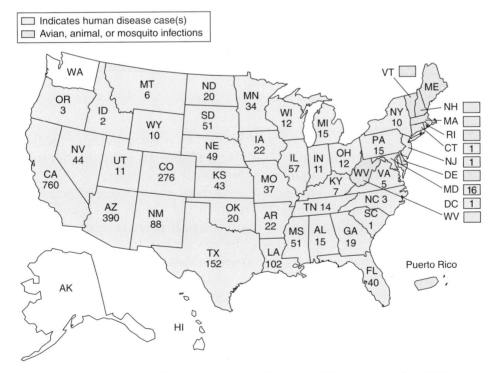

Figure 20-7 2004 West Nile virus activity in the United States reported to CDC.

Box 20-5   New Insect Repellents Recommended

In 2005 the CDC released new guidelines for mosquito repellents to protect against mosquito bites and the potential transmission of West Nile virus. Previously, only products containing the chemical DEET were recommended by the CDC, which continues to support the use of DEET products when used appropriately. The U.S. Environmental Protection Agency (EPA) has approved the use of DEET, which has been generally shown to be safe in tests when used as directed. Because DEET has toxic properties and must be used carefully—you must avoid inhaling the vapors and must not apply it to areas of broken skin—many people have had concerns about its use. Scientific studies are not definitive about the minimum age at which it is safe to apply DEET to infants or young children, and there is some variation in published guidelines.

The new CDC guidelines endorse the use of two additional active ingredients found in some repellents: picaridin (also called KBR 3023) and oil of lemon eucalyptus. These repellents have been used in other countries and have been determined to be as effective as DEET in products of comparable concentration. The EPA has also determined that they are safe and effective. Many people say picaridin feels better on the skin and smells better than DEET, and others prefer oil of lemon eucalyptus because it is a natural substance and not a manufactured chemical.

BEE AND WASP STINGS

Bee, wasp, and other insect stings are not poisonous but can cause life-threatening allergic reactions, called anaphylaxis, in victims who have severe allergies to them. Venomous insects include honeybees, bumblebees, hornets, wasps, yellow jackets, and fire ants. There are no reliable statistics about how many stings occur every year, but an estimated two million people in the United States are allergic to stinging insects, although the extent of the allergic reaction varies. Many people have very serious or life-threatening reactions, and about 50 people die every year from allergic reactions to insect stings.

Chapter 10 discusses anaphylactic shock and the first aid to give. Often someone who knows he or she is allergic to bee or wasp stings carries an EpiPen® or other emergency medication to take if stung. **Chapter 10** also describes steps you can take to prevent insect stings.

In most cases, a bee or wasp sting causes pain but is not an emergency or serious problem. If present in the skin after the sting, the stinger can be scraped away with a rigid piece of plastic like a credit card. The area is washed to prevent infection, and a cold pack applied to reduce the pain and swelling. Always observe for the signs of an allergic reaction, and if they appear call 9-1-1 immediately and prepare to treat anaphylactic shock. Some sting victims who do not have allergic reactions may have other delayed symptoms that include fever, rash, joint pain, and swollen glands (see First Aid: "Bee and Wasp Stings").

First Aid   Bee and Wasp Stings

When You See

- Complaints of pain, burning, or itching at sting site
- Redness, swelling
- Stinger possibly still in skin

Do This First

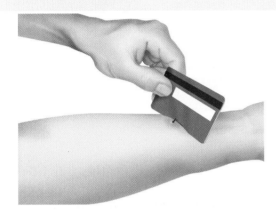

1 Remove stinger from skin by scraping it away gently with a piece of plastic (not a knife blade). Call 9-1-1 if victim has known allergy to stings.

2 Wash the area with soap and water.

3 Put ice or a cold pack on the sting site.

4 Watch the victim for 30 minutes for any signs or symptoms of allergic reaction (difficulty breathing, swelling in other areas, anxiety, nausea or vomiting); if there are any, call 9-1-1 and treat for shock.

Additional Care

- An over-the-counter oral antihistamine may help reduce discomfort.
- For an insect sting in the mouth, have the victim suck on ice to reduce swelling. Call 9-1-1 if breathing becomes difficult.
- Do not let the victim scratch the sting; this increases swelling and itching and the risk of infection.

SCORPION STINGS

In Southwestern and Southern states, thousands of scorpion stings occur every year, but few become emergencies (**Figure 20-8**). The great majority of scorpion species are not venomous. Even the sting of the poisonous bark scorpion, found in the Southwest, fortunately is seldom fatal. In one report only six deaths resulted from scorpion stings in a 10-year period in the United States. In other countries stings are more common; in Mexico, for example, hundreds are thought to die every year from scorpion stings. Scorpions are more active at night, and most stings occur during the warm summer months. People can avoid scorpions in areas where they are common by not walking barefoot or in sandals and by shaking out clothing and shoes before putting them on.

Scorpion stings are most dangerous for infants, young children, and the frail elderly. When death does occur, it is usually the result of anaphylactic shock caused by the victim's reaction to the venom. The victim of a sting

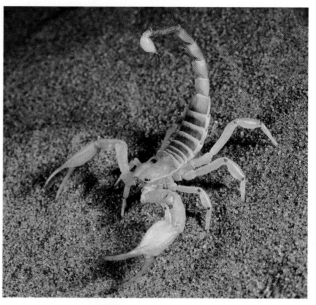

Figure 20-8 Scorpion.

should always be observed for this potential reaction. The more usual symptoms, however, consist of pain at the site along with numb-

---

First Aid   **Scorpion Stings**

When You See

- **The scorpion sting with its tail**
- **Complaints of severe burning pain at sting site, later numbness, tingling**
- **Possible nausea, vomiting**
- **Hyperactivity in a child**
- **Possible signs of shock, breathing difficulties**

Do This First

1 Call 9-1-1 if the victim has a problem breathing or severe symptoms.

2 Monitor the victim's breathing and give BLS as needed.

3 Carefully wash the sting area.

4 Put ice or a cold pack on the area.

5 Seek urgent medical attention unless the symptoms are very mild.

Additional Care

- **Keep the victim still.**

ness and tingling. More serious symptoms include nausea and vomiting, breathing difficulty, fever, convulsions, and in children, hyperactivity.

The first aid for a scorpion sting is similar to the first aid for a wasp or bee sting. The Arizona Poison and Drug Information Center, which manages thousands of stings a year, says most stings in healthy adults can be managed safely at home. Wash the area and apply a cold pack. Monitor the victim's symptoms, and seek medical attention for signs and symptoms beyond those at the sting site. Seek urgent medical attention for a sting in a child or elderly person. Antivenin for scorpion stings may be available in some areas (see First Aid: "Scorpion Stings").

Marine Bites and Stings

Biting marine animals include sharks, barracudas, and eels, although such bites are generally rare. The first aid for marine bites is essentially the same as for bleeding and wound care. For a bite that causes severe bleeding:

1. Stop the bleeding.
2. Care for shock.
3. Summon help from lifeguards.
4. Call 9-1-1.

Stings from marine life are much more common than bites. Stinging marine life include jellyfish, Portuguese man-of-war, corals, spiny sea urchins, anemones, and stingrays. Most stings are like bee or wasp stings: painful but not dangerous, except in the very rare few who may experience an allergic reaction or severe toxic reaction. Even the venomous sting of the Portuguese man-of-war, although it can be very painful and can cause other symptoms, is rarely an emergency or life threatening.

Most marine stings can be prevented by paying attention to your environment. Warnings are generally posted on public beaches when Portuguese man-of-wars are present in the water, or you may see their blue floats washed up on the beach or floating in the water (**Figure 20-9**). Long tentacles streaming from the floating body are the source of stings; these tentacles can break off and continue to cause stings in the water or on the beach. Do not touch a jellyfish or Portuguese man-of-war on the beach. In more isolated

areas, check the water around you frequently, and if there are known risks, wear a wetsuit for skin protection. Do not swim or snorkel in shallow water where you may bump into coral, urchins, or anemones. Watch the area in front of you when walking in shallow water where stingrays may be present, and do not let small children play in such areas. If you have ever had an allergic reaction to any marine sting, talk with your healthcare provider about having an allergy kit in case of a sting.

Jellyfish or Portuguese man-of-war stings cause an immediate intense pain and burning that may last for hours. Red welts usually appear on the skin, often in a row caused by a tentacle. In most cases these are the only symptoms. If a severe toxic or allergic reaction occurs after any marine sting, however, the victim may experience difficulty breathing, swelling of the throat, signs of shock, muscle

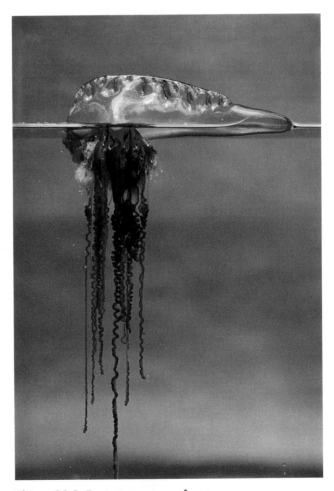

Figure 20-9 Portuguese man-of-war.

paralysis, seizures, or unresponsiveness. If any of these signs and symptoms occurs, or if the victim is a young child or is stung on the face or eyes, call 9-1-1.

Give this first aid for marine animal stings:

1. Scrape off any tentacles on the skin with a piece of rigid plastic like a credit card, or pick them off with tweezers or pliers. Be careful not to rub or squeeze the tentacles, which may continue to sting. Do not wash the skin with fresh water while tentacles remain because fresh water will stimulate additional stinging.
2. Apply a compress soaked in vinegar to the affected area. If vinegar is unavailable, apply a paste of baking soda and water just thick enough to not run off the skin. A warm or hot water pack may also help control pain.
3. Give standard wound care if there are breaks in the skin.
4. Seek medical attention if more serious signs or symptoms occur, if the victim is a young child or has ever had an allergic reaction to marine stings, or for significant stings on the face or eyes.

To care for urchin or stingray puncture wounds:

1. Relieve the pain by immersing the injured part in hot water for 30 minutes. Make sure the water is not so hot that it causes a burn.
2. Wash the wound with soap and water, and apply a dressing.
3. Seek medical attention.

Learning
Checkpoint 3

1. A bee's stinger can be removed from the skin using _____.

2. A co-worker was stung by a honeybee near the flower garden by your building's entrance. As she tells you about this, you see that her face is turning red, the skin around her eyes and mouth looks puffy, and she seems short of breath. What are the most important actions to take first? Why?

_____

3. What substance can be put on a jellyfish sting to help ease the pain?

a. Boiling water

b. Catsup or mayonnaise

c. Vinegar or baking soda

d. Any of the above

Concluding Thoughts

Bites and stings are common occurrences, but fortunately they seldom become emergencies. First aid in most cases is as simple as pain relief and wound care, along with observing for more serious signs and symptoms and then seeking medical care. For those who are often outdoors where most bites and stings occur, prevention is important. Most important, for those who are known to be allergic to bee or other stings or bites, is to carry an emergency epinephrine kit and follow precautions when in areas where stings or bites are likely.

Learning Outcomes

You should now be able to do the following:

1. List guidelines for preventing common bites and stings.

2. Explain the risk of infection from common types of bites and stings.

3. Describe the first aid care to give in cases of bites and stings that do not involve severe symptoms or an allergic reaction.

4. List signs and symptoms for which you should call 9-1-1 after a bite or sting.

5. Describe how to remove an embedded tick and the stinger from a bee or wasp.

Review Questions

1. Possible rabies infection should be a consideration with
   a. only wild animal bites.
   b. only dog bites if you do not know the owner.
   c. snakebites.
   d. all animal bites from mammals.

2. Seek immediate medical attention for
   a. a puncture wound from an animal bite.
   b. a bite to the head or neck.
   c. a bite wound from an animal that is not your own pet.
   d. All of the above

3. Why should all bites from a human be seen by a healthcare provider?
   a. Because many pathogens in the mouth can cause serious infection
   b. Because later bleeding is likely even if it is controlled at first
   c. Because many humans are carriers of the rabies virus
   d. Because saliva is acidic and may cause tissue damage

4. First aid for snakebite includes
   a. sucking the venom from the bite holes.
   b. applying a tourniquet.
   c. washing the wound with soap and water.
   d. applying a hot compress on the area.

5. When should you seek urgent medical care for a brown recluse spider bite?
   a. If the victim is known to be allergic
   b. With all victims bitten
   c. If the victim develops a breathing problem
   d. If the victim develops fever and chills

6. The best way to remove a tick embedded in the skin is to
   a. pull it out with tweezers.
   b. burn it with a needle sterilized in a flame.
   c. cover it with petroleum jelly.
   d. cover it with an alcohol-saturated dressing.

7. Which of the following is the most important reason to prevent mosquito bites?
   a. Mosquito bites are easily infected by scratching them.
   b. Many people have allergic reactions to mosquito bites.
   c. Mosquito bites can cause infection with West Nile virus.
   d. Multiple mosquito bites can add up to cause toxic effects.

8. When should 9-1-1 be called for a bee sting?
   a. Always
   b. When a child under age eight is stung
   c. When the victim has a known allergy
   d. When the bee was particularly aggressive before the sting

9. Which statement is true about scorpion stings?

    a. Almost all scorpion species are venomous.

    b. Scorpion stings are very rarely fatal.

    c. Scorpion stings are likely to cause anaphylaxis.

    d. The venom from a scorpion sting is easily washed out of the bite.

10. When can the tentacles of a Portuguese man-of-war sting?

    a. When the Portuguese man-of-war is floating in the water

    b. When the Portuguese man-of-war is washed up on the sand

    c. When the tentacles are detached from the body

    d. All of the above

References and Resources

American Academy of Orthopaedic Surgeons. Animal bites. http://orthoinfo.aaos.org

American College of Emergency Physicians. *First aid manual: a comprehensive guide to treating emergency victims of all ages in any situation.* New York: DK Publishing; 2001.

American Heart Association. 2005 International consensus on cardiopulmonary resuscitation (CPR) and emergency cardiovascular care (ECC) science with treatment recommendations. *Circulation*, 112(22). November 29, 2005.

American Medical Association. *Handbook of first aid and emergency care.* Revised ed. New York: Random House; 2000.

Arizona Poison and Drug Information Center. Snakes. www.pharmacy.arizona.edu/centers/apdic/snakes.shtml

Centers for Disease Control and Prevention. CDC adopts new repellent guidance for upcoming mosquito season. Press release, April 2005. www.cdc.gov

Centers for Disease Control and Prevention. Eastern equine encephalitis fact sheet. 2005. www.cdc.gov

Centers for Disease Control and Prevention. Nonfatal dog bite-related injuries treated in hospital emergency departments—United States, 2001. *MMWR Weekly* 2003 July 4; (52)26.

Centers for Disease Control and Prevention. West Nile virus: statistics, surveillance, and control. 2005. www.cdc.gov

Mayo Clinic staff. Spider bites. www.mayoclinic.com

National Library Medicine Medline Plus. Marine animal stings or bites. 2005. www.nlm.nih.gov/medlineplus/ency

National Safety Council. www.nsc.org

Chapter 21

Cold and Heat Emergencies

Chapter Preview

- Body Temperature
- Cold Emergencies
- Heat Emergencies

After several days of bitterly cold weather, you wonder how your elderly neighbor is coping with the cold and stop by his house. You have to ring the door several times before he answers, and when you step inside, it feels like 50 degrees inside his house. You ask why it is so cold, and he mumbles that with rising fuel prices, he can't afford to turn the thermostat any higher. You follow him into the living room where he stumbles before sitting on the sofa. You notice that he is shivering. You ask if you can get him a blanket, and he is slow to respond and his words slurred. Is he experiencing a problem? What should you do?

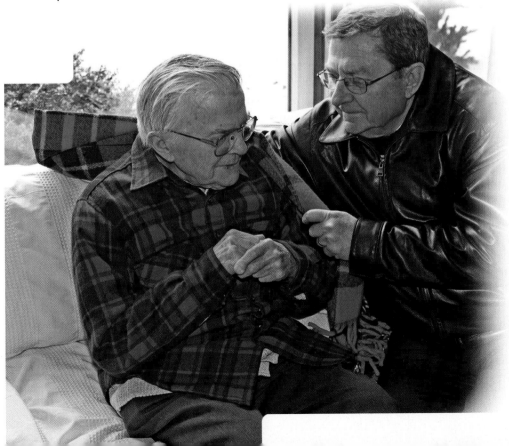

In temperature extremes or as a result of injury or illness, the body may not be able to successfully maintain its normal temperature, which can lead to medical problems. Often cold- and heat-related injuries begin gradually, but if a person remains exposed to an extreme temperature or engaged in strenuous activity, an emergency can develop. Untreated, either a cold or a heat emergency can lead to serious injury or death.

BODY TEMPERATURE

A fairly constant internal body temperature is necessary for body systems to function. The body has several mechanisms to create heat or to lose heat when necessary. In most environments these mechanisms, along with protective clothing and shelter from temperature extremes, work well, and body temperature is not a health issue. When exposed to environmental temperature extremes for an extended time, however, these mechanisms cannot maintain a constant internal temperature indefinitely, particularly if the victim is injured or in poor health. Infants and the elderly also are more susceptible to temperature extremes.

Mechanisms for Staying Warm

Most of the body's heat is produced by metabolic processes that break down nutrients to release energy for use by the body. About 60% of the energy in the food we eat is released as heat within the body, and this heat energy in most environments is sufficient to keep the body at the optimal temperature, averaging 98.6 degrees Fahrenheit. The contraction of muscle tissue also produces heat. Shivering is an involuntary movement of muscles to produce additional heat when the body needs it.

The body also has mechanisms to conserve heat when needed. Much of the body's heat is lost to a cooler environment through the process of radiation—heat radiates out from the skin in the same way that you can feel heat radiating from a hot surface. Skin temperature is normally much cooler than the body's internal temperature. If the body is losing too much heat by radiation, blood vessels in the skin contract (**vasoconstriction**) so that less internal heat is brought by the blood to the skin to radiate away. Minimizing heat loss helps the body to conserve its heat when necessary. We also have learned behaviors to minimize heat loss such as putting on more clothing or moving to a warmer environment.

Mechanisms for Staying Cool

Cold is the absence of heat, not a positive quality in itself—the body cannot *make* cold to cool the body when a very hot environment or prolonged exertion threatens to raise body temperature. Nor can the body shut down its own heat-producing processes, since cells continue to need energy to survive and function. Therefore, the body must lose internal heat when necessary to prevent overheating. A primary heat loss mechanism is dilation of blood vessels (**vasodilation**) to bring more blood to the skin. The skin becomes warmer as the blood carries heat out from the body's core, and more heat is then radiated from the body. Sweating is a second mechanism. Sweat evaporates from the skin's surface, cooling the skin and helping to dissipate the heat brought to the surface by the blood. We also have learned behaviors to promote heat loss when needed such as removing clothing to allow more heat to radiate away, getting out of the sun to avoid absorbing more radiated heat, spraying or wiping the body with water to help cool the skin by evaporation, or moving inside to a cooler environment where we can radiate heat more effectively.

The Body in Temperature Extremes

The body's normal heat production, heat conservation, and heat loss mechanisms, regulated by the nervous system, usually cope well with changes in environmental temperatures to maintain a constant internal temperature. With extended exposure to temperature extremes, however, these mechanisms are not enough to maintain a normal body temperature.

With prolonged exposure to cold, especially when wet (because water conducts heat away from the body much faster than does air), not enough heat can be conserved in the body and shivering cannot produce enough extra heat to keep the body warm. The person develops hypothermia, a potentially life-threatening condition. Because some cellular processes cannot occur at too low a temperature, organ systems gradually begin to fail, leading eventually to death.

With prolonged exposure to heat, the body eventually cannot lose enough heat to maintain a normal temperature. Profuse sweating in an attempt to cool the body frequently leads to dehydration, which reduces blood volume and blood pressure. Even when the environment is not very hot, a long period of physical exertion, such as that which accompanies endurance sports, can lead to dehydration caused by prolonged sweating. Without sufficient fluid, the body cannot cool itself adequately. Heatstroke occurs when the body temperature rises; sweating stops as the body tries to conserve its remaining fluid. Without treatment, organ damage eventually occurs, followed by death.

Hypothermia and heatstroke are the most dangerous temperature injuries. Because both develop gradually and worsen with continued exposure, the signs and symptoms of a develop-ing problem must be recognized early and the condition corrected before it becomes life threatening. The first aid for these and other cold and heat emergencies is described in this chapter.

Hypothermia and heatstroke can happen to anyone in certain conditions. Generally a healthy adult is most at risk after prolonged exposure to significant temperature extremes, such as being immersed in cold water or engaging in strenuous activities in the heat without drinking enough fluid. A number of factors, however, increase the risk for cold and heat injuries (**Box 21-1**).

Box 21-1   Risk Factors for Cold and Heat Injuries

- **Age:** Young children and the elderly are at greatest risk. Young children are at risk because their shivering produces less heat due to smaller muscle mass. They also have less body fat than others, making them more likely to lose heat. Older people are at a greater risk because their lower metabolic rate can result in a failure to maintain a normal body temperature, even indoors, when the air temperature falls under 64° F. It is also believed that older people may not perceive cold as well as younger people do, and they may be slower to act to compensate for the cold. Older adults are also more likely to have a chronic illness such as diabetes that increases the risk for hypothermia.

- **Illness or injury:** Many injuries and chronic health problems, particularly those affecting circulation or the heart, increase one's susceptibility to heat and cold injuries. For example, a victim in shock often produces insufficient body heat; for this reason shock treatment usually includes keeping the victim warm. The body responds less well to heat and cold with diabetes, infection, burns, head injuries, and other conditions.

- **Mental impairment:** People with cognitive disabilities are less likely to take action to prevent hypothermia when they are exposed to cold.

- **Dehydration:** Not drinking enough fluid makes one more susceptible to both heat and cold emergencies.

- **Body type:** People with little body fat have a greater risk of hypothermia, since body fat has an insulating effect to slow environmental cooling. People with much body fat have a greater risk of experiencing a heat emergency.

- **Activity:** Those who work outdoors in hot environments, such as construction workers or athletes in training, are more likely to experience a heat emergency if they do not take precautions such as resting and drinking fluids. People who work or participate in outdoor recreation in extreme cold are at greater risk for hypothermia, especially if they are not dressed properly or are in situations where they may not be able to reach shelter.

- **Drugs and medications:** Many medications and drugs increase the risk for heat and cold injuries. Alcohol dilates blood vessels, making hypothermia more likely

(continued)

Box 21-1   Risk Factors for Cold and Heat Injuries   *(continued)*

because heat is lost more quickly; alcohol is also a diuretic (increases urination), so the person becomes dehydrated more quickly and is more susceptible to heat-stroke. Caffeine is also a diuretic. Alcohol and some other abused drugs can suppress shivering, thereby reducing heat production, and can prevent surface blood vessels from constricting, thereby allowing more heat loss than normal. Many prescription medications also can increase a person's susceptibility to either heat or cold emergencies. Commonly used psychiatric medications, for example, predispose people to heat and cold emergencies because of the drug's physiological mechanisms. Finally, alcohol and drugs that affect the user's judgment and reasoning often lead to the person taking risks or entering situations where a heat or cold emergency is more likely, such as falling into cold water or

going into a freezing environment without adequate protection.

- **Environmental variables:** The risk of hypothermia is increased by becoming wet from rain or immersion in water. Water conducts heat away from the body much more quickly than heat can be radiated into the air. Wind also increases heat loss through the "wind chill" effect. The wind chill chart in **Figure 21-1** shows how the effects of cold increase with wind; for example, a temperature of 0° F with a wind of 20 mph has a wind chill effect of minus 22° F. High humidity increases the risk of heat emergencies because sweat evaporates more slowly and provides less cooling effect, as shown in the heat index chart (**Figure 21-2**). For example, an air temperature of 90° F with a humidity of 90% has the same effect on the body as an air temperature of 120 degrees.

COLD EMERGENCIES

Exposure to cold temperatures can cause either **frostbite,** which is localized freezing of skin and other tissues, or **hypothermia,** which is lowering of the whole body's temperature.

Frostbite

Frostbite is the freezing of skin or deeper tissues. Frostbite occurs when the temperature is 32° F or colder. It usually happens to exposed skin areas on the head or face, hands, or feet. Wind chill increases the risk of frostbite. Severe frostbite kills tissue and can result in gangrene and having to amputate the body part.

The first aid for frostbite involves removing the affected area from the cold as soon as possible and protecting the area until the victim receives

medical treatment. In special circumstances the body part may be rewarmed—but only under certain conditions. If the frostbitten area is at any risk of being refrozen, it should not be rewarmed, because warming followed by freezing increases the tissue damage. If the extrication, rescue, or transport of a frostbite victim may subject the area to cold again, do not warm it but let health-care or EMS professionals treat the frostbite. In a situation where help will be delayed, and only if refreezing can be prevented, then severe frostbite can be rewarmed by immersing the area in luke-warm—not hot—water (about 100 to 105° F) for at least 20 minutes or up to 45 minutes. Never apply a direct heat source to frostbitten skin, such as heat lamp, hot water bottle, or heating pad, because of the risk of additional tissue damage (see First Aid: "Frostbite").

	\multicolumn{19}{c}{Temperature (F)}																		
Calm	40	35	30	25	20	15	10	5	0	−5	−10	−15	−20	−25	−30	−35	−40	−45
5	36	31	25	19	13	7	1	−5	−11	−16	−22	−28	−34	−40	−46	−52	−57	−63
10	34	27	21	15	9	3	−4	−10	−16	−22	−28	−35	−41	−47	−53	−59	−66	−72
15	32	25	19	13	6	0	−7	−13	−19	−26	−32	−39	−45	−51	−58	−64	−71	−77
20	30	24	17	11	4	−2	−9	−15	−22	−29	−35	−42	−48	−55	−61	−68	−74	−81
25	29	23	16	9	3	−4	−11	−17	−24	−31	−37	−44	−51	−58	−64	−71	−78	−84
30	28	22	15	8	1	−5	−12	−19	−26	−33	−39	−46	−53	−60	−67	−73	−80	−87
35	28	21	14	7	0	−7	−14	−21	−27	−34	−41	−48	−55	−62	−69	−76	−82	−89
40	27	20	13	6	−1	−8	−15	−22	−29	−36	−43	−50	−57	−64	−71	−78	−84	−91
45	26	19	12	5	−2	−9	−16	−23	−30	−37	−44	−51	−58	−65	−72	−79	−86	−93
50	26	19	12	4	−3	−10	−17	−24	−31	−38	−45	−52	−60	−67	−74	−81	−88	−95
55	25	18	11	4	−3	−11	−18	−25	−32	−39	−46	−54	−61	−68	−75	−82	−89	−97
60	25	17	10	3	−4	−11	−19	−26	−33	−40	−48	−55	−62	−69	−76	−84	−91	−98

Wind (mph) — left axis

Wind Chill (F) = 35.74 + 0.6215T − 35.75($V^{0.16}$) + 0.4275T($V^{0.16}$)
Where, T = Air temperature (F)   V = Wind speed (mph)

Frostbite times: ☐ 30 minutes ☐ 10 minutes ☐ 5 minutes

Effective 11/01/01

Figure 21-1 Wind chill. (National Oceanic and Atmospheric Administration)

Temperature (F) versus Relative Humidity (%)

F	90%	80%	70%	60%	50%	40%
80	85	84	82	81	80	79
85	101	96	92	90	86	84
90	121	113	105	99	94	90
95		133	122	113	105	98
100			142	129	118	109
105				146	133	121
110						135

HI	Possible Heat Disorder
80F 90F	Fatigue possible with prolonged exposure and physical activity.
90F 105F	Sunstroke, heat cramps, and heat exhaustion possible.
105F 130F	Sunstroke, heat cramps, and heat exhaustion likely, and heatstroke possible.
130F or greater	−eatstroke highly likely with continued exposure.

Figure 21-2 Heat index. (National Weather Service)

Hypothermia

When the body cannot make heat as fast as it loses it in a cold environment, hypothermia develops. In hypothermia, body temperature drops below 95° F. It does not have to be freezing cold for hypothermia to occur. Hypothermia can occur at almost any cool temperature if the body is unprotected, especially if the victim is wet, exposed a long time, or unable to restore body heat because of a medical condition. An average of almost 700 individuals die each year in the United States of hypothermia, about half of them over age 65. Because hypothermia alters a person's mental status, an affected victim may not take corrective actions to avoid continued exposure to cold (**Box 21-2**).

Hypothermia is a progressive problem, as the victim transitions from simply feeling cold to mild hypothermia and, without the condition being relieved, to more serious symptoms and possibly to death. This progression may occur gradually, over

First Aid | Frostbite

When You See

- Skin looks waxy and white, gray, yellow, or bluish.
- The area is numb or feels tingly or aching.
- Severe frostbite:
  - The area feels hard.
  - May become painless.
  - After warming, the area becomes swollen and may blister.

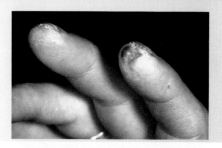

Do This First

1 Move the victim to a warm environment. Do not let the victim walk on frostbitten feet. Check the victim also for hypothermia.

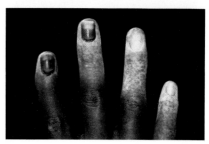

2 Remove any tight clothing or jewelry around the area.

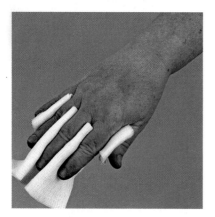

3 Put dry gauze or fluffy cloth between frostbitten fingers or toes. Protect the area from being touched or rubbed by clothing or objects.

4 Elevate the area if possible to reduce swelling.

5 Seek medical attention immediately.

ALERT

- Do not rub frostbitten skin because this can damage the skin.
- Do not rewarm frostbitten skin if it may be frozen again, which could worsen the injury.
- Do not use a fire, heat lamp, hot water bottle, or heating pad to warm the area.
- After rewarming, be careful not to break blisters.

Additional Care

- The victim may choose to take aspirin (adults only), acetaminophen, or ibuprofen for pain.
- Drink warm liquids but not alcohol.
- Prevent the area from refreezing.

Learning Checkpoint ①

1. True or False: Rubbing frostbitten fingers is the best way to warm them.

2. Frostbitten skin usually has what color(s)?

_____

3. A friend stops by your house after being outside for some time, complaining of being very cold. He has lost his hat, and his ears are white and hard and he says he has no feeling in them. Describe three actions to take for this man's frostbite.

_____

hours or even days, or very quickly, especially with a wind chill or if the victim is wet.

Preventing Hypothermia

When planning to be outdoors for a long time, be prepared for a cold emergency:

- Check the weather forecast before going outdoors for an extended period.
- Take along extra clothing, socks, sleeping bag, or a survival bag (see hypothermia blanket in **Chapter 24**).
- Have high-energy food bars and warm drinks.
- Do not consume alcohol or caffeine, both of which increase heat loss.

In addition, dress for the cold:

- Wear layers of clothing that do not retain moisture (wool or polypropylene).
- Choose a coat with wind- and waterproof outer layer.
- Wear a hat (up to 50% of body heat is lost from the head).

- Use rain gear to avoid becoming wet.

During cold periods, check on people who are at risk for hypothermia:

- Check on older family members, friends, and neighbors to ensure that the home is kept warm.
- Be familiar with the signs and symptoms of early hypothermia in order to recognize the problem and seek treatment.
- Employees of public health facilities, detoxification centers, shelters for the homeless, and similar facilities should be educated to recognize hypothermia so that victims receive appropriate treatment early.

First Aid for Hypothermia

Since hypothermia may begin gradually, it is crucial to recognize the first signs and symptoms in order to take early action. Shivering, numbness, lethargy, poor coordination, and slurred speech are early manifestations. Victims of early or mild hypothermia often experience the "umbles": mumbles, fumbles, stumbles. Infants may have bright red skin and little

Box 21-2 Facts About Hypothermia

- Hypothermia occurs more easily in elderly or ill people.
- People under the influence of alcohol or drugs are at greater risk for hypothermia.
- A person immersed in cold water cools 30 times faster than in cool air.

- Victims in cold water are more likely to die from hypothermia than to drown.
- Victims in cardiac arrest after immersion in cold water have been resuscitated after a long time underwater—don't give up!

First Aid   **Hypothermia**

When You See

- Shivering; may be uncontrollable (but stops in severe hypothermia)
- Victim seems apathetic, confused, or irrational; may be belligerent
- Lethargy, clumsy movements, drowsiness
- Pale, cool skin—even under clothing (check abdomen)
- Slow breathing
- Changing levels of responsiveness

Do This First

1 With an unresponsive victim, check for breathing and provide CPR as needed. Call 9-1-1 for all severe hypothermia victims.

2 Quickly get the victim out of the cold, and remove any wet clothing.

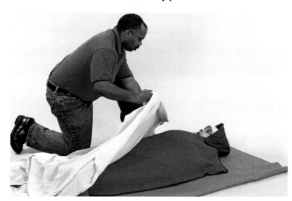

3 Have the victim lie down, and cover him or her with blankets or warm clothing. If outdoors, put a blanket or clothing under the victim as well. Do not let a responsive victim move around.

4 Except in mild cases, the victim needs immediate medical care.

))) ALERT)))

- Do not immerse a victim of hypothermia in hot water or use direct heat (hot water bottle, heat lamp, heating pad), because rapid warming can cause heart problems.
- Do not rub or massage the victim's skin. Be very gentle when handling the victim.

Additional Care

- Give warm (not hot) drinks to an alert victim who can easily swallow, but not alcohol or caffeine.
- Stay with the victim until he or she reaches a healthcare provider or help arrives.

Learning Checkpoint 2

1. True or False: Hypothermia occurs only when the air temperature is below freezing.

2. True or False: A hypothermia victim who is generating heat by shivering still needs first aid and warming.

3. A mildly hypothermic victim is brought into a ski lodge to be warmed. It will help to

   a. give him a warm rum drink.

   b. have him take off his outer clothes and sit close to the fire.

   c. send him to a hot shower.

   d. remove his damp clothing and warm him with a blanket.

4. You are on a backpacking camping trip in the mountains and are caught in an unexpected snowstorm. On the way back down the mountain, about four miles from your car, you encounter a teenager sitting in the snow. His clothes are snowy and damp. He is lethargic and seems very confused. You call for help on your cell phone, but it will be at least two hours before the rescue team arrives. Using typical camping gear, what first aid can you give this victim?

---

energy. As body temperature drops, hypothermia progresses and becomes more serious. Shivering typically stops, and the victim may not even feel cold. Check the victim's skin temperature under clothing at the abdomen; cool skin here often indicates hypothermia. Breathing becomes shallow, and mental status continues to deteriorate. In severe cases, the victim becomes unresponsive and may stop breathing.

First aid for hypothermia begins with removing the victim from the cold. Remove wet clothing and cover the victim with blankets or warm clothing. Call 9-1-1, and in severe cases be prepared to give basic life support. Do not try to warm the victim rapidly by immersing the body in warm water or by using a heat source except in a remote area far from healthcare (see **Chapter 24**), because a heart rhythm disturbance may result.

A hypothermia victim who is not breathing may still be resuscitated. Handle the victim gently, but provide CPR or other care as needed while waiting for help to arrive (see First Aid: "Hypothermia").

HEAT EMERGENCIES

Heat illnesses can result when people become overheated in a hot environment. Generally there are three types of heat illnesses:

- **Heat cramps** are the least serious and usually first to occur.
- **Heat exhaustion** develops when the body becomes dehydrated in a hot environment.
- **Heatstroke,** with a seriously high body temperature, may develop from heat exhaustion. It is a medical emergency and, if untreated, usually causes death.

Most heatstroke deaths occur from exposure to a high temperature for a sustained period. Most heat-related deaths occur during hot weather, but heatstroke also affects those in settings where heat is generated, such as furnace rooms, factories, or vehicles. Over the last two decades an average of 400 heat-related deaths a year have occurred in the United States, about half of these related to hot weather. In one heat wave alone, in Chicago in 1995, 485 people died of heat emergencies. Extreme heat is defined as temperatures that rise 10 degrees or more above the normal high temperature for the region and last several days to several weeks. As noted earlier in this chapter, many factors can increase the risk for developing a heat illness, including old age or infancy/youth, obesity, certain medical conditions such as heart disease, the use of certain medications, drinking alcohol, not drinking enough fluid, and strenuous activity in a hot environment.

Like hypothermia, heatstroke is a progressive disease. In the mild stage (heat exhaustion), the victim is becoming dehydrated and the body is unable to cool itself. If the condition is not corrected, with continuing exposure to heat the victim's body temperature begins to rise and more serious symptoms occur, potentially leading to death. Prevention of life-threatening heatstroke depends on recognizing the early signs and symptoms and providing care before the condition becomes more serious.

Preventing Heat Emergencies

Follow these guidelines to help prevent heat emergencies:

- In hot environments wear loose, lightweight clothing.
- Rest frequently in shady or cool areas.
- Drink adequate fluids before, during, and after activity, but avoid alcohol and caffeine. Prehydrating is especially important before an endurance sport activity.
- For sports and endurance activities that may last longer than short periods of time, sports drinks that replace depleted electrolytes are generally better than water, but in most other situations adequate water consumption will prevent heat exhaustion.
- Avoid exertion if you are overweight or elderly.
- When new to a hot area, take several days (up to a week to 10 days) to gradually acclimate to heat and humidity before engaging in strenuous activity.
- During heat waves, check on elderly friends, family, and neighbors, particularly those living alone or having any mental impairment, and if necessary move them to an air-conditioned area.
- Do not leave children alone in a vehicle. Make sure they cannot lock themselves into an enclosed space.
- Use sunscreen because sunburn causes a loss of body fluid as well as skin damage.

Heat Cramps

Activity in a hot environment may cause painful cramps in muscles, called **heat cramps,** often in the lower legs or abdominal muscles. The muscle cramps result when sweating lowers the body's sodium levels. Heat cramps may occur along with heat exhaustion and heatstroke (see First Aid: "Heat Cramps").

Heat Exhaustion

Activity in a hot environment usually causes heavy sweating, which may lead to dehydration and depletion of salt and electrolytes in the body if the person does not get enough fluids. This dehydration can lead to **heat exhaustion.**

The victim in heat exhaustion is usually sweating, and the skin is pale or ashen, moist, and often cool. Other signs and symptoms include thirst, fatigue, and muscle cramps. Late signs and symptoms include headache, dizziness, fainting, nausea, vomiting, and fast, shallow breathing.

First, move the victim from the heat to rest in a cool place. Loosen or remove unnecessary clothing and help cool the victim's body with wet cloths, sponging the skin with cool water, or spraying the skin with water and fanning the area. Give the victim a sports drink or water to drink. The victim's condition should improve within 30 minutes. If it does not, or if the victim has a heart condition or high blood pressure, seek medical attention immediately. Remember that if unrelieved, heat exhaustion may develop into heatstroke, a life-threatening emergency (see First Aid: "Heat Exhaustion").

Heatstroke

Heatstroke is a life-threatening emergency that is more common during hot summer periods. It may develop slowly over several days or more rapidly when engaged in strenuous activity in the heat. The victim may be dehydrated and not sweating when heatstroke gradually develops, or he or she may be sweating heavily from exertion. Heatstroke causes a body temperature of 104° F or higher and is different from heat exhaustion, although it may develop from untreated heat exhaustion (see First Aid: "Heatstroke"):

- In heatstroke the victim's skin is flushed and feels very hot to the touch; in heat exhaustion the skin may be pale or ashen and clammy.
- In heatstroke the victim becomes very confused and irrational and may become unresponsive or have convulsions; in heat exhaustion the victim is dizzy or tired or may be irritable or have a headache.

First Aid **Heat Cramps**

When You See

- Signs of muscle pain, cramping, spasms
- Heavy sweating

Do This First

1 Have the person stop the activity and sit quietly in a cool place.

2 Give a sports drink or water.

Additional Care

- For abdominal cramps, continue resting in a comfortable position.
- For leg cramps, stretch the muscle by extending the leg and flexing the ankle. Apply pressure to the cramped area.
- Seek medical attention for a victim who has heart problems or is on a low-sodium diet or if the cramps do not subside within an hour.

3 Have the person avoid strenuous activity for a few hours to prevent progression to heat exhaustion or heatstroke.

Learning Checkpoint ③

1. True or False: For abdominal heat cramps, the best care is vigorous massage and stomach kneading.

2. To treat heat cramps:

  a. Immerse the victim in a bathtub of cold water.

  b. Give a sports drink or water to drink.

  c. Keep the victim very active until the cramp works itself out.

  d. Do not let the victim eat or drink anything.

3. True or False: Give salt tablets to victims who have both heat cramps and heat exhaustion.

4. The problem of heat exhaustion begins when a person in a hot environment is not getting enough _____.

5. List three possible ways to cool a victim with heat exhaustion.

_____

6. On a hot day you join a friend on the athletic field who has been working out for a couple of hours. He is sitting on the grass in the sun. He is sweating heavily and says he has a headache and feels nauseous. Someone has already given him a sports drink. What should you do now? List in correct order the first four actions you would take.

_____

First Aid | **Heat Exhaustion**

When You See

- Sweating, pale or ashen, moist skin (often cool)
- Thirst
- Fatigue
- Muscle cramps

Later signs and symptoms:
- Headache, dizziness, fainting
- Nausea, vomiting
- Fast, shallow breathing

Do This First

1 Move the victim from the heat to rest in a cool place. Loosen or remove unnecessary clothing.

2 Give a sports drink or water to drink.

3 Raise the legs 8 to 12 inches.

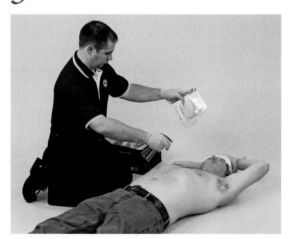

4 Cool the victim with one of these methods:
   - Put wet cloths on the forehead and body.
   - Sponge the skin with cool water.
   - Spray the skin with water from a spray bottle and then fan the area.

(ALERT)

- Do not give a heat exhaustion or heatstroke victim salt tablets. Use a sports drink instead (if the victim is awake and alert).
- Do not give liquids containing caffeine or alcohol.
- If the victim is lethargic, nauseous, or vomiting, do not give any liquids.

Additional Care

- Seek medical care if the victim's condition worsens or does not improve within 30 minutes.
- Seek urgent medical attention if the victim has a heart condition or high blood pressure.

First Aid | Heatstroke

When You See

- Skin flushed, dry, and hot to the touch; sweating usually has stopped
- Fast breathing
- Headache, dizziness, extreme confusion
- Irrational behavior
- Possible convulsions or unresponsiveness

Do This First

1 Call 9-1-1.

2 Move the victim to a cool place.

3 Remove outer clothing.

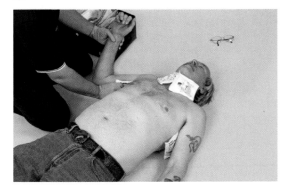

4 Cool the victim quickly with any means at hand:
- Wrap the victim in a wet sheet and keep it wet.
- Sponge the victim with cold water.
- Spray the skin with water from a spray bottle and then fan the area.
- Put ice bags or cool packs on the neck, armpits, and the groin.
- Partly submerge the victim in cool water and splash the skin (but do not immerse in cold water).

5 Keep cooling until the victim's temperature drops to about 101° F.

(ALERT)

- Do not apply rubbing alcohol to the victim's skin.
- The victim should not take pain relievers or salt tablets.
- Do not give any beverage containing caffeine or alcohol.
- If the victim is nauseous or vomiting or experiencing diminished mental status, do not give liquids.

Additional Care

- Monitor the victim and provide care as needed.
- Put an unresponsive victim in the recovery position and monitor breathing.
- Protect a victim having convulsions from injury (see **Chapter 17**).

Learning
Checkpoint (4)

1. True or False: It is safe to drive a heatstroke victim home after you have given first aid and cooled his or her body down to 100° F, as long as the victim is feeling better.

2. In what situation should you call 9-1-1 for a heatstroke victim?

_____

3. Describe how a heatstroke victim's behavior may be different from the way in which that person usually behaves.

_____

4. Your softball game happens to fall on the hottest day of the year. Your coach knows you have first aid training and asks you to help out to make sure none of the students has problems with heat exhaustion or heatstroke.

   a. To be prepared for these possibilities, what things should you make sure are present at the ball field?

   _____

   b. You decide to give a safety talk to your team before the game begins. What would you tell them about how to prevent heat emergencies? What signs and symptoms of a potential problem should players watch out for in others on their team?

   _____

   c. Despite these precautions, by the seventh inning the center fielder seems to be showing signs and symptoms of heatstroke. What is the first step you should take?

   _____

Concluding Thoughts

Heat and cold emergencies can be prevented by following commonsense guidelines and taking steps in extreme temperatures to maintain a normal body temperature. Recognizing the early signs and symptoms of both heat and cold emergencies is important to keep these conditions from worsening. When heat or cold illness does occur, act quickly to get medical attention before the emergency becomes life threatening. Be sure to take special precautions when engaged in activities in rural or wilderness areas where a victim cannot be easily or quickly reached by EMS professionals. **Chapter 24** describes these extra preparations to prevent these emergencies from occurring in such situations.

Learning Outcomes

You should now be able to do the following:

1. Describe the different types of cold and heat emergencies and what you can do to prevent them.

2. Explain factors that may make a person more susceptible to a cold or heat emergency.

3. List the signs and symptoms and first aid for:
   - Frostbite
   - Hypothermia
   - Heat cramps
   - Heat exhaustion
   - Heatstroke

Review Questions

1. Muscle contraction produces
   a. heat.
   b. heat loss.
   c. vasoconstriction.
   d. vasodilation.

2. Heat and cold emergencies are more likely to occur in
   a. the elderly.
   b. people with certain chronic diseases.
   c. infants.
   d. All of the above

3. First aid for frostbite includes
   a. rapid rewarming using a heat lamp or heating pad.
   b. protecting the area from rubbing or constricting jewelry.
   c. vigorously rubbing the area.
   d. running very hot water over the affected area for 10 minutes.

4. To help prevent hypothermia when outdoors in frigid temperatures,
   a. drink lots of coffee or hot tea.
   b. wear thick boots because most heat loss is through the feet.
   c. try to stay dry.
   d. drink alcohol to stay warm.

5. The signs and symptoms of hypothermia include
   a. apathy or confusion.
   b. red, blotchy skin.
   c. talkativeness.
   d. perceptions of being overly warm.

6. First aid for severe hypothermia includes
   a. putting the victim in a hot shower.
   b. massaging the victim all over.
   c. calling 9-1-1.
   d. giving CPR regardless of whether the victim is breathing.

7. In what order do heat illnesses typically progress with continued activity in a hot environment?
   a. Heat cramps → heatstroke → heat exhaustion
   b. Heat cramps → heat exhaustion → heatstroke
   c. Heat exhaustion → heat cramps → heatstroke
   d. Can occur in any order

8. First aid for heat cramps includes
   a. vigorously exercising the muscle.
   b. drinking a sports drink or water.
   c. applying a compression bandage.
   d. splinting the extremity until the cramps pass.

9. The late signs and symptoms of heat exhaustion include
   a. headache, dizziness, fainting.
   b. constipation or diarrhea.
   c. extreme excitability.
   d. cold, tingling fingers or toes.

10. How can you cool down someone who is experiencing heatstroke?
   a. Wrap the victim in a wet sheet and keep it wet.
   b. Sponge the victim with cold water.
   c. Put ice bags or cool packs beside the neck, armpits, and groin area.
   d. All of the above

References and Resources

American College of Emergency Physicians. *First aid manual: a comprehensive guide to treating emergency victims of all ages in any situation.* New York: DK Publishing; 2001.

American Heart Association. 2005 International consensus on cardiopulmonary resuscitation (CPR) and emergency cardiovascular care (ECC) science with treatment recommendations. *Circulation,* 112(22). November 29, 2005.

American Medical Association. *Handbook of first aid and emergency care.* Revised ed. New York: Random House; 2000.

Casa DJ., et al. National Athletic Trainers' Association position statement: fluid replacement for athletes. *Journal of Athletic Training,* 2000 June; 35(2).

Centers for Disease Control and Prevention. Extreme heat: a prevention guide to promote your personal health and safety. 2005. www.cdc.gov

Centers for Disease Control and Prevention. Hypothermia-related deaths—United States, 2003–2004. *MMWR Weekly* 2005. February 25; 54(07). www.cdc.gov

Inter-Association Task Force on Exertional Heat Illnesses. Consensus statement. The American Physiological Society. www.the-aps.org/news/consensus.pdf

National Oceanic and Atmosphere Administration. www.noaa.com

National Safety Council. www.nsc.org

National Weather Service. www.nws.noaa.gov

Chapter 22

Behavioral Emergencies

Chapter Preview

- Emotional and Behavioral Responses to Injury and Illness
- Victims with Emotional Problems
- Behavioral Emergencies
- Abuse
- Sexual Assault and Rape

Your boss has asked to meet with you and another employee, Meg, the woman in charge of order fulfillment. There have been several problems with important orders lately, and as the meeting explores ways to prevent future problems, Meg becomes increasingly emotional and defensive. You know she has been under a lot of stress lately, and you've overheard gossip that she has some personal problems, but that doesn't seem to account for how worked up she is becoming in this meeting. Finally, when the boss asks if she will be able to solve the order problems, Meg seems to explode, rising from her chair with her hands in fists. You are alarmed and wonder what you can do before the situation is completely out of control or even becomes violent.

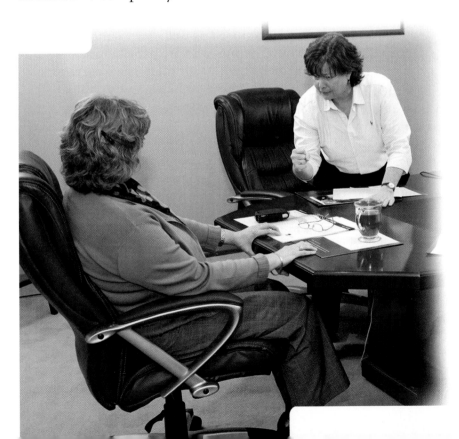

The process of giving first aid is sometimes complicated by the victim's behavior. Many injuries and medical emergencies may cause altered mental status, which can lead to a victim acting in unusual or unpredictable ways. Injury and illness also typically cause emotional responses that may affect how first aid must be given. Other victims may have emotional problems such as panic reactions or depression that also must be addressed when giving first aid. **Behavioral emergencies** involve situations in which the victim's behavior, whether caused by the injury or illness or by personality or mental health factors, results in or complicates an emergency situation. Abuse and rape are additional behavioral situations.

EMOTIONAL AND BEHAVIORAL RESPONSES TO INJURY AND ILLNESS

Injury, sudden illness, and other emergencies typically lead to strong emotional reactions in those involved. Normal reactions include fear, anxiety, and apprehensiveness. In addition to the physical effects of the injury or illness itself, which may include altered mental status, normal emotional reactions may cause other stress-related physical signs and symptoms such as trembling or shakiness, feelings of nausea, a fast heartbeat and breathing, and perspiration.

Victims with preexisting emotional problems or mental illness are more likely to have more severe reactions. They may overreact, panic and act wildly, speak incoherently, become argumentative or withdrawn, or become violent.

There is no clear-cut line between "normal" and "abnormal" responses to injury and sudden illness. Think of these responses as a continuum from normal to abnormal, with a wide range of behaviors in the middle. It is important not to judge a victim's behavior too quickly but to assess the situation. For example, a person who is usually calm and rational may become seemingly irrational and act inappropriately when in great pain. In such a case accept the victim's emotional state and address his or her concerns while providing first aid. At the other extreme, a person who is usually quick to anger and aggressive may respond to the stress of an injury with violent behavior. In this case it may become more important to protect yourself and others at the scene.

Your decision on how to approach a victim in a potential behavioral emergency depends on understanding normal versus abnormal reactions and an assessment of the victim's emotional and mental condition. Always remember your own safety: do not approach a victim who may become violent. Call 9-1-1 and stay at a safe distance until help arrives.

Altered Mental Status

As noted in previous chapters, altered mental status, or altered responsiveness, may result from many different injuries and illnesses. The brain requires a steady level of oxygen for normal functioning, and any injury or illness that affects oxygenation may affect the victim's mental status—and therefore his or her behavior. Lowered levels of responsiveness may result from significantly reduced oxygen levels. Mental status may suddenly or gradually diminish. The victim may first feel dizzy, drowsy, disoriented, or confused. The victim may suddenly or eventually become completely unresponsive. Often in such cases, the appropriate first aid is to care for the underlying cause of the altered mental status (**Box 22-1**).

Even small oxygen reductions can cause other reactions. A victim may respond to reduced brain oxygen with extreme anxiety and panic, even potential violence. In such cases, in addition to providing first aid, you also need to calm the victim and possibly prevent further injury caused by the victim's behavior. You may need to protect yourself as well. For example, near-drowning victims who are panicking as they desperately fight for air often behave irrationally and may grab onto a rescuer so forcefully that both lives are threatened.

Typical Emotional Reactions

As noted earlier, typical reactions to injury, sudden illness, and other emergencies include fear, anxiety, and apprehensiveness. The sight of their own blood makes many people panic. It is difficult to think clearly when in great pain. A victim with a serious injury may overreact and be fearful of dying. A victim may be unable to act, seemingly frozen by emotional shock, or may be acting irrationally and out of control. Any of these reactions can complicate the process of giving first aid for the victim's injury or illness.

Because emotional stress can have negative physical effects on the body, it may be just as important to address the victim's emotional reac-

Box 22-1   Causes of Altered Mental Status

- Respiratory emergencies
- Cardiac emergencies
- Poisoning
- Head injuries
- Seizures
- Diabetic emergencies

- Stroke
- High fever
- Substance abuse
- Drug overdose
- Heat or cold emergencies

tion as it is to care for the physical injury or illness. The victim needs to be calmed and reassured.

Reassuring and Calming Victims

How you act in the face of the victim's emergency can dramatically affect how the victim responds. If you react negatively, your words, gestures, or facial expressions may increase the victim's stressful response rather than diminish it. You may show your own concern or fear about the emergency. You may act impatiently if the victim is not immediately cooperative. If you show a lack of self-confidence in your ability to manage the emergency and provide first aid, the victim's level of stress may increase. Any of these reactions will only increase the problem.

Instead, take steps to calm and reassure the victim, following these guidelines (**Figure 22-1**):

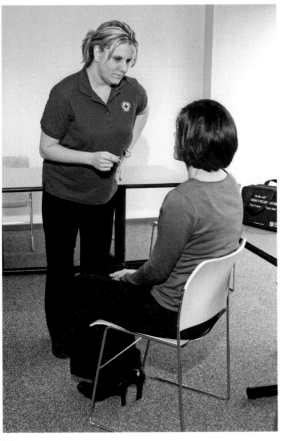
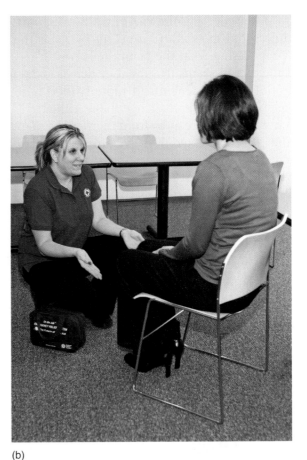

(a)   (b)

Figure 22-1 (a) When trying to calm an emotional victim, be careful not to assume a position that may seem threatening. (b) Stay a comfortable distance away and use accepting, nonthreatening body language.

1. Tell the victim who you are and say you are there to help. Avoid seeming judgmental.

2. Do not assume the victim is intoxicated, using drugs, or otherwise impaired, since the victim's behavior may result from a medical condition. Even if you smell alcohol on the victim's breath, do not assume a problem is due only to intoxication—you could overlook a serious injury.

3. Reassure the victim that help is on the way (after 9-1-1 has been called).

4. Ask the victim for his or her name, and use it when speaking to him or her.

5. If possible, try to involve any victim's friend or family member who is present at the scene.

6. Let the victim tell you what he or she thinks is wrong.

7. Let the victim know you understand his or her concerns.

8. Make eye contact with the victim, and stay at the victim's eye level.

9. Speak in a caring, reassuring voice, but do not give false assurances or lie about the victim's condition.

10. Do not argue with the victim. Show that you understand the victim's concerns by repeating or rephrasing what the victim tells you.

11. If the victim seems irrational or delusional, do not make statements to support their false beliefs, but do not challenge them, either.

12. Stay a safe distance away from the victim until your help is accepted. If the victim does not accept your help, do not try to restrain or force care on him or her. Withdraw if the scene seems unsafe and if the victim may become violent.

13. Tell the victim what you plan to do before doing it.

14. Move calmly and slowly, touching the victim only as necessary.

VICTIMS WITH EMOTIONAL PROBLEMS

Some victims have preexisting emotional problems that may present greater challenges than the emotions normally provoked by emergencies. Two common problems are anxiety/panic and depression.

Anxiety and Panic

While it is normal to feel fear and apprehension when injured or suddenly ill, some people are prone to extreme **anxiety** and may have a **panic attack.** A panic attack is a sudden, overwhelming fear that is excessive for the situation. Signs and symptoms of extreme anxiety include:

- Agitation, inability to hold still, rapid movements, pacing
- Speaking very fast, not making sense
- Inability to judge the situation accurately
- Rapid emotional changes, crying, hysteria, anger
- A desire to leave the scene or not wait for medical help
- Fast heartbeat and breathing
- Difficulty breathing, dizziness, trembling

With a victim exhibiting signs and symptoms of extreme anxiety or panic, it is important to remain calm and patient at all times. Any attempt you make to restrain the person or to shock the person out of this behavior will likely worsen the situation. Often the panic will begin to lessen in a few minutes because the physiological response of the body is self-limiting.

Follow the guidelines given earlier for calming and reassuring victims. Recognize that an individual prone to extreme anxiety or panic may need more time to calm down and may suddenly experience renewed anxiety. Continue to use the calming techniques while providing first aid. Be empathetic and gentle, and always explain what you are doing. Avoid touching the victim without first explaining what you are about to do and why. Allow these victims to keep talking about what they are feeling and to express their concerns.

Depression

Victims who experience depression also require special attention. Major **depression** is a common psychological illness, affecting an estimated 10% of Americans chronically and 20% to 25% of all adults at some time in their lives. It occurs in people of all ages, is common in the elderly, and is twice as common in women as in men. Common signs and symptoms of depression include:

- Frequent feelings of sadness
- Loss of energy
- Feelings of hopelessness or worthlessness
- Difficulty concentrating
- Difficulty making decisions

- Physical symptoms such as abdominal pain, insomnia, appetite loss, recurrent headaches
- Thoughts of death or suicide

Someone experiencing depression often acts withdrawn, apathetic, and subdued. Although the person may not resist your first aid care, he or she may not cooperate and may not offer information that would help you assess the situation. Therefore it is important to make an effort to communicate with a victim who seems depressed. Follow these guidelines:

1. Encourage the victim to talk. Acknowledge that the person seems sad and ask why.
2. Be reassuring and sympathetic.
3. Show the victim that you care about him or her as a person. Helping to make the person comfortable, offering a drink of water or a blanket, and providing other comforts can encourage the victim to open up and talk about the problem.
4. If the victim is crying, do not try to make him or her stop. Allow the person to work through the emotion.
5. If the victim complains about something in his or her life, listen sympathetically but do not offer false reassurances such as saying, "Everything will be just fine" or "I'm sure that problem won't last long." Instead, talk about resources you are aware of to help people with problems such as the victim's.
6. Be alert to the possibility of suicide (see later section on "Suicidal Feelings").

BEHAVIORAL EMERGENCIES

The previous sections have focused on interacting with victims of injury or sudden illness who are experiencing normal or abnormal emotional reactions. In most cases those reactions complicate the first aid problem but are not the primary problem. In some cases, however, the person's behavior constitutes the emergency. Behavioral emergencies include situations in which the victim has suicidal feelings or the potential to act violently in a way that may harm either him- or herself or others.

When a victim's behavior becomes obviously abnormal, remember not to assume simply that the person is intoxicated or under the influence of a drug. Many different factors can radically change a person's behavior, including:

- The stress of the situation
- Illnesses or injuries causing altered mental status
- Mental illnesses

Suicidal Feelings

The National Center for Injury Prevention and Control reports that more than 30,000 individuals committed suicide in the United States in a recent year. Suicide is the third leading cause of death among people aged 15 to 24. Men are four times more likely to commit suicide than women, although women report attempting suicide three times more often than men. Suicide is the eighth leading cause of death for adult men. Drug overdose (see **Chapter 19**) is the most common method used in attempted suicides, but firearms are used in most successful suicides.

The risk factors and signs of potential suicides are listed in **Box 22-2**. Research has shown that most people who commit suicide communicated their desire to others, although not always in an obvious way. Anyone who makes comments suggestive of suicidal feelings should be taken seriously.

Follow these guidelines if you are caring for a person who may be suicidal or whose injury may have been self-inflicted:

1. Take the person seriously, and listen to what he or she is saying. Ask what the person is planning to do. Talk calmly and supportively.
2. Do not try to argue the person out of committing suicide, but let him or her know that you understand and care. Do not give false reassurances.
3. Seek help. Call 9-1-1 if appropriate, and involve friends or family members if possible in any care given.
4. Do not leave the person alone unless your own safety is threatened.
5. Remove any weapons, drugs, or medications that might be used in a suicide attempt. Do not let the person drive.
6. If the person has a firearm and is threatening violence, withdraw, call 9-1-1, and wait for help to arrive and handle the situation. (See following section on "Violent Behavior.")
7. Give first aid and other care as appropriate.

Violent Behavior

In any behavioral emergency, consider the potential for violence. The person may threaten violence

Box 22-2 Suicide Risk Factors and Warning Signs

Risk Factors

- Mental disorders, including depression
- History of substance abuse
- Feelings of hopelessness
- Recent emotional crisis or painful illness
- Impulsive or aggressive tendencies
- Past attempts at suicide

Warning Signs

- Talking about suicide (it is a myth that people who talk about it rarely do it)
- Comments about feeling hopeless or worthless
- Taking risks that could cause death, such as driving too fast
- Loss of interest in one's past activities
- Suddenly and unexpectedly seeming calm or happy after being sad

to self or others on the scene. Following are signs that violent behavior may occur:

- The person is holding a weapon or any object that might be used as a weapon.
- The person is in a threatening or bullying posture or has his or her hands in fists, or is pacing and waving his or her arms around (**Figure 22-2**).
- The person is threatening, verbally abusing, or yelling at you or someone else.
- The person is uncontrollably angry, kicking or throwing things.
- The person seems to be hallucinating or yelling at someone not present.
- The person is known to have committed violent acts in the past.

If you think the person may commit an act of violence, follow these guidelines:

1. Do not enter the scene if there is a risk to your safety. Encourage others present in the scene to withdraw.
2. Call 9-1-1.
3. Do not try to restrain the person unless you have had special training and have assistance from others. Monitor the situation from a safe distance and wait for help to arrive.
4. While waiting for help, do the following if it is safe to remain with the person:
   - Talk to the person calmly and quietly, and listen to what he or she has to say. Do not argue or be falsely reassuring, which the person may

perceive as condescending or patronizing behavior. Try to divert the person from any violent action by keeping him or her talking.
- Do not move about or do anything the person may perceive as threatening.

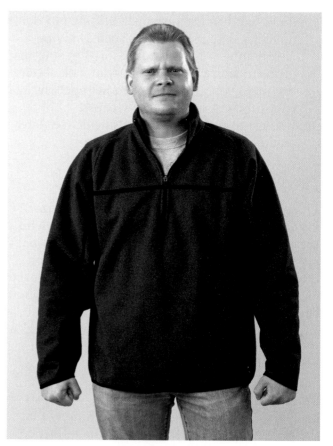

Figure 22-2 An emotional person is potentially violent.

Learning
Checkpoint ①

1. Normal responses to many injuries and sudden illnesses include

   a. trembling or shakiness.   **c.** altered mental status.

   b. fear, anxiety.   **d.** All of the above

2. Check off any of the following conditions that may cause altered mental status:

   ___ Respiratory emergencies   ___ Cardiac emergencies

   ___ Poisoning   ___ Head injuries

   ___ Seizures   ___ Diabetic emergencies

   ___ Stroke   ___ High fever

   ___ Drug overdose   ___ Heat or cold emergencies

3. Describe at least five things you can do to help calm an emotional victim.

_____

4. True or False: Never acknowledge that a depressed person seems sad, but be cheerful and pretend nothing is wrong.

5. True or False: People who talk about suicide rarely do it.

6. You see an injured victim who is shouting and making threatening gestures, and you realize he is potentially violent. Number the following actions in the order in which you should take them:

   ___ Talk to the person calmly and quietly, and try to divert the person from any violent action by keeping him or her talking.

   ___ Call 9-1-1.

   ___ Do not enter the scene if there is a risk to your safety. Encourage others at the scene to withdraw.

- Offer to give first aid if the person calms down, but do not try to do anything without the person's consent.
- Maintain an open exit from the room or scene; do not let a potentially violent person get between you and the door.

ABUSE

Abuse is the intentional inflicting of injury or suffering on someone under the abuser's power, such as a child, spouse, or elderly parent. In some cases a victim needs first aid for injuries sustained in an abuse incident. In other cases abuse may become apparent when a victim is being treated for another injury or sudden illness. In still other cases you may encounter a victim of abuse who does not have a present injury requiring first aid. In all situations, and in incidents of sexual abuse or rape, you need to be sensitive to the victim's emotional status and aware of special issues for handling the situation.

Prevention of Abuse

Many individual and cultural factors are involved in the causes of abuse. Tension, anger, and frustration can grow to the point where the person in a rage commits an act of violence. In most cases this leads to a cycle of regret and promises to change, but the cycle repeats as stresses again build and lead to often increasingly violent acts.

What originally causes a person to become an abuser? Many abusers were abused themselves as children or observed abuse in their homes. Some people never develop ways to manage stress and control their feelings. Many different psychological factors are involved in why some people easily lose their temper and become violent. Unfortunately there is no simple way to predict who may become an abuser, and therefore no simple way to prevent abuse from happening the first time. The cycle of repeated abuse, however, can be broken. Laws have become more protective of victims, shelters and hotlines are increasingly available for victims to break away from their abusers, and programs have been developed to help abusers learn to control impulses toward violence. Preventing abuse, therefore, begins with recognizing and acknowledging it when it occurs and understanding that resources are available for both victims and abusers. The following sections on child abuse, domestic violence, elder abuse, and rape include telephone hotline numbers for finding such resources throughout the United States.

Child Abuse

Child abuse and neglect are major problems in our society. Each week, child protective service agencies throughout the United States receive more than 50,000 reports of suspected child abuse or neglect. Every year over 800,000 children are found to have been victims of abuse or neglect. About two-thirds of these children are experiencing neglect, meaning that a caretaker failed to provide for their basic needs. Almost 20% are found to have been physically abused, and about 10% sexually abused. An average of three children die every day as a result of child abuse or neglect.

Any child may be abused. Boys and girls are almost equally likely to experience neglect and physical abuse. Girls are four times more likely to experience sexual abuse. Children of all races and ethnicities and all socioeconomic levels experience child abuse. Children of all ages experience abuse and neglect, but younger children are most vulnerable. Infants under one year old account for nearly one-half of deaths resulting from child abuse and neglect, and about 85% of children who die are younger than six years of age.

Mothers acting alone are responsible for almost half the cases of neglect and about one-third of the cases of physical abuse. Fathers acting alone are responsible for about one-fourth of cases of sexual abuse, and unrelated perpetrators commit about one-third of cases of sexual abuse. In about 80% of cases of sexual abuse, the perpetrator is known by the child. Often sexual abuse occurs in a pattern rather than as a single incident.

Physical Abuse

Physical abuse is physical injury (ranging from minor bruises to severe fractures or death) as a result of punching, beating, kicking, biting, shaking, throwing, stabbing, choking, hitting (with a hand, stick, strap, or other object), burning, or otherwise harming a child. These injuries are considered abuse regardless of whether the caretaker intended to hurt the child. Shaken baby syndrome is an example of usually unintended abuse: a parent or other caretaker, including babysitters, becomes frustrated with a crying infant and shakes the infant, potentially causing severe brain or spinal injury or death.

Following are signs of physical abuse:

The child:

- Has unexplained scalding or burns, rope burns, lacerations, bites, bruises, broken bones, or black eyes
- Has fading bruises or other marks after an absence from school or childcare
- Seems frightened of parents and protests or cries when it is time to go home
- Shrinks at the approach of adults
- Reports being injured by a parent or another adult caregiver
- Appears withdrawn or depressed and cries often—or is aggressive and disruptive
- Seems tired often and complains of frequent nightmares

The parent or other adult caregiver:

- Offers conflicting, unconvincing, or no explanation for the child's injury

- Describes the child with words such as "evil" or other negative terms
- Uses harsh physical discipline with the child
- Is known to have a history of abuse as a child

Sexual Abuse

Sexual abuse includes any kind of sexual activity by a parent or caretaker, such as fondling a child's genitals, penetration, incest, rape, sodomy, indecent exposure, or exploitation through prostitution or the production of pornographic materials. Following are signs of sexual abuse:

The child:

- Has difficulty walking or sitting
- Suddenly refuses to change clothing when necessary or to participate in physical activities
- Reports nightmares or bedwetting
- Experiences a sudden change in appetite
- Demonstrates bizarre, sophisticated, or unusual sexual knowledge or behavior
- Becomes pregnant or contracts a venereal disease, particularly if under age 14
- Runs away from home
- Reports sexual abuse by a parent or other adult caregiver
- Seems afraid of a particular person or of being alone with that person

The parent or other adult caregiver:

- Is unduly protective of the child or severely limits the child's contact with other children, especially those of the opposite sex
- Is secretive and isolated
- Is jealous or controlling with family members

Reporting Child Abuse

Parents or other caregivers who abuse or neglect a child need help. Programs are available in most communities to provide professional help.

You should not, however, try to talk by yourself to suspected abusers in an effort to get them to seek help. Almost always the abuser will deny the problem, and the situation may become worse than if you had said nothing. Instead, the single most important thing you can do, if you suspect a child is being abused or neglected, is to report it to the proper authorities. Your report will help protect the child and get help for the family.

If you care for children as part of your job, you may be legally required to report suspected cases of child abuse or neglect. State laws vary in the specifics of who must make a report and to what agency. If this is required in your job, follow your employer's policy.

The law provides ways for private citizens to report suspected abuse or neglect as well, and it is important for the child's welfare that you do this even if not required to do so. Contact your local child protective services agency or police department. For more information about where and how to file a report, call the Childhelp USA® National Child Abuse Hotline (1-800-4-A-CHILD).

When you call to report child abuse, you will be asked for specific information, which may include:

- The child's name
- The suspected perpetrator's name (if known)
- A description of what you have seen or heard
- The names of any other people having knowledge of the abuse
- Your name and phone number

Your name will not be given to the family of the child you suspect is being abused or neglected. If you are making the report as a private citizen, you may ask to make the report anonymously, but your report may be considered more credible and can be more helpful to the child protective services agency if you give your name. Remember: your suspicion of child abuse or neglect is enough to make a report. You do not have to provide proof. Almost every state has a law to protect people who make good-faith reports of child abuse from prosecution or liability.

Care for an Apparently Abused Child

If you suspect an injured child you are caring for has been abused or neglected, do not confront the parents or ask the child direct questions about abuse. If the child needs first aid for an illness or injury, provide it as you would for any child, following standard guidelines. If you are giving first aid as part of your job, follow your employer's guidelines for documenting the care and any other actions you take. If the child tells you an injury was caused by a parent or other adult, include this information when making your report.

Spouse Abuse

Like child abuse, spouse abuse, or domestic violence, is a major problem in our society:

- 31% of women in the United States report being physically or sexually abused by a husband or boyfriend at some time in their lives.
- Estimates of domestic violence suggest that up to four million women a year are physically abused by their husbands or live-in partners.
- 76% of women who report being physically assaulted or raped were victimized by a current or former husband, cohabiting partner, date, or boyfriend.
- One in five female high school students report being physically or sexually abused by a dating partner.
- Women are five to eight times more likely than men to be victimized by an intimate partner. But men, too, are victims of spouse abuse.

Domestic violence and spouse abuse affect people from all races, nationalities, economic levels, and religions. The three primary types of domestic violence are physical abuse, sexual abuse and rape, and verbal/emotional abuse. Physical abuse may involve hitting, slapping, punching, kicking, choking, biting, and assault with objects.

Many abusive relationships continue for some time without the victim reporting the abuse to authorities. Commonly the victim stays with the abusing spouse or partner for several reasons:

- They love their partner—they only want the abuse to stop.
- They are afraid of their partner.
- They feel guilty and may blame themselves for the violence.
- They often have low self-esteem.
- They are isolated from family and friends.
- They depend emotionally and/or financially on their partner.
- They do not know their rights not to be abused or that help is available.

Care for a Victim of Domestic Violence

It is seldom obvious that a victim's injuries resulted from physical abuse. Because there is often a history of abuse and physical injury, the victim may be experienced in covering up the cause of injuries. Certain signs, however, may raise a suspicion of domestic violence:

- The victim seems unusually fearful.
- The victim's account of the injury seems inconsistent or unlikely.

- The victim is uneasy in the presence of a spouse or partner.
- The victim's spouse or partner aggressively blames the woman for being injured.

If these or other signs of possible domestic violence are present, consider the possibility that the injury resulted from abuse. Follow these guidelines:

1. Provide first aid as usual for the injury. Call 9-1-1 for significant injuries, and tell responding EMS personnel in private about your suspicions; they will know the correct steps to take.
2. Ensure privacy for the victim while providing care.
3. Do not directly confront the victim with your suspicions, especially if the victim's spouse or partner is present.
4. Try to involve a friend or family member of the victim in your caregiving.
5. If you are giving first aid as part of your employment responsibilities, you may be required to report suspected cases of domestic violence to the authorities. Many healthcare workers generally are required by law to report suspected abuse. Check with your supervisor.
6. If the victim communicates information to you that suggests abuse, or if it is appropriate in your relationship with the victim to raise the issue yourself, you may choose to tell the victim that domestic violence is against the law and that help is available.
7. If you see physical abuse occurring or are certain a crime has been committed, or if the victim's partner is threatening and potentially violent, call law enforcement personnel. Withdraw from the scene to ensure your own safety.

Local and state agencies are present in all 50 states to assist victims of domestic violence in many ways. Often help can be provided to the abuser so that the relationship can continue, if that is the wish of both partners. Many support groups are available to help both victims and abusers. Other assistance is available for spouses who choose to end the relationship. Victims should never feel they have no choice but to remain in an abusive relationship.

The National Domestic Violence Hotline can provide information and local contacts for those seeking help: 1-800-799-SAFE (1-800-799-7233) and www.ndvd.org.

Table 22-1

National Estimates of the Incidence of Abuse, Neglect, and Self-Neglect of Persons 60 Years and Older

Type of Maltreatment	Number of Victims
Abuse	402,287
Neglect	182,368
Self-neglect	138,980
Total abuse and neglect	449,924
Total abuse, neglect, and self-neglect	551,011

Source: The National Elder Abuse Incidence Study. The Administration on Aging, U.S. Department of Health and Human Services. 1998.

Elder Abuse

Elder abuse is another common type of domestic violence. Typically **elder abuse** refers to physical, emotional, or financial abuse or neglect inflicted on someone over age 60, often by someone else in the home. Over half a million elders in the United States are abused or neglected each year **(Table 22-1)**.

This problem has become more common as the numbers of the elderly grow and as more elderly people live with, and are often cared for by, family members. In 90% of cases, the abusing person is a family member, usually an adult child or spouse of the victim. Generally, the older a person is, the greater the risk of elder abuse **(Figure 22-3)**. An older adult who needs help with daily activities, who has lost bladder control, or who behaves unusually because of altered mental status is more likely to be abused or neglected.

Because older adults are often more frail, physical abuse is more likely to result in injury. Physical elder abuse is defined as the willful infliction of physical pain or injury, such as slapping, hitting with an object, shoving, shaking, kicking, burning, sexually molesting, force-feeding, administering of unwanted drugs, or restraining the person.

The most important signs of elder maltreatment are:

- Frequent, unexplained crying
- Unexplained fear of or suspicion of particular person(s) in the home

The signs and symptoms of elder abuse are listed in **Box 22-3**.

Care for a Victim of Elder Abuse

If the signs of possible elder abuse are present, consider the possibility that the injury resulted from abuse. Follow the same general guidelines as for a

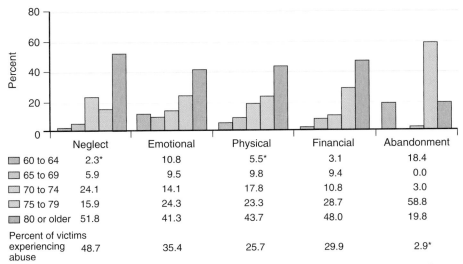

	Neglect	Emotional	Physical	Financial	Abandonment
60 to 64	2.3*	10.8	5.5*	3.1	18.4
65 to 69	5.9	9.5	9.8	9.4	0.0
70 to 74	24.1	14.1	17.8	10.8	3.0
75 to 79	15.9	24.3	23.3	28.7	58.8
80 or older	51.8	41.3	43.7	48.0	19.8
Percent of victims experiencing abuse	48.7	35.4	25.7	29.9	2.9*

Based on estimated 70,556 substantiated incidents of elder abuse. Some entries have missing values.

*The confidence band for these numbers is wide, relative to the size of the estimate. The true number may be close to zero or much larger than the estimate.

Figure 22-3 Ages of elder abuse victims for selected types of maltreatment. (From "The National Elder Abuse Incidence Study," The Administration on Aging, U.S. Department of Health and Human Services, 1998.)

Box 22-3   Signs and Symptoms of Elder Abuse and Neglect

Physical Abuse

- Bruises, black eyes, welts, lacerations, and rope marks
- Bone fractures, skull fractures
- Open wounds, cuts, punctures, untreated injuries, and injuries in various stages of healing
- Strains, dislocations, and internal injuries/bleeding
- Broken eyeglasses, physical signs of being subjected to punishment, and signs of being restrained
- Laboratory findings of medication overdose or under-utilization of prescribed drugs
- An elder's report of being hit, slapped, kicked, or mistreated
- An elder's sudden change in behavior
- A caregiver's refusal to allow visitors to see an elder alone

Sexual Abuse

- Bruises around the breasts or genital area
- Unexplained venereal disease or genital infections
- Unexplained vaginal or anal bleeding
- Torn, stained, or bloody underclothing
- An elder's report of being sexually assaulted or raped

Emotional/Psychological Abuse

- Emotional upset or agitation
- Extreme withdrawal, lack of communication and responsiveness
- An elder's report of being verbally or emotionally mistreated

Neglect

- Dehydration, malnutrition, untreated bedsores, and poor personal hygiene
- Unattended or untreated health problems
- Hazardous or unsafe living conditions (e.g., improper wiring, no heat or no running water)
- Unsanitary or unclean living conditions (e.g., dirt, fleas, lice on person, soiled bedding, fecal/urine smell, inadequate clothing)
- An elder's report of being neglected

Abandonment

- The desertion of an elder at a hospital, nursing facility, or other similar institution
- The desertion of an elder at a shopping center or other public location
- An elder's own report of being abandoned

Self-Neglect

- Dehydration, malnutrition, untreated or improperly attended medical conditions, and poor personal hygiene
- Hazardous or unsafe living conditions (e.g., improper wiring, no indoor plumbing, no heat or no running water)
- Unsanitary or unclean living quarters (e.g., animal/insect infestation, no functioning toilet, fecal/urine smell)
- Inappropriate and/or inadequate clothing, lack of necessary medical aids (e.g., eyeglasses, hearing aid, dentures)
- Grossly inadequate housing or homelessness

From "The National Elder Abuse Incidence Study," The Administration on Aging, U.S. Department of Health and Human Services, 1998.

victim of spouse abuse or other domestic violence. All 50 states have specific elder abuse laws. Suspected elder abuse should be reported to your state's adult protective service agency. As with reports of suspected child abuse, the information you report will be kept confidential. The state agency will investigate the case and will provide services as needed for the elder and family members.

SEXUAL ASSAULT AND RAPE

The following definitions of rape and sexual assault are from the U.S. Department of Justice's annual National Crime Victimization Survey:

Rape is forced sexual intercourse, including both psychological coercion and physical force. Forced sexual intercourse means vaginal, anal, or oral penetration by the offender(s). This category includes incidents where the penetration is from a foreign object such as a bottle. This definition includes attempted rapes, male and female victims, and heterosexual and homosexual rape.

Sexual assault includes a wide range of victimizations, distinct from rape or attempted rape. These crimes include completed or attempted attacks generally involving unwanted sexual contact between the victim and offender. Sexual assaults may or may not involve force and include such things as grabbing or fondling. Sexual assault also includes verbal threats.

In about two-thirds of cases of rape and sexual assault, the victim knows the person who commits the act. Date rape and acquaintance rape are more common than rape by strangers. Rape and sexual assault are serious problems in our society:

- In 2002, there were 247,730 victims of rape, attempted rape, or sexual assault. Of these, about 87,000 were victims of completed rape, 70,000 were victims of attempted rape, and 91,000 were victims of sexual assault.
- Up to 4315 pregnancies may have resulted from these attacks.
- One of every six women in the United States has been the victim of an attempted or completed rape in her lifetime. Over 17 million women have been victims of these crimes.
- In 2002, seven of every eight rape victims were female.
- About 3% of men in the United States—a total of 2.78 million men—have been victims of an attempted or completed rape in their lifetime.

- About 44% of rape victims are under age 18. Three of every 20 victims (15%) are under age 12.

Prevention of Rape and Sexual Assault

To reduce the risk of rape and sexual assault, the Rape, Abuse, and Incest National Network (RAINN) recommends these precautions:

- In a social setting, don't leave your beverage unattended or accept a drink from an open container because the drink may be drugged.
- When you go to a party, go with a group of friends. Arrive together, watch out for each other, and leave together.
- Be aware of your surroundings at all times.
- Don't allow yourself to be isolated with someone you don't know or trust.
- Think about the level of intimacy you want in a relationship, and clearly state your limits.

Care for a Victim of Rape or Sexual Assault

1. Be sensitive to the victim's psychological trauma. After a rape the victim may be hysterical, crying, hyperventilating, or in a dazed, unresponsive state. Provide emotional support as appropriate.
2. Ensure that 9-1-1 has been called. Rape requires a coordinated response of law enforcement and EMS personnel.
3. Ensure privacy for the victim.
4. Try to involve a friend or family member of the victim in your caregiving. A first aider of the same sex may be more comforting.
5. Provide first aid as needed for any injury. Someone should stay with the victim until help arrives.
6. For legal reasons, it is important to preserve evidence of a rape. Ask the victim not to urinate, bathe, or wash any area involved in the rape or assault before EMS personnel arrive.

Follow-up care of rape victims usually includes a full physical examination as well as possible later testing for sexually transmitted diseases and pregnancy.

Because rape can lead to later traumatic stress and psychological problems, victims benefit from counseling provided by rape crisis centers and support groups. To find a center in your area, call the National Sexual Assault Hotline at 1-800-656-HOPE (4673) or visit the RAINN website: www.rainn.org.

Learning
Checkpoint ②

1. If you suspect a child is being abused by a parent, the most important thing to do is
   a. talk to the parent so that he or she can get help.
   b. remove the child from the home.
   c. report the situation to authorities.
   d. talk to the spouse of the abusing parent and let him or her decide what to do.

2. Check off common characteristics of victims of domestic violence.
   ___ They love their partners.
   ___ They are not afraid of their partners.
   ___ They feel guilty and may blame themselves for the violence.
   ___ They often have low self-esteem.
   ___ They feel close to family and friends.
   ___ They depend emotionally and/or financially on their partners.

3. Elder abuse includes
   a. sexual abuse.   c. neglect.
   b. abandonment.   d. All of the above

4. List six important first aid actions for a victim injured in a rape.
   _____

Concluding Thoughts

Behavioral emergencies and abuse situations are generally stressful for first aiders because of the unpredictable behavior and difficult emotions of those involved. Remember that in most cases these situations last only a few minutes before EMS professionals, or sometimes law enforcement personnel, arrive and take over. These professionals have the training to manage the situation safely and appropriately. For the few minutes you may be with a victim, be sensitive to the situation and alert for your own safety. In almost all cases you can use common sense and the general guidelines in this chapter to avoid any confrontation while providing first aid.

Learning Outcomes

You should now be able to do the following:

1. Describe common emotional and behavioral responses to injury and illness.

2. Explain how to reassure and calm an emotional victim.

3. Describe how to interact with a victim who is experiencing anxiety or depression.

4. List actions to take when dealing with a suicidal or potentially violent victim.

5. Describe appropriate care for victims of child abuse, spouse abuse, elder abuse, and sexual assault and rape.

Review Questions

1. Normal physical signs and symptoms of injury-related stress include
   a. dry skin.
   b. nausea.
   c. slow breathing.
   d. drowsiness.

2. Altered mental status may result from any injury that causes
   a. reduced oxygen levels.
   b. increased oxygen levels.
   c. faster heartbeat.
   d. fluid loss.

3. Why is it important to calm and reassure an emotional victim?
   a. Emotional stress has negative physical effects on the body.
   b. It is difficult to give first aid to an emotional, uncooperative victim.
   c. Calming may help prevent a victim from becoming violent.
   d. All of the above

4. True or False: Making eye contact with a victim who is irrational, delusional, or potentially violent will likely upset the person and make the situation worse.
   a. True
   b. False

5. You should try to reassure an injured victim who is depressed by saying things like,
   a. "Don't worry, everything will be just fine."
   b. "Don't cry. Let's talk about more positive things in your life."
   c. "There are programs available to help you deal with problems like this."
   d. "I'm sure this problem won't last long."

6. Call 9-1-1 for
   a. a potentially violent victim of any kind of injury.
   b. someone talking about suicide who has a bottle of pills.
   c. an injured person who is shouting at a hallucination.
   d. All of the above

7. A parent who abuses his or her child, when confronted with an accusation, is most likely to
   a. deny the problem.
   b. admit the problem and feel relief that now he or she will get treatment.
   c. become violent and attack the accuser.
   d. blame his or her spouse for the problem.

8. Which of these statements is true?
   a. Authorities want proof of child abuse before they will take your report.
   b. A reasonable suspicion of child abuse is sufficient grounds to report to the authorities.
   c. After you report suspected child abuse, the authorities will ask you to help them "trap" the abuser to get a confession.
   d. You may be sued for making a report if your accusation turns out to be false.

9. Suspected cases of child abuse or domestic violence should be reported only by
   a. those who have cause to suspect abuse or violence.
   b. those whose jobs require it.
   c. the victims.
   d. family members of the victims.

10. Preserving evidence of a rape includes
   a. asking the victim not to wash until examined by a healthcare provider.
   b. asking the victim to avoid urinating until examined by a healthcare provider.
   c. not allowing the victim to move at all from the position in which he or she was found.
   d. not touching the victim when giving first aid for any injuries.

References and Resources

Childhelp USA® National Child Abuse Hotline 1-800-4-A-CHILD (1-800-422-4453)

National Domestic Violence Hotline 1-800-799-SAFE (1-800-799-7233)

National Sexual Assault Hotline 1-800-656-HOPE (1-800-656-4673)

The Administration on Aging. The National Elder Abuse Incidence Study. U.S. Department of Health and Human Services. 1998; www.aoa.gov 2004.

National Center for Injury Prevention and Control. Suicide fact sheet. 2004. www.cdc.gov

National Clearinghouse on Child Abuse and Neglect Information. U.S. Department of Health and Human Services Administration for Children & Families. 2004. http://nccanch.acf.hhs.gov

National Committee for the Prevention of Elder Abuse. www.preventelderabuse.org

National Domestic Violence Hotline. www.ndvh.org

National SAFE KIDS Campaign 2005. www.safekids.org

National Safety Council. www.nsc.org

National Women's Health Information Center. U.S. Department of Health and Human Services. www.4woman.gov

Rape, Abuse, and Incest National Network (RAINN). www.rainn.org

Stop Abuse for Everyone (SAFE). Resource list. 2004. www.safet4all.org

Chapter 23

Pregnancy and Childbirth

Chapter Preview

- Prevention of Problems in Pregnancy
- Pregnancy and Labor
- First Aid in Pregnancy
- Childbirth

Melanie is almost nine months pregnant with her first baby but still a week away from her due date. You have just trimmed her hair and are blowing it dry when she suddenly gets a funny look on her face and says, "Oh, no!" Then she tells you her "water just broke." What do you do?

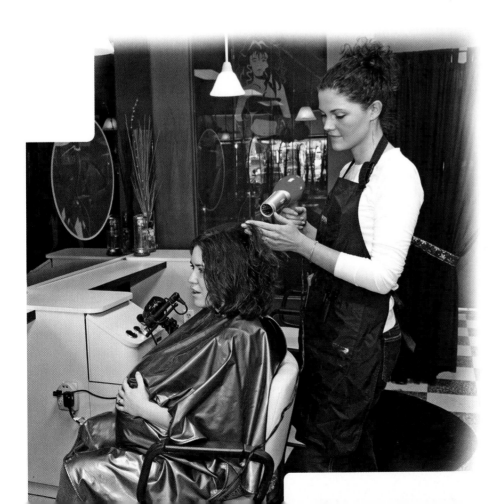

Although rare, certain health problems may occur during pregnancy that require first aid. In addition, childbirth sometimes occurs outside a planned setting. Because no one can predict in every case when labor will begin or how long it will last before the infant is delivered, a pregnant woman may find herself unable to reach the planned setting for childbirth and unattended by a doctor, midwife, or other person trained in childbirth. In such a situation a first aider may be called upon to assist. This is very rarely a medical emergency because childbirth is a normal, natural process that usually takes place without problems or complications—and with only minimal assistance from others.

PREVENTION OF PROBLEMS IN PREGNANCY

Preventing problems in pregnancy and maintaining good health for both the woman and the fetus begins with regular **prenatal** (before birth) care. Healthcare practitioners generally recommend that a woman see her healthcare provider as soon as she knows or suspects that she is pregnant. The healthcare provider thereafter will schedule a series of regular visits to ensure that the pregnancy is progressing well and to treat any complications that may arise.

Following are general guidelines many healthcare practitioners will recommend for pregnant women. *With any guideline, however, always follow the healthcare provider's specific instructions because all guidelines do not automatically apply to all pregnant women.*

- **Eat a healthy diet throughout pregnancy.** Good nutrition is important for both the woman and the developing fetus. A higher-than-usual caloric intake is usually advised along with specific recommendations for balanced nutrition and daily supplements. Most pregnant women are advised to take folic acid (vitamin B) and iron supplements and to ensure that their diet contains sufficient calcium, protein, carbohydrates, fluids, and other vitamins as well as moderate salt.
- **Accept normal weight gain.** Pregnant women should follow their healthcare provider's recommendations, but generally a woman of normal prepregnancy weight should gain 25 to 35 pounds gradually during pregnancy. Attempts to diet or exercise too much in an attempt to prevent weight gain are generally unhealthy for the fetus.
- **Minimize caffeine from coffee, tea, and soft drinks.** Although studies do not clearly show exactly how much caffeine is safe, it has been demonstrated that high levels of caffeine are associated with higher rates of **miscarriage** and can cause other problems for the fetus.
- **Avoid alcohol entirely.** Even very small amounts of alcohol have been shown to affect fetal growth, and higher levels can cause **fetal alcohol syndrome,** which causes growth deficiencies, mental retardation, and other problems.
- **Stop smoking.** Cigarette smoking in pregnancy has been associated with lowered birth weight and preterm delivery.
- **Do not use illicit drugs.** Some studies suggest that marijuana use in pregnancy may have harmful effects on the fetus, and drugs such as crack cocaine are known to have serious detrimental effects.
- **Get exercise.** The American College of Obstetricians and Gynecologists generally recommends 30 minutes of moderate exercise a day for most healthy pregnant women. The healthcare provider can recommend the most effective and safest types of exercise.
- **Get enough rest.** Sufficient sleep is important during pregnancy, as are frequent rest breaks during the day. The healthcare practitioner may also recommend avoidance of certain kinds of activities.
- **Prevent injury.** Avoid situations that may lead to falls, such as climbing a ladder or standing on a chair to reach a high shelf. Get help when needed, such as getting out of a bathtub during the last weeks of pregnancy. Avoid risky sports and recreational activities.

PREGNANCY AND LABOR

Pregnancy begins with fertilization of the woman's ovum, or egg cell, by a sperm cell, in the process often called conception. Growth and development proceed in an orderly manner for about 40 weeks, when childbirth typically occurs. The pregnancy is usually considered in three stages, followed by labor and delivery.

Stages of Pregnancy

Pregnancy is often divided into three trimesters of roughly three months each. Within the first few days, the single cell that results from fertilization divides into a mass of many cells. After it implants in the uterus at five to seven days, and thereafter for the first eight weeks, the developing human is called an **embryo;** thereafter it is called a **fetus.** The embryo develops inside the **amniotic sac,** which contains **amniotic fluid** (often called "water"). The embryo is attached to the woman's **placenta,** an organ that develops in pregnancy to supply the embryo and fetus with oxygen and nutrients, by the **umbilical cord (Figure 23-1).** By eight weeks the embryo has developed all major organ systems. Through the rest of the pregnancy it continues to grow and develop to the point where the infant can live independently outside the mother's body.

During the first trimester, although the fetus has recognizable human features and is about 2½ inches long, the pregnant woman experiences few visible changes. Her heart rate has increased by about eight beats per minute, and she may experience some normal results of hormonal changes in her body, such as nausea (**morning sickness**) and breast tenderness.

During the second trimester, weeks 13 to 28, the fetus grows to a length of 12 inches. At about 18 to 20 weeks the woman may feel it moving. The woman's abdomen gradually swells, and she may experience discharge from the nipples caused by changes in the milk-producing glands.

In the third trimester (weeks 29 to 40), the fetus grows rapidly. By week 36 it is fully formed, weighs about 6½ pounds, and can live outside the mother without advanced medical intervention. The head of the fetus is positioned downward in the woman's pelvis. The woman's uterus has expanded high into the abdomen and presses on the lungs, possibly causing a slight shortness of breath. The pregnant woman may also experience backache, heartburn, constipation, and frequent urination.

Stages of Labor and Delivery

Labor and delivery occur in three stages, beginning with the first uterine contractions. Up to 10 days before the beginning of contractions, the mucous plug from the cervix, which had blocked the uterus from possible infection from the vagina, is released; this is sometimes called "the show" or "bloody show" but is often unnoticed. Uterine contractions begin and eventually push the infant's head into the cervix, which is dilating (opening). The **cervix** is the lower part of the uterus opening into the vagina. Contractions gradually become stronger and more frequent. The amniotic sac ruptures either shortly before or during the first stage of labor, causing the fluid to either rush or trickle out the vaginal opening; this is often called the "water breaking." The first stage may last from a few hours to a day in a woman who has not given birth before, but sometimes occurs in only a few minutes in a woman who has given birth before. Contractions at first are usually 10 to 15 minutes apart, and shortly before childbirth they may be only 2 to 3 minutes apart.

In the second stage the infant is delivered. This stage typically lasts one to two hours but may happen more quickly in women who have given birth previously. The cervix has fully dilated, and contractions are powerful and often painful. The infant's head presses on the floor of the pelvis, and the woman feels a strong urge to push down. The vagina, or birth canal, stretches open as the infant's head moves out of the uterus, and the top of the infant's head can now be seen; this is called **crowning (Figure 23-2).** The vagina stretches more as the head emerges, often quickly, and rest of the infant's body is typically pushed out very quickly

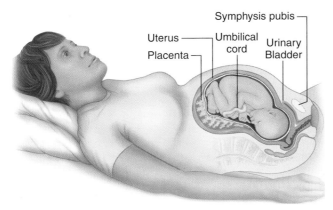

Symphysis pubis

Uterus — Umbilical cord

Placenta — Urinary Bladder

Figure 23-1 The fetus at eight months.

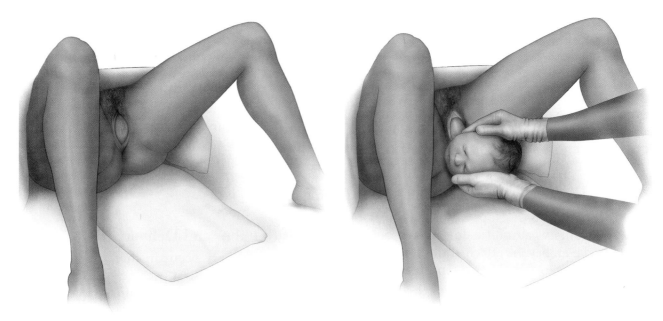

Figure 23-2 Crowning: the infant's head begins to show.

Figure 23-3 The infant moves through the birth canal.

(Figure 23-3). The person assisting with the delivery supports the infant's head as it emerges and ensures that the umbilical cord is not wrapped around the infant's neck.

In the third stage, the placenta separates from the uterus and is delivered, usually within 30 minutes after childbirth. The uterus then contracts and seals off bleeding vessels.

Learning
Checkpoint (1)

1. Put a check mark before the accepted guidelines for a healthy pregnancy:

____ Walk at least a mile a day.   ____ Eliminate salt from the diet.

____ Minimize caffeine and alcohol   ____ Take dietary supplements as
consumption.   recommended.

____ Exercise to prevent weight gain.   ____ Adopt a low-carbohydrate diet.

2. The first stage of labor begins with

a. crowning.   **c.** cervical dilation.

b. uterine contractions.   **d.** rupture of the amniotic sac.

3. Shortly before birth occurs, contractions usually occur

a. every 30 seconds.   **c.** every 5 to 10 minutes.

b. every 2 to 3 minutes.   **d.** irregularly, varying from 1 to 10 minutes.

FIRST AID IN PREGNANCY

Most pregnant women receive regular care and are advised by their healthcare providers about potential problems to watch for. Although rare, problems may occur that require medical care and possibly first aid before the woman receives medical attention.

Vaginal Bleeding

Vaginal bleeding during pregnancy is abnormal. Bleeding may be caused by cervical growths or erosion, by a problem with the placenta, or by miscarriage. In the third trimester, vaginal bleeding may be a sign of potential preterm birth. The woman should see her healthcare provider immediately. Call 9-1-1 for heavy bleeding. While waiting for help, calm the woman and help her into a comfortable position. Have a female assistant present if possible. Give the woman a towel or sanitary napkins to absorb the blood, but do not try to pack the vagina. Save the blood and any expelled material to give to arriving medical personnel.

Miscarriage

Miscarriage, also called spontaneous abortion, is loss of the embryo or fetus, usually during the first 14 weeks of pregnancy. An estimated 20% to 25% of all pregnancies end in miscarriage, which is a natural way that the body manages a potential problem in the pregnancy. It may result from a genetic disorder or fetal abnormality, some factor related to the woman's health, or to no known cause. Smoking and the use of alcohol or drugs are also risk factors. Most women who have a miscarriage do not have problems with later pregnancies.

The early signs of a possible miscarriage are vaginal bleeding and abdominal pain or cramping. The woman needs immediate medical attention. Give first aid for bleeding, and call 9-1-1 if the bleeding is heavy. Take steps to minimize shock if bleeding is heavy (see **Chapter 10**). Because the possibility of miscarriage is usually very distressing, be calm and reassuring.

Other Signs of Possible Problems

Bleeding is one of the most serious problems during pregnancy, but other signs and symptoms may also indicate a problem. The woman should see her healthcare provider if she experiences any of the following:

- **Abdominal pain** may result from miscarriage or a problem with the placenta. The woman should rest until she receives medical advice.
- **Persistent or severe headache,** especially in the last trimester, may be a sign of a serious condition called **toxemia.** Toxemia may also cause unusual weight gain, blurred vision, and swollen fingers or face.

Learning
Checkpoint ②

1. Describe first aid to give a pregnant woman who has heavy vaginal bleeding.

_____

2. The early signs of a possible miscarriage include

   a. vaginal bleeding.   **c.** altered mental status.

   b. high fever.   **d.** All of the above

3. Check off the signs and symptoms that may indicate a possible problem during pregnancy:

   ___ Abdominal pain   ___ Persistent headache

   ___ Chills and fever   ___ Convulsions

   ___ Difficulty breathing   ___ Water leaking from vagina in 20th week

- **Sudden leaking of water from the vagina,** unless the woman is close to the time of labor, may indicate premature rupture of the amniotic sac. The woman should see her healthcare provider.
- **Other serious signs and symptoms include persistent vomiting, chills and fever, convulsions, and difficulty breathing.** All should be reported immediately to the healthcare provider.

Choking Care for Pregnant Woman

Do not use abdominal thrusts on a responsive pregnant woman who is choking. Instead give chest thrusts as described in **Chapter 7**.

CHILDBIRTH

In our society, childbirth has occurred predominantly in hospitals for so long that people may assume it is so difficult or dangerous that hospitals are needed. In reality, childbirth is a natural process that seldom involves complications or requires elaborate medical care. It is true that some complications are possible and that medical steps are then necessary for the health of the mother or infant. But if a woman is unable to reach medical care when contractions suggest childbirth may be imminent, this should not be a cause for panic. *The childbirth itself is not an emergency.* Nonetheless, a pregnant woman who realizes she may have her baby before reaching her planned location, and perhaps without healthcare providers present, is likely to be fearful and distressed. If you are helping the woman and realize that it may be you who helps deliver the infant, you are likely to experience similar emotions. Coping with these stresses may be more difficult than assisting with the childbirth itself.

Remember that once you have called 9-1-1, help is usually only minutes away. It is very unlikely that a woman close to childbirth will actually give birth before advanced care personnel arrive. Remember also that even if help is delayed or her labor advances very quickly to childbirth, in the great majority of cases there are no complications and you will be able to assist her through this process for the short time needed. It is crucial that you remain calm in order to reassure and assist the woman. Although you may be concerned about doing something wrong, try to relax and focus on the woman's need for your calm guidance to help manage her fears and the pain of labor.

Is Delivery Imminent?

Depending on how the woman's labor is progressing and the time before EMS personnel are expected to arrive, you may be assisting the woman only with labor or also with delivery. An important initial step in first aid, therefore, is assessing whether delivery may occur soon.

Remember that labor usually lasts for several hours, allowing plenty of time for the woman to be transported to the hospital or other planned childbirth location or for other assistance to arrive. In rare cases, however, labor may proceed very quickly or transportation may be delayed. Even an expert cannot predict exactly when childbirth will occur, but the following assessments can help determine whether delivery may be imminent. If so, do not try to transport the woman but prepare for childbirth.

- **Assess the contractions.** How close together are they, and how long does each last? Contractions generally become stronger, last longer, and come more frequently as labor progresses. If contractions are less than five minutes apart and each lasts 45 to 60 seconds, delivery may occur soon, and you should be making preparations.
- **Ask the woman if she has given birth before.** First childbirths usually take longer than later ones. If she has given birth in the past, labor is likely to proceed more quickly this time. Also ask if she knows whether she may be having twins or triplets—most women have learned this during their prenatal care.
- **Check whether the amniotic sac has ruptured.** Ask the woman if her water has broken. Since this often occurs hours before delivery, however, it is not a reliable sign that childbirth is imminent.
- **Ask whether the woman feels a strong urge to push.** This may mean delivery is approaching. Similarly, a feeling that she needs to have a bowel movement may indicate the infant's head has moved to a position close to delivery.
- **If other signs are suggestive, check whether the infant's head is crowning.** If possible, ask another woman present to check this. Once the top of the head is visible through the vaginal opening, be prepared for delivery very soon.

Note that labor may begin potentially many weeks before the woman is due, resulting in a premature birth. Since a premature infant is more likely to need medical care after birth, it is important to recognize the first signs of labor at any point in the pregnancy and take appropriate action.

Assisting During Labor

If labor has begun but delivery is not imminent, give supportive care to the expectant mother. Follow these guidelines:

- Ensure that a plan is in place for the woman's transport to the planned childbirth location or for the arrival of the planned attendant.
- Help the woman to rest in whatever position is most comfortable for her.
- Provide any desired comfort measures, such as massaging the lower back (which may help reduce pain). Although the woman should not eat or drink, she may suck on small ice chips or have her lips moistened if her mouth is dry.
- Do not let the woman have a bath if the amniotic sac has ruptured, because of the risk of infection.
- Time the length of contractions and the interval between them, and write this information down.
- Help remind the woman to control her breathing: short, quick breaths (panting) during contractions, and deep, slow breaths between.
- Continue to help the woman to stay calm, and provide reassurance. Anxiety and fear will only add to her pain. Regular, deep breathing in through the nose and out through the mouth may help her to relax. (Using the same technique yourself, in synch along with the woman, may help you to relax, too.)

Assisting with Delivery

If signs are present that delivery may be imminent, prepare to assist with the delivery. Remember that childbirth is a natural process that will occur essentially by itself. Your role is simply to prepare the environment to maintain cleanliness for the mother and child, and to support both during and after the birth.

Preparations

Ensure that someone stays with the woman while preparations are being made. If possible, another woman should be present, preferably a friend or family member.

First, gather the items needed or helpful for the delivery:

- A clean blanket or coverlet
- Several pillows
- A plastic sheet (or shower curtain) or a stack of newspapers
- Clean towels and washcloths
- Sanitary napkins or pads made of clean, folded cloth
- Medical exam gloves (use plastic bags on your hands if gloves are unavailable)
- Plastic bags (for afterbirth and cleanup)
- Bowl of hot water (for washing)
- Empty bowl or bucket (in case of vomiting)
- Clean handkerchief (to wear as face mask)
- Clean, soft towel, sheet, or blanket (to wrap the newborn)
- Bulb syringe if available (to suction infant's nose and mouth), or sterile gauze
- If help may be delayed: clean, strong string, shoelaces, or cloth strips to tie the cord
- If help may be delayed: sharp scissors or knife sterilized in boiling water for five minutes or held over a flame for 30 seconds, to cut the cord

Prepare the birthing bed with clean sheets over a rubber or plastic sheet (or shower curtain or thicknesses of newspaper) to protect the mattress. If a bed is not present, prepare a clean place on the floor or ground, making a padded area of newspapers, clothes, or blankets. Roll up your sleeves, wash your hands thoroughly for five minutes, and put on medical exam gloves. If possible, protect your eyes, mouth, and nose from likely splashes of blood and other fluids; a handkerchief can be tied over your mouth and nose.

When childbirth seems imminent, follow the steps listed in the First Aid: "Assisting with Delivery." If a telephone is available at the scene, have someone call the woman's healthcare provider or 9-1-1 so that additional instructions can be given over the phone during or after the childbirth if necessary.

Care of the Mother After Delivery

After the delivery, continue to support and comfort the mother. Ensure that she is warm and comfortable. She may drink water now and may find it

First Aid   Assisting with Delivery

When You See

- Contractions occurring two to three minutes apart
- The woman feels a strong urge to push
- Crowning of the infant's head

Do This First

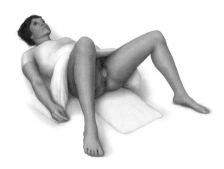

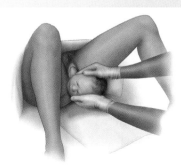

1 Help the woman to lie on her back with knees bent and apart and feet flat on the bed. Note that she may have been trained already in other birthing positions, which are acceptable. Ensure that she is not wearing undergarments or other clothing that may get in the way. If she prefers, cover her above the knees with a blanket or sheet. Have folded towels or a blanket under her buttocks.

2 As the infant's head appears, have your gloved hands ready to receive and support the head, which may emerge very quickly. Check that the head is not covered by the amniotic sac; if so, pull it away as the mouth and nose emerge.

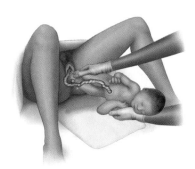

3 As the head emerges (usually face down), support the head. Check that the umbilical cord is not wrapped around the infant's neck; if it is, see if it is loose enough to slip over the head or shoulder to prevent strangulation. Use a bulb syringe to gently suck secretions from the nose and mouth, or wipe both with sterile gauze. Compress the bulb syringe before insertion.

4 After the head is out, have the woman stop pushing and breathe in a panting manner. Support the infant as its body emerges, often very quickly after the head. Usually the infant turns to the side as the shoulder emerges. Newborns are usually very slippery and should be handled carefully. If the mother is having multiple births, prepare for the delivery of the second infant. Note the time of delivery to tell medical personnel later.

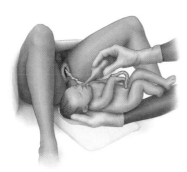

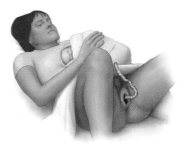

5 The newborn normally begins to cry. Hold it with head lower than the feet for secretions to drain from the nose and mouth. Use a bulb syringe to gently suck secretions from the nose and mouth, or wipe both with sterile gauze. If the infant is not crying, gently flick the bottom of its feet with a finger or gently rub its back. If he or she is still not crying, check for breathing and start CPR if needed (see **Chapter 6**).

6 Gently dry and wrap the infant in a towel or blanket to prevent heat loss, keeping the cord loose. Place the infant on its side with its head low for the nose and mouth to drain. Place the infant on the mother's abdomen only after the umbilical cord has been clampled or tied.

7 Stay with the mother and infant while waiting for the delivery of the afterbirth, the placenta and umbilical cord, which usually occurs with milder contractions in 10 to 30 minutes. Typically there will be a gush of blood as the placenta detaches from the uterus. Save the placenta in a plastic bag or towel because it is important for healthcare providers to examine it.

8 In most situations it is not necessary to tie or cut the umbilical cord, even after the placenta has been delivered, because medical help will be arriving very soon. If help may be delayed in a remote location, tie and cut the cord before delivery of the afterbirth. Wait until the cord stops pulsating. Then tie a tight knot around the cord about ten inches from the infant, using string, clean shoelaces, or thin strips of cloth. Tie a second knot about seven inches from the infant, and cut the cord between the two ties with sterilized scissors or knife.

First Aid   **Assisting with Delivery** *(continued)*

ALERT

- Do not try to delay the birth by having the woman hold her legs together or any other maneuver.
- Do not place your hands or anything else in the woman's vagina.
- Do not interfere with the childbirth or touch the infant until the head is completely out.
- Do not pull on the head or shoulders.
- Do not try to wash the infant's skin, eyes, or ears.
- Do not pull on the umbilical cord in an effort to pull out the afterbirth.

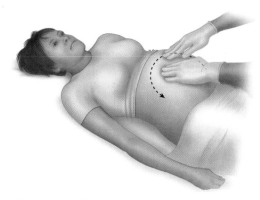

Additional Care

- The mother may continue to bleed for a time, normally up to a pint following delivery. Place sanitary napkins or folded clean cloths against the vaginal opening but do not push. Gently massage the mother's abdomen just below the navel to help the uterus contract to stop the bleeding.
- Ensure that the infant stays warm and continues to breathe. Skin-to-skin contact between mother and infant helps the infant to stay warm. The mother can begin nursing the infant immediately, which will help the uterus to contract and stop bleeding.

comforting to have her face wiped with cool water. Even with a successful delivery, she and the infant should still see a healthcare provider because problems sometimes occur within the first 24 hours.

Care of the Newborn

Once you are assured that the newborn is breathing well, little specific care is needed. Dry but do not try to wash the newborn, whose skin may be covered with a protective, white, cheesy coating called vernix. Ensure that the infant stays wrapped, including the head, to stay warm. Support the newborn's head if it must be moved for any reason. Continue to check the newborn's breathing.

A very small or premature infant born a significant time before the mother's due date is at greater risk for complications after birth. It is crucial to keep a small newborn warm. There is also a greater likelihood that resuscitation may be needed.

Childbirth Problems

Most deliveries occur without problems or complications, but you should be prepared to manage a problem if one does occur. The most common problems involve the **presentation** of the infant (its position at emergence) or maternal bleeding after delivery.

Breech Birth

A **breech presentation** occurs when the infant's buttocks or feet appear in the birth canal rather than the head (**Figure 23-4**). This can become an emergency because as the head enters the birth canal, the umbilical cord is squeezed and blood flow may stop. Also, if the infant's head becomes lodged in the birth canal and the infant tries to breathe, it may suffocate because the face is pressed against the vaginal wall. Medical attention may be urgently needed.

When you first see a breech presentation, move the woman to a kneeling position with her head and chest down (**Figure 23-5**). This helps to minimize pressure on the cord and is generally the preferred childbirth position in this situation. Support the infant's body as it emerges, but do not try to pull the head out, which may cause injury and will not speed up the birth. If the head does not emerge soon after the body, you may need to open a breathing space for the infant. Carefully insert one hand alongside the infant's head, palm against the face, and make a V with two fingers positioned on each side of the infant's

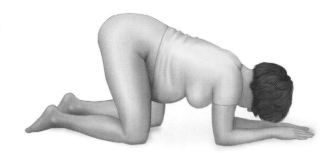

Figure 23-5 Position for breech presentation.

nose. Press against the birth canal to allow air to reach the infant's nose while waiting for the head to be delivered. Check the infant immediately and be prepared to give CPR if needed.

Limb Presentation

Very rarely one arm or leg may emerge first from the birth canal. This is an emergency requiring immediate medical assistance. Position the woman in the same knee-chest position as for a breech birth while waiting for help. Do not try to pull the infant out or push the arm or leg back inside the woman.

Prolapsed Cord

The umbilical cord is said to be **prolapsed** when a segment of it protrudes through the birth canal before childbirth (**Figure 23-6**). This is an emergency because the cord will be compressed as the infant begins to move through the birth canal, cutting off blood flow. Position the woman in the knee-chest position to reduce pressure on the cord. Do not try to push the cord back inside the mother. If medical personnel have not arrived when the infant

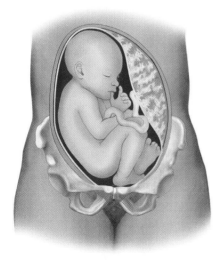

Figure 23-4 Breech presentation.

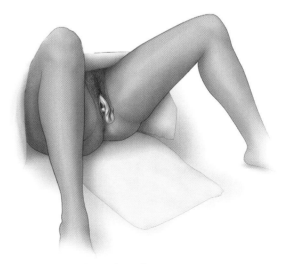

Figure 23-6 Prolapsed cord.

presents and begins to emerge, carefully insert your hand into the birth canal and try to separate the cord and presenting part while allowing the birth to continue. Check the infant immediately and be prepared to give CPR if needed.

Cord Around Neck

If the umbilical cord is wrapped around the infant's neck when the head emerges, you can slip it over the head or shoulder to allow the infant to emerge without strangling on the cord. Rarely, it may be wrapped so tight that you cannot release the infant's head and the cord is strangling the infant and preventing emergence of the body. This is a life-threatening emergency. If medical personnel are not present, you must tie off the cord in two places and cut the cord between the two.

Bleeding After Delivery

It is normal for bleeding to occur with childbirth and with delivery of the placenta. Use sanitary pads or clean, folded cloths to absorb the blood. Usually bleeding stops soon after the placenta is delivered. As described earlier, massage the mother's abdomen below the level of the navel, where you should feel the uterus as a mass about the size of a softball. Massage with your palms using a kneading motion.

Bleeding that persists can become an emergency. Keep the mother still and try to calm her while waiting for help to arrive. Give first aid to minimize shock (see **Chapter 10**).

Learning Checkpoint ③

1. True or False: Childbirth is a difficult process that frequently involves complications and the need for medical treatment.

2. Put a check mark next to signs and symptoms that childbirth may occur soon:

   ___ Contractions every 10 minutes   ___ Woman feels urge to push

   ___ Amniotic sac has ruptured   ___ Infant's head is crowning

   ___ Cervix is starting to dilate   ___ Contractions are painful

3. Assisting a woman with childbirth may include

   a. helping position the woman.

   b. supporting the infant as it emerges from the birth canal.

   c. helping secretions drain from the infant's nose and mouth.

   d. All of the above

4. List at least three things you should *not* do when assisting with childbirth.

   _____

5. When the umbilical cord can be seen protruding from the birth canal before childbirth occurs, what should you do?

   a. Cut the cord and wait for childbirth.

   b. Push the cord back inside the mother.

   c. Position the mother to reduce pressure on the cord.

   d. Pull on the cord to speed up the birth.

6. True or False: Some bleeding normally occurs with childbirth and delivery of the placenta.

Concluding Thoughts

Although problems sometimes do occur during childbirth, and in such cases it is important to know what to do, remember that the overwhelming majority of births occur naturally and without problems, even when outside healthcare settings. Countless numbers of healthy infants have been born in taxis caught in traffic en route to hospitals, and other similar places. Should you ever find yourself in such a situation, stay calm and remember the simple basics of supporting the mother and newborn through this natural process.

Learning Outcomes

You should now be able to do the following:

1. List healthy behaviors during pregnancy to prevent problems for the woman and fetus.

2. Describe the stages of pregnancy and the stages of labor and delivery.

3. Explain the first aid to give for vaginal bleeding during pregnancy and for possible miscarriage.

4. Describe how to assist during childbirth and care for the mother and newborn after the birth.

5. Explain actions to take in case of complications: breech presentation, prolapsed cord, the cord wrapped around the infant's head, and bleeding after delivery.

Review Questions

1. During pregnancy a woman should avoid or minimize the consumption of
   a. unsaturated fats.
   b. alcohol.
   c. artificial sweeteners.
   d. beta carotene.

2. Which sign or symptom is abnormal during pregnancy?
   a. Backache
   b. Vaginal bleeding
   c. Heartburn
   d. More frequent urination

3. When the amniotic sac ruptures after contractions begin, which of these statements is true?
   a. Childbirth may occur soon.
   b. The infant must be delivered immediately before suffocation occurs.
   c. The infant's lungs are likely to become infected if childbirth does not occur soon.
   d. The mother needs care to prevent dehydration.

4. Crowning occurs
   a. in breech presentations.
   b. when the cord is prolapsed.
   c. when the woman pushes too hard before the delivery begins.
   d. in all normal head-first births.

5. First aid for a pregnant woman with vaginal bleeding includes
   a. massaging the abdomen with a kneading motion.
   b. packing the vagina with a pad made from sterile dressings.
   c. absorbing the blood with a towel or sanitary napkin.
   d. controlling the bleeding with direct pressure on the abdomen.

6. A pregnant woman should see her healthcare provider for which of these signs and symptoms?
   a. Severe headache
   b. Difficulty breathing
   c. Abdominal pain
   d. All of the above

7. Choking care for a pregnant woman includes
   a. abdominal thrusts.
   b. chest thrusts.
   c. back blows.
   d. abdominal thrusts and back blows.

8. During labor you can support the woman by
   a. urging her to push with each contraction.
   b. massaging her uterus.
   c. helping her to control her breathing.
   d. holding an ice pack against her abdomen.

9. If the newborn is not crying or breathing after birth,
   a. start care for an airway obstruction.
   b. blow air into his or her mouth using the bulb syringe.
   c. flick the bottom of his or her feet with your finger.
   d. give back blows.

10. Care of the newborn includes
    a. supporting the head when holding or moving the newborn.
    b. keeping the newborn warm.
    c. monitoring the newborn's breathing.
    d. All of the above

References and Resources

American College of Obstetricians and Gynecologists. www.acog.org

Mistovich JJ. *Prehospital emergency care.* 7th ed. Upper Saddle River, New Jersey: Pearson Prentice Hall; 2004.

National Safety Council. www.nsc.org

Chapter 24

Remote Location First Aid

Chapter Preview

- Remote Locations
- Situations When Help May Be Delayed
- General Principles When Help Is Delayed
- Special Care for Emergencies When Help Is Delayed
- Special Wilderness Emergencies

You are on a hike with several friends and family members. About 5 miles along the trail you stopped for lunch beside a river, where a friend's daughter is climbing on rocks at the water's edge. Her foot slips on a mossy patch, and she falls and strikes her head on a rock. Immediately an adult in the party helps her away from the water. Her head did not go under water, but she has a welt on her forehead and she seems groggy and mildly confused. A few minutes later she seems better, although she has a slight headache. You allow her to rest, but now you face the decision whether it is safe for her to hike back out. Unfortunately you have no means to call for help, and the terrain is too steep and rough to consider carrying her out. What should you do?

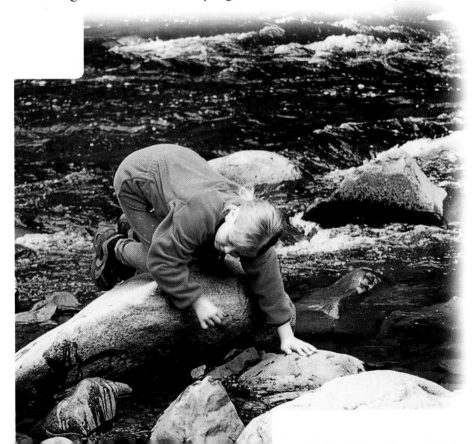

The principles of first aid described earlier in this text are based on the fact that in most locations in the United States medical help will arrive in 10 to 20 minutes after a call is made to 9-1-1 or the local emergency number. That means that the care first aiders give in emergencies is intended primarily to meet *short-term* goals until advanced medical personnel arrive and take over. In remote locations, however, advanced medical care may not be available for many hours or longer. In such situations you should be prepared to give additional care and, when necessary, to make decisions regarding evacuating and transporting the victim, going for help, and preparing to assist in special rescues.

REMOTE LOCATIONS

Being prepared for the possibility of injury or illness in a remote location is crucial. It is important to plan ahead to prevent emergencies from occurring, to be able to communicate the need for help, to have additional first aid supplies when needed, and to know how to care for a victim with common injuries and illness when more advanced medical help may be delayed. First aiders should also be prepared to manage certain types of emergencies that are more likely in remote locations, often involving extreme environmental conditions such as cold or heat or other special circumstances.

The specific issues involved in seeking medical care and caring for the victim depend on the setting where the emergency occurs, but the same general principles apply in most situations. This chapter cannot detail all procedures to follow in every possible emergency, since so many different variables are involved. For example, if a hiker in the mountains breaks his leg 20 miles from the nearest road and his only companion discovers his cell phone has no signal, the situation is different from that of an electrical power line worker who falls and breaks his leg on a rural road 40 miles from the nearest town with his partner nearby. First aiders who live, work, or engage in recreational activities in remote areas should take a special remote location or wilderness first aid course and prepare for the situations in which they may find themselves.

This chapter focuses on how general principles of first aid may need to be modified when help is delayed and on other issues first aiders face in remote locations.

SITUATIONS WHEN HELP MAY BE DELAYED

Rural Areas

Rural areas include open countryside, isolated farms and ranches, and even some very small towns at a distance from medical services. The primary issue is usually only the length of time before help arrives, since roads and telephones are typically present. Any type of emergency may occur, although those working with certain types of farm equipment or in other specialized activities may face special risks. Injury prevention is especially important because an injury that may be more easily cared for in an urban area where help can be expected to arrive within minutes may become life threatening if it takes an hour or more for help to arrive.

Hiking, Camping, Boating

Millions of people enjoy a wide range of recreational activities in natural settings far from roads, land-line telephones, and shelter. If an emergency occurs in such a wilderness area, you may not be able to contact EMS immediately, and rescue vehicles may not be able to reach the victim. In addition to providing first aid for what may be an extended time, you may need to decide how best to shelter the victim from harsh weather and whether to send someone for help or to evacuate the victim. Again, being prepared for emergencies is crucial, but psychological and emotional issues may also become important.

Emergencies that occur when boating on remote lakes and rivers present issues similar to hiking and camping emergencies. Transportation and communication problems are likely. Boating in the ocean offshore or in remote coastal areas often involves different communication and rescue issues, generally involving the Coast Guard in addition to land-based EMS agencies. Like others entering remote areas, boaters need to think and plan ahead for possible emergencies and carry the appropriate first aid, communication, and signaling equipment.

Learning Checkpoint ①

1. Name at least three different emergency situations in which rescue and medical help may be delayed.

_____

2. Being prepared for emergencies in remote locations includes

   a. knowing how to give first aid for an extended period.

   b. planning how to contact EMS if needed.

   c. having appropriate first aid supplies at hand.

   d. All of the above

Natural and Other Disasters

Those who live in areas that are prone to natural disasters such as hurricanes or earthquakes are generally aware of the need to be prepared. But other types of natural disasters can strike many other places, such as wildfires, floods, tornadoes, and unanticipated ice storms that may close roads and cut off electricity for days. Since many natural disasters cause widespread damage and injuries, even if a hospital is not far away you may need to provide first aid in an emergency when help will be delayed. Widespread injuries may stretch emergency resources thin, increasing the time before a victim receives care. An airliner crash, industrial explosion, or terrorist act may have similar effects (see **Chapter 26**).

GENERAL PRINCIPLES WHEN HELP IS DELAYED

Preventing injury and illness when help may be delayed is especially important. This book has emphasized specific actions and guidelines for prevention, and all of these apply in remote locations. Those who live or work in rural areas, and those entering remote locations for recreational or other purposes, should be thinking about safety issues at all times because of the risk that serious problems may develop if EMS cannot respond within minutes.

Regardless of the specific rural or remote location, five general principles apply whenever medical help may be delayed:

1. Be prepared for the situation. Plan for emergencies, and have the right equipment and supplies.
2. Understand the psychological and emotional issues involved in a remote location emergency, and be prepared to use leadership skills.
3. Know how to contact EMS or call for help by alternative means, or know how to use distress signals.
4. Know how to decide when to send someone for help versus evacuating the victim.
5. Know how to protect the victim until help arrives.

The following sections discuss these principles as they apply in different situations.

Being Prepared for the Situation

Like those who live or work in rural or remote locations, those planning a trip to remote locations should be prepared for emergencies. What will you do if someone in your group is injured and you are unable to telephone for help? Will you have the right equipment and supplies with you? Anticipating problems not only can help you to prevent them but can also help to ensure that you are ready to act if they do occur.

Being prepared involves several guidelines that should be followed in all situations, as well as making specific preparations for the location.

1. **Do not enter remote locations alone.** All wilderness agencies and experts advise against this. Even a simple injury, such as a sprained ankle that

prevents walking, can become life threatening if you are unable to reach help. Do not assume your cell telephone will bring help instantly. You may not have a signal, or rescuers may not be able to find you or reach you in time. Even a small wound can bleed severely, for example, and if you are unresponsive or unable to stop the bleeding, you may go into shock rapidly and die before help arrives. Ideally, go in a group of three or more; if there are only two of you and one is injured, no one is left to help the injured person if the other has to go for help.

2. **Tell someone where you are going and when you plan to return.** If an emergency does happen and you are unable to call for help, your contact person should be able to send help to you if you do not return as scheduled.

3. **Take a first aid kit equipped for possible emergencies you may face. Chapter 1** describes a general first aid kit. If you anticipate other types of injuries or illness because of the location you are entering, you should include additional items in your kit, including survival supplies and signaling devices.

4. **Take more food and water than you expect to need.** Any kind of emergency may delay your return, and running out of food or water would only worsen the situation. Although most people can survive a long time without food, becoming weak with hunger complicates the emergency. Anyone can rapidly become dehydrated without adequate water intake, and this can become an emergency within hours depending on the environment and the person's health status. Severe fluid loss caused by the injury, vomiting, diarrhea, excessive sweating, or other conditions is a medical emergency.

5. **Expect weather emergencies.** Take extra clothing and some means to stay dry. Remember that being wet greatly increases heat loss from the body, making hypothermia a risk even at temperatures you do not consider "cold."

6. **Know where you are at all times.** Take a map along and know where you are on it. A **GPS**, a handheld location device using the satellite-based global positioning system, can show you where you are on a topographical map or water chart. If you can call for help in an emergency, you will need to be able to tell rescuers exactly where you are.

7. **Do not use alcohol or other drugs.** Alcohol and other drugs affect your physical perfor-

mance and judgment, increasing the risk of injury and other emergencies.

8. **Study the location.** Be sure you are not trying to do something beyond your physical abilities. Becoming fatigued puts you at a greater risk for injury. Learn the conditions of the trail, find out whether any dangerous animals may be present, and so on. Talk to local recreational groups, park rangers, the Coast Guard, or other appropriate agencies.

In addition to these general principles, being prepared involves trip planning and having the right equipment and supplies, as described in the next sections.

Trip Planning

Trip planning begins with the eight general principles described in the previous section. Following are additional suggestions that depend on the specific locale.

1. Ensure that you are in good physical condition for the trip.
2. Choose the equipment you need for the setting.
3. Plan an appropriate menu with enough nutritious foods.
4. Learn the specifics of the area you plan to enter, including weather, presence of water, fire history and conditions, etc.
5. Obtain maps and guidebooks for the route you plan to take.
6. Refresh your first aid and CPR skills, if needed.
7. Plan for communications needs.

The Essential Equipment

The Wilderness Medical Society recommends a list of "10 Essentials for Outdoor Adventures." For those traveling through very isolated areas, these items should also be kept in your vehicle.

1. Map and compass
2. Flashlight, extra batteries and bulb
3. Extra clothing including hat, gloves, rain gear
4. Sunglasses
5. Extra food and water
6. Waterproof matches in sealed container
7. Candle or fire-starter
8. Knife
9. First aid kit
10. Space blanket

Additional items that may prove useful when driving through isolated areas, especially in temperature extremes:

- Emergency flares or bright orange help sign
- Sleeping bag
- Cell phone or CB radio
- Extra engine oil
- Toolkit
- Jumper cables
- Tire chains
- Shovel
- Sand (for tire traction)
- Deicer for fuel line

Remote Location First Aid Kit

If an emergency occurs in a remote location, despite the best planning and having all the appropriate equipment, the single most important item may be your first aid kit. In addition to the items listed in **Chapter 1** for a standard first aid kit, a kit carried into remote locations should have the items listed in **Box 24-1**. These should be kept also in rural location first aid kits.

Water Disinfection

Always take more water than you anticipate needing in a remote location. If you are a long distance from help or in an emergency where you may have to wait for some time, you may still run out of water. You should be prepared to disinfect the water found in your location. Surface water is often contaminated with bacteria, viruses, or protozoa that may cause serious or life-threatening illness.

The three most common methods of disinfecting water for drinking are boiling, filtering, and treating with chemicals. Boiling water effectively kills bacteria, viruses, and protozoa and is often the best solution, but boiling is not always possible or practical. Many different filters are now sold in camping and specialty stores for filtering surface water. Most remove bacteria and protozoa from water but do not remove viruses. Viruses are generally rare in water that is found in wilderness areas.

Several different chemical treatments are available for disinfecting water, commonly using iodine or chlorine in tablet or liquid form. Both are generally effective for killing bacteria, viruses, and some protozoa. These products must be used as directed. Before planning to use any product to obtain drinking water, it is best to learn about the characteristics of the surface water you are likely to find where you are going (**Figure 24-1**).

In an emergency, if you have no method of disinfecting water, a difficult decision may have to be

Box 24-1 First Aid Kit for Remote Locations

- First aid book
- Pain medication/anti-inflammatory
- Antihistamine
- Laxative
- Antidiarrhea tablets
- Safety pins
- Calamine lotion
- Oral decongestant
- Eye drops
- Motion sickness/antinausea medication
- Antifungal cream
- Antacid tablets
- Oral rehydration solution (especially for small children)
- Hemorrhoid treatment

- Moleskin or Spenco® 2nd Skin® (for burns or open blisters)
- Oral hypothermia thermometer (to 85° F)
- Oil of cloves or other product for dental pain
- Temporary dental filling kit
- Throat lozenges
- Sunscreen and lip protection
- Sunburn lotion (aloe vera)
- Insect repellent
- SAM® splint
- Penlight
- Irrigation syringe
- Water purification tablets
- Sports drink containing sodium for endurance activities

Prescription Medications in Remote Location First Aid

Experts debate whether first aiders should have prescription medications for use in remote locations. One side argues that when medical help may be one or several days away, prescription medications such as a narcotic pain medication or systemic antibiotics have great value for a victim's health and well-being, and may even save a life. A responsible adult can be instructed in the safe use of certain prescription medications and trusted not to misuse or abuse them. On the other side, others argue that the situations in which such medications are genuinely needed are rare and do not justify the potential for misuse or abuse.

Those planning long trips to remote locations that involve activities that put them at risk for medical emergencies are advised to talk with their healthcare provider about this issue. Medications that have been prescribed in such situations include cardiac emergency medications, pain medications, antibiotics, treatments for gastrointestinal infections, allergic reaction medications, and others. When such prescribed medications are added to the first aid kit for remote locations, care must be taken to ensure that they are used only as directed and only in controlled circumstances.

made between the risk of drinking untreated water and the risk of dehydration. Certainly it is better to be prepared and to have a disinfecting method along with other supplies and first aid items.

Psychological Issues

Emergencies are always stressful, and in remote locations mental and emotional issues can become much more significant. The victim may not receive advanced care for many hours or days, and many decisions may be required about how best to care

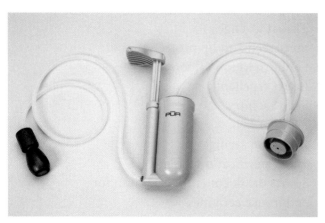

Figure 24-1 Commercially available water purification kit and filter.

for the victim, whether to attempt **evacuation** or wait for help, how to provide shelter, and so on. An outdoor environment often adds further stresses, such as coping with weather, temperature extremes, shortages of food or water, and other problems and uncertainties. The victim or other members of the party may not be able to cope with such stresses and may experience panic attacks, depression, denial, emotional shock, or other problems that worsen the situation. In a worst-case scenario, just when cool heads and clear thinking are needed to address the emergency and first aid needs, there is a risk of the situation deteriorating because of panic, fear, confusion, or indecision. Experts in wilderness survival and crisis management emphasize the importance of mental preparedness and leadership skills to be ready to act effectively in an emergency.

Mental Preparedness

Being mentally prepared for an emergency in a remote location begins with first aid training and learning how best to provide care when help will be delayed. Self-confidence is important, but so is a realistic attitude about what you can and cannot do. With a life-threatening injury or illness far from help, you may need to accept that you do not have the tools needed to give the victim all the help he or she needs. Yet it is equally important not to give up hope and fail to take actions that may help a victim.

Six aspects of mental preparedness are important for wilderness survival situations. They apply as well in many other emergency situations.

1. Stay confident and remember your training.
2. Do not deny the seriousness of the situation, but calmly think through what you need to do.
3. Consider all your equipment and supplies as well as human resources. Be creative and improvise as necessary.
4. Stay focused on the goal and not on the hardships of the situation. Help others in the group to stay calm and act productively.
5. Remain positive but realistic.
6. Keep the faith—in yourself, and in your spiritual beliefs.

Staying calm can be difficult in an emergency but is one of the most important actions one can take. If necessary, take time to control your own stress before beginning to act. Breathe deeply and slowly and try to relax. Help others to control their fears also in order to prevent panic, and then use your leadership skills to develop and carry out a plan.

Leadership Skills

Whenever two or more people are with a victim in an emergency, someone needs to be in charge. Often one person has more experience or training and naturally assumes leadership. In other situations, such as a group of friends going on a week-long backpacking trip, the group should discuss this before the trip begins. Who is packing the first aid kit? Who has thought about emergency communications? Advance conversations about emergency preparedness often lead naturally to consensus about who should take charge.

The most important leadership skill involves mental preparedness. Be confident and calm, and help others to focus on the goal. Other leadership strategies include calmly talking through all actions with other members of the group and asking for suggestions when appropriate. Remember that you are caring not only for the victim but for other group members. Avoid rushing into decisions. The Outdoor Action Program of Princeton University describes five leadership steps when responding in an emergency:

1. Assess the situation and the victim's needs.
2. Make a plan for first aid and other needs related to rescue or obtaining medical care.
3. Delegate responsibilities to others for victim

care, building shelter, handling communication or distress signals, and so on.
4. Initiate first aid care, set up camp, and carry out other needed actions. Everyone in the group should participate in some useful way.
5. Continually reassess the situation and change the plan as needed. Always maintain the focus on the overall goal of getting the victim to medical care.

Remember, hours or days may pass before the victim receives advanced help. During this period many decisions may be required, and emotional difficulties are likely. An effective leader needs to be aware of the needs of the whole group and must work to keep up morale and prevent panic.

Calling for Help

In any emergency, one of the highest priorities is to call for help. With serious injuries or illness, medical care is needed beyond first aid. In remote locations or wilderness areas it may be more difficult to contact EMS, but with advanced planning and the appropriate equipment, help can be summoned in most situations. Communication options include cellular or satellite telephones, radios, and emergency rescue beacons.

Cell Phones

Some hikers and other users of wilderness areas refuse to carry a cell phone, preferring to "get away from it all." Others take their cell phones along and assume they can simply call for help if they get lost or have any problems. Many forest rangers and park officials have received calls from hikers who were tired and lost and who expected instant help even though they had no idea where they were.

Between these two extremes, cell phones obviously have value in emergencies, although because of their limitations no one should depend entirely on a cell phone in an emergency. Cell phones are relatively fragile devices that may stop working due to temperature extremes, moisture, physical shocks, or simply a dead battery. Many remote areas lack a signal. Follow these guidelines for using a cell phone in a remote area:

- Protect the phone from extreme cold, moisture, and shocks.
- Pack the phone in a way that it cannot accidentally turn on and discharge the battery.
- Ensure that the battery is strong by saving the phone for emergency use.
- If you need the phone in an emergency and do

not have a signal, try to get to a higher location such as a ridge top; even climbing a tree may help. Point the antenna upward, and move the phone around your body, as even your own body can block a weak signal. Switch the phone from digital to analog, if you have this choice.

- Be sure you know where you are before making the call. Inexpensive handheld GPS units can provide exact longitude and latitude coordinates for rescuers.

Satellite Phones

Although still relatively expensive, satellite telephones are now available for communication anywhere in the world and can be rented for special trips to very remote locations. Their use is similar to using cell phones, but signal strength is not usually an issue.

Radios

Different types of radios are available for various specialized or general uses (**Figure 24-2**). In some areas, a handheld citizen's band (CB) radio may be able to reach authorities or other CB users, although cell phones have led to the declining use of CBs. Channel 9 is the emergency frequency for calling for help.

The new **family radio service (FRS)** is a citizen's band frequency used by relatively new, inexpensive handheld radios. Even in the best conditions, however, these radios generally transmit less than three miles, giving them limited use in remote locations. In areas where numbers of people are likely to be close by, however, such as ski areas, FRS radios may allow contact with others for help. They may also be useful for staying in touch when members of a group split up.

Amateur (ham) radio is another option. Portable units generally reach a significantly wider area, and more people are likely to monitor common frequencies. An FCC license is required to use ham equipment, which is also generally more expensive.

VHF radios are used on boats. Because of the lack of signal obstructions on the water, VHF (very high frequency) radios can cover up to 30 miles. Most U.S. coastal areas have coverage by Coast Guard towers. The Coast Guard monitors channel 16 and can send a rescue ship or helicopter in an emergency. Although less powerful, handheld units used in smaller watercraft have enough power to summon help from the Coast Guard or other boaters in the vicinity. Larger boats often use single sideband (SSB) radio. These units use a frequency that travels greater distances beyond coastal areas.

Rescue Beacons

Emergency beacons send out a signal that is picked up by an international system of satellites. All commercial and most civil airplanes carry these beacons, known as emergency locator transmitters (ELTs), which automatically send out a signal if the aircraft crashes or has an emergency landing.

Using the same system, marine rescue beacons called **emergency position indicating radio beacons (EPIRBs)** are available for boats that leave coastal areas and cannot depend on radio transmission in an emergency. Some units are manually operated, while others automatically begin sending rescue signals upon being immersed if the boat capsizes.

In 2003 the FCC authorized the use of **personal locator beacons (PLBs).** Hikers and other wilderness users now have the same ability to summon help from any remote location. As these units become more popular, they will become more widely available and inexpensive.

All types of rescue beacons are one-way communication devices: they function only to send an emergency signal that is received by satellites. Only the device's location is communicated. No information can be sent about the nature of the emergency, nor can the user know for certain that the signal is being received. Rescue beacons must be used only in a true emergency requiring rescue. In addition, users must register beacons, each of which sends out a unique signal, to help rescuers determine if an emergency has occurred when a signal is received. In 2003, of the over 50 activations of PLBs in the lower 48 states, none was for a valid emergency, most having been activated by accident. Nonetheless, satellite beacons have already led to the rescue

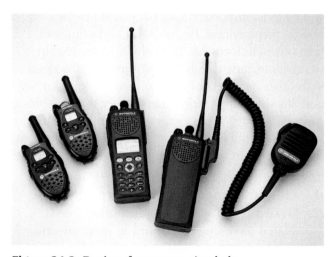

Figure 24-2 Devices for summoning help.

of over 17,000 people worldwide, including almost 5000 rescues in the United States.

Distress Signals

If help cannot be summoned by telephone, radio, or other means when rescue is required, distress signals may be used to catch the attention of passing aircraft. Following are recognized distress signals for different situations:

- At night, build three small campfires in a triangle up to 100 feet apart. Three flares can also be used, or series of three flashes from a flashlight.
- In the daytime, make a large campfire and put green branches or leaves on it to create smoke. Do this in a clearing or on a hilltop. A standard signal is to create three puffs of smoke in a row by covering and uncovering a campfire by any means available.
- Make a large X of markings in the snow or on clear ground. Green branches or bright clothing may be used. Use any material available that will contrast with the ground.
- If a passing aircraft is close enough to see you, raise both (not just one) arms above your head.
- If you have a firearm, fire three shots in a row, or try three whistle blasts.
- In sunlight, use a signal mirror to flash light at a passing aircraft. The reflected beam can be aimed at the aircraft by sighting the beam past a nearby object or your own hand (**Figure 24-3**). If you do not have a mirror, use any shiny object such as the lid from a can or a piece of glass with mud coating the back side.

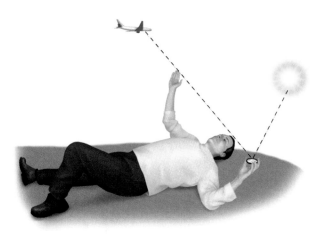

Figure 24-3 To send a distress signal to an aircraft, aim the mirror's reflected sunlight past your fingers or a stationary object.

Many commercial distress signals are available, including such things as flares and aerial flare guns, strobe lights, signal flags and banners, and orange smoke signals.

Sending Someone for Help

In a situation in which an injured or ill victim cannot easily be transported to medical care and it is impossible to call for help, one or more people may need to go for help while others remain with the victim. Difficult decisions are involved, particularly in small groups with only one leader experienced in the area. Should that person be the one to go for help, if he or she may get there faster or more safely, or is he or she better equipped to deal with building a camp and caring for the victim? There are no simple rules that apply in all situations, since so many different variables are involved. Most importantly, before decisions are made, the group should talk through the issues so that everyone understands what may be involved in both staying and going.

The person going for help must be able to communicate the group's location to rescuers. This information should be written down and carried. Unless this location is a well-known place, the person going for help must also be confident about his or her ability to lead rescuers back to the victim.

Sheltering the Victim

While awaiting rescuers, a victim of injury or sudden illness needs to be protected from the environment. Unless you have camping equipment with you, you need to create an emergency shelter to keep the victim (and you) warm and dry. The type of shelter depends on the characteristics of the area and what materials you have with you. Look for natural shelters such as a cave or rock overhang. If you need to make a shelter, use a poncho or tarp hung over a rope or pole to make a lean-to or tent (**Figure 24-4a and b**). If you have no waterproof material, make a lean-to from branches or poles and cover the framework with leaves, grass, or other material (**Figure 24-4c**). In swampy areas where the victim must be elevated to stay dry, cut saplings to build a "swamp bed" (**Figure 24-4d**). A "debris hut," like a tent made of branches piled over with brush, twigs, and leaves, can keep you and the victim dry and warm (**Figure 24-4e**). In a heavy snowfall, dig a pit in the snow around the base of an evergreen tree with low boughs, piling boughs against the trunk to form a snow roof as more snow falls (**Figure 24-4f**).

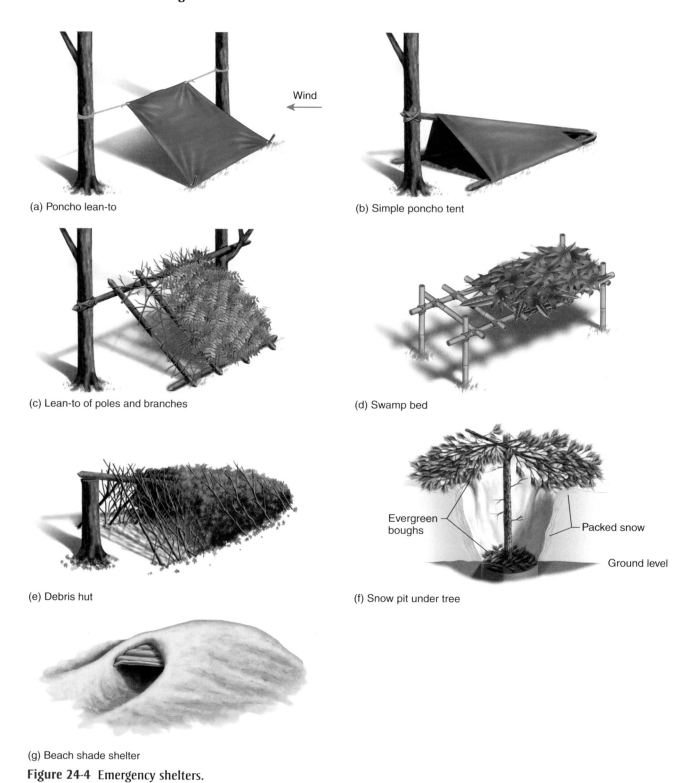

(a) Poncho lean-to

(b) Simple poncho tent

(c) Lean-to of poles and branches

(d) Swamp bed

(e) Debris hut

Evergreen boughs

Packed snow

Ground level

(f) Snow pit under tree

(g) Beach shade shelter

Figure 24-4 Emergency shelters.

In a desert or on a shadeless beach, where the victim needs to be sheltered from the sun and heat, construct a shade shelter by digging a trench in cooler sand, stretching clothing or other material between mounds on each side, and anchoring the material with more sand on top at its edges (**Figure 24-4g**).

Leaving the Victim Alone

Consider leaving a victim alone to go for help only if you are alone, you cannot communicate your need for help, and it is unlikely that someone will pass your location. Because a victim's condition may deteriorate without further care, take this action only if there is no alternative. Prepare the victim as well as possible before leaving, attending to shelter and food and water needs. Leave a written note with the victim explaining when you anticipate returning with help.

With three or more in the group, never leave the victim alone, even when you feel sure the victim will be okay—and even if the victim agrees. Conditions may change, or unanticipated things may happen.

Preparing for Rescue

Once an emergency has been communicated from the remote location to authorities such as EMS, search and rescue operations, or the Coast Guard, it is critical to remain in the same location until help arrives. You may need to help rescuers find you as they approach the area, signaling with a fire or flashlight, smoke, or a whistle. Depending on the urgency of the situation and the terrain, rescuers may arrive by vehicle, on foot, or by other means.

Helicopter rescues are often used in remote areas to get a victim to advanced medical care most quickly. Following are safety principles when a helicopter is arriving at your location (**Figure 24-5**):

- A large, clear area is needed for a safe landing. Stay far back from any clearing where the helicopter is likely to land.
- The rotor wash "wind" from the helicopter typically exceeds 100 mph. Protect your face and the victim from injury caused by flying debris.
- Once the helicopter has landed, do not approach it until signaled to do so. The spinning tail rotor cannot be seen, and you may inadvertently walk into it. Approach only in a crouch, and never from an uphill side where the blade is closer to the ground.
- When making a rescue at sea, or in a wilderness area where landing is impossible, the helicopter may lower a basket on a cable. Sometimes the helicopter crew lower a two-way radio first to enable communication and give instructions for the rescue.

Evacuation of Victim

Generally it is better to wait for help to come to you rather than to try to evacuate the victim yourself from a remote location. Moving the victim may worsen the victim's condition and is likely to cause additional pain. The decision to evacuate a victim depends on several key factors:

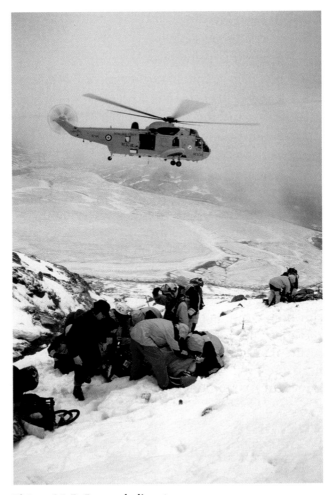

Figure 24-5 Rescue helicopter.

- The length of time before help can be expected to arrive
- Whether the victim's condition will be aggravated more by waiting for help than by moving the victim
- The number of people present and their ability to safely carry the victim out
- How much daylight remains, and whether the weather may deteriorate
- Whether it is possible to continue giving first aid during evacuation

According to the Wilderness Medical Society, victims with the following conditions may be evacuated if help will be delayed and group members can safely carry the victim:

- A worsening condition such as a breathing problem, deteriorating mental status, shock, or recurring diarrhea or vomiting
- Severe pain
- Inability to walk

- Persistent bleeding
- Severe altitude sickness
- An infection getting worse
- Chest pain symptomatic of a cardiac condition
- Mental or behavioral disorder that threatens the safety of the victim or others
- Near drowning
- Severe burns or wounds
- Severe traumatic injury

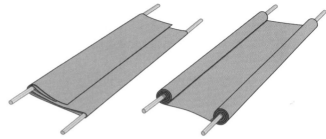

Litter made of poles and blanket

If enough people are present, someone should be sent ahead for help, since those carrying the victim will travel more slowly.

Four or six people can carry the victim on an improvised stretcher or litter. Cut two poles from saplings and create a litter from a blanket or sleeping bag, or even two jackets or shirts as shown in **Figure 24-6**. Use other clothing to pad the litter under the victim. Use belts or rope to secure the victim in the litter and support the head and neck. During the evacuation, monitor the victim's condition and stay alert for vomiting,

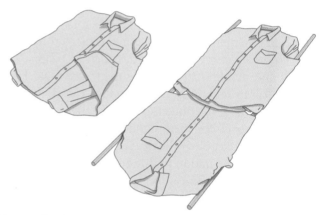

Litter made of poles and two jackets or shirts (sleeves inside)

Figure 24-6 Emergency litters for evacuating an injured victim.

Learning
Checkpoint ②

1. Check off important principles for planning a trip into a wilderness location:

   ___ Do not go alone.

   ___ Do not go longer than three to four days.

   ___ Tell someone where you are going and when you will return.

   ___ Take more food and water than you expect to need.

   ___ Split up the first aid kit among three or four in the group in case someone gets lost.

   ___ Do not drink more alcohol than usual.

2. True or False: When dealing with a complex emergency in a remote location, the group's leader must set the plan and resist any temptation to change it along the way.

3. Name three reasons why you should not depend on a cell phone in a wilderness location.

   _____

4. Never leave a victim alone to go for help when

   a. you cannot communicate your need for help.

   b. it is unlikely that someone will pass by your location.

   c. there are three or four people in the group.

   d. All of the above

which can threaten the airway of a victim lying on his or her back.

Other emergency carries such as the hammock carry (see **Chapter 25**) are ineffective for the distances typically involved in remote location evacuations. In certain circumstances the two-person walking assist may be appropriate for a short distance.

SPECIAL CARE FOR EMERGENCIES WHEN HELP IS DELAYED

Earlier chapters describe the standard first aid for injuries and sudden illness. **This chapter describes only special considerations when help may be delayed.**

Bleeding, Wounds, and Shock

Special care for bleeding may be needed in a remote location for these reasons:

- Bleeding can soon become life threatening if not stopped and medical care will not be provided soon.
- A contaminated wound that a first aider may leave for medical personnel in normal situations can become seriously infected if medical care is not provided soon.
- A victim in shock caused by blood loss requires special care if medical attention is delayed, such as providing fluids if possible.

Special remote location care for bleeding, wounds, and shock includes the following steps *in addition to the care described in earlier chapters.*

1. Control external bleeding as soon as possible. Maintain direct pressure as long as needed with a pressure bandage, but check for circulation below the bleeding site to avoid cutting off circulation to the limb unless absolutely necessary to control bleeding.
2. A **tourniquet** is used *only as an extreme last resort* to stop bleeding from an arm or leg to save the victim's life when medical attention will be delayed. The victim will then likely face amputation of the limb. To apply a tourniquet:

   - Wrap a wide belt or bandage around the limb just above the bleeding site, and knot it.
   - Knot a metal rod or strong stick over the first knot and twist it to tighten the constricting band until bleeding stops (**Figure 24-7**). Note that considerable pressure may be necessary to squeeze closed the bleeding artery deep within the limb.

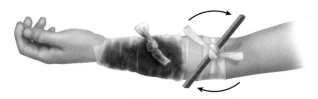

Figure 24-7 An emergency tourniquet is used only as the last resort to stop bleeding.

   - Tape or fasten the rod in place to hold the pressure.
   - Note the time of application to inform medical personnel.
   - After 15 minutes slowly release the tourniquet pressure to see if bleeding has stopped; reapply the tourniquet if bleeding begins.

3. After stopping bleeding from a wound, you should clean the wound to prevent infection. Wash the wound with soap and water; then apply a sterile dressing and bandage over the wound to keep dirt out. For a deeper wound or one visibly contaminated with dirt or foreign matter, use an irrigation syringe to forcefully rinse the wound clean; if necessary, part the wound edges to allow the water to reach the bottom of the wound. Then apply a sterile dressing and bandage, applying pressure again if necessary to stop bleeding. For gaping wounds, use "butterfly" bandage strips or strips of clean tape to hold the wound closed, or pack a deep wound that will not close with a dressing.
4. There is one exception to the usual care for shock caused by bleeding as described in **Chapter 10**. Normally a shock victim is not given anything to drink in the brief time before medical help arrives, but when help is delayed, the victim needs fluid. If the victim is responsive and can swallow, give water, a clear fluid, or an oral rehydration solution in small drinks, frequently but only as tolerated. If the victim vomits, wait a while before giving another drink.
5. If the victim's shock resulted from dehydration, keep giving fluids slowly but steadily.

Musculoskeletal Injuries

As explained in **Chapter 16**, an injured extremity normally is splinted only if the victim is at risk for moving the injured area before help arrives. When help is delayed, especially if the victim is to be evacuated, splinting is often necessary. You may need to improvise the splint with materials

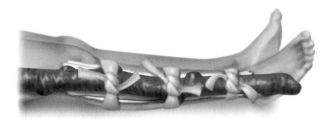

Figure 24-8 Improvising a splint with materials at hand.

at hand, such as a ski pole or a sturdy piece of wood broken from a tree branch (**Figure 24-8**). Ideally, a first aid kit used in remote locations should include a SAM® splint. When the splint will be in place for an extended time, it is essential to check circulation below the injury and to periodically loosen the splint to improve blood flow.

In very rare cases of an extremity fracture, circulation may be cut off below the injury site. If medical care is hours away and you are certain there is no circulation in the extremity below the injury, then you may try to carefully straighten the extremity to restore circulation unless this would increase bleeding. Never try to straighten a fractured limb if the victim may receive medical care within 30 minutes or if there is some circulation below the injury site.

In some cases a dislocation may impair circulation to an extremity. If you have been trained to reduce a dislocation (return bones to their normal position in the joint), and if you are sure that circulation to the extremity is cut off and the victim will not receive medical care within 30 minutes, you may then try to reduce the dislocation.

Spinal Injuries

In remote locations, three aspects of first aid in cases of suspected spinal injuries are somewhat different from the usual care described in **Chapter 13**. First, if the victim is thought to have a possible spinal injury, it may be difficult to keep the spine immobilized for an extended time. You may need to improvise with materials at hand, such as using large pieces of wood or stones padded with clothing positioned on both sides of the head to immobilize the spine of a victim who is lying down. If the victim is on the ground, you may need to put clothing or other material under the victim's body to prevent heat loss; do this by holding the head in line with the body as others roll the body to one side long enough for an insulated material to be put under the victim's body. A victim with a spinal injury should not be evacuated.

Second, although it is generally best to immobilize a victim in the position found when help will arrive soon, in remote locations it is generally better to gently place the victim in the normal position with head straight and eyes forward to prevent further injury to the spine. Do not move the victim's head, however, if it causes more pain or you feel resistance to movement.

Finally, great care is needed in assessing a possible spinal injury. When help will arrive soon, it is better to be safe than sorry, and a conservative approach is generally advised: immobilize the victim's head and neck in line with the body, keep the victim still, and wait for advanced medical personnel to determine how best to manage the possible spinal injury. In a remote location, however, other risks may be involved in waiting a long time for help, and in such cases if the presence of a spinal injury is not obvious, the victim may be further assessed to determine whether immobilization is in fact necessary. The Wilderness Medical Associates have developed a protocol for spinal injuries in which a spine injury can be ruled out if *all* the following criteria are met:

1. The victim is alert, sober, and cooperative.
2. The victim does not feel neck or back tenderness when you press with fingers along the spine.
3. The victim does not have other injuries that mask or distract him or her from feeling the pain or tenderness of a spinal injury.
4. The victim has normal function in all four limbs:
   - The fingers of both hands can be opened and closed and the wrist moved up and down.
   - Both feet can be moved up and down and the big toe moved up and down.
   - The victim has no tingling sensation but has normal sensation in all four limbs, as determined by being able to feel a light touch and a painful pinch in all areas. One specific area may have reduced function if the cause is clearly not related to a spinal injury, such as occurs with a sprained wrist.

Head Injuries

Chapter 13 describes how when help is expected to arrive soon, it is generally best to call 9-1-1 and give supportive care while waiting for help. In a delayed help situation, especially if you cannot communicate with EMS to ask advice, you may need to make difficult decisions about whether to evacuate the victim.

A victim with a concussion caused by a blow to the head may be able to safely walk out of a remote location. The victim should be closely monitored for the signs and symptoms of a more serious brain injury, however, and should be awakened and checked every two to three hours.

A victim with a more serious head injury may have swelling or bleeding in the brain, a potentially life-threatening condition. The signs and symptoms of a brain injury are described in **Chapter 13**. A serious brain injury is unlikely to improve by itself; the victim needs immediate medical attention. If possible, call for emergency evacuation, by helicopter if available. If communication is impossible, you may face the difficult decision of whether to attempt to evacuate the victim yourself. The sooner the victim receives medical care, the better his or her chances for survival, but moving the victim over difficult terrain may worsen the condition. Either way, the victim may die. Evacuate the victim only if necessary to prevent a dangerous delay and you can do so safely.

Abdominal Injury or Illness

A victim with an abdominal injury or severe abdominal pain needs to receive medical attention as soon as possible. As with a head injury, if communication with EMS is impossible, you must balance the risk of the victim's condition being worsened by evacuation with the risk of waiting for delayed help. A closed or open abdominal wound may progress to life-threatening shock, and abdominal pain may be a sign of appendicitis that can rapidly become an emergency.

Burns

The care for burns when help is delayed is similar to standard burn care. In addition, because a severe or large burn may cause a significant loss of body fluids, a victim who is alert should be given large amounts of water or clear fluids slowly and a little at a time to prevent or minimize shock.

Burn prevention is especially important in outdoor recreational activities such as camping. Fire is a greater risk with an outdoor campfire because of the risk of windblown sparks and the flammability of tents, sleeping bags, and other camp gear. Because many of the synthetic fabrics used in such camping equipment and clothing melt when on fire, causing deeper and more serious burns when in contact with skin, water should be immediately available for dousing flames.

Sudden Illness

Special considerations may be necessary for diabetic emergencies or anaphylactic shock when help may be delayed.

A diabetic who regularly self-injects insulin or takes medication should inform others in the remote environment how to administer insulin or medication in an emergency. It is especially important that diabetics monitor their blood sugar levels and inform others of the signs and symptoms of hypoglycemia and hyperglycemia as well as what to do. Prevention is critical, but others should be prepared to take action by giving a sugar substance. If diabetic shock develops, give water and other shock care. Evacuate a victim in a diabetic crisis as quickly as possible.

Similarly, someone who has severe allergies should inform others in the group, and the first aid kit should contain emergency epinephrine such as an EpiPen® if possible. Someone with severe allergies entering a wilderness location may carry up to three emergency epinephrine doses. Be sure others know where the EpiPen® is kept and how to use it. A victim who develops anaphylaxis should be evacuated as quickly as possible. The protocol of the Wilderness Medical Associates calls for administering epinephrine to victims with a definite reaction marked by difficulty breathing and generalized skin redness or swelling. Although usually only one dose is needed, up to three doses may be administered if required, every five minutes if the condition is worsening or every 15 minutes if the victim's condition is not improving.

Hypothermia

Hypothermia is more likely to occur during outdoor activities in cold environments, especially if one is wet or a wind is blowing. Because the body loses heat 25 to 30 times faster when immersed in cold water, hypothermia is even more likely if a victim falls into cold water.

A responsive victim of mild hypothermia, with a body temperature above 90° F may recover with adequate warming. Follow the standard guidelines to warm the victim. With sufficient rest and warming, in time this person may be able to walk out from the remote location.

A body temperature below 90° F indicates severe hypothermia. At this point the victim is usually no longer shivering and often has changing levels of responsiveness. This is a life-threatening emergency. It is unlikely that you will be able to fully rewarm the victim in the remote location, but make every effort to prevent further heat loss and to warm the victim as much as possible while waiting for help. Do not try to evacuate the victim by foot, as it will be difficult or impossible to keep the victim warm while being transported through a cold environment. Send someone for help immediately. Put the victim in dry clothing and inside a sleeping bag protected by shelter. The victim should be wrapped fully to prevent heat loss, including the use of a space blanket if available (**Figure 24-9**). Avoid rough handling. Add heat with bodily contact, heating pads, or hot water bottles beside the neck, armpits, or groin. Whereas a hypothermia victim should not be actively rewarmed with heat sources when close to medical care, in a remote location you may actively warm the victim with a heat source and by putting containers of warm (not hot) water against the victim's skin.

A victim in very severe hypothermia may seem to be dead. The skin is cold and blue, and the victim is totally unresponsive. The internal body temperature may be below 85° F. Do not rush to provide CPR, however, which can lead to a life-threatening heart dysrhythmia if the victim still has a heartbeat. Assess the victim carefully. The victim may be breathing only once every 30 seconds or so. Rewarm the victim as described previously, and provide CPR if the victim is not breathing.

Hypothermia caused by immersion in cold water may occur very rapidly and is often severe. These victims generally need both rewarming and CPR. Because the body's need for oxygen decreases when very cold, resuscitation may occur even after significant time in the water. Although

CPR is generally not given for longer than 30 minutes in normal temperatures, victims with severe hypothermia have been given CPR for as long as three hours and recovered fully. The saying "a victim is never cold and dead, only warm and dead" reminds us not to assume a victim is dead until rewarming has occurred, because often severe hypothermic victims do survive.

Heat Emergencies

Like cold emergencies, heat emergencies such as heatstroke are more common during outdoor activities in remote locations where no relief may be possible from extreme temperatures. Prevent heat emergencies by staying out of direct sunlight, minimizing activity, and staying well hydrated.

For heat exhaustion or heatstroke, cool the victim as soon as possible. If the victim is alert and not vomiting, give water or fluid a little at a time. A victim with heat exhaustion may be able to travel from the location after cooling and resting. The victim may remain in a weakened condition, however, and walking out in continued heat may renew the problem and become an emergency.

Heatstroke is a life-threatening emergency. Cool the victim and evacuate if possible rather than waiting for delayed medical attention. Even if the victim seems to recover, there may be damage to internal organs.

Snakebites

Unless you are certain the bite was from a non-poisonous snake, assume a snakebite is poisonous. Splint the limb to reduce movement and keep the area below the level of the heart.

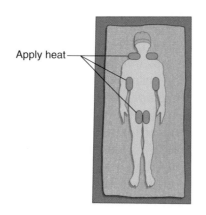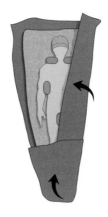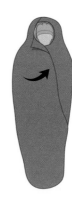

Apply heat

Figure 24-9 Hypothermia wrap.

Check the fingers or toes periodically to ensure that circulation is not impeded. Evacuate the victim as soon as possible. To be effective, antivenin must be administered within four to six hours after the bite. Other medical care may be needed.

CPR

Chapter 6 describes the standard procedures for CPR. Follow the same approach for a victim in cardiac arrest in a remote location, although in some cases the victim has smaller chances for recovery when advanced medical care cannot be given soon. CPR was developed as a short-term treatment to keep the victim alive until treated by medical professionals. Depending on the cause of the cardiac arrest, resuscitation in a remote location may be unlikely, as when cardiac arrest is caused by a heart attack or traumatic injuries. Nonetheless, always give CPR for 30 minutes. If the victim is far from medical care and does not revive within 30 minutes *except in certain special situations,* you can stop CPR after 30 minutes.

In three situations victims have been successfully resuscitated after CPR for longer than 30 minutes: hypothermia, drowning, and lightning strike. As noted earlier, victims with severe hypothermia have survived after hours of CPR. In these cases follow the standard protocol to give CPR until another trained rescuer takes over or you are too exhausted to continue.

Learning Checkpoint ③

1. What is important about first aid for bleeding in a remote location?

    a. Control bleeding as quickly as possible.

    b. Use a tourniquet only as a last resort.

    c. A responsive victim in shock can drink water.

    d. All of the above

2. True or False: If you suspect a victim in a remote location may have a spinal injury, do not move him or her no matter how long you may have to wait for help.

3. True or False: In a remote location, the best thing to do for a victim thought to have a brain injury is to wait and see if the victim's condition improves.

4. On a cold day, a hiker in your group of four falls into an icy stream about a three-hour walk from the car. After being pulled out, he develops the signs and symptoms of severe hypothermia. Which is the best action to take?

    a. Immediately start hiking out—keep the person moving and he'll be okay.

    b. Send someone to get help while rest of the group works to warm the victim.

    c. Put the victim in a hypothermia wrap and carry him out.

    d. None of the above

5. Except in cases of hypothermia, drowning, and lightning strike, CPR can be stopped in a remote location if the victim does not revive within ____ minutes.

SPECIAL WILDERNESS EMERGENCIES

In addition to being prepared for an emergency in a remote location and knowing what first aid to give when help will be delayed, those entering wilderness locations where there is a risk of certain kinds of emergencies need special preparations. These special situations include:

- Ice rescue
- Snow emergencies
- Desert survival
- Lightning strikes
- Wildfires
- Altitude sickness
- SCUBA diving incidents

This text only introduces the issues involved in these situations. Special training programs are available for those planning a trip into locations where these emergencies may occur, including preparations, equipment, and first aid and survival techniques.

Ice Rescue

In circumstances where EMS can be called and trained rescuers arrive within minutes, you should never go onto ice yourself to rescue a victim. In a remote location, however, a rescuer may choose to go onto the ice as a last resort. Lie flat with arms and legs spread to distribute your weight, and push a tree limb or other object ahead of you for the victim to grab. If at all possible, others should hold onto your legs, or use clothing to fashion a rescue line if rope is not available, in case the ice breaks under you as well.

Snow Emergencies

Avalanches

Avalanches are a risk for backcountry trekkers and skiers. Try to avoid areas that are prone to avalanches, and talk with local officials before entering the area. Avalanche transceivers are available that emit signals from a trapped person to transceivers carried by others in the group to help them to locate the victim. Most avalanche deaths occur by suffocation; the snow packs tightly around the victim, preventing breathing or digging out. The victim's chances of survival rapidly diminish as time passes after burial.

Call for help if someone in your group is buried by an avalanche, but time is critical and those present should begin searching for the person immediately. Start at the point where the victim was last seen and work down the slope, using a ski pole or tree branch to probe into the snow. CPR will likely be necessary.

Snow Blindness

Snow blindness is a burn on the cornea of the eyes caused by intense sunlight reflected from snow. It can be prevented by wearing dark sunglasses or goggles with UV protection. At first the eyes feel scratchy and burning and become more sensitive to light. Headache may develop. Eventually the victim loses vision. First aid involves bandaging the eyes to prevent any further exposure to light. Cold compresses may ease the pain. The victim usually recovers sight in 12 to 18 hours, but if symptoms linger, medical care should be sought.

Desert Survival

Desert hiking and trekking have become more popular, exposing more people to the risks of very harsh climates. As when entering very cold climates, preparation and training are essential. Appropriate clothing is necessary for sun and heat protection, as are the right camping equipment and first aid supplies. Perhaps most important is water. Few people realize that the daily intake of water can increase up to three to five gallons per person in extreme dry heat. Since water weighs eight pounds per gallon, it is impractical to carry enough to sustain life for days in an emergency. Desert survival training therefore includes skills in finding and purifying water as well as techniques for building shelter, communications and distress signals, direction finding, and traveling at night to avoid the worst heat.

Lightning Strikes

Chapter 12 lists tips to avoid being struck by lightning. About one-third of victims of lightning strike die, usually as a result of cardiac arrest. Immediate CPR is therefore critical to increase the victim's chances for survival. Remember that lightning strikes are one of the three situations (along with drowning and hypothermia) in which CPR should be continued past the 30-minute wilderness limit.

Altitude Sickness

Hikers at altitudes over 8000 to 10,000 feet are at risk for different forms of **altitude sickness** caused by the lower concentration of oxygen. Know what symptoms to watch for and what actions to take. As many as one-fourth of people may experience altitude sickness, and it is impossible to predict in advance whether one is susceptible.

Acute mountain sickness (AMS) is most common, and up to 75% of people will have mild symptoms after one or two days at over 10,000 feet. Others may experience more severe symptoms as low as 8000 feet. Symptoms include headache, dizziness, fatigue, shortness of breath, nausea and lack of appetite, and general malaise. Moderate AMS causes more severe headache not relieved by medication, nausea and vomiting, decreased coordination, and worsening of the mild symptoms. Severe AMS causes shortness of breath even at rest, decreasing mental status, and inability to walk. Mild AMS may be overcome with acclimatization, but descent to lower altitude is the only cure for more severe symptoms. The Outdoor Action Program advises this test of a person experiencing AMS symptoms: Try to walk a straight line heel to toe (like a sobriety test). A person who has difficulty doing this should start the descent immediately before symptoms worsen.

Medication is available to treat mild to moderate symptoms in those who have experienced AMS in the past. Hikers should also maintain good hydration, since body fluid is lost more rapidly at high altitudes. New research also suggests that a high-carbohydrate diet before and during the high-altitude period may reduce the symptoms of AMS.

Two other types of altitude sickness, **high altitude pulmonary edema (HAPE)** and **high altitude cerebral edema (HACE),** are rare but more serious. Both occur after more time at altitude and involve a fluid buildup—in the lungs in HAPE, or the brain in HACE—that becomes life threatening. A victim of HAPE experiences shortness of breath even at rest, a feeling of tightness in the chest, significant fatigue and weakness, a persistent, productive cough, and confusion or irrational behavior. A victim of HACE has significant mental signs and symptoms including headache, loss of coordination, memory loss, possible hallucinations and psychotic confusion, and coma. Any victim thought to be experiencing HAPE or HACE must be evacuated immediately down the mountain to a medical facility.

SCUBA Diving

Underwater divers, as part of their SCUBA training and certification, learn about the risks of staying

Learning Checkpoint (4)

1. To rescue someone in deep water, what actions should you take? Number these in the order in which you should try them (from safest to least safe):

____ Throw a rope or floating object to the victim.

____ Swim to the victim.

____ Reach to the victim with a stick or long object.

____ Go to the victim in a boat or other craft.

2. In a desert or other extremely dry, hot environment, a person's daily intake of water may rise to ____ gallons.

3. Put a check mark next to the typical signs and symptoms of acute mountain sickness:

____ Headache   ____ Cold, dry skin

____ Dizziness   ____ Fatigue

____ Diarrhea   ____ Nausea

down too long or surfacing too quickly. Operators of dive boats and facilities know what signs and symptoms to look for and typically have the communications equipment and resources to call for professional medical help when it is needed. Some divers, however, may dive on their own or accompanied by others without this training. EMS should be contacted immediately for any diver experiencing breathing difficulty, pain in joints or extremities, feelings of paralysis, tingling or numbness, significant fatigue and generalized weakness, convulsions, coma, or nonresponsiveness. Decompression treatment and other specialized care may be needed.

Concluding Thoughts

For those living or working in rural areas or visiting remote locations for any reason, the most important thing is to be aware that if an injury or sudden illness strikes, you may be on your own for a time before being rescued or reaching advanced care. This makes injury and illness prevention crucial, as is being prepared for the kinds of emergencies that are more likely to occur in the specific setting. With these preparations and a healthy attitude to minimize the risks, you will likely be among the millions who live in remote locations or visit wilderness areas every year without incident.

Learning Outcomes

You should now be able to do the following:

1. Explain what is different about first aid principles when help may be delayed.

2. Describe common situations in which help is likely to be delayed.

3. List actions to take to be prepared for injury and illness emergencies in remote locations.

4. Describe methods by which EMS can be contacted from isolated areas.

5. Explain how to protect a victim until help arrives or how to safely transport a victim if help cannot reach the victim.

6. Describe special care for victims with common injuries and illnesses when help will be delayed.

7. Explain what to do in special wilderness emergencies such as avalanche or ice rescue, lightning strikes, wildfires, altitude sickness, and SCUBA diving illness.

Review Questions

1. If you will be in the wilderness for several days, consider bringing along
   a. more water than you expect to need.
   b. special medications you might need.
   c. a device for emergency communication.
   d. All of the above

2. If you need to use your cell phone to call for help while in a remote location and the signal is weak, what can you try in order to get a stronger signal?
   a. Point the antenna directly at the horizon.
   b. Move the phone around your body.
   c. Try to get near a body of water.
   d. Wrap a damp cloth around the antenna.

3. Standard distress signals involve making ____ sounds, lights, or visual signals that may be heard or seen by others.
   a. two
   b. three
   c. four
   d. as many as possible

4. In a remote location, leave a victim alone to go for help only if
   a. you are alone with the victim.
   b. you cannot communicate your need for help.
   c. it is unlikely someone will pass your location soon.
   d. Only if all of the above are true.

5. Your group in a wilderness area decides to use a litter to carry an unresponsive injured victim back to safety. Which of the following is the most dangerous possibility to stay alert to as you carry the victim?
   a. Vomiting
   b. Heat exhaustion
   c. Pain caused by jiggling the litter
   d. Dehydration

6. What is different about wound care if medical attention may be delayed a day or two?
   a. Try to insert antibiotic cream into a puncture wound by any method, even cutting open the wound if necessary.
   b. Rather than covering the wound with a dressing, leave it open to "breathe" and to be able to check it frequently for signs of infection.
   c. Clean the wound after the bleeding stops, even at the risk of bleeding starting again.
   d. Use your sewing kit, if available, to stitch any wound closed.

7. A hiker in your group has experienced a blow to the head. The group cannot decide whether to send someone immediately to call for emergency evacuation or to wait and see if the victim is well enough in a few hours to walk out. Which of the following signs and symptoms may indicate a more serious brain injury requiring medical treatment as soon as possible?
   a. Unequal pupils not responding to light
   b. Headache
   c. Warm, flushed skin
   d. Bleeding of the scalp

8. Guidelines for burn prevention when camping are based in part on which of the following?
   a. Lightning strikes are very common at campsites.
   b. Tents, sleeping bags, and other camping gear are often highly flammable.
   c. Campfires usually flare up several hours after going "out."
   d. Burns by boiling water are more likely when cooking over a campfire.

9. A person with diabetes who is in a group of campers in a remote location should
   a. tell others the signs and symptoms of a diabetic emergency and what to do.
   b. bring glucose or a sugar substance to take in case of hypoglycemia.
   c. monitor his or her blood sugar levels carefully.
   d. All of the above

10. Which of these victims in cardiac arrest have been revived when CPR lasts longer than 30 minutes?
    a. Heart attack victims
    b. Trauma victims
    c. Drowning victims
    d. Stroke victims

References and Resources

American Heart Association. 2005 International consensus on cardiopulmonary resuscitation (CPR) and emergency cardiovascular care (ECC) science with treatment recommendations. *Circulation*, 112(22). November 29, 2005.

Curtis R (director, Outdoor Action Program). Outdoor action guide. Princeton, New Jersey: Princeton University; 2004. www.princeton.edu/~oa/safety

Liffrig J. Mental preparedness and leadership in wilderness survival. 2004. wms.org/pubs/survival.html

National Safety Council. www.nsc.org

National Environmental Satellite, Data, and Information Service. Emergency Beacons. 2004. www.sarsat.noaa.gov/emerbcns.html

Pelton RW. *The official urban and wilderness emergency survival guide.* West Conshohocker, Pennsylvania: Infinity Publishing; 2002.

Wilderness Medical Associates. Emergency training for outdoor professionals. 2001. www.wildmed.com

Wilderness Medical Society. www.wms.org

Wilderness Survival. www.wilderness-survival.net

Chapter 25

Rescuing and Moving Victims

Chapter Preview

- Rescuing a Victim
- Multiple Victims
- Moving Victims

You are called to the equipment room where an employee has been found unresponsive. He is lying on the floor beneath a rack of electrical equipment which he apparently was working on. Thinking he may have been electrocuted, you first make sure the power is turned off to this equipment, and then you check his breathing. He is not breathing. Because he is lying on his side underneath the shelf of equipment, however, you cannot give him chest compressions. What should you do?

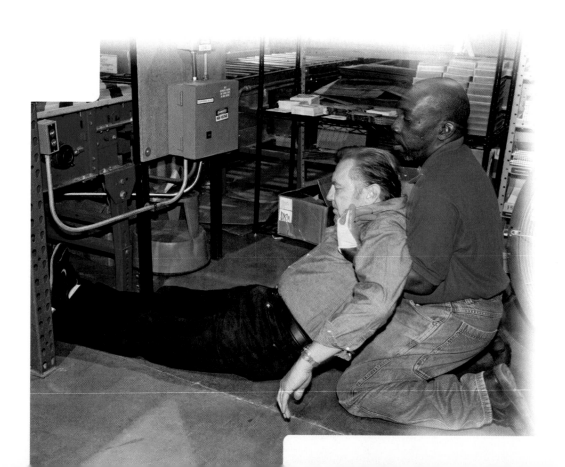

Before you can give first aid and basic life support (BLS), you have to reach the victim. If the scene is dangerous, you must stay away or take special precautions. Sometimes there is more than one victim and you have to decide whom to care for first. Sometimes the victim must be moved, if it is safe to do so, before you can give first aid. Never attempt any rescue or move a victim unless it is safe for both you and the victim.

RESCUING A VICTIM

Common situations involving victim rescue are fires, hazardous materials incidents, motor vehicle crashes, and water rescues. Before entering any of these situations, however, be sure that it is safe to do so. If the scene is dangerous and you cannot safely approach the victim, *stay away and call for help.* The 9-1-1 dispatcher will send a crew with the appropriate training and equipment to safely reach and care for the victim. **Chapter 2** discusses scene safety in more detail. Safe rescues in most situations described in this chapter require specialized training and gear. It is essential that you do only what you have been trained to do

because otherwise you may only become another victim others will have to rescue.

Fire

If a victim needs rescue from a fire scene, do not approach unless you are certain it is safe to reach the victim. Smoke or fumes are usually present in fire situations and can easily overcome anyone entering the scene. Invisible gases resulting from the fire pose a threat in both indoor and outdoor locations.

If a fire breaks out in your location, quick action is essential. Most important, evacuate others present and call 9-1-1. Do not enter an area of smoke or flames to search for victims, however, because of the high risk that you will be overcome by smoke or fumes. Do not remain in the area in an attempt to fight the fire unless the fire is very small, you have and know how to use a fire extinguisher, and you can flee safely if the fire gets out of control. If caught indoors in a smoky area, take action to avoid the smoke as much as possible by staying close to the floor (smoke rises), not opening doors, and preventing the entry of smoke through vents or door cracks (**Figure 25-1** and First Aid: "Fire"). See other guidelines in **Chapter 12**.

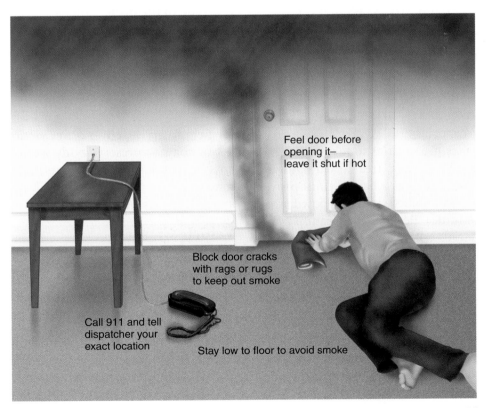

Feel door before opening it— leave it shut if hot

Block door cracks with rags or rugs to keep out smoke

Call 911 and tell dispatcher your exact location

Stay low to floor to avoid smoke

Figure 25-1 If trapped in a building where there is a fire, take precautions to avoid smoke inhalation.

First Aid　Fire

When You See

- Flames or smoke
- A fire alarm sounding

Do This First

1 Remove everyone from the area. Close doors behind you as you leave.

2 Call 9-1-1, set off alarms, or follow other workplace protocols.

3 Use a fire extinguisher to combat a fire only if:
- The fire is small.
- You can easily and quickly escape the area.
- You know how to use the fire extinguisher.
- You can stay between the exit and the fire, so that you can always safely get out.

4 Do not enter an area of flames and smoke in an attempt to rescue others.

5 If trapped inside:
- In a smoky room, crawl along the floor where there is breathable air.
- Do not open a door that feels hot.
- Do not use elevators.
- If stuck inside, turn off the ventilation system, stuff towels or rags (wet if possible) into door cracks and vents, and use a phone to report your location.

ALERT

- **Never put yourself at risk to rescue a victim.**
- **When hazards are present, leave the rescue to the professionals.**
- **Never try to perform any rescue technique you have not been trained to do.**

Hazardous Materials

Chapter 2 describes precautions to take around a spill of hazardous materials. Treat any unknown substance you see spilled as a hazard until proven otherwise. Avoid any spilled liquid or powder as well as possible fumes. Because the cleanup of hazardous materials takes special training, knowledge, and equipment, leave this to "hazmat" professionals. Do not enter a scene contaminated by hazardous materials in order to reach a victim. If a victim emerges from the spill area with potentially hazardous substances on clothing or skin, do not touch the victim because of the risk of contaminating yourself as well. If possible, use a water hose to wash the victim's skin and clothing before providing first aid. **Chapter 12** describes the first aid for chemicals on the skin. While waiting

for help to arrive, cover a wet victim with a blanket or coats to preserve body warmth. Do not let anyone who has contacted a potentially hazardous material leave the area before EMS professionals arrive (see First Aid: "Hazardous Materials").

Vehicle Crashes

Vehicle crash scenes can be extremely dangerous for rescuers because of the risks of passing traffic, fire, vehicle instability, and other factors. Rescuers have been injured by accidentally setting off an automatic airbag while trying to reach a victim. For all these reasons it is crucial to ensure that the scene is safe before approaching the vehicle and providing care for the victim.

If it is safe to reach the vehicle, do not try to remove a victim unless fire or another threat to

First Aid   Hazardous Materials

When You See

- Warning signs or placards (with "flammable" or other warning terms) (see Chapter 2)
- Any spilled substance
- Vapors you can see or fumes you can smell

Do This First

1 Stay out of the area and keep bystanders away.

2 Outside, stay upwind of the area to avoid possible fumes.

3 Call 9-1-1.

4 Approach the victim only if you are sure it is safe to do so. With a large exposure to hazardous materials, guide the victim to an emergency shower or rinse skin and clothing with a hose. Do only what you have been trained to do.

Additional Care

- If it is safe to reach the person, move the victim away from the hazard and give first aid for a chemical burn or smoke inhalation (see Chapter 12).

---

life is likely. Call 9-1-1 as soon as you recognize a victim is present, and describe the circumstances to the dispatcher so that the appropriate rescue team is sent. Crash victims often have spinal or other injuries that could be made worse by moving the victim unnecessarily. Provide needed first aid through the door or window or from behind the driver's seat if the vehicle is stable and it is safe to approach (see First Aid: "Vehicle Crashes"). Since an unresponsive victim is likely to have a spinal injury, support the head and neck with your hands while waiting for help to arrive (see Chapter 13).

Water Rescues

Water rescues are often needed to prevent drowning. A nonswimmer may have gotten into deep water, or a swimmer may have sustained an injury or sudden illness, such as a heart attack or seizure, that prevents the person from reaching safety. Regardless of the reason, if someone in deep water cannot reach safety, immediate rescue may be required.

Preventing Drownings

Drowning is a common cause of accidental death in the United States, resulting in 3482 deaths in a recent year and about three times that many visits to emergency rooms for near-drowning treatment. Near drowning can result in brain damage and other permanent disabilities. Drowning remains the second-leading cause of injury-related death for children ages 1 to 14 years. The CDC reports that the following are the most common risk factors for drowning:

First Aid   **Vehicle Crashes**

When You See

- A victim inside a motor vehicle after a crash

Do This First

1 Stop a safe distance past the crash and turn on your vehicle's hazard lights.

2 Call 9-1-1 if you have a cell phone, or ask someone else to call.

3 If available, set up warning triangles well back from the scene to warn oncoming traffic. Flares should be used only when there are no spilled chemicals and no chance of grass fire.

4 Ensure that the scene is safe before you approach the crashed vehicle. Stay away if there are risks from passing traffic, downed electrical wires, fire, or vehicle instability. Do not try to stabilize the vehicle unless you have special training.

5 If the vehicle is still running, ask the driver to turn off the ignition. If the driver is unresponsive and you can do so safely, reach in and turn the ignition off.

6 Do not try to remove a victim trapped inside a vehicle; wait for professional rescuers.

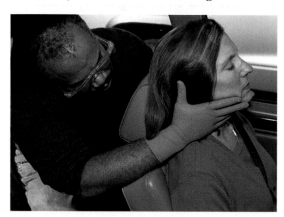

7 Assume that an unresponsive victim may have a neck injury. If the scene is safe, support the victim's head and neck with your hands.

8 Do not move the victim unless there is an immediate threat of fire. If so, get several bystanders to help to move the victim while you support the victim's head in line with the body the whole time.

9 Provide BLS and care for any serious injuries while waiting for help.

- Children under age one most often drown in bathtubs, buckets, or toilets.
- Among children aged one to four years, most drownings occur in residential swimming pools. Most young children who drowned in pools were last seen in the home, had been out of sight less than five minutes, and were in the care of one or both parents at the time.
- Alcohol use is involved in about 25% to 50% of adolescent and adult deaths associated with water recreation. Alcohol influences balance, coordination, and judgment, and its effects are heightened by sun exposure and heat.
- Boating carries risks for injury. In 2002, the U.S. Coast Guard received reports for 5705 boating incidents; 4062 participants were reported injured and 750 killed in boating incidents. Most boating fatalities from 2002 (70%) were caused by drowning, and the remainder were due to trauma, hypothermia, carbon monoxide poisoning, or other causes. Alcohol was involved in 39% of reported boating fatalities. Open motor boats were involved in 41% of all reported incidents, and personal watercraft were involved in another 28%.

Following are guidelines to help prevent drowning by children:

- Never leave children alone near water. Do not leave small children alone in a bathtub or wading pool.
- Do not let children dive in shallow, murky, or unknown water.
- At open waterfronts, keep children away from areas with big waves, undertows, and boats.
- Both children and adults should use personal flotation devices (PFDs) or lifejackets on boats and around water.
- In public swimming areas, let children enter the water only where lifeguards are present.
- Make sure rescue floats and other devices are present at pools and other water areas.
- Children at appropriate ages should learn from a qualified instructor to swim and to be safe in the water.
- Adult supervisors should realize that even children who can swim are not "drown-proof."
- Do not let older siblings or babysitters supervise children in the water.

- Most important, when supervising children in or near water, avoid all distractions: do not read, eat, or socialize with others. Most children drown when being "supervised" by someone not paying close attention.
- Childproof home pools with appropriate fencing, gates, floating pool alarms, and other safety devices (**Figure 25-2**).

Adults too should practice water safety principles to prevent drowning:

- Never drink or use other drugs when in or on the water. This includes when boating.
- Always wear a PFD when boating, even when in calm water and well away from the edge of the boat. No one ever plans to fall into the water—drowning usually occurs when the victim feels sure that a PFD is not needed.
- Dive into water only in depths of nine feet or more when the water is clear and no obstructions are present.
- Do not swim alone.
- Consider your swimming ability before attempting a swim out to a float or boat to ensure that you are not exhausted before reaching safety. Consider waves and other conditions.

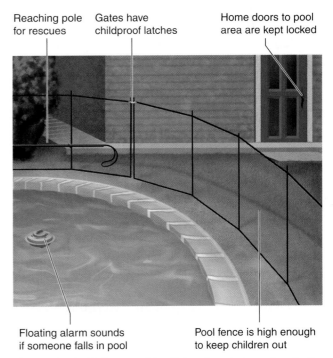

Reaching pole for rescues

Gates have childproof latches

Home doors to pool area are kept locked

Floating alarm sounds if someone falls in pool

Pool fence is high enough to keep children out

Figure 25-2 Make a residential swimming pool safe for children with preventive devices.

- Be aware that swimming in cold water can lead to hypothermia, which may lead to drowning.
- Be prepared for an emergency. Keep CPR skills fresh, and have a telephone handy when supervising others in the water.

Safe Techniques for Water Rescue

Rescuing someone at risk of drowning in deep water first requires recognizing that the person needs help. There are common misconceptions about how drowning victims act: you should not expect the victim to shout for help, nor is it true that "going down for the third time" is a prelude to drowning.

Recognizing a drowning situation depends on understanding three general scenarios of how people drown:

- **People who can swim,** or "dog paddle" or float well enough to keep their head above water at least for a time, may gradually or suddenly be at risk for drowning. A swimmer may become too tired to keep swimming, or hypothermia may set in and weaken the victim. If the problem develops gradually, the person may be in trouble but not yet actively drowning. This type of victim may call for help in some circumstances or may be able to keep his or her head above water but unable to make progress to safety. Since it can be difficult sometimes to know whether someone like this in the water needs help, it is better to offer assistance than to wait until it is obvious that the person is drowning.
- **A responsive drowning victim** cannot swim, float, or tread water effectively and is at immediate risk for drowning. This victim is struggling just to keep his or her head out of the water and is in a panic state. This victim is very unlikely to call for help. You may see the victim's face just above the surface or bobbing in and out, and the victim's arms may be flailing. The victim is clearly struggling, however, rather than treading water or moving forward at all.
- **An unresponsive drowning victim** is no longer breathing. This victim may be (1) a swimmer who became too exhausted to tread water or even float, (2) a nonswimmer who can no longer keep his or her face up to breathe and

has stopped struggling, or (3) a swimmer or nonswimmer who has experienced an injury or sudden illness (such as heart attack or hypothermia) that prevented him or her from swimming or staying at the surface, resulting in submersion and respiratory arrest. Breathing stops either when water enters the lungs or when water in the larynx causes a spasm that closes the airway. When breathing stops, the victim soon becomes unresponsive. Depending on the victim's body composition and the presence or absence of air in the lungs, this victim may be floating face-down at the surface or may be underwater.

When you recognize any of these scenarios, quick action is needed to rescue the victim. Your choice of rescue technique depends on the type of situation, the equipment or objects at hand, and the circumstances. Resist the temptation to jump immediately into the water to save the victim. An actively drowning victim is in a state of panic that often leads to the victim grabbing you so forcefully and desperately that you may become a drowning victim yourself. The victim may grab your head or arms in a way that you can neither swim back to safety nor tread water to keep both of you afloat. Lifeguards receive special training in how to manage such victims: they are trained to keep a rescue tube between themselves and the victim to avoid being grabbed and also to break a victim's hold underwater should it become necessary.

Even a tired swimmer who is not yet struggling and panicking may become panicked before you reach him or her. Therefore it is a poor choice to swim out to assist this kind of victim as well.

It may be appropriate to swim to an unresponsive victim, however, if you have no other means to get the victim quickly out of the water so that you can give CPR if needed. Similarly, a responsive small child may be rescued by an adult who is a good swimmer—although even children may cling tenaciously to one's head or arms when panicked, making a swimming rescue difficult or dangerous for the adult.

The safest and often most effective rescue technique is to reach to the victim with some object that the victim can grasp while you pull him or her to safety. The second-most safe and effective technique is to throw something that floats to the victim, preferably with a rope attached for pulling the victim to safety. Third, and least safe and effective, is to go to the victim yourself. This is called the **reach-throw-go** priority, which emphasizes which techniques to try first.

"Reach" Rescue

Most public and some private pools have a rescue pole, which often has a hook at the end (called a **shepherd's crook**). This pole is usually long enough to reach a victim from the edge of the pool. Let a responsive victim hold onto it while you slowly pull the victim to the edge (**Figure 25-3**). If the victim is unresponsive, you can hook the victim's body to pull the victim to the edge or shallow water. Unless the unresponsive victim is a small child, pulling an unresponsive victim to the edge will be faster than jumping in to tow the victim to the pool's edge.

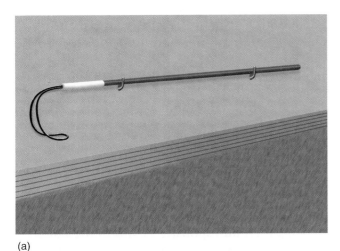

(a)

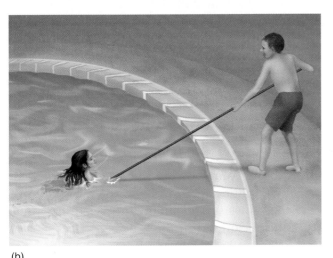

(b)

Figure 25-3 (a) Shepherd's crook. (b) Pulling a victim to safety with a reaching rescue.

Use anything available to reach to the victim. A residential pool may not have a reaching pole, but a broom or rake handle may work just as well. In open water settings you may use a fishing pole, a boat's oar, or even a long branch. If the victim is close enough to the pool's edge, a dock, or shore, you may also reach with your own body; for example, you could hold onto something secure with your arms and extend your legs on the surface to the victim.

In a natural water setting in which the water gradually gets deeper from the shore, you may be able to reach to the victim with an object after wading a short distance into the water. If possible, stay in water shallow enough for you to stand on the bottom while reaching to the victim.

"Throw" Rescue

If you cannot reach to the victim, look for anything that floats that you can throw. Swimming pool or boating equipment may include a life ring, rescue tube, lifejacket, or other devices (**Figure 25-4**). Some boats carry a throw bag, which has a coiled rope inside that uncoils when the bag is thrown to a victim while you hold the other end. If no throwable rescue device is available, look around for anything that will float—such as a buoyant seat cushion, a water jug that can be mostly emptied (keep some water inside to give it weight for throwing), or even an empty soft drink cooler.

If a rope is already attached to the throwable device (or can quickly be tied on), hold it in one hand, coil the rope loosely, and throw with your stronger arm. Try to throw it over the victim so that the line comes down beside the person and can be easily grasped (**Figure 25-5**).

If you have no rope handy for the throw device, throw it to the victim anyway if it is buoyant enough to help the victim keep his or her head above water. A victim who can float by holding onto something can breathe more easily and may have the strength to kick to shore while holding the object. Even if the victim is too weak to do anything but just hold on, the thrown object can keep the victim safely afloat while you find a rope or something to reach with. Even if you must enter the water to go to the victim, a victim who is holding onto something that floats is much less likely to panic and grab you, and you can more easily tow the object and victim to safety.

In a natural water setting in which the water gradually gets deeper from the shore, you may be better able to throw a rope or floating object to

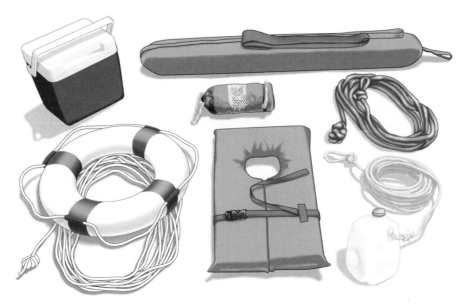

Figure 25-4 Rescue devices and objects that can be thrown to a drowning victim.

the victim after wading out into the water to get closer to the victim. If possible, stay in water shallow enough for you to stand on the bottom while throwing to the victim.

"Go" Rescue

As noted earlier, swimming to rescue a responsive victim is very dangerous—so much so that unless you have training, you should not attempt this except with a small child or unresponsive victim. Look for other ways to go to the victim. At a waterfront you may find a surfboard, kayak, or other watercraft in which to go to the victim. Even if it is too small to support both of you, it likely has enough buoyancy to keep you both

afloat until help arrives, or the victim may be able to hold onto it for buoyancy while you tow him or her to shore. Wear a lifejacket when entering the water or going in a boat to the victim. Remember that the victim is likely panicking, and keep the object between you and the victim so that you cannot be grabbed and pulled underwater. The same is true if you decide to swim to a responsive victim: if at all possible take something with you that the victim can hold onto, and that you can release if the victim tries to grab you, and keep the object between you and the victim.

Note: if an unresponsive victim in the water may have a spinal injury (e.g., a diving incident), take care to stabilize the head and neck before removing the victim from the water, if possible.

Walking Assist

Many natural bodies of water gradually get deeper away from the shore. If a responsive victim in the water is at a depth where he or she can stand, or if you can assist the victim to that depth, you can help the victim to exit the water with a **walking assist (Figure 25-6)**. Put the victim's arm around your shoulder and hold it at the wrist with your hand. Put your other arm around the victim's waist, and support the victim as you walk the person out of the water.

Beach Drag

An unresponsive victim who is in or can be brought to shallow water with a gradual shoreline can be taken from the water using a **beach drag (Figure 25-7)**.

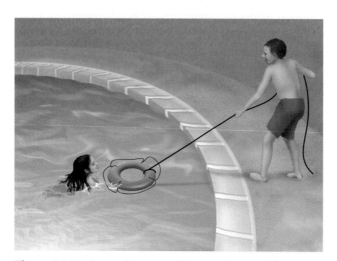

Figure 25-5 Throw the rescue device where the victim can grab it or the rope.

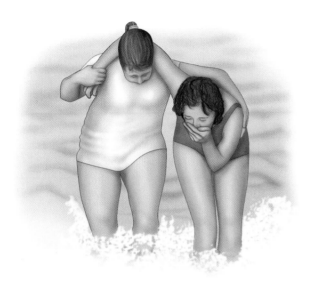

Figure 25-6 Walking assist.

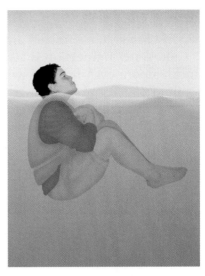

Figure 25-8 The HELP position to minimize body heat loss.

Reach under the victim's shoulders and hold the victim at the armpits, resting the victim's head on your forearms (and preventing head or neck movement in case of a possible spinal injury). Then slowly back out of the water, dragging the victim out. This rescue technique is similar to the shoulder drag used to move an unresponsive victim on land from a hazardous scene, shown later in this chapter.

If Stranded in Cold Water

If you are immersed in cold water and cannot swim to safety or climb out of the water onto an overturned boat or other floating object, try to minimize heat loss from your body while awaiting rescue. If alone, use the heat escape lessening position (HELP): hold your arms close to your

sides and raise your knees to your chest, and remain as still as possible **(Figure 25-8)**.

Two or more people together in cold water should use the huddle position to conserve heat: everyone puts arms around each others' shoulders to bring the sides of your chests together (if three or more) in a tight circle **(Figure 25-9)**. Sandwich a child between adults.

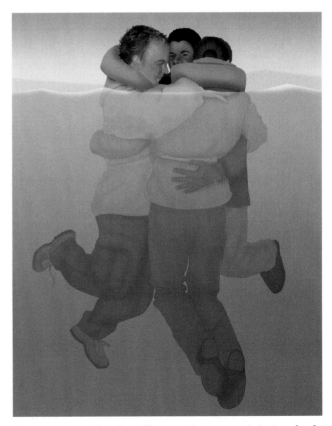

Figure 25-9 The huddle position to minimize body heat loss.

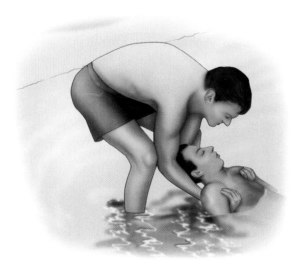

Figure 25-7 Beach drag.

Ice Rescue

As described in **Chapter 2**, ice rescues are very dangerous. Cold-water immersion is very serious and can quickly doom even the best swimmers. Ice rescue should be left for specially trained personnel who have the necessary safety equipment. Call 9-1-1 immediately to summon emergency personnel.

If safe to do so and emergency personnel will not arrive in time, you may attempt an ice rescue using the same priorities as a water rescue: reach-throw-go. Try first to reach to the victim who has broken through ice using a pole or tree limb (**Figure 25-10**). If you cannot reach to the victim, throw a rope or any buoyant object tied to a rope. As a last resort, throw any object that will float to help the victim stay afloat, but be aware that in icy water hypothermia sets in very quickly and the victim will not be able to hold onto an object very long. Only as an extreme last resort should you try to go to the

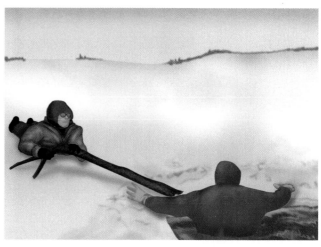

Figure 25-10 Try to reach to a victim who has fallen through ice.

victim yourself. Realize that the ice may not hold your weight and that you too may become a victim. If you must go on the ice, lie down to distribute your weight over a larger surface

Learning
Checkpoint (1)

1. With a fire, the first action to take is

    a. get everyone out and call 9-1-1.   **b.** throw water on the fire immediately.

    c. use a fire extinguisher.   **d.** close all doors and windows.

2. If you are caught in a building that is on fire,

    a. stay low to the floor.   **b.** feel doors before opening them.

    c. use stairs, not the elevator.   **d.** All of the above

3. True or False: OSHA requires fire prevention and safety guidelines in the workplace.

4. True or False: The first action to take with a spilled dry chemical is to vacuum it up.

5. True or False: Spilled liquids may produce poisonous fumes.

6. You are the first on the scene where a car has crashed into a telephone pole. After you make sure that the scene is safe, you approach the car and find the driver alone, slumped forward against the steering wheel, unresponsive. What can you do to help?

_____

7. The safest order in which to attempt a water rescue is

    a. throw-reach-go.   **b.** go-throw-reach.

    c. reach-throw-go.   **d.** reach-go-throw.

area. Another person should hold your feet and be prepared to pull you out if the ice under you breaks. If possible, push a branch or other object ahead of you to the victim to minimize the distance you must go onto the ice.

Following ice rescue, the victim is likely to need treatment for hypothermia (**Chapter 21**).

MULTIPLE VICTIMS

An incident such as a car crash or a workplace explosion may involve multiple victims who need first aid care. In such a case the first thing you must do, after calling 9-1-1 to get help on the way, is decide who needs your care most and who can wait until others can help. This process of setting priorities is called **triage** (**Figure 25-11**).

Triage systems usually put each victim into one of four categories (**Table 25-1**). Since the goal of triage is to determine which victim(s) require immediate care, this process should be done very quickly. As you check the scene for safety and approach, ask who can walk and have these victims move to one side—they are the third priority. Try to assess each of the remaining victims in less than a minute by checking for responsiveness, breathing, and severe bleeding; do not start to give care to any victim until you have quickly checked all. If a victim is very severely injured and is not breathing, and there are other victims requiring your immediate care, you should attend to others who you judge can be saved. This situation can require a difficult decision, but remember that giving BLS to an obviously dying victim may mean that someone who could have been saved may not be.

Because a victim's condition may change during the process of triage or giving care, you may have to change priorities. For example, if you are treating a second-priority victim with a fracture, another victim who at first seemed to have only minor injuries (third priority) may suddenly become unresponsive and require your immediate attention (first priority) to maintain an open airway (see First Aid: "Multiple Victims").

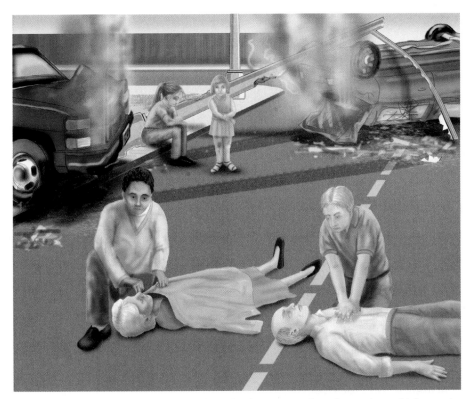

Figure 25-11 In an emergency with multiple victims, first determine which are the highest priority for first aid.

Table 25-1

Triage Priorities for Multiple Victims

Priority	Victim's Condition	Severity	Examples
First	Critical	Victims with life-threatening injuries who cannot wait for help	Airway or breathing problems Severe bleeding Shock Severe burn
Second	Serious	Victims with injuries that need care very soon but may be able to wait for help	Burns Broken bones Other injuries not severely bleeding
Third	Stable	Victims who can wait for some time	Minor injuries Victims who can walk
Fourth	Obviously dead or dying	Victims who cannot be saved	Not breathing after an attempt to open the airway (unless there are no first-priority victims)

First Aid   Multiple Victims

When You See

- **Two or more victims needing care**

Do This First

1 Call 9-1-1 immediately. Tell the dispatcher there are multiple victims.

2 Ask any victims who can walk (third priority) to move to one side. These victims do not have immediately life-threatening problems.

3 With the remaining victims, starting with unresponsive victims, quickly check for breathing and severe bleeding looking for life-threatening injuries in victims who can be saved (first priority). Spend a minute or less with each victim, and do not start giving care until you have checked all victims.

4 Start providing BLS to first-priority victims first. Move to second-priority victims only when the first-priority victims are stable. Ask any bystanders with first aid training to help you with other victims.

5 When help arrives, quickly tell the EMS professionals about the victims present. Offer to help them care for victims.

Learning
Checkpoint ②

1. True or False: A victim with a broken arm is a second priority in a multiple-victim incident.

2. True or False: Victims with life-threatening injuries are first priority in a multiple-victim incident.

3. You are alone at a construction site where a collapsed wall has injured four workers. Using standard triage priorities, rank these four in terms of who gets care first, second, third, and fourth:

   ____ **a.** A woman with a bruised face and abrasions on her arms, who is walking around holding her bleeding forehead.

   ____ **b.** A man on the ground with no apparent external injuries but who is unresponsive.

   ____ **c.** A man who is not breathing, whose chest has caved in under a steel beam, and who is surrounded by a pool of blood.

   ____ **d.** A man sitting up and leaning against the rubble, looking very pale, who says he feels nauseous.

MOVING VICTIMS

Moving an injured victim is more likely to cause further injury than not. In most cases you should wait for professionals who have training and equipment to transport the victim to advanced medical care.

In some instances, however, you must move a victim to protect him or her from a danger at the scene, such as a spreading fire, the chance of an explosion, or to escape a structure at risk of collapse (**Figure 25-12**). *Remember: never enter a scene unless you can do so safely.* You may also have to move a victim to a firm, flat surface in order to provide CPR. If you decide to move a victim, several factors are involved in choosing the best method (see First Aid: "Moving Victims"):

• How quickly must the victim be moved?
• Does the victim's condition affect the move (nature of injury, responsiveness, potential spinal injury, etc.)?

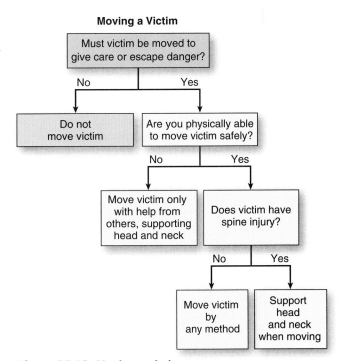

Figure 25-12 Moving a victim.

First Aid   First Aid: Moving Victims

When You See

Consider moving a victim only if:

- Fire or explosion is likely.
- Poisonous fumes may be present.
- The structure may collapse.
- The victim needs to be moved into position for life-saving care such as CPR.
- The victim is in the way of another seriously injured victim.

Do This First

1 Try to move the victim only if you are physically able and can do it safely.

2 Get help from others at the scene.

3 With an unresponsive victim or a victim with a spinal injury, support the head and neck in line with the body during the move.

4 Use good body mechanics.

5 **If alone:**
For an unresponsive victim with suspected spinal injury:

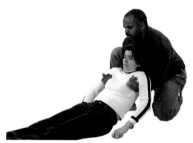

- For a short distance, use the **shoulder drag** (supporting the victim's head against your chest) or the **clothes drag** (supporting the victim's head with clothing taut between your hands).

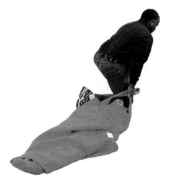

- Use the **blanket drag** to support the victim's head for a longer distance.

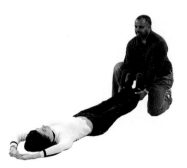

For an unresponsive victim without a spinal injury:
- The **ankle drag** is easier to use for short distances over a smooth surface.

First Aid   **First Aid: Moving Victims** *(continued)*

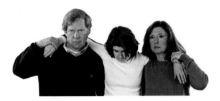

For a responsive victim who can walk with help:
- Use the one- or two-person **walking assist.**

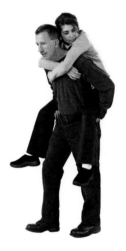

- Use a **piggyback carry** for responsive victims.

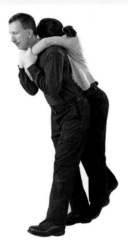

For an unresponsive victim who cannot safely be moved with a drag (if you are strong enough to lift the victim):
- Use the **packstrap carry.**

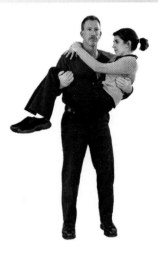

For a lighter victim or child:
- Use a **cradle carry** for responsive or unresponsive victims.

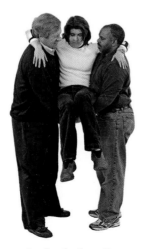

6 **With the help of one or more others:**
For a responsive victim:
- Use the two-person assist or **two-handed seat carry.**

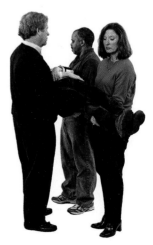

For an unresponsive victim:
- Use three to six rescuers with the **hammock carry.**

- Are others present who can help with the move?
- Is any equipment (e.g., stretcher) or other object (e.g., blanket) needed?
- Do you have the physical strength needed to move the victim?

Whenever you lift a victim, be sure to use good body mechanics. This means:

- Do not try to lift more weight than you can lift without straining.
- Lift with your legs instead of your back. Keep your feet shoulder-width apart with one foot in front of the other. Keep your back straight and crouch down, then lift by straightening your legs.
- Do not turn or twist your back while bearing weight.
- Bear the victim's weight as close to your trunk as possible.
- Take short steps, and move forward rather than backward.

Learning Checkpoint 3

1. Check situations in which you should consider moving a victim:

___ Fire is present   ___ Bleeding victim inside a car

___ Cold environment   ___ Strong smell of natural gas in the room

___ Small child with severe burns   ___ The hospital is only a short drive

___ A victim going into shock   ___ A victim is lying on top of another

2. If you have to move an unresponsive injured victim by yourself, an effective method would be

a. sling the victim over your shoulder.

b. roll the victim over the ground like a log.

c. grab both of the victim's wrists and pull him or her along.

d. use a blanket drag to support the victim's head.

Concluding Thoughts

Remember that your own safety must be assured before rescuing or moving a victim in any situation. Pause to think and plan before acting, and then move carefully to protect both yourself and the victim from further injury.

Learning Outcomes

You should now be able to do the following:

1. Describe how to rescue or care for a victim in each of the following emergencies:
   - A fire scene
   - A hazardous materials incident
   - A vehicle crash
   - A potential drowning situation
   - Broken ice

2. Describe how to prioritize the care for multiple victims with different types of injuries.

3. Explain when it may be necessary to move a victim.

4. Demonstrate the following emergency moves:
   - Shoulder drag
   - Clothes drag
   - Ankle drag
   - Blanket drag
   - Walking assist
   - Packstrap carry
   - Cradle carry
   - Piggyback carry
   - Two-handed seat carry
   - Hammock carry with multiple rescuers

Review Questions

1. If the emergency scene is very dangerous, you should
   a. run in quickly and give lifesaving care to the victim.
   b. run in quickly and pull the victim to safety.
   c. call 9-1-1 and wait for professionals with appropriate training and equipment.
   d. rescue the victim if help has not arrived five minutes after calling 9-1-1.

2. It is safe to enter the scene of a fire when
   a. you can keep at least 15 feet away from flames.
   b. you can crouch below the smoke to breathe.
   c. you know a victim inside needs help.
   d. It is never safe to enter a fire scene.

3. Which of these statements is true?
   a. Poisonous fumes from a spilled substance are always visible.
   b. Poisonous fumes are not present if you see "normal" black smoke at a fire.
   c. Dangerous fumes are lighter than air and always rise to the ceiling.
   d. Invisible dangerous fumes may be present at any fire or hazardous materials spill.

4. Which action is appropriate for a victim of a vehicle crash with suspected spinal injury?
   a. Support the victim's head in place with your hands, remaining in the vehicle.
   b. Support the victim's head in place with your hands while you help the victim to exit the vehicle.
   c. Use a splint to support the victim's head while you help the victim to exit the vehicle.
   d. Use the clothes drag to support the victim's head while you pull the victim from the vehicle.

5. How can you tell if someone in the water may be drowning?
   a. The person is swimming only slowly toward a destination.
   b. The person is struggling to keep his or her mouth above the water.
   c. The person always calls out for help.
   d. The person waves both arms high above his or her head.

6. Which water rescue technique should you try first?
   a. Throwing a rope to the victim
   b. Throwing the victim a ring buoy with a rope tied to it
   c. Reaching to the victim with a pole or tree branch
   d. Swimming to the victim with a flotation device

7. When you are alone and encounter a vehicle crash scene with four victims, which of these victims should you help first?
   a. The driver, who is slumped over the wheel and not breathing, his chest bloody, with a pool of blood on the seat beside him
   b. A front-seat passenger who has a cut on the forehead and a sprained wrist, who gets out of the vehicle as you approach
   c. An unresponsive rear-seat passenger who is not breathing
   d. A responsive rear-seat passenger who says she thinks her leg is broken

8. How you move a victim in an emergency may depend on
   a. whether the victim is in shock.
   b. whether others are present.
   c. whether you have medical exam gloves with you.
   d. whether the victim is wearing a medical ID.

9. Which of these emergency moves provides the best head and neck support for an unresponsive victim with a suspected spinal injury?
   a. Clothes drag
   b. Ankle drag
   c. Cradle carry
   d. Piggyback carry

10. Good body mechanics includes
    a. lifting with your legs rather than your back.
    b. not twisting your back when carrying weight.
    c. taking short steps.
    d. All of the above

References and Resources

American Academy of Pediatrics. Prevention of drowning in infants, children, and adolescents. www.aap.org

American Heart Association. 2005 International consensus on cardiopulmonary resuscitation (CPR) and emergency cardio-vascular care (ECC) science with treatment recommendations. *Circulation*, 112(22). November 29, 2005.

National Center for Injury Prevention and Control. Water-related injuries fact sheet. 2005. www.cdc.gov/ncipc/factsheets/drown.htm

National Safety Council. www.nsc.org

Office of Hazardous Materials Safety, U.S. Department of Transportation. http://hazmat.dot.gov

Chapter 26

Are You Prepared?

Chapter Preview

- Before an Emergency Strikes
- After an Emergency Strikes
- Evacuation
- Natural Disasters
- Biological Threats
- Chemical Threats
- Nuclear Explosions and Radiological Contamination
- Recovering from an Emergency

It is late Saturday afternoon and you have been so busy doing household chores that you have barely noticed the thunderstorm moving in from the west. You glance out a window and see the sky is turning black. You remember you left the car windows open and go out to raise them before the rain starts, and as you come around the corner of the house you see a funnel cloud apparently less than a mile away. What should you do?

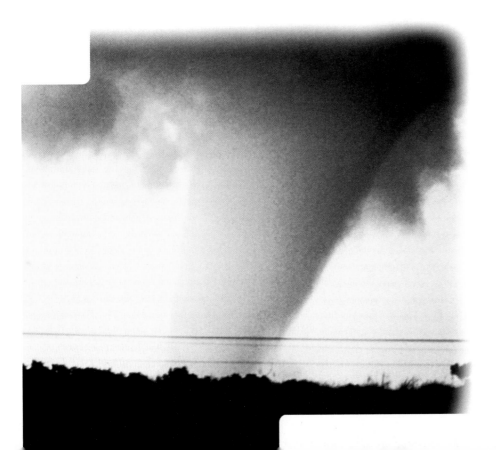

This guide will help you to*

- learn what to do before, during, and after an emergency.
- create an emergency plan for your family.
- prepare an Emergency Go Kit.

BEFORE AN EMERGENCY STRIKES

During an emergency, you and your family may have little or no time to plan what to do next. You must learn about the things you can do to be prepared before an emergency occurs. Two actions that will help you to do this are to develop an emergency plan and to prepare an Emergency Go Kit.

Create an Emergency Plan

Part of creating your household emergency plan is to learn about the types of emergencies that may affect your community, how you will be notified of an emergency, and plans that may already be in place to deal with emergencies. Determine if your community has a warning system—via television, radio, or another signal—and learn what it sounds like and what to do when you hear it. Emergencies may strike when your family members are away from home, so find out about plans at your workplace, school, or anywhere else you and your family spend time. Steps to take in creating a household emergency plan include:

1. Meeting with household members to discuss the dangers of possible emergency events, including fire, severe weather, hazardous spills, and terrorism.
2. Discussing how you and your family will respond to each possible emergency.
3. Discussing what to do in case of power outages or personal injuries.
4. Drawing a floor plan of your home. Mark two escape routes from each room.
5. Teaching adults how to turn off the water, gas, and electricity at main switches. If for any reason you do turn off natural gas service to your home, call your gas utility company to

restore service. *Do not attempt to restore gas service yourself.*

6. Posting emergency contact numbers near all telephones, and pre-program emergency numbers into phones with autodial capabilities.
7. Teaching children how and when to dial 9-1-1 to get emergency assistance.
8. Teaching children how to make long-distance telephone calls and/or to use a cell phone.
9. Choosing a friend or relative that all family members will call if separated (it is often easier to call out-of-state during an emergency than within the affected areas).
10. Instructing household members to turn on the radio for emergency information.
11. Picking two meeting places:
    - A place near your home
    - A place outside your neighborhood in case you cannot return home after an emergency
12. Taking a first aid and CPR class.
13. Keeping family records in a waterproof and fireproof safe. Inexpensive models can be purchased at most hardware stores.

Prepare an Emergency Go Kit

Often during an emergency, electricity, water, heat, air conditioning, or telephone service may not work. Preparing an Emergency Go Kit ahead of time can save precious time in the event you must evacuate or go without electricity, heat, or water for an extended period of time. You should consider including the following items in an Emergency Go Kit:

1. At least a three-day supply of water (one gallon per person per day). Store water in sealed, unbreakable containers. Replace every six months.
2. A three- to five-day supply of nonperishable packaged or canned food and a nonelectric can opener.
3. A change of clothing, rain gear, and sturdy shoes.
4. Blankets, bedding, or sleeping bags.
5. A first aid kit and prescription medications (be sure to check the expiration dates).
6. An extra pair of glasses or contact lenses and solution (be sure to check the expiration dates).
7. A list of family physicians, important medical information, and the style and serial number of medical devices such as pacemakers.
8. Special items for infants, the elderly, or family members with disabilities.

*This chapter is adapted from the "Federal Employees' Family Preparedness Guide" prepared by the United States Office of Personnel Management.

9. A battery-powered radio, flashlight, and plenty of extra batteries (or hand-cranked radio and flashlight).
10. Identification, credit cards, cash, and photocopies of important family documents, including home insurance information.
11. An extra set of car and house keys.
12. Tools such as screwdrivers, cutters, and scissors, duct tape, waterproof matches, a fire extinguisher, flares, plastic storage containers, needle and thread, pen and paper, a compass, garbage bags, and regular household bleach.

Know the Plans of Your School System

If you have a child who attends school, it is important for you to contact your school system administrators to understand fully what plans are in place to protect your child in the event of an emergency.

Be sure to keep the contact information for your child up to date. Provide your school administrators with a list of family members or caregivers who you authorize to pick up your child or children at school.

If a dangerous substance were released in the atmosphere and posed a threat to students during the school day, it is very likely that the schools affected would shelter-in-place and protect children and staff by keeping them inside and moving them to safer areas within the school building.

Prescriptions

Store three to five days of medications that are important to your health.

Include any medications that are used to stabilize a medical condition or keep a condition from worsening or resulting in hospitalization, such as medications for asthma, seizures, cardiovascular disorders, diabetes, psychiatric conditions, HIV, and thyroid disorders.

Carry these with you, if possible, in a purse or briefcase in labeled containers. Rotate these medications whenever you get your prescriptions refilled. If your child takes medications, communicate with the school to discuss their emergency preparedness plans.

People with complex medication regimens should talk to their physician and pharmacist to help with emergency preparation plans. Such regimens include: injectable medications, including those delivered by pumps (e.g., insulin, analgesics, chemotherapy, parenteral nutrition); medications delivered by a nebulizer (e.g., antibiotics, bronchodilators); and dialysis.

Neighbors Helping Neighbors

Working with neighbors in an emergency can save lives and property. Meet with your community members to plan how you could work together until help arrives. If you are a member of a neighborhood organization, such as a home association or crime watch group, introduce emergency preparedness as a new activity.

If You Have Pets

If you evacuate, avoid leaving family pets behind. However, keep in mind that with the exception of service animals, pets are generally not permitted in emergency shelters for health reasons.

For this reason, find out before a disaster occurs which hotels or motels (both within and outside your local area) allow pets. Determine where pet boarding facilities are located.

Create an emergency kit for your pet. This should include:

- Identification tag and rabies tags worn on a collar at all times
- Carrier or cage
- Leash
- Any medications (be sure to check expiration date)
- Newspapers and plastic bags for handling waste
- A supply of food, bottled water, and food bowls
- Veterinary records (most animal boarding facilities do not allow pets without proof of vaccination)

For complete information, the American Society for the Prevention of Cruelty to Animals has an emergency preparedness guide designed

THINGS TO THINK ABOUT . . .

If any members of your household have disabilities or are elderly, find out what services may be available to aid in their care or evacuation in the event of an emergency.

specifically for pets at http://www.aspca.org/site/PageServer?pagename=emergency.

AFTER AN EMERGENCY STRIKES

Shelter-in-Place

In the event of an emergency such as the release of a hazardous material, it is not always recommended that you immediately evacuate because leaving your house might expose you to harmful agents that have been dispersed into the air. "Sheltering-in-place," which means simply staying in your house or current location, may be the best means to avoid harm. Federal agencies have protocols in place at every agency to shelter-in-place at the workplace if circumstances warrant that action. Federal employees can ask their managers for more information about the procedures in place at their agency.

If Your Power Goes Out

1. Remain calm, and assist family members or neighbors who may be vulnerable if exposed to extreme heat or cold.
2. Locate a flashlight with batteries to use until power comes back on. Do not use candles—this can cause a fire.
3. Turn off sensitive electric equipment such as computers, VCRs, and televisions.
4. Turn off major electric appliances that were on when the power went off. This will help prevent power surges when electricity is restored.
5. Keep your refrigerator and freezer doors closed as much as possible to keep cold in and heat out.
6. Do not use the stove to heat your home.
7. Use extreme caution when driving. If traffic signals are out, treat each signal as a stop sign—come to a complete stop at every intersection and look before you proceed.
8. Do not call 9-1-1 to ask about the power outage.
9. Listen to the news radio stations for updates.

If You Need Clean Water

Flooding can cause contamination of water supplies. Contaminated water can contain microorganisms that cause diseases such as dysentery, typhoid, and hepatitis. If you think your water may be contaminated, you should purify it before using it. This includes water used for drinking, cooking, cleaning dishes, or bathing. The best way to purify water is to boil it.

Boiling

Boiling is considered the safest method of purifying water. Bring water to a boil for three to five minutes, and then allow it to cool before drinking. Pouring water back and forth between two containers will improve the taste by putting oxygen back into the water.

EVACUATION

If you are notified or become aware of a technological hazards emergency such as a hazardous spill/release, fire, or explosion, do not panic. If you need to get out of the surrounding area or are directed to evacuate, do so immediately and:

- Take your Emergency Go Kit.
- Lock your home.
- Cover your nose and mouth with a wet cloth.
- Travel on routes specified by local authorities.
- Head upwind of the incident.

If you are sure you have time:

- Shut off water, gas, and electricity before leaving.
- Post a note telling others when you left and where you are going.
- Make arrangements for your pets.

If you are instructed to stay inside and not to evacuate:

- Close and lock windows and doors.
- Seal gaps under doorways and windows with wet towels or seal with plastic and duct tape.
- Turn off ventilation systems.

Prepare Your Evacuation Routes in Advance

Many major cities have established evacuation routes that can be used to effectively move people from heavily populated areas in the event of an emergency. For instance, the city of Washington, D.C. has identified 14 major arterials that will be used for outbound traffic only. During a major event or emergency situation, radial evacuation routes featuring traffic signals will be timed. In addition, critical intersections on evacuation routes will be manned with uniformed police officers to expedite the flow of traffic and to prevent bottlenecks. Officers will be able to direct drivers to alternate routes should an emergency warrant the closing of current event/evacuation routes.

If you work or live in a heavily populated area, you should prepare in advance the best available routes for you to use in the event that you need to quickly leave the area. Contact your local police or other local emergency preparedness offices for protocols that will be in place in your area during an evacuation.

NATURAL DISASTERS

Many areas are vulnerable to a variety of types of severe weather, including thunderstorms, hurricanes, flash floods, snowstorms, and tornadoes (see **Appendices C, D, E, F**).

It is important for you to understand the difference between a watch and a warning for severe weather. A severe storm watch means that severe weather may develop. A severe weather warning means a storm has developed and is on its way—take cover immediately!

The safest place to ride out any storm is inside a secure building or well-built home. Even in a well-built apartment building, you should

- listen to weather updates and stay informed.
- be ready to evacuate if necessary.
- keep away from windows and doors.
- have your Emergency Go Kit handy.

Tornadoes are dangerous because of their high winds and ability to lift and move heavy objects. If you receive a tornado warning, seek shelter immediately. If you are in your car:

- *Stop!* Get out and lie flat face down in a low area.
- Cover your head and wait for the tornado to pass.

If you are at home:

- Go to the basement or storm shelter, or rooms near the center of the house.

In a high-rise or other public building:

- Move to the interior, preferably a stairwell or hallway.

Flash flooding can be very dangerous because of strong, swift currents.

- Move immediately and quickly to higher ground. The force of six inches of swiftly moving water can knock people off their feet!
- If flood waters rise around your car, get out and move to higher ground immediately. Cars can be easily swept away in just two feet of moving water.

BIOLOGICAL THREATS

A biological attack is the deliberate release of germs or related substances. To affect individuals adversely, these substances must usually be inhaled, be ingested, or enter through cuts in the skin. Some biological agents such as smallpox can be spread from person to person, while others like anthrax do not cause contagious diseases.

Different than a conventional explosive or attack, biological attacks may not be immediately evident. Some of the normal indicators of this type of attack would be an increase in the number of illnesses reported by local healthcare workers or a large number of dead or sick animals throughout your area. These attacks are normally discovered by emergency response personnel in reaction to the indicators listed previously.

What Should You Do?

In the event that you witness a suspicious attack using an unknown substance, there are a number of things you can do to protect yourself and your family. First, leave the immediate area as quickly as possible and protect yourself by finding something to place over your nose and mouth. Any layered material like a T-shirt, handkerchief, or towel may help prevent particles of the substance from entering your respiratory system. If you have a long-sleeved shirt or jacket, they would be useful in covering exposed skin. They may also prevent bacteria from entering cuts you may have. If you are indoors and the suspected attack takes place outdoors, remain inside unless told otherwise by authorities. Report the attack to emergency personnel.

You can also take precautionary measures such as keeping shots up to date and making sure you practice good personal hygiene. A healthy body will be able to better fight any potential contamination by biological agents. In the event that anyone around you becomes ill, do not automatically assume that it is from the suspected attack because many of the symptoms from these attacks resemble common illnesses. Seek the medical advice of your physician.

CHEMICAL THREATS

Chemical attacks differ from biological attacks in that a toxic gas or liquid is used to contaminate people or the environment. The prevalent symptoms you would experience from a chemical attack are tightness in the chest, difficulty breathing, blurred vision, stinging of the eyes, or loss of coordination. It is worth noting that the public routinely accepts the risks posed by accidental release of chemicals. The response to an emergency event involving chemicals, however, is the same regardless of whether the emergency is a result of intentional or unintentional actions.

What Should You Do?

If you witness a suspected chemical attack outdoors, move laterally or upwind from the area as quickly as possible. If you cannot leave the area, try to get inside, away from direct exposure and follow your instructions to shelter-in-place. If you are inside and an attack occurs in your building, try to leave the area if possible. If you cannot, move to a safe location in the building and shelter-in-place.

If you experience any of the symptoms mentioned previously, try to remove any clothing you can and wash your body with water or soap and water if available. Do not scrub the area, as this may wash the chemical into the skin. Seek medical assistance as soon as possible. If you see someone experiencing these symptoms, keep them away from others as much as possible, and try to keep them comfortable.

While extensive decontamination requiring disrobing is a possibility, this will normally only occur if you become a casualty of the agent or are evacuated and require medical treatment in a "clean" medical facility. This procedure may be required to prevent the spread of contamination.

NUCLEAR EXPLOSIONS AND RADIOLOGICAL CONTAMINATION

A nuclear blast consists of tremendous thermal (heat), light, and blast energy. The blast can spread radioactive waste capable of contaminating the air and surrounding landscape. While this type of attack is less likely than a biological or chemical attack, the remote possibility of its occurrence means you should be prepared.

What Should You Do?

If a nuclear explosion occurs, immediately drop and stay down until any blast wave passes over you and it is safe to get up. Debris can often cause injuries from a nuclear explosion, so it is often safer to remain down until debris stops falling. Do not look at the blast. When it is safe to do so, seek shelter inside a building or basement. Since dirt or earth is one of the best forms of protection from radiation, put as much shelter between you and the potential contamination as possible. If it is safe to leave without going in the direction from which the blast came, you should decide whether to leave the area to minimize the amount of time you spend exposed to radiological contamination. You should always try to place as much shielding and distance between yourself and the contamination as possible and limit the amount of your exposure by leaving laterally or upwind from the area when it is safe to do so.

Dirty Bombs

Dirty bombs are regular explosives that have been combined with either radiation-causing material or chemical weapons. While most news reports talk about radiological dirty bombs, chemical agents may be used as well. Blasts from these types of weapons normally look more like a regular explosion, and the contamination spread is not often immediately noticeable. While this type of attack normally spreads contamination over a more localized area, you should be prepared to follow many of the same procedures as listed previously.

After experiencing any of these types of attacks, tune to your local channels for information and instructions. Emergency responders are trained and equipped to evaluate and react to threats arising from these incidents. After a nuclear blast, you may be unable to get a signal from radio or television stations for a period of time. This is expected; so be persistent.

While radioactive, biological, and chemical weapons do pose a threat, they are attacks that you and your family or fellow employees can survive if you keep a cool head and follow the instructions given by your local responders.

RECOVERING FROM AN EMERGENCY

Recovery continues even after you return home, as you and your family face the emotional and psychological effects of the event. Reactions vary from person to person, but may include:

- Restless sleep or nightmares
- Anger or desire for revenge
- Numbness or lack of emotion

- Needing to keep active, restlessness
- Needing to talk about your experiences
- Loss of appetite
- Weight loss or gain
- Headaches
- Mood swings

All of these are normal reactions to stressful events, and it is important to let people react in their own way. It may be helpful to:

- Talk with your family and friends about what happened and how you feel about it, and try

to evaluate and plan for the chance that it could happen again.

- Volunteer at a local shelter, blood bank, or food pantry to assist emergency victims.
- Consult with your minister or faith advisor.

In particular, children may need reassurance and extra attention. It is best to encourage them to share their feelings, even if you must listen to their stories repeatedly—this is a common way for children to grasp what they have experienced. You may also want to share your feelings about the event with them.

Concluding Thoughts

Events in recent years have made us all more aware of the possibilities of natural disasters, terrorist attacks, and other emergencies involving large-scale destruction. It is important to consider the risks for disasters in your own region and to take appropriate precautions. Simple preparations can make a huge difference for your safety and well-being should such a disaster strike.

Learning Outcomes

You should now be able to do the following:

1. List general steps for what to do before, during, and after an emergency.

2. Create an emergency plan for your family.

3. Prepare an Emergency Go Kit.

4. Describe specific actions to take in case of a natural disaster, chemical threat, or nuclear explosion.

5. List actions to help recover from an emergency.

Review Questions

1. Being prepared for an emergency includes knowing how to
   a. turn off the main electricity switch in your house.
   b. inspect a backpack found in a public place for a possible bomb.
   c. defend yourself in case of personal attack.
   d. restore your natural gas service when the emergency is over.

2. Whom should family members plan to call to locate each other if separated in an emergency?
   a. A nearby neighbor
   b. A local public official
   c. A distant friend or relative
   d. FEMA

3. When storing water for use after an emergency, calculate the amount needed per person per day:
   a. 1 gallon
   b. 2 gallons
   c. 3 gallons
   d. 4 gallons

4. If an emergency strikes, you should always
  a. stay in your home except in cases of rising water or fire.
  b. drive away from your home as soon as possible following an authorized evacuation route.
  c. go to the nearest nuclear fallout shelter in your community.
  d. follow instructions from emergency officials whether and when to evacuate.

5. The safest place to be if a severe storm strikes is
  a. inside your car in a garage.
  b. in the basement or in a room near the center of the building.
  c. near a doorway or exit for quick evacuation.
  d. in the attic or highest part of the home.

References and Resources

Department of Homeland Security: 1-800-BE-READY

FBI Joint Terrorism Task Force (24-hour line for reporting suspicious activity): (202) 278-2000

Federal Emergency Management Agency (FEMA): (202) 566-1600

National Weather Service: (301) 713-4000

Poison Control Center: (800) 222-1222

Department of Homeland Security. *Preparing makes sense. Get ready now.* 2005. www.ready.gov/readygov_brochurev2.pdf

Federal Emergency Management Agency. *Are you ready? A guide for citizen preparedness.* 2005. www.fema.gov/areyouready

Federal Office of Personnel Management. *Federal employee's emergency guide.* 2005. www.opm.gov/emergency

Federal Office of Personnel Management. *Manager's handbook on handling traumatic events.* 2005. www.opm.gov/emergency

Chapter 27

Moving Foward

Chapter Preview

- Acting with Confidence
- Key Principles of First Aid
- Prevention of Injury and Illness
- Going Forward

You are checking a co-worker's young son, who fell and hurt his arm while playing in the reception area near your office. The boy is calmer now, as you check for bleeding and potential musculoskeletal injury. When you first saw the boy crying in pain, you were worried you might not know what to do or might cause him more pain when you checked his arm, but you remembered your first aid training and realized you know what to do and can act confidently.

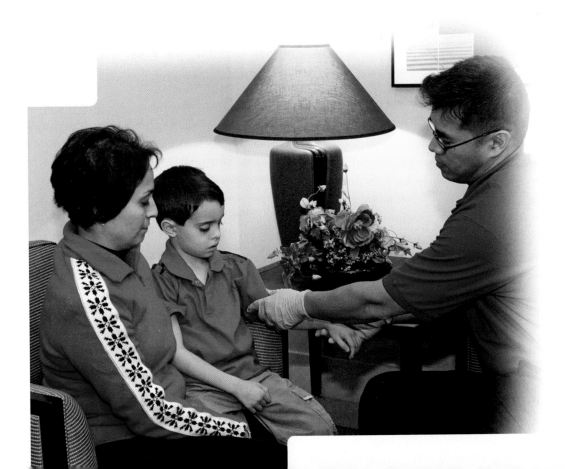

Having reached the end of this text and your first aid course, you should now feel confident that you know what to do in an emergency involving an injury or sudden illness. What is important now, as you move forward, is to remember the key principles of first aid so that you are ready to act without delay when needed.

ACTING WITH CONFIDENCE

It is only human to be concerned that when actually confronted with an emergency, a situation that is stressful for everyone involved, you may hesitate or feel unsure exactly what to do. You may worry that you have forgotten some of the details of certain kinds of first aid. You may be fearful of or reluctant to deal with an injury involving blood or other body fluids or with an emotional victim in pain. These are natural feelings we all share.

Nonetheless, you should feel confident in your abilities to provide first aid after completing this course. Experience has shown that even first aiders with less training than you very competently provide first aid when they encounter an emergency. There are many stories in the media about lay people saving a heart attack victim, stopping life-threatening bleeding, or pulling a drowning victim from the water. First aiders are often surprised how well they remember their training and are able to put their knowledge into action when suddenly called upon. Even if at some point in the future you forget some minor point, following the key principles of first aid is usually sufficient to help the victim for the few minutes before emergency medical personnel arrive.

KEY PRINCIPLES OF FIRST AID

Although this text has described in some detail the first aid for all common injuries and sudden illnesses, a simple set of key principles guides one's actions in all emergencies. Remember to follow these basic principles and you will be able to render valuable aid to all victims:

- **Stay calm.** Emergencies happen without warning, not giving us time to prepare ourselves emotionally or to carefully plan out our actions. The victim's pain and fears about what is happening, as well as the emotions of others at the scene, can cause panicky feelings that might lead to hasty or careless actions. It is very important to be calm when you respond to an emergency. Take a moment if necessary to gather your thoughts and energies. The victim and others at the scene will be reassured by your calm actions and will cope better with the situation. Remember: you have the training and know what to do until help arrives—be confident of your ability to help.

- **Call 9-1-1 for all serious emergencies and whenever in doubt.** In most areas in the United States, help is only a few minutes away once you call 9-1-1 or your local emergency number. Even if you are not near a telephone you can shout for help, and likely someone nearby will have a cell phone to call 9-1-1. Arriving EMS personnel will take over the care of the victim. If you are not sure how serious an injury or sudden illness is, call 9-1-1 anyway and tell the dispatcher the situation. Often the dispatcher can also advise you what care to give in case you are unsure what first aid is appropriate in this situation.

- **Remember your own safety.** As you take a moment to assess the situation and calm yourself before acting, remember to check the scene for any dangers before going to a help a victim. Avoid any temptation to act heroically if the scene is dangerous. Once you have called 9-1-1, personnel with special training and equipment will soon arrive who can better manage the dangers of the scene. If it is safe to give first aid, remember also to take steps to protect yourself from infectious disease.

- **Act quickly.** Although it is important to take a moment to calm yourself and plan your actions, remember that in many situations it is crucial not to delay before starting care for a life-threatening emergency. For example, a victim of cardiac arrest after a heart attack needs CPR and defibrillation immediately—every second counts once breathing and the heart stop. Call for an AED and call 9-1-1 and start CPR immediately if the victim is not breathing normally.

- **Check the victim.** Remember: first check for responsiveness, breathing, and severe bleeding, and give care immediately for life-threatening problems. If there are no immediate threats, perform a physical examination and take a SAMPLE history. This information will help you to know what first aid to give and will be valuable for responding EMS professionals.

- **Do no harm.** Do only what you have learned to do. Trying some first aid technique you heard about somewhere is risky, as people often are misinformed about what first aid is safe and effective. Call 9-1-1 and give basic first aid as you have learned in this course, and nothing you do will harm the victim. Recognize your limits as a lay first aider and do not try something you have not learned to do, such as trying to rescue a victim from a hazardous situation.

- **Ask others for help.** You may be the only one at the scene of an emergency with first aid training, but bystanders are often present and will help you if asked. You may need someone to keep pressure on a wound to control bleeding, for example, while you attend to another injury. Others can call 9-1-1 or bring a first aid kit or AED. Do not hesitate to ask.

PREVENTION OF INJURY AND ILLNESS

This text has emphasized the importance of acting to prevent injury and sudden illness. Effective prevention depends on understanding that most injuries and sudden illnesses *can* be prevented and on adopting an attitude that motivates acting on safety principles and adopting a healthy lifestyle.

The problem in injury and illness prevention is that knowledge alone does not always translate directly into action. Everyone from school-age children to adults knows that cigarette smoking causes cancer and heart disease, yet almost one-fourth of the population still smokes. Everyone knows that safety belts and shoulder harnesses help prevent injuries in automobiles, yet every year hundreds die or are seriously injured in vehicular crashes because they were not properly restrained. The statistics go on and on. Taking the time to act safely, and making the commitment to break unhealthy habits and adopt a healthy lifestyle, requires motivation. At this point you *know* what you need to do to invest in your future health and well-being—but it is also up to you to *care* enough to make the effort.

GOING FORWARD

As you conclude your first aid course, you probably are not thinking about future follow-up activities and refreshing your skills. It is important, however, to understand the need to stay current in your skills and knowledge, for two reasons. First, it is only human that over time we forget things and our skills become rusty. Second, new information often becomes available that changes how first aid should be given. For example, every five years an international group of emergency medical care professionals gathers to analyze the most recent research data and make recommendations for improvements in basic life support protocols. CPR techniques have changed over time and may change again in the future—and you may not learn about more effective techniques if you do not refresh your knowledge and skills.

Staying current in your knowledge and skills starts today. To help you remember what to do in different kinds of emergencies, keep this book in an appropriate place where you can consult it when needed.

You may also need additional first aid information at some future time. The Internet is an excellent source for current information, but be sure to trust only reputable websites. Much outdated or controversial information, as well as simply incorrect information, remains on private websites, but the sites for healthcare associations and governmental agencies generally have updated information. The agencies frequently referred to in this text, such as the Centers for Disease Control and Prevention (CDC), are excellent sources for new information; see the websites listed in the references and resources at the end of each chapter.

Depending on your field of study and career plans, you may also choose to take additional advanced or specialized first aid or emergency care courses. People working in settings where they are likely to be the first trained person on the scene of an injury or sudden illness, such as law enforcement or fire personnel, healthcare workers, and many others may take a First Responder or Professional Rescuer course. The National Safety Council has more information about these and other courses (www.nsc.org).

Even if you do not move on to more advanced courses, you should still periodically renew your essential skills by taking a refresher course. Everyone needs a CPR/AED refresher course periodically. Studies have shown that lay people who do not use their CPR skills often will not be as effective when called upon to give CPR long after their training. The information and techniques may also have changed.

Concluding Thoughts

Congratulations on the completion of your first aid course! You can now be confident that at work or at play, in the privacy of your home or when interacting with others in public places, you know what to do when an emergency occurs.

Learning Outcomes

You should now be able to do the following:

1. Act with confidence if needed in an emergency.

2. List seven key principles of first aid.

3. Take steps to prevent injury and illness— both for you and for your family.

4. Describe the actions needed to stay current in your first aid knowledge and skills.

Review Questions

1. Remember that a primary goal of first aid is to
   a. get a victim to a healthcare provider as quickly as possible.
   b. provide definitive medical care.
   c. provide care only for the few minutes it takes for help to arrive.
   d. administer medications as needed in an emergency.

2. When in doubt about how serious an injury or sudden illness is,
   a. always do as the victim wishes.
   b. call 9-1-1.
   c. perform an extensive physical examination.
   d. wait a few minutes to watch for changes in signs and symptoms.

3. Check the scene
   a. as soon as you arrive at the victim's side.
   b. as you approach the victim.
   c. as soon as you have checked the victim's breathing.
   d. before you go to the victim.

4. Perform the initial assessment of a victim
   a. for any immediate threats to life.
   b. after performing a physical examination.
   c. as you collect the SAMPLE history.
   d. by asking bystanders what happened.

5. The most important element for preventing injury and illness is
   a. memorizing all the rules about what to do or not do.
   b. being motivated for safety and a healthy lifestyle.
   c. frequently researching the latest medical studies.
   d. taking annual courses in injury prevention.

References and Resources

American Heart Association. 2005 International consensus on cardiopulmonary resuscitation (CPR) and emergency cardio-vascular care (ECC) science with treatment recommendations. *Circulation*, 112(22). November 29, 2005.

National Safety Council. www.nsc.org

Appendix

A Advanced Resuscitation Techniques

The skills included in this appendix are typically not taught to lay rescuers. Healthcare providers and rescuers at higher levels of training may be trained in some or all of these skills. As always, never attempt a skill in which you have not been appropriately trained. This appendix discusses the following topics:

- Definition of pediatric victims
- Assessment skills
  - Call first vs. call fast
  - Jaw thrust
  - Assessing breathing
  - Pulse check for circulation
- Ventilation skills
  - Rescue breathing without chest compressions
  - Resuscitation masks
  - Cricoid pressure
  - Airway suctioning
  - Bag-valve masks
  - Supplemental oxygen
  - Oral and nasal airways
- CPR skills
  - Hand position for chest compressions
  - Compressions for bradycardia in child
  - CPR
  - Two-rescuer CPR
- AED skills
- Special resuscitation situations
  - Trauma
  - Hypothermia
  - Near-drowning
  - Electric shock
  - Pregnancy

DEFINITION OF PEDIATRIC VICTIMS

Lay rescuers define a child as 1 to 8 years of age (to about 55 lbs and a height of about 50 inches) for all BLS skills including AED use. For purposes of using an AED, healthcare providers also consider a child to be age 8 or younger. For rescue breathing and CPR, however, healthcare providers should consider a victim a child from age 1 up to the onset of adolescence or puberty (defined by the occurrence of secondary sex characteristics such as armpit hair in boys and breast development in girls).

ASSESSMENT SKILLS

Healthcare providers and professional rescuers with higher training follow different BLS protocols from lay first aiders, and may use specialized equipment and supplies beyond basic personal protective equipment such as gloves and a resuscitation mask. Other equipment that may be of value in resuscitation situations includes suction devices, bag-valve-mask units, supplemental oxygen, and airways.

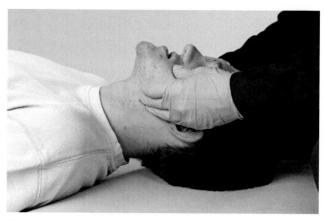

Figure A-1 The jaw thrust.

Call First vs. Call Fast

As a general rule, a healthcare provider alone with an adult victim should **call first** for help and an AED before providing CPR. For a child victim, **call fast** after providing about 5 cycles of CPR (about 2 minutes).

The rescue response should depend on the most likely cause of the victim's problem. **Call first** for a victim *of any age seen to collapse suddenly.* These victims are more likely to have a dysrhythmia and to require defibrillation. Calling EMS immediately starts the process of getting an AED to the victim sooner.

For unresponsive victims in cardiac arrest because of a likely asphyxial arrest, such as a downing victim or a child likely to have an airway obstruction, **call fast.** Give about 5 cycles of CPR (about 2 minutes) before stopping to call EMS.

The Jaw Thrust

Lay rescuers are generally taught to use the head tilt-chin lift technique to open the airway of an unresponsive victim lying on the back, regardless of whether there may be a spinal injury. The jaw thrust technique, which is less likely to cause additional injury in a victim with a spinal injury, is no longer recommended to be taught to lay rescuers because it is somewhat more difficult to perform. Healthcare providers, however, are often taught to use this technique.

With the jaw thrust, you do not tilt the head back to open the airway. Instead, only lift the jaw upward using both hands (**Figure A-1**). If you cannot successfully open the airway with the jaw

thrust, however, then switch to the head tilt, chin lift method.

Assessing Breathing

Lay rescuers are trained to look for "normal" breathing in adult victims. BLS healthcare providers, however, should look for "adequate" breathing in adults and the "presence or absence of breathing" in children and infants. In an adult who is not breathing adequately, therefore, do not wait for respiratory arrest before beginning to provide rescue breaths. If an adult victim is breathing at a rate less than 10 breaths per minute, take this as a sign of inadequate breathing. In an infant or child it is difficult for BLS rescuers to assess breathing adequacy, and abnormal breathing patterns may be adequate. Provide rescue breaths, therefore, to an infant or child who is not breathing.

Pulse Check

Lay rescuers are not recommended to check victims for circulation in the initial assessment but to start CPR for a victim who is not breathing. Healthcare providers, with a higher level of training, should in the initial assessment palpate for a pulse.

Remember the steps of the initial assessment as the ABCs: open the airway, check for breathing, and check for circulation. A victim with an obstructed airway needs care for choking. A victim who is not breathing but who has a pulse needs rescue breathing. A victim who is not breathing and does not have a pulse or signs of circulation needs CPR.

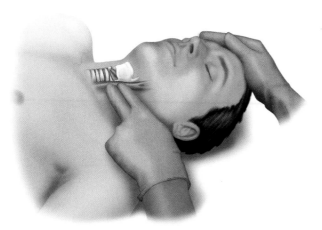

Figure A-2. Checking the carotid pulse in an adult or child.

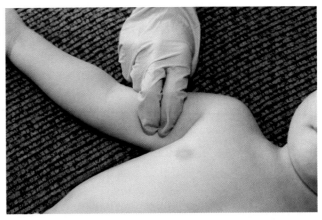

Figure A-4 Checking the brachial pulse in an infant.

To check the pulse in an adult or child, use the **carotid pulse** in the neck. Holding the victim's forehead with one hand to keep the airway open, put the index and middle fingers of your other hand on the side of the victim's neck nearer to you. Find the Adam's apple and then slide your fingertips toward you and down the neck to the groove at the side of the neck **(Figure A-2)**. Pressing gently, feel for a pulse for at least 5 but no more than 10 seconds. If a pulse cannot be definitely detected within 10 seconds, start CPR beginning with chest compressions. In a child, check either the carotid or femoral pulse. The femoral pulse is located in the center of the groin crease **(Figure A-3)**.

To check the pulse in an infant, use the **brachial pulse** in the inside of the upper arm instead of the carotid pulse. With one hand on the infant's forehead to maintain head position for an open airway, put the fingers of your other hand about midway between the shoulder and elbow on the inside of the arm and press gently, feeling for no more than 10 seconds **(Figure A-4)**.

Lack of a definite pulse along with the absence of other signs of circulation signifies that the heart has stopped or is not beating effectively enough to circulate blood.

If the victim lacks a pulse and other signs of circulation, start CPR and call for an AED to be brought to the scene.

An infant or child may have a pulse under 60 beats/minute and lack adequate perfusion. This victim also needs CPR (see later section "Compressions for Bradycardia in Child").

VENTILATION SKILLS

Rescue Breathing Without Chest Compressions

In some situations a victim may not be breathing adequately but still have a heartbeat. Someone pulled from the water in a near-drowning, for example, may have stopped breathing but still have a heartbeat. Healthcare providers trained in assessing for signs of circulation, when checking the ABCs in the initial assessment, may find a pulse in a nonbreathing victim. In this situation, chest compressions are not given while rescue breaths are provided, as described in the Skill: "Rescue Breathing."

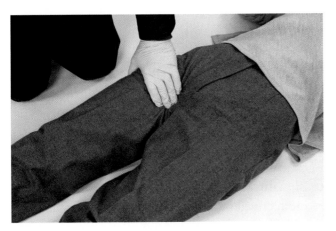

Figure A-3 Checking the femoral pulse.

Skill | Rescue Breathing

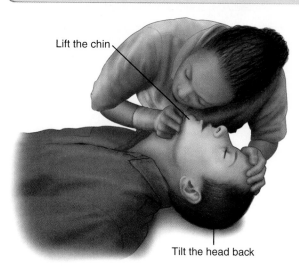

Lift the chin

Tilt the head back

1 Open the airway. Look, listen, and feel for adequate breathing for up to 10 seconds.

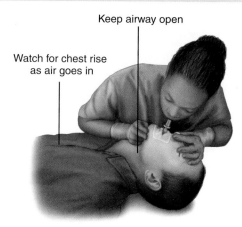

Keep airway open

Watch for chest rise as air goes in

2 If not breathing adequately, give 2 breaths over 1 second each, watching the chest rise and letting it fall.

3 If the first breath does not go in, try again to open the airway and give another rescue breath. If it still does not go in, the victim may be choking. Proceed to CPR for choking.

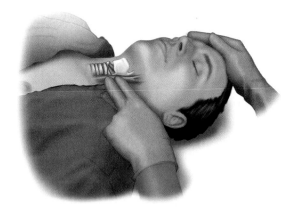

4 If your first 2 breaths go in, check the victim for no more than 10 seconds for a pulse and other signs of circulation. If there is a pulse but no adequate breathing, continue rescue breathing at rate of 10 to 12 breaths per minute (1 breath every 5–6 seconds) for an adult (or about 12 to 20 breaths per minute for a infant or child: 1 breath every 3–5 seconds), rechecking for a pulse about every minute. If there is no pulse, start CPR beginning with chest compressions.

((ALERT))

- Do not blow harder than is needed to make the chest rise.
- After each breath remember to let the air escape and the chest fall.
- Blowing in too forcefully or for too long is ineffective and may put air in the stomach, which may cause vomiting.
- Be careful not to tilt an infant's head too far back.

Resuscitation Masks

The resuscitation mask, often called a pocket face mask or simply a face mask, seals over the victim's mouth and nose and has a port through which the rescuer blows air to give rescue breaths. A one-way valve allows the rescuer's air in through the mouthpiece, but the victim's exhaled air exits the mask through a different opening.

When using a face mask, it is essential to seal the mask well to the victim's face while maintaining an open airway. How you hold the mask depends on your position by the victim, whether the head tilt-chin lift or jaw thrust technique is used to open the airway, and whether you have one or two hands free to seal the mask. The following hand positions assume you have both hands free to seal the mask, whether alone at the victim's side while performing CPR or at the victim's head (alone giving only rescue breathing, or with another rescuer who is providing chest compressions). When using a bag-valve-mask unit alone, you have only one hand free to seal the mask and therefore use a different hand position as described later.

From a position at the victim's side (when giving CPR) using the head tilt-chin lift:

1. With the thumb and index finger of your hand closer to the top of the victim's head, seal the top and sides of the mask to the victim's head as shown in **Figure A-5,a**.
2. Put the thumb of your second hand on the lower edge of the mask.
3. Put the remaining fingers of your second hand under the jaw to lift the chin.
4. Press the mask down firmly to make a seal as you perform a head tilt-chin lift to open the airway.

From a position at the top of the victim's head (with two rescuers or when not giving CPR) using the head tilt-chin lift:

1. Put your thumbs and index fingers on both sides of the mask as shown in **Figure A-5,b**.
2. Put the remaining fingers of both hands under the angles of the victim's jaw on both sides.

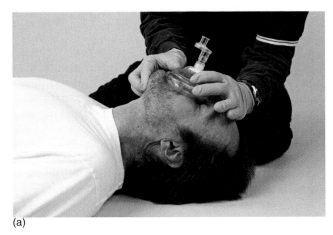
(a)

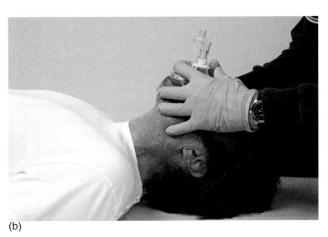
(b)

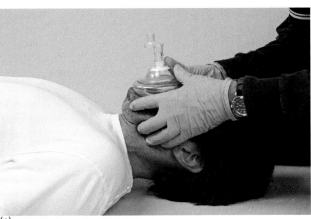
(c)

Figure A-5 (a) Face mask hand position with rescuer at victim's side. (b) Face mask hand position with rescuer at victim's head. (c) Do not tilt the head when using the jaw thrust technique for a victim with spinal injury.

3. As you tilt the head back, press the mask down firmly to make a seal as you lift the chin with your fingers.

From a position at the top of the victim's head using the jaw thrust:

1. Without tilting the victim's head back, position your thumbs on the mask the same as for the head tilt-chin lift from the top of the victim's head, with fingers under the angles of the jaw.
2. Lift the jaw to open the airway as you press down with your thumbs to seal the mask, without tilting the head back **(Figure A-5,c).**

Cricoid Pressure

Cricoid pressure, also called the Sellick maneuver, is a technique that prevents the air given during rescue breathing from passing through the esophagus to the stomach. Air in the stomach can cause vomiting, which interrupts rescue breathing and carries the risk of **aspiration,** the movement of vomit or other fluids or solids into the lungs, which can cause a serious infection and other problems. Cricoid pressure put on the trachea squeezes the esophagus closed, preventing air from traveling to the stomach **(Figure A-6).**

Cricoid pressure is performed only on unresponsive victims, only by a rescuer trained in this technique, and only by an additional rescuer who uses the technique while other rescuer(s) perform rescue breathing and CPR chest compressions if needed. Cricoid pressure can be used with an adult, child, or infant, using less pressure for smaller victims. Follow these steps:

1. With your index finger, locate the victim's Adam's apple (thyroid cartilage).
2. Slowly slide your finger down the neck. Feel the indentation just past the bottom of the thyroid cartilage and, just below this, the higher cricoid cartilage.
3. With index finger and thumb, apply moderate pressure down on the cricoid cartilage. Maintain this pressure continuously while rescue breathing is being given.

Suction Devices

A **suction device** is used to clear blood, vomit, and other substances from a victim's airway. These devices are generally safe and easy to use. Although different types of suction devices are available, they are similar in their use. Manual devices develop suction with a hand-pumping action, and other devices are powered by a battery or pressurized oxygen. Soft rubber bulb syringes are used for suctioning infants.

Suction devices for adults and children have a clear plastic tip that is inserted into the mouth or nostrils to suck out fluids and small solids. Different suction tips are available, varying from small, soft plastic tips that are more effective with fluids to larger, more rigid tips that are more effective for vomit and particulates. Some devices have a suction control port at the base of the tip that you cover with your finger to produce suction. As

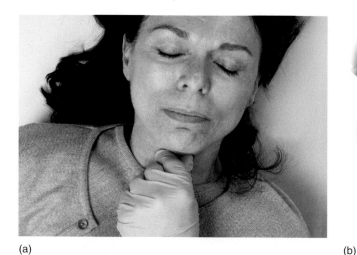
(a)

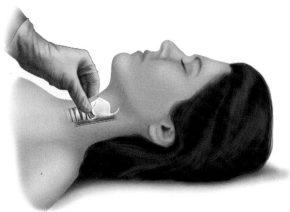
(b)

Figure A-6 (a) The hand position for cricoid pressure. (b) Cricoid pressure compresses the esophagus against the spine.

always, you should be familiar in advance with the specific equipment you may use in an emergency.

Suction is useful whenever a victim's airway may be obstructed—fully or in part—by body fluids, food substances, or other matter. If the victim vomits when rescue breathing or CPR is underway, or if secretions or blood accumulate and impede ventilation, stop and quickly suction the mouth and/or nose and then continue the resuscitation. An unresponsive breathing victim may also need suctioning to maintain an open airway. Usually you know the airway needs suctioning when you hear gurgling sounds during breathing or ventilation.

The victim's head is turned to the side to help drain vomit or fluids before suctioning. If the victim may have a spinal injury, the victim must be turned on the side with the head and body inline as a unit, with the help of other rescuers See Skill: "Suctioning (Adult or Child)" and Skill: "Suctioning (Infant)."

Safety precautions are necessary when suctioning. Because many suction devices generate strong suction pressures, be careful with the suction tip. Prolonged contact with mucous membranes in the mouth and nose can cause bruising, swelling, and even bleeding. Never insert the suction tip farther than you can see. Prolonged suctioning can also decrease the volume of air reaching the victim's lungs. Vigorous suctioning may stimulate the victim's gag reflex, causing additional vomiting. Be especially careful not to suction too deeply in an infant. Always suction an infant's mouth before the nostrils, because suctioning the nose may stimulate the infant to breathe in and thereby inhale fluid or secretions from the mouth.

Remember standard precautions against disease transmission through body fluids. After the emergency, dispose of any contents in the reservoir of the suction device and clean the device according to the manufacturer's recommendations.

Bag-Valve-Mask

Bag-valve-mask (BVM) units, like regular face masks, protect the first aider from disease transmission, and they are also more effective for providing ventilations to nonbreathing victims. With the BVM the victim receives air from the atmosphere (21% oxygen) rather than air the rescuer exhales (16% oxygen). The more oxygen delivered to the lungs, the more oxygen that will reach the victim's vital organs to maintain life. Several different types of BVM units are available, but each has at least three components (**Figure A-7**):

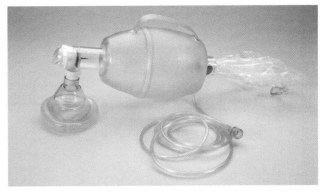

Figure A-7 Bag-valve-mask (BVM).

- The self-inflating bag holds the air or oxygen that is delivered to the victim when the bag is squeezed.
- The one-way valve allows air or oxygen to flow from the bag to the victim but prevents exhaled air from returning from the victim to the bag.
- The mask is similar to a resuscitation mask and is connected to the bag and valve; the proper size mask must be used for a proper fit.

An oxygen reservoir bag may be attached to the other end of the bag when supplemental oxygen is used.

To use the BVM on a nonbreathing victim, position yourself above the victim's head. Perform a head tilt, and then position the mask on the victim's face. If you are alone, you need to hold the mask with one hand and squeeze the bag with the other, as shown in **Figure A-8**. To hold the mask in place with one hand, use the C-clamp

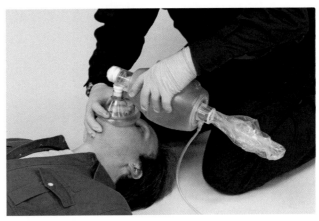

Figure A-8 A single rescuer using a BVM for rescue breathing.

S k i l l | **Suctioning (Adult or Child)**

1 Confirm that the suction device is working and produces suction.

2 Turn the victim's head to one side and open the mouth (with spinal injury, support the head and turn with body as one unit).

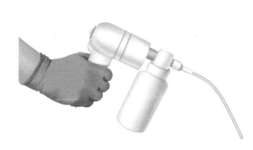

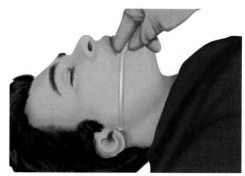

3 Sweep out solids and larger amounts of fluid with your finger.

4 Determine maximum depth of insertion by measuring catheter tip from earlobe to corner of mouth.

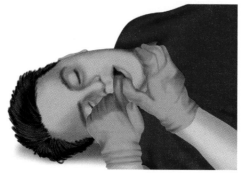

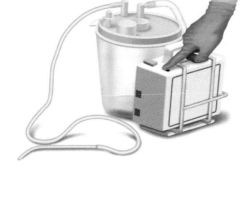

5 Turn on suction or pump handle to create suction.

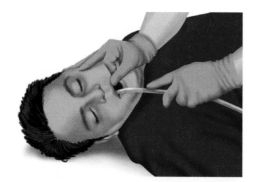

6 With suction on, insert catheter tip carefully into mouth, moving the tip about as you withdraw it.

7 Reposition the victim's head with airway open, and resume rescue breathing or CPR.

Skill **Suctioning (Infant)**

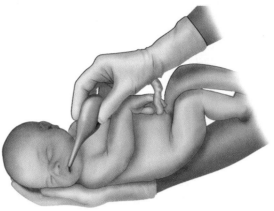

1 Hold infant in position for suctioning, with head lower than body and turned to one side.

2 Squeeze suction bulb first and then gently insert the tip into infant's mouth.

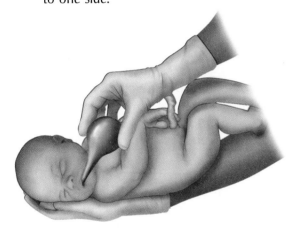

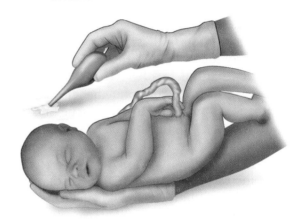

3 Gradually release the bulb to create suction as you withdraw tip from mouth.

4 Move the bulb aside and squeeze it with tip down to empty it.

5 Repeat steps 2–4 until airway seems clear, up to three times.

6 Repeat suctioning steps for each nostril.

7 Resume rescue breathing or CPR.

technique, with thumb and index finger on the edges of the mask while the other fingers lift the jaw into the mask. When a second rescuer is available to help with the BVM, one rescuer holds the mask in place using both hands as described earlier, as shown in the Skill: "Bag-Valve-Mask for Rescue Breathing (2 Rescuers)." Two-rescuer use of the BVM is recommended whenever possible because of the difficulty one person may have sealing the mask on the victim's face with one hand while squeezing the bag with the other.

With the mask sealed in place, rescue breaths are delivered to the victim by squeezing the bag. Squeeze a 1-liter adult bag about $^{1}/_{2}$–$^{2}/_{3}$ of its volume. Squeeze a 2-liter adult bag about $^{1}/_{3}$ its volume. Squeeze the bag over 1 second, watching the victim's chest rise. Give a ventilation every 5 to 6 seconds in an adult (or every 3 to 5 seconds in an infant or child), the same as with rescue breathing by mouth or resuscitation mask. If supplemental oxygen is being provided through the BVM, slightly smaller ventilations can be given.

When using a BVM, monitor the effectiveness of ventilations. Be careful to give rescue breaths at the usual rate and not to over-ventilate the victim. Watch for the rise and fall of the victim's chest, and feel for resistance as you squeeze the bag. An increased resistance may mean that there is blood or vomit in the airway or that the airway is no longer open. A problem can also occur with sealing the mask to the victim's face, especially when a single rescuer must do this with one hand. If air is escaping around the mask, try repositioning the mask and your fingers. If you cannot obtain an adequate seal and the victim's chest does not rise with ventilations, or there are any other problems with using the BVM, then use an alternate technique, such as a resuscitation mask, instead. (See Skill: "Bag-Valve-Mask for Rescue Breathing [2 Rescuers].")

If available, supplemental oxygen should be used with the BVM (see next section). An oxygen reservoir bag is attached to the valve on the bag, and the oxygen tubing attached to the bag. The device is used the same way to give ventilations, only now it is oxygen rather than air being delivered to the victim. The reservoir holds oxygen being delivered to the device so that the bag always fills with oxygen to be delivered in the next ventilation. When two res-

cuers are present, the second sets up the oxygen equipment and prepares to connect it to the BVM while the first begins providing rescue breathing with the BVM alone.

The BVM can be used with a nonbreathing infant in the same manner as with an adult or child. Be sure to choose the correct size mask. A smaller bag is also used: typically about 500 mL for newborns, 750 mL for infants and small children, and 1200 mL for large children and adolescents, compared to 1600 mL for adults. Squeeze the bag only enough to make the chest rise, avoiding forceful squeezing or overinflation that may lead to vomiting.

Supplemental Oxygen

In many emergency situations the victim will benefit from receiving **supplemental oxygen,** if available. Victims receiving basic life support are often receiving insufficient oxygen because of respiratory or cardiovascular problems. The air around us is about 21% oxygen, and the air we breathe out (and into a victim's lungs during rescue breathing) is about 16% oxygen. Depending on the supplemental oxygen delivery device, the victim can receive oxygen at concentrations up to 100%.

Supplemental oxygen, when available, should be used along with other basic life support techniques, including rescue breathing and CPR. In addition, victims with serious medical conditions, including heart attack, stroke, seizures, or serious injury, will potentially benefit from supplemental oxygen (see **Chapter 17**).

The equipment involved in giving supplemental oxygen includes:

- The **oxygen source** is typically a pressurized cylinder. When full, cylinders have a pressure of 2000 pounds per square inch (psi). They come in various sizes and are usually painted green, although some stainless steel cylinders are not.

- The **pressure regulator** reduces the pressure of oxygen leaving the tank to a safe level and has a gauge that shows the pressure remaining within the cylinder. If the gauge reads 2000 psi, the tank is full; if it reads 1000 psi, it is half full, and so on. The pressure regulator is designed so that it works only with oxygen tanks.

- The **flowmeter,** used to adjust the rate of oxygen delivery, is usually built into the pressure

Skill **Bag-Valve-Mask for Rescue Breathing (2 Rescuers)**

1 Rescuer 1 assembles the BVM with correct size mask and puts the mask over the victim's mouth and nose.

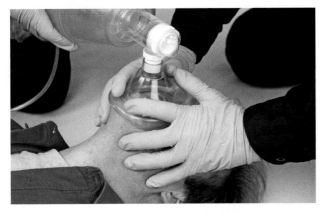

2 Rescuer 2 positions hands: thumbs and index fingers circling each side of mask, other three fingers behind lower jawbone. Pull the jaw up into the mask rather than pushing the mask down on the jaw.

3 Rescuer 2 opens the airway and seals the mask to the victim's face.

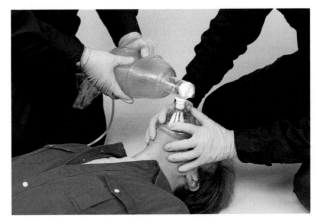

4 Rescuer 1 squeezes the bag to provide ventilations:
   a. 1 ventilation over 1 second in adult, every 5 to 6 seconds.
   b. 1 ventilation over 1 second in child or infant, every 3 to 5 seconds.

5 Recheck pulse and other signs of circulation about every 2 minutes. If no signs of circulation, call for an AED and start CPR.

regulator. The flow of oxygen reaching the victim is set by turning the calibrated flow valve.

- **Oxygen tubing** connects the cylinder to the delivery device. Connecting tubes are typically 4 to 5 feet long and have an adapter at each end.

- **An oxygen delivery device,** such as a face mask or nasal cannula, provides the flowing oxygen to the victim.

Safety Around Oxygen

Although oxygen itself does not burn, it vigorously supports combustion and creates a hazardous situation if used near an ignition source. Follow these guidelines around oxygen:

- Never allow smoking or an open flame near the oxygen source.

- Never use grease, oil, or adhesive tape on the cylinder, pressure regulator, or delivery device, because these are combustible.

- Never expose an oxygen cylinder to a temperature over 120 degrees F.

- Never drop a cylinder or let it fall against another object. If the valve is dislodged, the cylinder can become a dangerous projectile powered by the compressed gas.

- Never try to use a nonoxygen regulator on an oxygen cylinder.

Oxygen Delivery Devices

Many different oxygen delivery devices are available, each with certain advantages and disadvantages. The following devices are most frequently used in emergency situations:

- **Nasal cannulas,** sometimes called nasal prongs, are used with breathing victims who do not require a high concentration of oxygen. The device has two small prongs that fit shallowly into the nostrils. The nasal cannula is easy to use and comfortable for the victim. The oxygen concentration delivered depends on the flow rate (1 to 6 L/min) and the victim's breathing rate, varying from about 24% to 50% **(Figure A-9).**

- **Resuscitation face masks** cover the mouth and nose and can be used for nonbreathing victims receiving rescue breaths. Some masks have a special port for oxygen, which can be used for breathing victims who need oxygen. The mask then can be

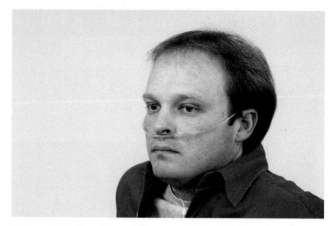

Figure A-9 Nasal cannula.

secured to the victim's head by an elastic band. A typical plastic face mask provides an oxygen concentration of 30% to 60% with a flow rate of 10 liters per minute **(Figure A-10).**

- **Nonrebreathing masks** have a mask and a reservoir bag and are used with breathing victims. The oxygen fills the reservoir, which empties partially as the victim inhales. The victim's exhaled air escapes through a valve. With a minimum oxygen flow rate of 8 liters per minute, the oxygen concentration ranges from 80% to 95%. The flow rate is adjusted to prevent the reservoir from completely collapsing when the victim inhales. A firm mask fit is needed to prevent room air from entering the mask **(Figure A-11).**

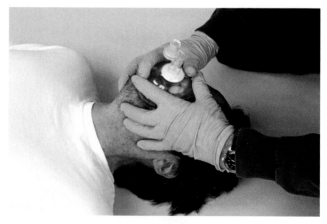

Figure A-10 Resuscitation mask.

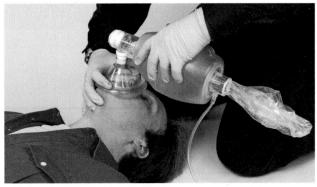

Figure A-12 BVM with oxygen reservoir.

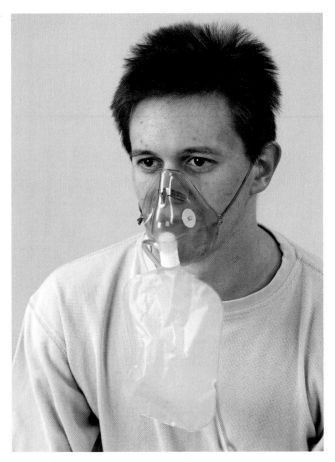

Figure A-11 Nonrebreather mask.

- **Bag-valve-mask units,** as described earlier, can also deliver oxygen either through a simple connecting tube to the bag or with an oxygen reservoir. Oxygen concentrations delivered to a nonbreathing victim by a BVM with a reservoir can approach 100%. A breathing victim can also use a BVM with a reservoir to receive oxygen; unless the victim is having difficulty breathing, the bag is not squeezed (**Figure A-12**).

Administration of Oxygen

The Skill: "Oxygen Administration" describes the steps for setting up the oxygen equipment and administering oxygen to the victim. Remember to follow safety principles when working with oxygen. If you are alone with a victim, do not stop providing basic life support to set up oxygen equipment. Give rescue breathing or CPR as needed, use the AED if present and appropriate, and care for other life-threatening problems first. Wait until the

victim is relatively stable and breathing independently or until another rescuer can help with the oxygen equipment. Once the victim is receiving oxygen, continue to monitor the flow of oxygen, tank pressure, and flow rate, as well as the victim's condition.

Airway Adjuncts

Oral and nasal **airway adjuncts** are devices that help keep a victim's airway open during resuscitation or until the victim receives advanced medical attention. The most common cause of airway obstruction in unresponsive victims is the tongue. An airway device prevents this problem and keeps the airway open more easily than head position alone while using resuscitation techniques or caring for a breathing victim. Supplemental oxygen can be given through a resuscitation mask or bag-valve-mask with an oral or nasal airway in place.

Oral Airways

Oral airways, also called **oropharyngeal airways,** are used only in unresponsive victims who do not have a gag reflex. If inserted into a responsive victim, or one who still has a gag reflex, the airway adjunct can cause vomiting. The victim's airway must be opened before the airway device is inserted; the device does not open the airway itself but will help to keep it open. An oral airway can be used in an unresponsive victim who is breathing or who is receiving rescue breaths.

Proper placement of the oral airway is essential. An improperly placed airway device can compress the tongue into the back of the throat and further block the airway. Oral airways are

Skill **Oxygen Administration**

1 Check equipment: oxygen labels on the cylinder and regulator; tubing and delivery device ready.

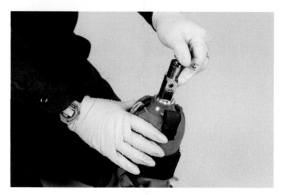

2 Remove any protective seal, point cylinder away, and open main valve for 1 second.

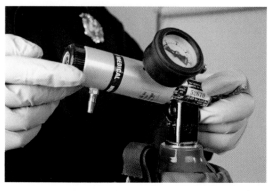

3 Remove any protective seals and attach regulator to oxygen cylinder.

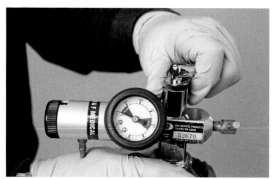

4 Open the main cylinder valve.

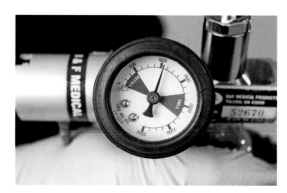

5 Check the pressure regulator gauge.

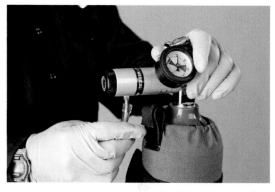

6 Attach the tubing to the flowmeter and the oxygen delivery device.

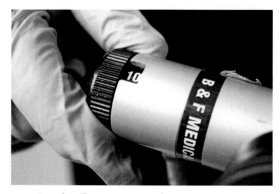

7 Set the flowmeter at the correct oxygen flow rate.
   a. 1 to 6 lpm for nasal cannula
   b. 10 lpm for face mask
   c. 10 to 15 lpm for BVM or nonrebreather mask

Skill **Oxygen Administration** *(continued)*

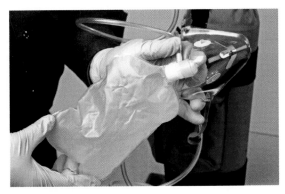

8 Confirm oxygen is flowing.

9 Position the delivery device on the victim and continue rescue breathing (or allow victim to breathe spontaneously).

10 Monitor the pressure regulator gauge and be prepared to remove the delivery device and change tanks if the pressure drops below 500 psi. Observe oxygen safety precautions.

---

curved so that they fit the natural contour of the mouth and are available in various sizes to assure a proper fit **(Figure A-13)**. An airway adjunct that is too big can cause vomiting and may prevent the resuscitation mask from sealing well. An airway adjunct that is too small can slide into the back of the pharynx and obstruct the airway **(Figure A-14)**. Remember to open the victim's airway before inserting the oral airway, as described in the Skill: "Oral Airway Insertion." Periodically reassess the airway adjunct to confirm that it remains in proper position. A victim can be suctioned with an oral airway in place.

Nasal Airways

A nasal airway, like an oral airway, helps maintain an open airway **(Figure A-15)**. A nasal airway **(nasopharyngeal airway)** can be used in a victim who is responsive or who, although unresponsive, has a gag reflex. Nasal airways are also effective for unresponsive victims with mouth or jaw injuries or tightly clenched teeth that prevent the use of an oral airway. Nasal airways

are less likely to cause gagging and vomiting than oral airways, but a disadvantage is that they are too narrow to suction. Insert a nasal airway as described in the Skill: "Nasal Airway Insertion," and continue to keep the victim's airway open with the head tilt-chin lift or jaw thrust. If needed, suction through a nasal airway using a small, flexible suction catheter.

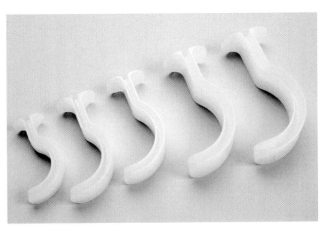

Figure A-13 Oral airways.

Skill   **Oral Airway Insertion**

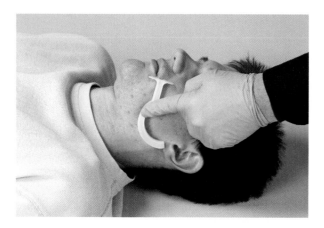

1 Choose the correct airway device size.

2 Open the victim's airway with head tilt-chin lift or jaw thrust, and open the mouth.

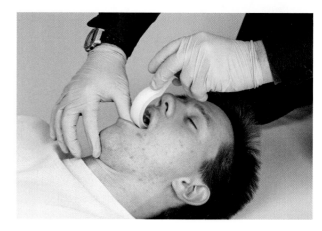

3 Insert the airway device with the tip pointing toward the roof of the mouth.

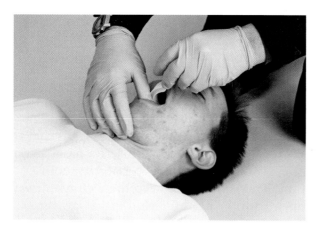

4 When tip reaches back of mouth and you feel resistance, rotate the airway 180 degrees.

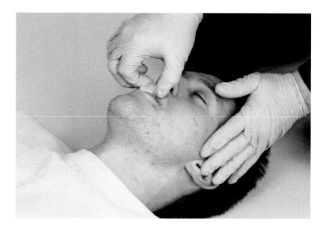

5 Continue to insert the airway device to final position (the flange resting on the lips).

Skill   **Nasal Airway Insertion**

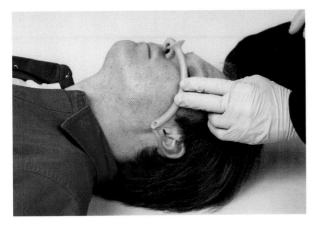

1   Choose the correct nasal airway size.

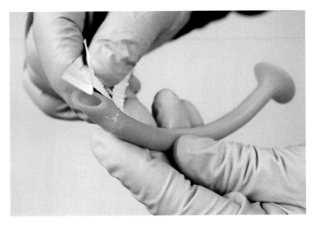

2   Coat the nasal airway with lubricant.

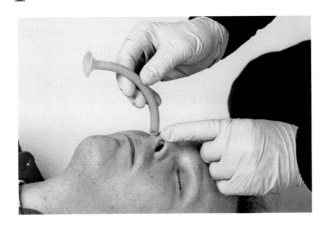

3   Insert the nasal airway in the right nostril with the bevel toward the septum.

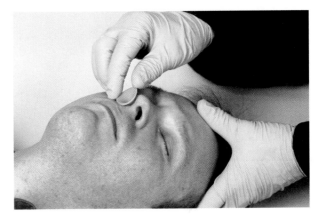

4   Insert the nasal airway straight back, sliding it along the floor of the nostril.

5   Insert the nasal airway until the flange rests against the nose.

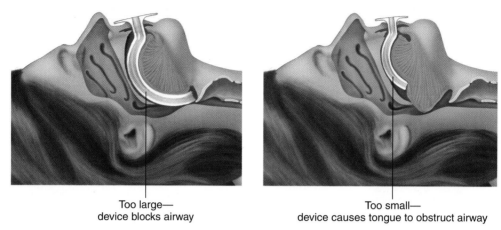

Too large—
device blocks airway

Too small—
device causes tongue to obstruct airway

Figure A-14 An oral airway that is too large or too small will obstruct the airway.

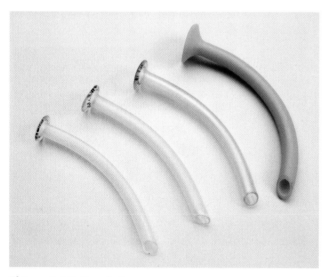

Figure A-15 Nasal airways.

CPR Skills

Compressions for Bradycardia in Child

An infant or child being given rescue breaths or oxygen may have a pulse but still have inadequate perfusion. If the pulse is under 60 beats/minute and the infant or child has signs of poor systemic perfusion, the healthcare provider should provide CPR with chest compressions. Do not wait for the victim to become pulseless if perfusion is poor even with ventilation with or without supplemental oxygen.

CPR

The protocol for CPR for more highly trained healthcare providers differs somewhat from that for CPR by lay rescuers. Healthcare providers check for a pulse and other signs of circulation before beginning chest compressions.

A lone healthcare provider uses the same 30:2 ratio of compressions and rescue breaths for all victims. Two-rescuer CPR provided by healthcare providers, however, uses a 15:2 ratio for children up to the onset of puberty.

Healthcare providers like lay rescuers should give chest compressions at a rate of 100 a minute—push hard, push fast—letting the chest come all the way up between compressions. In an adult, compress to a depth of $1\frac{1}{2}$–2 inches; in an infant or child, compress $\frac{1}{3}$ to $\frac{1}{2}$ the depth of the chest. Interruptions to give rescue breaths or check the pulse should take less than 10 seconds.

Two-Rescuer CPR for Adults and Children

When two rescuers at the scene are trained in CPR, resuscitation performed by both together offers several advantages. Two-rescuer CPR

- minimizes the time between rescue breaths and compressions, making CPR more effective.
- allows for more quickly setting up an AED (**Chapter 8**).
- reduces rescuer fatigue.

The first rescuer, who will be giving rescue breaths, begins by checking the victim for responsiveness and breathing. If the victim is not breathing adequately, this rescuer gives two rescue breaths as usual, and then checks for a pulse. Meanwhile, the second rescuer ensures 9-1-1 has been called and moves into position on the opposite side of the victim to give chest compressions.

Two-rescuer CPR is performed in the same cycles of 30 compressions and 2 breaths for an adult (15 compressions and 2 breaths for an infant or child). The first rescuer provides rescue breaths, and the second rescuer gives the chest compressions at a rate of 100 compressions per minute. The second rescuer should count aloud during the compressions and pause after the last compression to let the first rescuer give two breaths.

The rescuers should switch positions about every 2 minutes (after 5 cycles of 30 compressions and 2 breaths) to prevent the compressing rescuer from becoming fatigued and giving ineffective compressions. This change should be done at the end of a full CPR cycle after breaths are given, and should be accomplished in less than 5 seconds.

If an AED is present at the scene, the first rescuer gives both breaths and chest compressions while the second rescuer sets up the unit and attaches the pads (see **Chapter 8**). If the AED unit advises continuing CPR, the rescuers then give CPR together.

Note: A third rescuer, if present, can give cricoid pressure to help ensure that rescue breaths do not go into the stomach and possibly cause vomiting.

Note: You may be assisting an EMT or other professional with a higher level of training who places an advanced airway in the victim for ventilation. With an advanced airway in place, chest compressions are given continually, without pauses for rescue breaths. Ventilation (8 to 10 breaths per minute) is provided while compressions are ongoing.

Transitioning from One-Rescuer CPR to Two-Rescuer CPR

In some situations a rescuer is already giving CPR when a second rescuer arrives on the scene. The rescuers should coordinate their actions for a smooth transition from one-rescuer CPR to two-rescuer CPR. The second rescuer moves into position on the other side of the victim to prepare to take over chest compressions. The first rescuer completes a cycle of compressions and breaths. While the first rescuer then pauses to check for a pulse, the second rescuer finds the correct hand position for compressions. When the first rescuer says, "No circulation, continue CPR," the second rescuer begins chest compressions and the first rescuer then gives only rescue breaths. See Skill: "CPR for Adult or Child (2 Rescuers)."

Note: If you are the first rescuer who started CPR, the arriving second rescuer may be a rescuer or EMT with a higher level of training. In such a case this rescuer assumes authority for how CPR should best be continued. If this rescuer determines your breathing or compression technique is inadequate, he or she may ask you to take on the other role—or may take over the CPR alone.

Two-Rescuer CPR for Infants

Two-rescuer CPR for an infant uses a different hand position for giving chest compressions. The rescuer giving compressions places the thumbs of both hands together in the correct position on the infant's sternum (just below a line between the nipples). The fingers of both hands encircle the infant's chest **(Figure A-16)**. The breastbone is compressed with both thumbs while the chest is squeezed with the fingers, as described in the Skill: "CPR for Infant (2 Rescuers)."

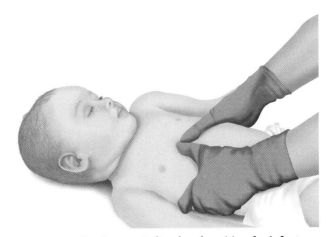

Figure A-16 The chest-encircling hand position for infant chest compressions when two professional rescuers are giving CPR.

Skill   **CPR for Adult or Child (2 Rescuers)**

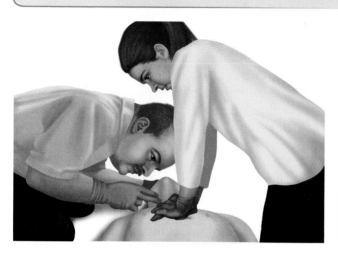

1 At the victim's head, Rescuer 1 checks the victim's ABCs. An AED has been summoned. At the victim's side, Rescuer 2 locates the site for chest compressions.

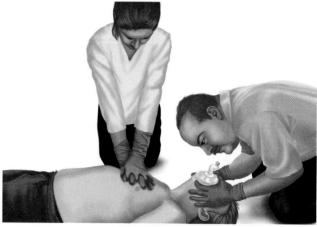

2 Rescuer 1 indicates "No circulation." Rescuer 2 gives 30 compressions for an adult (15 for a child) at rate of 100 per minute, counting aloud for a fast, steady rate, then pauses.

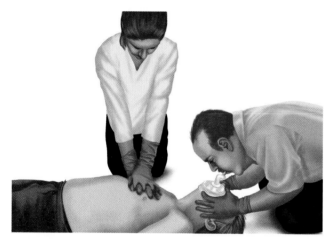

3 Rescuer 1 gives 2 breaths.

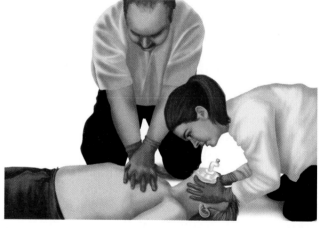

4 Rescuers continue cycles of 30 compressions in an adult (15 in a child) and 2 breaths for about 2 minutes (or after 5 cycles of compressions and ventilations at a ratio of 30:2) before switching compressor and ventilator roles. The switch should be done quickly (in less than 5 seconds).

5 Rescuers continue CPR until:
   a. The victim moves
   b. An AED is brought to the scene and is ready to use
   c. Help arrives and takes over

6 If the victim starts breathing and has a pulse, put in the recovery position and monitor the ABCs.

7 If an AED is brought to the scene, start the AED sequence.

Skill | **CPR for Infant (2 rescuers)**

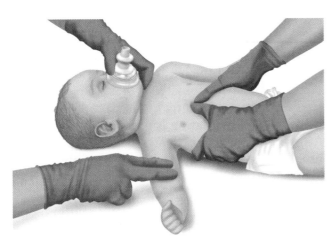

1 At the infant's head, Rescuer 1 checks the ABCs. At the infant's feet, Rescuer 2 locates the site for chest compressions with both thumbs.

2 If absent, Rescuer 1 says, "No pulse." Rescuer 2 gives 15 chest compressions at a rate of 100 per minute, counting aloud for a fast, steady rate, then pauses.

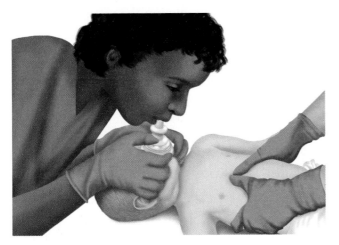

3 Rescuer 1 gives 2 breaths.

4 Rescuers continue cycles of 15 compressions and 2 breaths for about 2 minutes before switching compressor and ventilator roles. The switch should be done quickly (in less than 5 seconds). Rescuers continue CPR until:
a. Infant moves
b. Help arrives and takes over

5 If the infant starts breathing, hold infant in the recovery position and monitor the ABCs.

AED Skills

Lay rescuers are taught to use the AED on any nonbreathing adult as soon as the unit is available. When two lay rescuers are present, one should give CPR while the other sets up the AED. Lay rescuers are taught to give 5 cycles of CPR (2 minutes), without a pause to check circulation, for a child found unresponsive (not observed to have collapsed suddenly).

Healthcare providers in out-of-hospital settings should also use the AED as soon as it is ready *except in two situations:*

- For a pulseless child who was not observed to have collapsed suddenly, provide 5 uninterrupted cycles of CPR (about 2 minutes) before using the AED.
- For an adult found pulseless on your arrival, when more than 4–5 minutes have passed since you were called to respond, provide 5 uninterrupted cycles of CPR (about 2 minutes) before using the AED.

Healthcare providers, like lay rescuers, after giving a shock should immediately provide CPR for uninterrupted 5 cycles (about 2 minutes) before the AED again analyzes the victim's rhythm and advises another shock if needed.

Special Resuscitation Situations

In most emergencies, basic life support skills are used in the same way. A few situations, however, involve special considerations in the use of these skills or in the approach to the victim.

Trauma

In most situations in which the victim is severely injured by blunt or penetrating trauma, problems with the airway, breathing, or circulation are the result of the trauma rather than a coinciding problem. Do not assume, however, that a trauma victim has experienced *only* trauma, because another problem may have occurred first or at the same time. For example, a victim may have a heart attack and sudden cardiac arrest while on a ladder, resulting in a fall and possible fractures. A victim of drug overdose or poisoning may develop a severe breathing problem while operating machinery, causing an accident and traumatic injury. As a general rule, treat a trauma victim like any

other: check the ABCs and give basic life support as needed.

Trauma victims generally have a *call first* rather than *call fast* status. Since trauma that is severe enough to cause cardiac arrest usually requires surgical correction, the victim needs to be transported for definitive care as quickly as possible.

Depending on the nature of the trauma, the victim may have a spinal injury as well. Any blow to the body severe enough to impact the airway, breathing, or circulation is likely also to potentially injure the spine. Remember to keep the head in line with the body when positioning the victim, and use the jaw thrust technique rather than head tilt–chin lift to open the airway.

Trauma to the head or face may result in blood or other fluid blocking the airway. Check the mouth when opening the airway, and if necessary wipe out any blood or vomit. With more extensive amounts of fluid, you may have to turn the victim onto one side to let it drain from the mouth. If the equipment is available and you are trained in its use, suction the victim's mouth when opening the airway.

In cases of cardiac arrest in victims with very severe trauma, local protocol may include not using the AED, since these victims seldom have a heart rhythm that can be corrected. Always follow your local protocol, and if the AED is not used, give CPR as usual while waiting for advanced help.

Hypothermia

Hypothermia is a lowering of the body's core temperature as a result of exposure to a cold environment, often caused by immersion in cold water. Hypothermia requires special consideration because breathing and pulse may be difficult to find, because the victim is susceptible to heart rhythm problems, and because victims have been successfully resuscitated after a long period of hypothermia or immersion.

In severe hypothermia, the victim's heart may be beating very slowly or may be in arrest, and the respiratory rate may be very slow or may have stopped. Because the victim's skin is cold and pale, the victim may appear to be dead. Take extra time as needed to check for breathing and up to 30 to 45 seconds to find a pulse. If the victim has no pulse, start CPR as usual. Follow local protocol for the use of an AED with a hypothermia victim. Typically only one shock is given while the victim is cold; CPR and rewarming continue, and the AED may be used again when the core temperature has risen to 86 to 90 degrees F (30 to 32 degrees C).

Do not delay or stop resuscitation efforts in order to rewarm the victim, but if possible prevent further heat loss from the victim's body. Other rescuers can remove wet clothing, for example, or cover the victim with a blanket while basic life support is ongoing. Be gentle when handling or moving a hypothermic victim because the heart is susceptible to dysrhythmias precipitated by motion or jarring.

Near-Drowning

In any situation in which a victim is in the water, ensure your own safety before attempting a rescue. It is very dangerous for an untrained rescuer to enter the water to rescue a responsive victim, who may grab the rescuer and make rescue difficult or impossible. Reach to the victim with a pole or long object, throw a rope or floating object, or go to the victim in a watercraft if possible. Beginning rescue breaths as soon as possible is a high priority for drowning victims. If you can do so, begin rescue breaths (after confirming respiratory arrest) even before removing the victim from shallow water. It is necessary to remove the victim from water, however, to give CPR.

With an unresponsive victim removed from the water, consider whether the nature of the incident suggests a possible spinal injury, such as diving in shallow or murky water or being thrown against the shore in surf conditions. If the cause of the submersion is unknown, assume the victim may have a spinal injury. Keep the head in line with the body when moving or positioning the victim, and use the jaw thrust technique rather than head tilt-chin lift to open the airway.

Check the ABCs as usual. Remember that this is a *call fast* rather than *call first* situation. If you are alone, give 5 cycles of CPR (about 2 minutes) before stopping to telephone for help.

The victim may need rescue breathing or CPR. Give basic life support as usual—do not try to remove water from the victim first. If the victim is not breathing and your rescue breaths do not make the chest rise, a foreign body may be obstructing the airway. Check inside the mouth and remove any foreign body. Open the airway again and try to give two breaths. If your breaths still do not go in, give chest compressions for an airway obstruction. Do not try to take other actions to remove suspected water from the lungs.

If supplemental oxygen is available and you are trained in its use, administer oxygen to the victim. When an AED is available and is ready to use, use it as usual. Victims have been resuscitated after being submerged in cold water for some time. If the victim may be hypothermic, follow the special considerations described earlier.

Electric Shock

Electric shock may result from a lightning strike or from contact with a source of household current or high-voltage power lines. The shock may cause breathing to stop because of paralyzed respiratory muscles and may cause cardiac arrest by disrupting the heart's electrical controls.

Remember scene safety before approaching the victim. Downed power lines or household or industrial electrical appliances or cords may still be "live" and pose a threat to rescuers. Call 9-1-1 for downed power lines, and do not try to move them yourself or to move the victim away from them. With electrical appliances, first shut the power off at the circuit breaker box or unplug the power cord if it is safe to do so.

The electrical shock may cause a range of injuries in addition to effects on respiration and circulation. Especially with a high-voltage shock such as that caused by lightning, the victim may have severe burns and possible fractures due to strong muscular contractions caused by the electrical shock. With a lightning strike victim, assume a possible spinal injury.

When it is safe to approach the victim, check his or her ABCs and provide care as needed. If the victim has a pulse but is not breathing, provide rescue breathing and continue to monitor signs of circulation. If the victim has no pulse; provide CPR and call for an AED. Often an electrical shock causes ventricular fibrillation, in which case the AED may return the heart to a normal rhythm. If you are alone, shout for help and for an AED to be brought, but give 5 cycles of CPR (about 2 minutes) before stopping to telephone for help.

Pregnancy

A woman in late stages of pregnancy with an airway obstruction should be given chest thrusts rather than abdominal thrusts to expel an obstructing object. A responsive victim can be given chest thrusts from behind while standing, and an unresponsive victim is given chest thrusts in the same manner as the chest compressions of CPR. Note that chest compressions should be given slightly higher on the sternum in a pregnant woman.

When a pregnant woman at a gestational age beyond 20 weeks lies on her back, the enlarged uterus may press against the inferior vena cava, the vein that returns blood to the heart from the lower half of the body. This pressure may decrease the blood flow to the heart and affect circulation to vital organs. When possible, there-fore, position an injured pregnant woman lying on her left side, which reduces pressure from the uterus on the vena cava. Gently move the uterus to the left to help alleviate the pressure.

When giving CPR to a pregnant woman at a gestational age beyond 20 weeks, if possible position her for chest compressions on a firm surface that can be tilted so that her back is angled back 15 to 30 degrees from the left lateral position (lying on left side).

Otherwise, perform basic life support skills on a pregnant woman in the same manner as for other victims, including the use of an AED in cases of cardiac arrest.

Appendix

B Performance Checklists for Key Skills

Participant Name _____   Date _____

Instructor Name _____

Performance Checklist: AED

Skill Step	Initial Practice		Final Performance	
	Needs Practice	Proficient	Remediate	Proficient
1. Position victim away from water and metal. Place unit by victim's shoulder and turn it on.				
2. Expose victim's chest, and dry or shave the area if necessary.				
3. Apply pads to victim's chest. If needed, plug cables into unit.				
4. Stand clear during rhythm analysis.				
5. Follow prompts from AED unit to (a) press the shock button or (b) do not shock but immediately give CPR with the pads remaining in place, starting with chest compressions.				
6. Follow the AED's prompts to analyze the rhythm again after 5 cycles of CPR (about 2 minutes).				
7. Continue Steps 4 to 6 until the victim moves or professional rescuers arrive and take over.				
8. If the victim recovers (moves), check for breathing and put a breathing unresponsive victim in the recovery position (with pads remaining in place) and continue to monitor breathing.				
Complete Skill				

Participant Name _____   Date _____
Instructor Name _____

Performance Checklist: Arm Sling and Binder

Skill Step	Initial Practice		Final Performance	
	Needs Practice	**Proficient**	**Remediate**	**Proficient**
1. Secure the point of the bandage at the elbow.				
2. Position the triangular bandage.				
3. Bring up the lower end of the bandage to the opposite side of the neck.				
4. Tie the ends.				
5. Tie a binder bandage over the sling and around the chest.				
Complete Skill				

Participant Name _____   Date _____
Instructor Name _____

Performance Checklist: Bleeding Control

Skill Step	Initial Practice		Final Performance	
	Needs Practice	**Proficient**	**Remediate**	**Proficient**
1. Put on gloves. *Use your bare hands only if no barrier is available, and then wash immediately.*				
2. Place a sterile dressing on the wound and apply direct pressure with your hand. *Do not put pressure on an object in a wound. Do not put pressure on the scalp if the skull may be injured.*				
3. If needed, put another dressing or cloth pad on top of the first and keep applying pressure.				
4. Apply a roller bandage to keep pressure on the wound. *Do not use a tourniquet to stop bleeding except as an extreme last resort because the limb will likely be lost.*				
5. If appropriate, treat the victim for shock, and call 9-1-1.				
Complete Skill				

Participant Name _____   Date _____
Instructor Name _____

Performance Checklist: Choking Care for Responsive Adult or Child

Skill Step	Initial Practice		Final Performance	
	Needs Practice	Proficient	Remediate	Proficient
1. Stand behind an adult victim with one leg forward between the victim's legs. Keep your head slightly to one side. With a small child, kneel behind the child. Reach around the abdomen.				
2. Make a fist with one hand and place the thumb side of the fist against the victim's abdomen just above the navel.				
3. Grasp your fist with your other hand and thrust inward and upward into the victim's abdomen with quick jerks. Continue abdominal thrusts until the victim can expel the object or becomes unresponsive. If abdominal thrusts do not succeed in clearing the object from the airway, you may try chest thrusts and back blows as well.				
4. For a responsive pregnant victim, or any victim you cannot get your arms around, give chest thrusts from behind the victim. Take care not to squeeze the ribs with your arms. If chest thrusts do not clear the obstructing object, support the woman's chest with one hand and give back blows with the other.				
Complete Skill				

Participant Name _____   Date _____

Instructor Name _____

Performance Checklist: Choking Care for Responsive Infant

Skill Step	Initial Practice		Final Performance	
	Needs Practice	Proficient	Remediate	Proficient
1. Support the infant's head in one hand, with the torso on your forearm and your thigh. Give up to 5 back blows between the shoulder blades.				
2. Check for expelled object. If not present, continue with next step.				
3. With other hand on back of infant's head, roll the infant faceup.				
4. Give up to 5 chest thrusts with two fingers on sternum. Check mouth for expelled object.				
5. Repeat Steps 1 through 4, alternating back blows and chest thrusts and checking the mouth. If alone, call 9-1-1 after 1 minute. Continue until the object is expelled or the infant becomes unresponsive. If the infant becomes unresponsive, give CPR. Look inside the mouth when opening the mouth to give breaths, and remove any object you see.				
Complete Skill				

Participant Name _____   Date _____

Instructor Name _____

Performance Checklist: Choking Care for Unresponsive Adult or Child

Skill Step	Initial Practice		Final Performance	
	Needs Practice	Proficient	Remediate	Proficient
1. Open airway and determine the victim is not breathing.				
2. Give 2 rescue breaths, each lasting 1 second. If the first breath does not go in and the chest does not rise, position the head again to open the airway, and try again.				
3. If breaths still do not go in, give chest compressions. Put hand(s) in correct position for chest compressions. *Be careful with your hand position for chest compressions. Keep fingers off the chest. Do not give compressions over the bottom tip of the breastbone. When compressing, keep your elbows straight and keep your hands in contact with the chest at all times.*				
4. Give 30 chest compressions at rate of 100 per minute. Count aloud for a steady, fast rate: "One, two, three . . . ." Then give 2 breaths. Look inside the mouth when opening the mouth to give breaths, and remove any object you see.				
5. Continue CPR until: • Victim begins to move • Professional help arrives and takes over • You are too exhausted to continue				
Complete Skill				

Participant Name _____ Date _____

Instructor Name _____

Performance Checklist: CPR

Skill Step	Initial Practice		Final Performance	
	Needs Practice	Proficient	Remediate	Proficient
1. Open airway and determine if the victim is not breathing normally.				
2. Give 2 rescue breaths, each lasting 1 second. (If the first breath does not go in, reposition the head and try again; if the second breath still does not go in, give choking care.)				
3. Put hands in correct position for chest compressions. *Do not give compressions over the bottom tip of the breastbone. Keep fingers off the chest. When compressing, keep your elbows straight and keep your hands in contact with the chest at all times.*				
4. Give 30 chest compressions at a rate of 100 per minute. Count aloud for a steady, fast rate: "One, two, three . . . ." Then give 2 breaths.				
5. Continue cycles of 30 compressions and 2 breaths.				
6. Continue CPR until: • Victim begins to move • An AED is brought to the scene and is ready to use • Professional help arrives and takes over • You are too exhausted to continue				
7. a. If the victim starts moving, check for normal breathing. If the victim is breathing normally, put the victim in the recovery position and monitor breathing. **b.** When an AED arrives, start the AED sequence.				
Complete Skill				

Participant Name _____   Date _____
Instructor Name _____

Performance Checklist: Figure-Eight Bandage

Skill Step	Initial Practice		Final Performance	
	Needs Practice	Proficient	Remediate	Proficient
1. Anchor the starting end of the roller bandage.				
2. Turn bandage diagonally across the wrist and back around the hand.				
3. Continue with overlapping figure-eight turns.				
4. Fasten end of bandage by tying it or using clips, tape, or safety pins.				
Complete Skill				

Participant Name _____   Date _____
Instructor Name _____

Performance Checklist: Glove Removal

Skill Step	Initial Practice		Final Performance	
	Needs Practice	Proficient	Remediate	Proficient
1. With one hand, grasp your other glove at the wrist or palm and pull it away from your hand.				
2. Pull the glove the rest of the way off.				
3. Holding the removed glove balled up in the palm of your gloved hand, insert two fingers under the cuff of the remaining glove.				
4. Remove the glove by stretching it up and away from the hand and turning it inside out as you pull it off.				
5. Dispose of gloves in a biohazard container and wash your hands.				
Complete Skill				

Participant Name _____   Date _____

Instructor Name _____

Performance Checklist: Initial Assessment

Skill Step	Initial Practice		Final Performance	
	Needs Practice	**Proficient**	**Remediate**	**Proficient**
1. Check responsiveness.				
2. Open the airway with the head tilt-chin lift.				
3. Check for breathing.				
4. Check for severe bleeding.				
Complete Skill				

Participant Name _____   Date _____

Instructor Name _____

Performance Checklist: Inline Stabilization

Skill Step	Initial Practice		Final Performance	
	Needs Practice	**Proficient**	**Remediate**	**Proficient**
1. Assess a responsive victim for spinal injury.				
2. Hold the victim's head with both hands to prevent movement of neck or spine.				
3. Monitor the victim's breathing.				
4. If needed, use objects to maintain head support.				
Complete Skill				

Participant Name _____   Date _____

Instructor Name _____

Performance Checklist: Physical Examination

Skill Step	Initial Practice		Final Performance	
	Needs Practice	Proficient	Remediate	Proficient
If you find any problems in any body area, do not let the victim move. Wait for help.				
1. Being careful not to move the victim's head or neck, check the head.				
2. Check neck area for medical alert necklace, deformity or swelling, and pain. Do not move the neck.				
3. Check skin appearance, temperature, moisture.				
4. Check chest. Ask victim to breathe deeply.				
5. Check abdomen.				
6. Check pelvis and hips.				
7. Check upper extremities. Look for medical alert bracelet.				
8. Check lower extremities.				
Complete Skill				

Participant Name _____   Date _____

Instructor Name _____

Performance Checklist: Pressure Bandage

Skill Step	Initial Practice		Final Performance	
	Needs Practice	Proficient	Remediate	Proficient
1. Anchor the starting end of the bandage below the wound dressing.				
2. Make several circular turns, then overlap turns.				
3. Work up the limb.				
4. Tape or tie the end of the bandage in place.				
Complete Skill				

Participant Name _____   Date _____

Instructor Name _____

Performance Checklist: Recovery Position (Modified HAINES)

Skill Step	Initial Practice		Final Performance	
	Needs Practice	**Proficient**	**Remediate**	**Proficient**
1. Extend the victim's arm that is farther from you above the victim's head.				
2. Position the victim's other arm across the chest.				
3. Bend the victim's nearer leg at the knee.				
4. Put your forearm that is nearer the victim's head under the victim's nearer shoulder with your hand under the hollow of the neck.				
5. Carefully roll the victim away from you by pushing on the victim's flexed knee and lifting with your forearm while your hand stabilizes the head and neck. The victim's head is now supported on the raised arm.				
6. While continuing to support the head and neck, position the victim's hand palm down with fingers under the armpit of the raised arm, with forearm flat on the surface at 90 degrees to the body.				
7. With victim now in position, check the airway and open the mouth to allow drainage.				
Complete Skill				

Participant Name _____   Date _____

Instructor Name _____

Performance Checklist: Shock Position

Skill Step	Initial Practice		Final Performance	
	Needs Practice	Proficient	Remediate	Proficient
1. Check for normal breathing and severe bleeding, and care for life-threatening injuries.				
2. Call 9-1-1.				
3. a. Position a responsive victim on his or her back. Raise the legs about 8 to 12 inches (unless the victim may have a spinal injury). **b.** Put an unresponsive victim (if no suspected spinal injury) in the modified HAINES recovery position.				
4. Loosen any tight clothing.				
5. Maintain the victim's normal body temperature. If the victim is lying on the ground, put a coat or blanket under the victim. Keep the victim warm with a blanket or coat over the victim. *Do not let a shock victim eat, drink, or smoke.*				
6. If the victim vomits, turn the head to drain the mouth.				
Complete Skill				

Participant Name _____   Date _____

Instructor Name _____

Performance Checklist: Splinting the Forearm

Skill step	Initial Practice		Final Performance	
	Needs Practice	Proficient	Remediate	Proficient
1. Support the arm. Check circulation.				
2. Position the arm on a rigid splint.				
3. Secure the splint.				
4. Check circulation.				
5. Put the arm in a sling, and tie a binder over the sling and around the chest.				
Complete Skill				

Participant Name _____   Date _____

Instructor Name _____

Performance Checklist (Appendix A): Bag-Valve-Mask for Rescue Breathing (Two Rescuers)

Skill Step	Initial Practice		Final Performance	
	Needs Practice	**Proficient**	**Remediate**	**Proficient**
1. Rescuer 1 assembles BVM with correct-size mask and puts mask over victim's mouth and nose.				
2. Rescuer 2 positions hands: thumbs and index fingers circling each side of mask, other three fingers behind lower jawbone. Pull the jaw up into the mask rather than pushing the mask down on the jaw.				
3. Rescuer 2 opens airway and seals mask to victim's face.				

4. Rescuer 1 squeezes bag to provide ventilations:
   a. 1 ventilation over 1 second in adult, every 5 to 6 seconds.
   b. 1 ventilation over 1 second in child or infant, every 3 to 5 seconds.				

5. Recheck for a pulse about every two minutes. If no pulse, call for AED and start CPR.				
Complete Skill				

Participant Name _____   Date _____

Instructor Name _____

Performance Checklist (Appendix A): CPR for Adult or Child (Two Rescuers)

Skill Step	Initial Practice		Final Performance	
	Needs Practice	**Proficient**	**Remediate**	**Proficient**
1. At the victim's head, Rescuer 1 checks the victim's ABCs. An AED has been summoned. At the victim's side, Rescuer 2 locates the site for chest compressions.				
2. Rescuer 1 indicates "No circulation." Rescuer 2 gives 30 compressions for an adult (15 for a child) at rate of 100 per minute, counting aloud for a fast, steady rate, then pauses.				
3. Rescuer 1 gives 2 breaths.				
4. Rescuers continue cycles of 30 compressions in an adult (15 in a child) and 2 breaths for about 2 minutes (or after 5 cycles of compressions and ventilations at a ratio of 30:2) before switching compressor and ventilator roles. The switch should be done quickly (in less than 5 seconds).				
5. Rescuers continue CPR until: • Victim shows signs of circulation or breathing • An AED is brought to the scene and is ready to use • Help arrives and takes over				
6. If the victim starts breathing and has signs of circulation, put in the recovery position and monitor the ABCs.				
7. If an AED is brought to the scene, start the AED sequence.				
Complete Skill				

Participant Name _____   Date _____

Instructor Name _____

Performance Checklist (Appendix A): CPR for Infant (Two rescuers)

Skill step	Initial Practice		Final Performance	
	Needs Practice	**Proficient**	**Remediate**	**Proficient**
1. At the infant's head, Rescuer 1 checks the ABCs. At the infant's feet, Rescuer 2 locates the site for chest compressions with both thumbs.				
2. If absent, Rescuer 1 says, "No circulation." Rescuer 2 gives 15 chest compressions at a rate of 100 per minute, counting aloud for a fast, steady rate, then pauses.				
3. Rescuer 1 gives 2 breaths.				
4. Rescuers continue cycles of 15 compressions and 2 breaths for about 2 minutes before switching compressor and ventilator roles. The switch should be done quickly (in less than 5 seconds). Rescuers continue CPR until: • Infant shows signs of circulation or breathing • Help arrives and takes over				
5. If the infant starts breathing, hold infant in the recovery position and monitor the ABCs.				
Complete Skill				

Participant Name _____   Date _____

Instructor Name _____

Performance Checklist (Appendix A): Nasal Airway Insertion

Skill Step	Initial Practice		Final Performance	
	Needs Practice	Proficient	Remediate	Proficient
1. Choose the correct nasal airway size.				
2. Coat the nasal airway with lubricant.				
3. Insert the nasal airway in the right nostril with the bevel toward the septum.				
4. Insert the nasal airway straight back, sliding it along the floor of the nostril.				
5. Insert nasal airway until flange rests against the nose.				
Complete Skill				

Participant Name _____   Date _____

Instructor Name _____

Performance Checklist (Appendix A): Oral Airway Insertion

Skill Step	Initial Practice		Final Performance	
	Needs Practice	Proficient	Remediate	Proficient
1. Choose the correct airway device size.				
2. Open the victim's airway with head tilt-chin lift or jaw thrust, and open the mouth.				
3. Insert the airway device with the tip pointing toward the roof of the mouth.				
4. When tip reaches back of mouth and you feel resistance, rotate the airway 180 degrees.				
5. Continue to insert the airway device to final position (the flange resting on the lips).				
Complete Skill				

Participant Name _____   Date _____

Instructor Name _____

Performance Checklist (Appendix A): Oxygen Administration

Skill Step	Initial Practice		Final Performance	
	Needs Practice	Proficient	Remediate	Proficient
1. Check equipment: oxygen labels on the cylinder and regulator; tubing and delivery device ready.				
2. Remove any protective seal, point cylinder away, and open main valve for 1 second.				
3. Remove any protective seals and attach regulator to oxygen cylinder.				
4. Open the main cylinder valve.				
5. Check the pressure regulator gauge.				
6. Attach the tubing to the flowmeter and the oxygen delivery device.				

7. Set the flowmeter at the correct oxygen flow rate.
   a. 1–6 Lpm for nasal cannula
   b. 10 Lpm for face mask
   c. 10–15 Lpm for BVM or nonrebreather mask				

8. Confirm that oxygen is flowing.				
9. Position the delivery device on the victim and continue rescue breathing (or allow victim to breathe spontaneously).				
10. Monitor the pressure regulator gauge and be prepared to remove the delivery device and change tanks if the pressure drops below 500 psi. Observe oxygen safety precautions.				
Complete Skill				

Participant Name _____   Date _____

Instructor Name _____

Performance Checklist (Appendix A): Rescue Breathing

Skill step	Initial Practice		Final Performance	
	Needs Practice	**Proficient**	**Remediate**	**Proficient**
1. Open the airway. Look, listen, and feel for adequate breathing for up to 10 seconds. *Be careful not to tilt an infant's head too far back.*				
2. If not breathing adequately, give 2 breaths over 1 second each, watching the chest rise and letting it fall. *Do not blow harder than is needed to make the victim's chest rise.*				
3. If the first breath does not go in, try again to open the airway and give another rescue breath. If it still does not go in, the victim may be choking. Proceed to CPR for choking.				
4. If your first 2 breaths go in, check the victim for no more than 10 seconds for a pulse and other signs of circulation. If there is a pulse but no adequate breathing, continue rescue breathing at rate of 10 to 12 breaths per minute (1 breath every 5–6 seconds) for an adult (or about 12 to 20 breaths per minute for an infant or child: 1 breath every 3–5 seconds), rechecking for a pulse about every 2 minutes. If there is no pulse, start CPR beginning with chest compressions.				
Complete Skill				

Participant Name _____   Date _____

Instructor Name _____

Performance Checklist (Appendix A): Suctioning (Adult or Child)

Skill Step	Initial Practice		Final Performance	
	Needs Practice	**Proficient**	**Remediate**	**Proficient**
1. Confirm that the suction device is working and produces suction.				
2. Turn the victim's head to one side and open the mouth (with spinal injury, support the head and turn with body as one unit).				
3. Sweep out solids and larger amounts of fluid with your finger.				
4. Determine maximum depth of insertion by measuring catheter tip from earlobe to corner of mouth.				
5. Turn on suction or pump handle to create suction.				
6. With suction on, insert catheter tip carefully into mouth, moving the tip about as you withdraw it.				
7. Reposition the victim's head with airway open, and resume rescue breathing or CPR.				
Complete Skill				

Participant Name _____   Date _____

Instructor Name _____

Performance Checklist (Appendix A): Suctioning (Infant)

Skill Step	Initial Practice		Final Performance	
	Needs Practice	**Proficient**	**Remediate**	**Proficient**
1. Hold infant in position for suctioning, with head lower than body and turned to one side.				
2. Squeeze suction bulb first and then gently insert the tip into infant's mouth.				
3. Gradually release the bulb to create suction as you withdraw tip from mouth.				
4. Move the bulb aside and squeeze it with tip down to empty it.				
5. Repeat Steps 2 through 4 until airway seems clear, up to 3 times.				
6. Repeat suctioning steps for each nostril.				
7. Resume rescue breathing or CPR.				
Complete Skill				

Appendix

C Natural Disasters: Earthquakes

Surviving an earthquake and reducing its health impact requires preparation, planning, and practice. Far in advance, you can gather emergency supplies, identify and reduce possible hazards in your home, and practice what to do during and after an earthquake. Learning what actions to take can help you and your family to remain safe and healthy in the event of an earthquake.

BEING PREPARED

While California has been the state most prone to serious earthquakes in recent years, there are many other fault zones in other areas of the United States. For example, geologists and seismologists have predicted a 97% chance of a major earthquake occurring in the New Madrid seismic zone of the central United States (including Arkansas, Missouri, Tennessee, and Kentucky) between now and the year 2035. While earthquakes with the power of the one that hit the greater Los Angeles area in January 1994 are fairly rare, less severe earthquakes can interrupt your normal living patterns and cause substantial injury.

During a major earthquake, you may hear a roaring or rumbling sound that gradually grows louder. You may feel a rolling sensation that starts out gently and, within a second or two, grows violent. Or you may first be jarred by a violent jolt. A second or two later, you may feel shaking and find it difficult to stand up or move from one room to another.

The key to surviving an earthquake and reducing your risk of injury lies in planning, preparing, and practicing what you and your family will do if it happens.

Practice Drills

By planning and practicing what to do if an earthquake strikes, you and your family can learn to react correctly and automatically when the shaking begins. During an earthquake, most deaths and injuries are caused by collapsing building materials and heavy falling objects, such as bookcases, cabinets, and heating units. Learn the safe spots in each room of your home. If you have children, get the entire family to practice going to these locations. Participating in an earthquake drill will help children to understand what to do in case you are not with them during an earthquake.

Make sure you and your child also understand the school's emergency procedures for disasters. This will help you to coordinate where, when, and how to reunite with your child after an earthquake.

During your earthquake drill:

- Get under a sturdy table or desk and hold onto it.
- If you're not near a table or desk, cover your face and head with your arms and stand or crouch in a strongly supported doorway or brace yourself in an inside corner of the house or building.
- Stay clear of windows or glass that could shatter or objects that could fall on you.
- Remember: If you are inside, stay inside. Many people are injured at entrances of buildings by falling debris.

Evacuation Plans

After an earthquake occurs, you may need to evacuate a damaged area. By planning and practicing for evacuation, you will be better prepared to respond appropriately and efficiently to signs of danger or to directions by civil authorities.

- Take a few minutes with your family to discuss a home evacuation plan. Sketch a floor plan of your home; walk through each room and discuss evacuation details.
- Plan a second way to exit from each room or area, if possible. If you need special equipment, such as a rope ladder, mark where it is located.
- Mark where your emergency food, water, first aid kits, and fire extinguishers are located.
- Mark where the utility switches or valves are located so that they can be turned off, if possible.

Source for information is the Centers for Disease Control and Prevention (http://www.bt.cdc.gov/disasters).

- Indicate the location of your family's emergency outdoor meeting place.

Establish Priorities

Take time before an earthquake strikes to write an emergency priority list, including

- important items to be hand-carried by you.
- other items, in order of importance to you and your family.
- items to be removed by car or truck if one is available.
- things to do if time permits, such as locking doors and windows, turning off the utilities, etc.

Write Down Important Information

Make a list of important information and put it in a secure location. Include on your list

- important telephone numbers, such as police, fire, EMS, and medical centers.
- the names, addresses, and telephone numbers of your insurance agents, including policy types and numbers.
- the telephone numbers of the electric, gas, and water companies.
- the names and telephone numbers of neighbors.
- the name and telephone number of your landlord or property manager.
- important medical information (i.e., allergies, regular medications).
- the vehicle identification number, year, model, and license number of your automobile, boat, RV, etc.
- your financial institution's telephone number, account types, and numbers.
- radio and television broadcast stations to tune to for emergency broadcast information.

Gather and Store Important Documents in a Fireproof Safe

- Birth certificates
- Ownership certificates (automobiles, boats, etc.)
- Social Security cards
- Insurance policies
- Wills
- Household inventory, including:
  - List of contents
  - Photographs of contents of every room
  - Photographs of items of high value, such as jewelry, paintings, collectors' items

EMERGENCY SUPPLIES

Stock up now on emergency supplies that can be used after an earthquake. These supplies should include a first aid kit, survival kits for the home, automobile, and workplace, and emergency water and food. Store enough supplies to last at least three days.

First Aid Kit

Store your first aid supplies in a toolbox or fishing tackle box so they will be easy to carry and protect from water. Inspect your kit regularly and keep it freshly stocked. *Note:* Important medical information and most prescriptions can be stored in the refrigerator, which also provides excellent protection from fires.

Survival Kit for Your Home

Assemble a survival kit for your home with the following items:

Tools and Supplies

- Axe, shovel, broom
- Screwdriver, pliers, hammer, adjustable wrench
- Rope for towing or rescue
- Plastic sheeting and tape

Items for Safety and Comfort

- Sturdy shoes that can provide protection from broken glass, nails, and other debris
- Gloves (heavy and durable for cleaning up debris)
- Candles
- Waterproof matches
- Change of clothing
- Knife
- Garden hose (for siphoning and firefighting)
- Tent
- Recreational supplies for children and adults
- Blankets or sleeping bags
- Portable radio, flashlight, and extra batteries
- Essential medications and eyeglasses
- Fire extinguisher—multipurpose, dry chemical type
- Food and water for pets
- Toilet tissue
- Cash

Survival Kit for Your Automobile

Assemble a survival kit for your automobile with the following items. Storing some of these supplies in a small bag or backpack will make them more convenient to carry if you need to walk.

- Blankets
- Bottled water
- Change of clothes
- Coins for telephone calls
- Fire extinguisher—multipurpose, dry chemical type
- First aid kit and manual
- Emergency signal device (light sticks, battery-type flasher, reflector, etc.)
- Flashlight with fresh batteries
- Food (nonperishable—nutrition bars, trail mix, etc.)
- Gloves
- Local map and compass
- Rope for towing, rescue, etc.
- Paper and pencils
- Premoistened towelettes
- Prescription medicines
- Battery-operated radio with fresh batteries
- Small mirror for signaling
- Toilet tissue
- Tools (pliers, adjustable wrench, screwdriver, etc.)
- Whistle for signaling
- Jumper cables
- Duct tape

Survival Kit for Your Workplace

Assemble a survival kit for the workplace with the following supplies:

- Food (nonperishable—nutrition bars, trail mix, etc.)
- Bottled water
- Jacket or sweatshirt
- Pair of sturdy shoes
- Flashlight with fresh batteries
- Battery-operated radio with fresh batteries
- Essential medications
- Blanket
- Small first aid kit

- Extra pair of eyeglasses and/or contact lens solution
- Whistle or other signaling device

EMERGENCY WATER STORAGE AND PURIFICATION

Following are recommendations for storing and purifying water supplies:

- The minimum drinking water supply is one gallon per person per day. You will also need water for food preparation, bathing, brushing teeth, and dishwashing. Store a three- to five-day supply of water (at least five gallons for each person).
- Water should be stored in sturdy plastic bottles with tight-fitting lids. Rinsed chlorine bleach bottles work well. Plastic containers for juice and milk do not work as well because they tend to crack and leak more readily.
- Stored water should be changed every six months.
- Avoid placing water containers in areas where toxic substances, such as gasoline and pesticides, are present. Vapors may penetrate the plastic over time.
- Do not store water containers in direct sunlight. Select a place with a fairly constant, cool temperature.

Safe Water Sources in the Home

If you do not have enough water stored, there are sources in your home that may provide safe, clean water for drinking purposes.

- Water drained from the water heater faucet, if the water heater has not been damaged
- Water dipped from the tank of the toilet (not the bowl). The water in the bowl can be used for pets. Do not use water that has been chemically treated or "blue" water.
- Melted ice cubes
- Canned fruit, vegetable juice, and liquids from other canned goods
- Water from the swimming pool. Use this water only after other sources of pure water are exhausted.

Unsafe Water Sources

Never use water from the following sources for drinking:

- Radiators
- Hot water boilers (home heating system)
- Water beds (fungicides added to the water or chemicals in the vinyl may make water unsafe for use)

Note: Remember that carbonated beverages do not meet drinking water requirements. Caffeinated drinks and alcohol dehydrate the body, which increases the need for drinking water.

Water for Drinking and Cooking

Safe drinking water includes bottled, boiled, or treated water. Your state or local health department can make specific recommendations for boiling or treating drinking water in your area. Here are some general rules about water for drinking and cooking. Remember:

- Do not use contaminated water to wash dishes, brush your teeth, wash and prepare food, or make ice.
- If you use bottled water, make sure the seal has not been broken. Otherwise, water should be boiled or treated before use. Drink only bottled, boiled, or treated water until your supply is tested and found safe.
- Boiling water kills harmful bacteria and parasites. Bringing water to a rolling boil for one minute will kill most organisms.
- Treat water with chlorine or iodine tablets or mix six drops ($^1/_8$ teaspoon) of unscented, ordinary household chlorine bleach per gallon of water. Mix the solution thoroughly, and let stand for about 30 minutes. However, this treatment will not kill parasitic organisms.

Containers for water should be rinsed with a bleach solution before using and reusing. Use water storage tanks and other types of containers with caution. For example, fire truck storage tanks, as well as previously used cans or bottles, can be contaminated with microbes or chemicals.

EMERGENCY FOOD

Keep foods that

- have a long storage life.
- require little or no cooking, water, or refrigeration, in case utilities are disrupted.
- meet the needs of babies or other family members who are on special diets.

- meet pets' needs.
- are not very salty or spicy, as these foods increase the need for drinking water, which may be in short supply.

How to Store Emergency Food

- A disaster can easily disrupt the food supply at any time, so plan to have at least a three-day supply of food on hand.
- When storing food, it is not necessary to buy dehydrated or other types of emergency food. Canned foods and dry mixes will remain fresh for about two years.
- Certain storage conditions can enhance the shelf life of canned or dried foods. The ideal location is a cool, dry, dark place. The best temperature is 40 to 60° F. Keep foods away from ranges or refrigerator exhausts. Heat causes many foods to spoil more quickly.
- Keep food away from petroleum products, such as gasoline, oil, paints, and solvents. Some food products absorb their smell.
- Protect food from rodents and insects. Items stored in boxes or in paper cartons will keep longer if they are heavily wrapped or stored in airtight containers.
- Date all food items. Use and replace food before it loses freshness.

How to Use Emergency Food

- Use perishable food in your refrigerator or freezer before using food in your emergency supplies.
- Discard cooked, unrefrigerated foods after two hours at room temperature, regardless of appearance.
- Eat only foods that have a normal color, texture, and odor.
- Discard cans that bulge at the ends or that are leaking.

Preparing Food

Your ability to prepare food after an earthquake may be complicated by damage to your home and loss of electricity, gas, and water. The following items will help you to prepare meals safely:

- Cooking utensils
- Knives, forks, and spoons

- Paper plates, cups, and towels
- A manual can- and bottle-opener
- Heavy-duty aluminum foil
- Gas or charcoal grill; camp stove
- Fuel for cooking, such as charcoal. (*Caution:* Never burn charcoal indoors. The fumes are deadly when concentrated indoors.)

Note: Do not use your fireplace for cooking until the chimney has been inspected for cracks and damage. Sparks may escape into your attic through an undetected crack and start a fire.

INSPECTING FOR POSSIBLE HOME HAZARDS

An important step in earthquake preparedness is to inspect your home and its surroundings for possible hazards and then take action to lessen those hazards. Remember: anything can move, fall, or break during an earthquake or its aftershocks.

The following is a basic checklist to help you identify and correct possible home hazards.

Rooms in the Home

Look for the following hazards in each room:
- Windows and other glass that might shatter
- Unanchored bookcases, cabinets, refrigerators, water heaters, and other furniture that might topple
- Heating units, fireplaces, chimneys, and stoves that could move or fall
- Areas that could be blocked by falling debris

Securing Appliances

- Secure your large appliances with flexible cable, braided wire, or metal strapping.
- Install flexible gas and water connections on all gas appliances. This will significantly reduce your chances of having a major fire after an earthquake.
- Brace and support air conditioners, particularly those on rooftops.

A typical water heater weighs about 450 pounds when full. In an earthquake, the floor on which it is standing tends to move out from under the heater, often causing it to topple. The movement can also break the gas, electric, and water-line connectors, posing fire or electric

shock hazards, and can shatter the glass lining within the water heater. The water tank should be well secured with bolts to wall studs.

Securing Items in the Bathroom

Replace glass bottles from your medicine cabinet and around the bathtub with plastic containers.

Hanging and Overhead Items

- Inspect and anchor overhead light fixtures, such as chandeliers.
- Move heavy mirrors and pictures hanging above beds, chairs, and other places where you sit or sleep. Otherwise, anchor these items with wire through eyescrews bolted into wall studs. Or place screws on both sides, top, and bottom of the frame and screw these into the studs.
- Determine whether the full swing of your hanging lamps or plants will strike a window. If so, move them.
- Secure hanging objects by closing the opening of the hook.
- Replace heavy ceramic or glass hanging planters with lightweight plastic or wicker baskets.

Shelves, Cabinets, and Furniture

- Identify top-heavy, freestanding furniture, such as bookcases and china cabinets, that could topple in an earthquake.
- Secure your furniture by using:
  - L brackets, corner brackets, or aluminum molding to attach tall or top-heavy furniture to the wall
  - Eyebolts to secure items located a short distance from the wall
- Attach a wooden or metal guardrail on open shelves to keep items from sliding or falling off. Fishing line can also be used as a less-visible means of securing an item.
- Place heavy or large objects on lower shelves.
- Use Velcro®-type fastenings to secure some items to their shelves.
- Secure your cabinet doors by installing sliding bolts or childproof latches.

Hazardous Materials

Identify poisons, solvents, or toxic materials in breakable containers and move these containers to a safe, well-ventilated storage area. Keep them away from your water storage and out of reach of children and pets.

INSPECTING AND SECURING YOUR HOME'S STRUCTURE

Examine the structural safety of your house. If your house is of conventional wood construction, it will probably be relatively resistant to earthquake damage, particularly if it is a single-story structure.

For information on structural safety standards and qualified contractors in your area, contact your city or county government office on community development or building code enforcement.

The following suggestions will take an investment of time and money but will add stability to your home. If you want to do the work yourself, many hardware or home-improvement stores will assist you with information and instructions.

Foundation

Check to see if your house or garage is securely fastened to the foundation. (If your house was built before 1950, it probably does not have bolts securing the wood structure to the concrete foundation.) If your house is not secured to the foundation, talk to a building contractor.

Beams, Posts, Joists, and Plates

Strengthen the areas of connection between beams, posts, joists, and plates using such hardware as T and L straps, mending plates, and joist hangers. Pay particular attention to exposed framing in garages, basements, porches, and patio covers.

Roof and Chimney

- Check your chimney or roof for loose tiles and bricks that could fall in an earthquake. Repair loose tiles or bricks as needed.
- Protect yourself from falling chimney bricks that might penetrate the roof by reinforcing the ceiling immediately surrounding the chimney with $3/4$-inch plywood nailed to ceiling joists.

LEARNING TO SHUT OFF UTILITIES

- Know where and how to shut off utilities at the main switches or valves. Check with your local utility companies for instructions.

- Teach all family members how and when to shut off utilities.

Gas

- An automatic valve (Earthquake Command System) is commercially available that will turn the gas off for you in the event of an earthquake.
- After an earthquake, *do not use* matches, lighters, or appliances, and do not operate light switches until you are sure there are no gas leaks. Sparks from electrical switches could ignite gas, causing an explosion.
- If you smell the odor of gas, or if you notice a large consumption of gas being registered on the gas meter, shut off the gas immediately. First, find the main shutoff valve, located on a pipe next to the gas meter. Use an adjustable wrench to turn the valve to the Off position.

Electricity

After a major disaster, shut off the electricity. Sparks from electrical switches could pose a shock or fire hazard. Carefully turn off the electricity at the main electrical breaker in your home.

Water

Water may be turned off at either of two locations:

- At the main meter, which controls the water flow to the entire property; or
- At the water main leading into the home. (Shutting off the water here retains the water supply to your water heater, which may be useful in an emergency.)

Attach a valve wrench to the water line. (This tool can be purchased at most hardware stores.) Also, label the water mains for quick identification.

DURING AN EARTHQUAKE

Indoor Safety

There are actions you can take, even while an earthquake is happening, that will reduce your chances of being hurt. Lights may be out, and hallways, stairs, and room exits may be blocked by fallen furniture, ceiling tiles, and other debris. Planning for these situations will help you to take action quickly.

- If an earthquake strikes, you may be able to take cover under a heavy desk or table. It can provide you with air space if the building collapses. If you get under a table and it moves, try to move with it.

- Inner walls or door frames are the least likely structures to collapse and may also shield you from falling objects. If other cover is not available, go to an inner corner or doorway, away from windows or glass panels.
- Stay away from glass and hanging objects, and bookcases, china cabinets, or other large furniture that could fall. Watch for falling objects, such as bricks from fireplaces and chimneys, light fixtures, wall hangings, high shelves, and cabinets with doors that could swing open.
- Grab something to shield your head and face from falling debris and broken glass.
- If the lights go out, use a battery-operated flashlight. Don't use candles, matches, or lighters during or after the earthquake. If there is a gas leak, an explosion could result.
- If you are in the kitchen, quickly turn off the stove and take cover at the first sign of shaking.

High-Rise Buildings

Get under a desk and stay away from windows and outside walls. Stay in the building. The electricity may go out, and the sprinkler systems may come on. *Do not* use the elevators.

Crowded Indoor Public Places

If you are in a crowded public place, do not rush for the doorways. Others will have the same idea. Move away from display shelves containing objects that may fall. If you can, take cover and grab something to shield your head and face from falling debris and glass.

Outdoor Safety

If you are outdoors, move away from buildings and utility wires. The greatest danger from falling debris is just outside doorways and close to outer walls. Once you are in the open, stay there until the shaking stops.

Automobiles

If you are in a moving automobile, stop as quickly and safely as possible and move over to the shoulder or curb, away from utility poles, overhead wires, and under- or over-

passes. Stay in the vehicle, set the parking brake, and turn on the radio for emergency broadcast information. A car may jiggle violently on its springs, but it is a good place to stay until the shaking stops. If you are in a life-threatening situation, you may be able to reach someone with either a cellular or an emergency roadside assistance phone.

When you drive on, watch for hazards created by the earthquake, such as breaks in the pavement, downed utility poles and wires, and fallen overpasses and bridges.

AFTER AN EARTHQUAKE
Aftereffects

Be prepared for additional earth movements called aftershocks. Although most of these are smaller than the main earthquake, some may be large enough to cause additional damage or bring down weakened structures.

Because other aftereffects can include fires, chemical spills, landslides, dam breaks, and tidal waves, be sure to monitor your battery-operated radio or TV for additional emergency information.

Injuries

Check for injuries. Do not attempt to move injured or unconscious people unless they are in immediate danger from live electrical wires, flooding, or other hazards. Internal injuries may not be evident, but they may be serious or life-threatening. If someone has stopped breathing, call for medical or first aid assistance immediately and begin CPR if you are trained to do so. Stop a bleeding injury by applying direct pressure to the wound. If you are trapped, try to attract attention to your location.

Checking Utilities

An earthquake may break gas, electrical, and water lines. If you smell gas: (1) open windows, (2) shut off the main gas valve, (3) do not turn any electrical appliances or lights on or off, (4) go outside, (5) report the leak to authorities, and (6) do not reenter the building until a utility official says it is safe to do so.

- If electric wiring is shorting out, shut off the electric current at the main box.

- If water pipes are damaged, shut off the supply at the main valve.

Other Precautions

- Have chimneys inspected for cracks and damage. Do not use the fireplace if the chimney has any damage.
- Check to see if sewage lines are intact before using bathrooms or plumbing.
- Do not touch downed power lines or objects in contact with downed lines. Report electrical hazards to the authorities.
- Immediately clean up spilled medicines, drugs, flammable liquids, and other potentially hazardous materials.
- Stay off all telephones except to report an emergency. Replace telephone receivers that may have been knocked off by the earthquake.
- Stay away from damaged areas. Your presence could hamper relief efforts, and you could endanger yourself.
- Cooperate fully with public safety officials. Respond to requests for volunteer assistance from police, firefighters, emergency management officials, and relief organizations, but do not go into damaged areas unless assistance has been requested.

Evacuating Your Home

If you must evacuate your home:

- Post a message, in a prearranged location known only to family members, indicating where you have gone.
- Confine pets to the safest location possible and make sure they have plenty of food and water. Pets will not be allowed in designated public shelters.
- Take vital documents (such as wills and insurance policies), emergency supplies, and extra medications with you.

PEOPLE WITH SPECIAL NEEDS
People with Disabilities

Before an earthquake:

- Write down any specific needs, limitations, and capabilities that you have, and any

medications you take. Make a copy of the list and put it in your purse or wallet.
- Find someone (a spouse, roommate, friend, neighbor, relative, or co-worker) to help you in case of an emergency. Give them the list. You may wish to provide a spare key to your home, or let them know where they can find one in an emergency.

During an earthquake:

- If you are confined to a wheelchair, try to get under a doorway or into an inside corner, lock the wheels, and cover your head with your arms. Remove any items that are not securely attached to the wheelchair.
- If you are able, seek shelter under a sturdy table or desk. Stay away from outer walls, windows, fireplaces, and hanging objects.
- If you are unable to move from a bed or chair, protect yourself from falling objects by covering up with blankets and pillows.
- If you are outside, go to an open area away from trees, telephone poles, and buildings, and stay there.

After an earthquake:

- If you are trapped, try to attract attention to your location.
- Turn on your battery-operated TV or radio to receive emergency information and instructions.
- If you can, help others in need.

Children's Needs

Fear is a normal reaction to danger. Children may be afraid of recurrence, injury, or death after an earthquake. They may fear being separated from their family or being left alone. Children may even interpret disasters as punishment for real or imagined misdeeds. Children will be less likely to experience prolonged fear or anxiety if they know what to expect before, during, and after an earthquake. Talking to children openly will also help them to overcome fears.

Here are some suggestions:

- Explain that an earthquake is a natural event and not anyone's fault.
- Talk about your own experiences with natural disasters, or read aloud books about earthquakes.
- Encourage your child to express feelings of fear. Listen carefully and show understanding.

- Your child may need both verbal and physical reassurance that everything will be all right. Tell your child that the situation is not permanent.
- Include your child in cleanup activities. It is comforting to the child to watch the household begin to return to normal and to have a job to do.

Note: Symptoms of anxiety may not appear for weeks or even months after an earthquake, and they can affect people of any age. If anxiety disrupts daily activities for any member of your family, seek professional assistance through a school counselor, community religious organization, your physician, or a licensed mental health professional.

Appendix

D Natural Disasters: Floods

During a flood and its aftermath, there are some basic facts to remember that will help you to protect your personal health and safety.

PREPARING FOR A FLOOD

Here are some basic steps to take to prepare for the storm:

- Contact the local county geologist or county planning department to find out if your home is located in a flash flood–prone area or landslide-prone area.
- Learn about your community's emergency plans, warning signals, evacuation routes, and locations of emergency shelters.
- Plan and practice a flood evacuation route with your family. Ask an out-of-state relative or friend to be the "family contact" in case your family is separated during a flood. Make sure everyone in your family knows the name, address, and phone number of this contact person.
- Post emergency phone numbers at every phone.
- Inform local authorities about any special needs, such as elderly or bedridden people, or anyone with a disability.
- Identify potential home hazards and know how to secure or protect them before the flood strikes. Be prepared to turn off electrical power when there is standing water, fallen power lines, or before your evacuation. Turn off gas and water supplies before you evacuate. Secure structurally unstable building materials.
- Buy a fire extinguisher and make sure your family knows where it is and how to use it.
- Buy and install sump pumps with backup power.

- Have a licensed electrician raise electric components (switches, sockets, circuit breakers and wiring) at least 12-inches above your home's projected flood elevation.
- For drains, toilets, and other sewer connections, install backflow valves or plugs to prevent floodwaters from entering.
- Anchor fuel tanks that can contaminate your basement if torn free. An unanchored tank outside can be swept downstream and damage other houses.

If you are under a flood watch or warning:

- Gather the emergency supplies you previously stocked in your home and stay tuned to local radio or television stations for updates.
- Turn off all utilities at the main power switch and close the main gas valve if evacuation appears necessary.
- Have your immunization records handy or be aware of your last tetanus shot, in case you should receive a puncture wound or a wound becomes contaminated during or after the flood.
- Fill bathtubs, sinks, and plastic soda bottles with clean water. Sanitize the sinks and tubs first by using bleach. Rinse and fill with clean water.
- Bring outdoor possessions, such as lawn furniture, grills, and trash cans, inside or tie them down securely.

Emergency Supplies You Will Need

You should stock your home with supplies that may be needed during the emergency period. At a minimum, these supplies should include:

- Several clean containers for water, large enough for a three- to five-day supply of water (about five gallons for each person).
- A three- to five-day supply of nonperishable food and a nonelectric can opener.

Source for information is the Centers for Disease Control and Prevention (http://www.bt.cdc.gov/disasters).

- A first aid kit and first aid manual; prescription medicines and items for special medical needs.
- A battery-powered radio, flashlights, and extra batteries.
- Sleeping bags or extra blankets.
- Water-purifying supplies, such as chlorine or iodine tablets or unscented, ordinary household chlorine bleach.
- Baby food and/or prepared formula, diapers, and other baby supplies.
- Disposable cleaning cloths, such as "baby wipes," for the whole family to use in case bathing facilities are not available.
- Personal hygiene supplies, such as soap, toothpaste, and sanitary napkins.
- An emergency kit for your car with food, flares, booster cables, maps, tools, a first aid kit, fire extinguisher, and sleeping bags.
- Rubber boots, sturdy shoes, and waterproof gloves.
- Insect repellant containing DEET, window screens, and long-sleeved and long-legged clothing for protection from mosquitoes that may gather in pooled water remaining after the flood.

Preparing to Evacuate

Expect the need to evacuate and prepare for it. When a flood watch is issued, you should:

- Fill your vehicle's gas tank and make sure the emergency kit for your car is ready.
- If no vehicle is available, make arrangements with friends or family for transportation.
- Fill your clean water containers.
- Review your emergency plans and supplies, checking to see if any items are missing.
- Tune in the radio or television for weather updates.
- Listen for disaster sirens and warning signals.
- Put livestock and family pets in a safe area. Due to food and sanitation requirements, emergency shelters cannot accept animals.
- Adjust the thermostat on refrigerators and freezers to the coolest possible temperature.

If You Are Ordered to Evacuate

You should never ignore an evacuation order. Authorities will direct you to leave if you are in a low-lying area, or within the greatest potential path of the rising waters. If a flood warning is issued for your area or you are directed by authorities to evacuate the area:

- Take only essential items with you.
- If you have time, turn off the gas, electricity, and water.
- Disconnect appliances to prevent electrical shock when power is restored.
- Follow the designated evacuation routes and expect heavy traffic.
- Do not attempt to drive or walk across creeks or flooded roads.

If You Are Ordered *Not* to Evacuate

To get through the storm in the safest possible manner:

- Monitor the radio or television for weather updates.
- Prepare to evacuate to a shelter or to a neighbor's home if your home is damaged, or if you are instructed to do so by emergency personnel.

FLOOD RECOVERY

How to Avoid Illness

Always wash your hands with soap and water that has been boiled or disinfected before preparing or eating food, after toilet use, after participating in flood cleanup activities, and after handling articles contaminated with floodwater or sewage. If you receive a puncture wound or a wound contaminated with feces, soil, or saliva, have a doctor or health department determine whether a tetanus booster is necessary.

How to Make Sure Your Food Is Safe

Do not eat any food that may have come into contact with floodwater. For infants, use only pre-prepared canned baby formula that requires no added water, rather than powdered formulas prepared with treated water. Thawed food can usually be eaten or refrozen if it is still "refrigerator cold," or if it still contains ice crystals. To be safe, remember, "When in doubt, throw it out." Discard any refrigerated or frozen food that has been at room temperature for two hours or more and any food that has an unusual odor, color, or texture.

How to Make Sure Your Water Is Safe

Listen for public announcements on the safety of the municipal water supply. Flooded, private water wells will need to be tested and disinfected after floodwaters recede. Questions about testing should be directed to your local or state health departments.

Safe water for drinking, cooking, and personal hygiene includes bottled, boiled, or treated water. Your state or local health department can make specific recommendations for boiling or treating water in your area. Here are some general rules concerning water for drinking, cooking, and personal hygiene. Do not use contaminated water to wash dishes, brush your teeth, wash and prepare food, wash your hands, make ice, or make baby formula. If possible, use baby formula that does not need to have water added. You can use an alcohol-based hand sanitizer to wash your hands.

- If you use bottled water, be sure it came from a safe source. If you do not know that the water came from a safe source, you should boil or treat it before you use it. Use only bottled, boiled, or treated water until your supply is tested and found safe.
- Boiling water, when practical, is the preferred way to kill harmful bacteria and parasites. Bringing water to a rolling boil for one minute will kill most organisms.
- When boiling water is not practical, you can treat water with chlorine tablets, iodine tablets, or unscented household chlorine bleach (5.25% sodium hypochlorite):
  - If you use chlorine tablets or iodine tablets, follow the directions that come with the tablets.
  - If you use household chlorine bleach, add $1/8$ teaspoon (about 0.75 mL) of bleach per gallon of water if the water is clear. For cloudy water, add $1/4$ teaspoon (about 1.50 mL) of bleach per gallon. Mix the solution thoroughly and let it stand for about 30 minutes before using it.

Note: Treating water with chlorine tablets, iodine tablets, or liquid bleach will not kill parasitic organisms.

Use a bleach solution to rinse water containers before reusing them. Use water storage tanks and other types of containers with caution. For example, fire truck storage tanks and previously used cans or bottles may be contaminated with microbes or chemicals. Do not rely on untested devices for decontaminating water.

How to Handle Animals and Mosquitoes

Many wild animals have been forced from their natural habitats by flooding, and many domestic animals are also without homes after the flood. Take care to avoid these animals. Do not corner an animal. If an animal must be removed, contact your local animal control authorities. If you are bitten by any animal, seek immediate medical attention. If you are bitten by a snake, try to accurately identify the type of snake so that, if it is poisonous, the correct antivenom may be administered.

Contact local or state health and agricultural officials for state guidelines on the disposal of dead animals. Protect yourself from mosquitoes: use screens on dwellings, wear long-sleeved and long-legged clothing, and use insect repellents that contain DEET.

How to Deal with Chemical Hazards

Be aware of potential chemical hazards you may encounter during flood recovery. Floodwaters may have buried or moved hazardous chemical containers of solvents or other industrial chemicals from their normal storage places. If any propane tanks (whether 20-pound tanks from a gas grill or household propane tanks) are discovered, do not try to move them yourself. These represent a very real danger of fire or explosion, and if any are found, police or fire departments or your state fire marshal's office should be contacted immediately. Car batteries, even those in floodwater, may still contain an electrical charge and should be removed with extreme caution by using insulated gloves. Avoid coming in contact with any acid that may have spilled from a damaged car battery.

How to Deal with Electric and Gas Utilities

Electrical power and natural gas or propane tanks should be shut off to avoid fire, electrocution, or explosions until it is safe to use them. Use battery-powered flashlights and lanterns, rather than candles, gas lanterns, or torches. If you smell gas or suspect a leak, turn off the main gas valve, open all windows, and leave the house immediately. Notify the gas company or the police or fire departments or state fire marshal's office, and do not turn on the lights or do anything that could cause a spark. Avoid any downed power lines, particularly those in water. All electrical equipment and appliances must be completely dry before returning them to service. It is advisable to have a certified electrician check these items if there is any question. Also, remember not to operate any gas-powered equipment indoors.

How to Clean Up

Walls, hard-surfaced floors, and many other household surfaces should be cleaned with soap and water and disinfected with a solution of one cup of bleach to five gallons of water. Wash all linens and clothing in hot water, or dry clean them. For items that cannot be washed or dry cleaned, such as mattresses and upholstered furniture, air dry them in the sun and then spray them thoroughly with a disinfectant. Steam clean all carpeting. If there has been a backflow of sewage into the house, wear rubber boots and waterproof gloves during cleanup. Remove and discard contaminated household materials that cannot be disinfected, such as wall coverings, cloth, rugs, and drywall. Additional guidance is available from the Environmental Protection Agency at http://www.epa.gov/iaq/pubs/flood.html and the Federal Emergency Management Agency at http://www.fema.gov/hazards/floods/whatshouldidoafter.shtm.

Appendix

E — Natural Disasters: Hurricanes

PREPARING FOR A HURRICANE

If you are in an area that is susceptible to hurricanes, here are some basic steps to take to prepare:

- Learn about your community's emergency plans, warning signals, evacuation routes, and locations of emergency shelters.
- Identify potential home hazards and know how to secure or protect them before the hurricane strikes. Be prepared to turn off electrical power when there is standing water, fallen power lines, or before your evacuation. Turn off gas and water supplies before you evacuate. Secure structurally unstable building materials.
- Buy a fire extinguisher and make sure your family knows where to find it and how to use it.
- Locate and secure your important papers, such as insurance policies, wills, licenses, and stock certificates.
- Post emergency phone numbers at every phone.
- Inform local authorities about any special needs, such as elderly or bedridden people or anyone with a disability.

Emergency Supplies You Will Need

You should stock your home with supplies that may be needed during the emergency period. At a minimum, these supplies should include:

- Several clean containers for water, large enough for a three- to five-day supply of water (about five gallons for each person).
- A three- to five-day supply of nonperishable food.
- A first aid kit and manual.
- A battery-powered radio, flashlights, and extra batteries.
- Sleeping bags or extra blankets.

Source of information is the Centers for Disease Control and Prevention (http://www.bt.cdc.gov/disasters).

- Water-purifying supplies, such as chlorine or iodine tablets or unscented, ordinary household chlorine bleach.
- Prescription medicines and special medical needs.
- Baby food and/or prepared formula, diapers, and other baby supplies.
- Disposable cleaning cloths, such as "baby wipes," for the whole family to use in case bathing facilities are not available.
- Personal hygiene supplies, such as soap, toothpaste, and sanitary napkins.
- An emergency kit for your car with food, flares, booster cables, maps, tools, a first aid kit, fire extinguisher, and sleeping bags.

You can find more information on emergency plans and supply kits at http://www.ready.gov.

PREPARING TO EVACUATE

Expect the need to evacuate and prepare for it. The National Weather Service will issue a hurricane watch when there is a threat to coastal areas of hurricane conditions within 24 to 36 hours.

When a hurricane watch is issued, you should:

- Fill your automobile's gas tank.
- If no vehicle is available, make arrangements with friends or family for transportation.
- Fill your clean water containers.
- Review your emergency plans and supplies, checking to see if any items are missing.
- Tune in the radio or television for weather updates.
- Listen for disaster sirens and warning signals.
- Prepare an emergency kit for your car with food, flares, booster cables, maps, tools, a first aid kit, fire extinguisher, and sleeping bags.
- Secure any items outside that may damage property in a storm, such as bicycles, grills, and propane tanks.

- Cover windows and doors with plywood or boards or place large strips of masking tape or adhesive tape on the windows to reduce the risk of breakage and flying glass.
- Put livestock and family pets in a safe area. Due to food and sanitation requirements, emergency shelters cannot accept animals.
- Place vehicles under cover, if at all possible.
- Fill sinks and bathtubs with water as an extra supply for washing.
- Adjust the thermostat on refrigerators and freezers to the coolest possible temperature.

If You Are Ordered to Evacuate

Because of the destructive power of a hurricane, you should never ignore an evacuation order. Authorities will be most likely to direct you to leave if you are in a low-lying area, or within the storm's greatest potential path of destruction. If a hurricane warning is issued for your area or you are directed by authorities to evacuate the area:

- Take only essential items with you.
- Leave pets indoors in a safe, covered area with ample food and water.
- If you have time, turn off the gas, electricity, and water.
- Disconnect appliances to reduce the likelihood of electrical shock when power is restored.
- Make sure your automobile's emergency kit is ready.
- Follow the designated evacuation routes—others may be blocked—and expect heavy traffic.

If You Are Ordered *Not* to Evacuate

The great majority of injuries during a hurricane are cuts caused by flying glass or other debris. Other injuries include puncture wounds from debris and bone fractures.

To get through the storm in the safest possible manner:

- Monitor the radio or television for weather conditions, if possible.
- Stay indoors until the authorities declare the storm is over.
- Do not go outside, even if the weather appears to have calmed. The calm "eye" of the storm can pass quickly, leaving you outside when strong winds resume.

- Stay away from all windows and exterior doors, seeking shelter in a bathroom or basement. Bathtubs can provide some shelter if you cover yourself with plywood or other materials.
- Prepare to evacuate to a shelter or to a neighbor's home if your home is damaged, or if you are instructed to do so by emergency personnel.

HURRICANE RECOVERY

Hurricanes often cause power outages. Indoor use of portable generators, charcoal grills, or camp stoves can lead to carbon monoxide poisoning. Take steps to protect your family from carbon monoxide poisoning.

How to Store Food Safely

Your refrigerator will keep foods cool for about four hours without power if it is unopened. Add block or dry ice to your refrigerator if the electricity will be off longer than four hours.

Thawed food can usually be eaten if it is still "refrigerator cold," or refrozen if it still contains ice crystals. Discard any food that has been at temperatures greater than 40° F for two hours or more, and discard any food that has an unusual odor, color, or texture.

While the power is out, keep the refrigerator and freezer doors closed as much as possible to keep food cold for as long as possible.

If the power is out for longer than four hours, follow these guidelines:

- Use dry ice, if available. Twenty-five pounds of dry ice will keep a 10-cubic-foot freezer below freezing for three to four days. Use care when handling dry ice, and wear dry, heavy gloves to avoid injury.
- For the freezer section: A freezer that is half full will hold food safely for up to 24 hours. A full freezer will hold food safely for 48 hours. Do not open the freezer door if you can avoid it.
- For the refrigerated section: Pack milk, other dairy products, meat, fish, eggs, gravy, and spoilable leftovers into a cooler surrounded by ice. Discard this food if it is held at a temperature greater than 40° F for more than two hours.
- Use a digital quick-response thermometer to check the temperature of your food right before you cook or eat it. Throw away any food that has a temperature of more than 40° F.

For additional information on food safety concerns following hurricanes or floods, visit the FDA website.

How to Make Sure Your Water Is Safe

Hurricanes, especially when accompanied by a tidal surge or flooding, can contaminate the public water supply. Drinking contaminated water may cause illness. You cannot assume that the water in the hurricane-affected area is safe to drink.

Listen for public announcements about the safety of the municipal water supply. Safe water for drinking, cooking, and personal hygiene includes bottled, boiled, or treated water. Your state or local health department can make specific recommendations for boiling or treating water in your area. Here are some general rules concerning water for drinking, cooking, and personal hygiene. Remember:

- Do not use contaminated water to wash dishes, brush your teeth, wash and prepare food, wash your hands, make ice, or make baby formula. If possible, use baby formula that does not need to have water added. You can use an alcohol-based hand sanitizer to wash your hands.

- If you use bottled water, be sure it came from a safe source. If you do not know that the water came from a safe source, you should boil or treat it before you use it. Use only bottled, boiled, or treated water until your supply is tested and found safe.

- Boiling water, when practical, is the preferred way to kill harmful bacteria and parasites. Bringing water to a rolling boil for one minute will kill most organisms.

- When boiling water is not practical, you can treat water with chlorine tablets, iodine tablets, or unscented household chlorine bleach (5.25% sodium hypochlorite):
  - If you use chlorine tablets or iodine tablets, follow the directions that come with the tablets.
  - If you use household chlorine bleach, add $\frac{1}{8}$ teaspoon (about 0.75 mL) of bleach per gallon of water if the water is clear. For cloudy water, add $\frac{1}{4}$ teaspoon (about 1.50 mL) of bleach per gallon. Mix the solution thoroughly and let it stand for about 30 minutes before using it.

Note: Treating water with chlorine tablets, iodine tablets, or liquid bleach will not kill parasitic organisms.

Use a bleach solution to rinse water containers before reusing them. Use water storage tanks and other types of containers with caution. For example, fire truck storage tanks and previously used cans or bottles may be contaminated with microbes or chemicals. Do not rely on untested devices for decontaminating water.

If there is flooding along with a hurricane, the waters may contain fecal material from overflowing sewage systems and agricultural and industrial waste. Although skin contact with floodwater does not, by itself, pose a serious health risk, there is risk of disease from eating or drinking anything contaminated with floodwater.

Do not allow children to play in floodwater areas. Wash children's hands frequently (always before meals), and do not allow children to play with floodwater-contaminated toys that have not been disinfected. You can disinfect toys using a solution of one cup of bleach in five gallons of water.

For more information about water purification after a hurricane or other weather emergency, please visit CDC's Web page on "Hurricanes and Your Health and Safety."

How to Prevent Injury after a Hurricane

When the wind and waters recede, people in the areas affected by a hurricane will continue to face a number of hazards associated with cleanup activities. The National Institute for Occupational Safety and Health (NIOSH) offers the following guidelines for preventing injury:

Wear Protective Gear

For most work in flooded areas, wear hard hats, goggles, heavy work gloves, and watertight boots with steel toe and insole (not just steel shank).

Wear earplugs or protective headphones to reduce risk from equipment noise. Equipment such as chainsaws, backhoes, and dryers may cause ringing in the ears and subsequent hearing damage.

Beware of Electrical Hazards

- If water has been present anywhere near electrical circuits and electrical equipment, turn off the power at the main breaker or fuse on the service panel. Do not turn the power back on until electrical equipment has been inspected by a qualified electrician.

- Never enter flooded areas or touch electrical equipment if the ground is wet, unless you are certain that the power is off. *Never* handle a downed power line.

- When using gasoline and diesel generators to supply power to a building, switch the main breaker or fuse on the service panel to the Off position prior to starting the generator.

- If clearing or other work must be performed near a downed power line, contact the utility company to discuss de-energizing and grounding or shielding of power lines. Extreme caution is necessary when moving ladders and other equipment near overhead power lines to avoid inadvertent contact.

Avoid Carbon Monoxide

Carbon monoxide is an odorless, colorless gas that is poisonous to breathe. During flood cleanup, operate all gasoline-powered devices such as pumps, generators, and pressure washers outdoors and never bring them indoors. This will help to ensure your safety from carbon monoxide poisoning.

For additional information on carbon monoxide, see "Protecting Yourself from Carbon Monoxide Poisoning after an Emergency" and "Carbon Monoxide Poisoning" (from CDC's National Center for Environmental Health [NCEH]).

Prevent Musculoskeletal Injury

Special attention is needed to avoid back injuries associated with manual lifting and handling of debris and building materials.

To help prevent injury:

- Use teams of two or more to move bulky objects.

- Avoid lifting any material that weighs more than 50 pounds (per person)

- Use proper automated-assist lifting devices

Beware of Structural Instability

Never assume that water-damaged structures or ground are stable. Buildings that have been submerged or have withstood rushing floodwaters may have suffered structural damage and could be dangerous.

- Don't work in or around any flood-damaged building until it has been examined and certi-

fied as safe for work by a registered professional engineer or architect.

- Assume all stairs, floors, and roofs are unsafe until they are inspected.

- Leave immediately if shifting or unusual noises signal a possible collapse.

Avoid Hazardous Materials

Floodwaters can dislodge tanks, drums, pipes, and equipment, which may contain hazardous materials such as pesticides or propane.

- Do not attempt to move unidentified dislodged containers without first contacting the local fire department or hazardous materials team.

- If you are working in potentially contaminated areas, avoid skin contact or inhalation of vapors by wearing appropriate protective clothing and respirators.

- Frequently and thoroughly wash skin areas that may have been exposed to pesticides and other hazardous chemicals.

- Contact NIOSH for more information on the proper safety equipment.

Be Prepared for Fires

Fire can pose a major threat to an already badly damaged flood area for several reasons:

- Inoperative fire protection systems
- Hampered fire department response
- Inoperable firefighting water supplies
- Flood-damaged fire protection systems

At least two fire extinguishers, each with a UL rating of at least 10A, should be provided at every cleanup job.

Prevent Drowning

When entering moving water, you are at risk for drowning, regardless of your ability to swim. Because those in vehicles are at greatest risk of drowning, it is important to comply with all hazard warnings on roadways and to avoid driving vehicles or heavy equipment into water of an unknown depth. NIOSH recommends that you avoid working alone and wear a Coast Guard-approved lifejacket when working in or near floodwaters.

Reduce Risk of Thermal Stress

While cleaning up after the hurricane, you are at risk for developing health problems from working in hot or cold environments.

To reduce heat-related risks:

- Drink a glass of fluid every 15 to 20 minutes.
- Wear light-colored, loose-fitting clothing.
- Work during the cooler hours of the day.

To reduce cold–related risks when standing or working in water which is cooler than 75° F (24° C):

- Wear rubber boots.
- Ensure that clothing and boots have adequate insulation.
- Take frequent breaks out of the water.
- Change into dry clothing when possible.

Prevent Fatigue-Related Injuries

Continued long hours of work, combined with exhaustion, can create a highly stressful situation during cleanup. People working on hurricane and flood cleanup can reduce their risks of injury and illness in several ways:

- Set priorities for cleanup tasks and pace the work. Avoid physical exhaustion.
- Resume a normal sleep schedule as quickly as possible.
- Be alert to emotional exhaustion or strain. Consult family members, friends, or professionals for emotional support.

How to Cope with Stress after a Hurricane

The days and weeks after a hurricane are going to be rough. In addition to your physical health, you need to take some time to consider your mental health. Remember that some sleeplessness, anxiety, anger, hyperactivity, mild depression, or lethargy are normal, and may go away with time. If you feel any of these symptoms acutely, seek counseling.

Your state and local health departments will help you to find the local resources, including hospitals or healthcare providers, that you may need.

Individual responses to a threatening or potentially traumatic event may vary. Emotional reactions may include feelings of fear, grief, and depression. Physical and behavioral responses might include nausea, dizziness, and changes in appetite and sleep pattern, as well as withdrawal from daily activities. Responses to trauma can last for weeks to months before people start to feel normal again.

Seek medical care if you become injured, feel sick, or experience stress and anxiety.

There are many things you can do to cope with traumatic events, including:

- Keep as many elements of your normal routine incorporated into the disaster plans as possible, including activities to allay children's fears.
- Be aware that you may have fewer resources with which to attend to your day-to-day conflicts, so it is best to resolve what you can ahead of time.
- Turn to family, friends, and important social or religious contacts to set up support networks to help you to deal with the potential stressors.
- Let your children know that it is okay to feel upset when something bad or scary happens.
- Encourage your children to express feelings and thoughts, without making judgments.

Dealing with Wild and Domestic Animals in a Disaster

Be cautious if you encounter wild or stray animals. They may be disoriented and dangerous following a hurricane or flood. Try to confine the animal without putting yourself at risk of being bitten. Call the animal control agency in your county.

Wild and domestic animals may escape or be killed in disasters. Escaped animals may wander onto land where they could:

- contaminate water supplies.
- cause a buildup of manure.
- overgraze sensitive ecosystems.
- cause damage to crops.

Decaying carcasses create biologic waste and attract flies and rodents, which can spread disease. They may also contaminate groundwater and cause bad odors. Animal carcasses should be disposed of as soon as possible to avoid creating a health hazard to animals or humans. Contact your local animal control department or local health department for specific disposal guidance.

Handwashing in Emergency Situations

After an emergency, it can be difficult to find running water. However, it is still important to wash your hands to avoid illness. It is best to wash your hands with soap and water, but when water isn't available, you can use alcohol-based products made for washing hands.

Preventing West Nile virus (WNV)

After a hurricane, mosquitoes may breed in standing water during the summer and autumn months. The easiest and best way to avoid WNV is to prevent mosquito bites.

- When you are outdoors, use insect repellents containing DEET (N, N-diethyl-meta-toluamide). Follow the directions on the package.
- Many mosquitoes are most active at dusk and dawn. Be sure to use insect repellent and wear long sleeves and pants at these times or consider staying indoors during these hours. Light-colored clothing can help you to see mosquitoes that land on you.
- Make sure you have good screens on your windows and doors to keep mosquitoes out.
- Get rid of mosquito breeding sites by emptying standing water from flowerpots, buckets, and barrels. Change the water in pet dishes and replace the water in bird baths weekly. Drill holes in tire swings so that water drains out. Keep children's wading pools empty and on their sides when they aren't being used.

F Natural Disasters: Tornadoes

Knowing what to do when you see a tornado, or when you hear a tornado warning, can help protect you and your family. During a tornado, people face hazards from extremely high winds and risk being struck by flying and falling objects. After a tornado, the wreckage left behind poses additional injury risks. Although nothing can be done to prevent tornadoes, there are actions you can take for your health and safety.

BEING PREPARED

Stay Tuned for Storm Watches and Warnings

When there are thunderstorms in your area, turn on your radio or TV to get the latest emergency information from local authorities. Listen for announcements of a tornado watch or tornado warning.

Local Warning System

Learn about the tornado warning system of your county or locality. Most tornado-prone areas have a siren system. Know how to distinguish between the siren's warnings for a tornado watch and a tornado warning.

A tornado watch is issued when weather conditions favor the formation of tornadoes—for example, during a severe thunderstorm.

During a tornado watch:

- Stay tuned to local radio and TV stations or a National Oceanographic and Atmospheric Administration (NOAA) weather radio for further weather information.
- Watch the weather and be prepared to take shelter immediately if conditions worsen.

A tornado warning is issued when a tornado funnel is sighted or indicated by weather radar. *You should take shelter immediately.*

Thunderstorms

Because tornadoes often accompany thunderstorms, pay close attention to changing weather conditions when there is a severe thunderstorm watch or warning. A severe thunderstorm *watch* means severe thunderstorms are possible in your area. A severe thunderstorm *warning* means severe thunderstorms are occurring in your area.

Keep fresh batteries and a battery-powered radio or TV on hand. Electrical power is often interrupted during thunderstorms—just when information about weather warnings is most needed.

Important Measures to Take

- Take a few minutes with your family to develop a tornado emergency plan. Sketch a floor plan of where you live, or walk through each room and discuss where and how to seek shelter.
- Show a second way to exit from each room or area. If you need special equipment, such as a rope ladder, mark where it is located.
- Make sure everyone understands the siren warning system, if there is such a system in your area.
- Mark where your first aid kit and fire extinguishers are located.
- Mark where the utility switches or valves are located so they can be turned off—if time permits—in an emergency.
- Teach your family how to administer basic first aid, how to use a fire extinguisher, and how and when to turn off water, gas, and electricity in your home.
- Learn the emergency dismissal policy for your child's school.
- Make sure your children know
  - what a tornado is.
  - what tornado watches and warnings are.
  - what county or parish they live in (warnings are issued by county or parish).
  - how to take shelter, whether at home or at school.

Source of information is the Centers for Disease Control and Prevention (http://www.bt.cdc.gov/disasters).

Extra Measures for People with Special Needs

- Write down your specific needs, limitations, capabilities, and medications. Keep this list near you always—perhaps in your purse or wallet.
- Find someone nearby (a spouse, roommate, friend, neighbor, relative, or co-worker) who will agree to assist you in case of an emergency. Give him or her a copy of your list. You may also want to provide a spare key to your home, or directions to find a key.
- Keep aware of weather conditions through whatever means are accessible to you. Some options are closed captioning or scrolled warnings on TV, radio bulletins, or call-in weather information lines.

Practicing Your Emergency Plan

Conduct drills and ask questions to make sure your family remembers information on tornado safety, particularly how to recognize hazardous weather conditions and how to take shelter.

Writing Down Important Information

Make a list of important information. Include these on your list:

- Important telephone numbers, such as emergency (police and fire), paramedics, and medical centers
- Names, addresses, and telephone numbers of your insurance agents, including policy types and numbers
- Telephone numbers of the electric, gas, and water companies
- Names and telephone numbers of neighbors
- Name and telephone number of your landlord or property manager
- Important medical information (for example, allergies, regular medications, and brief medical history)
- Year, model, license, and identification numbers of your vehicles (automobiles, boats, and RVs)
- Financial institution's telephone number, and your account numbers
- Radio and television broadcast stations to tune to for emergency broadcast information

Storing Important Documents

Store the following documents in a fire- and waterproof safe:

- Birth certificates
- Ownership certificates (autos, boats, etc.)
- Social security cards
- Insurance policies
- Wills
- Household inventory
  - List of contents of household; include serial numbers, if applicable
  - Photographs or videotape of contents of every room
  - Photographs of items of high value, such as jewelry, paintings, collection items

Reducing Household Hazards

The following suggestions will reduce the risk for injury during or after a tornado. No amount of preparation will eliminate every risk.

Possible Hazards

Inspect your home for possible hazards, including the following:

- Are walls securely bolted to the foundation?
- Are wall studs attached to the roof rafters with metal hurricane clips, not nails?

Utilities

- Do you know where and how to shut off utilities at the main switches or valves?

Home Contents

- Are chairs or beds near windows, mirrors, or large pictures?
- Are heavy items stored on shelves more than 30-inches high?
- Are there large, unsecured items that might topple over or fall?
- Are poisons, solvents, or toxic materials stored safely?

Securing Your Home's Structure

No home is completely safe in a tornado. However, attention to construction details can reduce damage and provide better protection for you and your family if a tornado should strike your house. If an inspection reveals a possible hazard in the way your home is built, contact your local city or county building inspectors for more information about structural safety. They may also offer suggestions on finding a qualified contractor to do any needed work for you.

Walls and Roof Rafters

Strengthen the areas of connection between the wall studs and roof rafters with hurricane clips.

Shutting Off Utilities

Gas

After a tornado, *do not use* matches, lighters, or appliances or operate light switches until you are sure there are no gas leaks. Sparks from electrical switches could ignite gas and cause an explosion.

If you smell the odor of gas or if you notice a large consumption of gas being registered on the gas meter, shut off the gas immediately. First, find the main shut-off valve located on a pipe next to the gas meter. Use an adjustable wrench to turn the valve to the Off position.

Electricity

After a major disaster, shut off the electricity. Sparks from electrical switches could ignite leaking gas and cause an explosion.

Water

- Water may be turned off at either of two locations:
  1. At the main meter, which controls the water flow to the entire property.
  2. At the water main leading into the home. If you may need an emergency source of fresh water, it is better to shut off your water here because it will conserve the water in your water heater.
- Attach a valve wrench to the water line. (This tool can be purchased at most hardware stores.)
- Label the water mains for quick identification.

Arranging and Securing Household Items

- Arrange furniture so that chairs and beds are away from windows, mirrors, and picture frames.
- Place heavy or large items on lower shelves.
- Secure your large appliances, especially your water heater, with flexible cable, braided wire, or metal strapping.

- Identify top-heavy, freestanding furniture, such as bookcases and china cabinets, that could topple over.
- Secure your furniture by using one of two methods.
  1. L brackets, corner brackets, or aluminum molding, to attach tall or top-heavy furniture to the wall.
  2. Eyebolts, to secure items located a short distance from the wall.
- Install sliding bolts or childproof latches on all cabinet doors.
- Store all hazardous materials such as poisons and solvents
  - in a sturdy, latched or locked cabinet.
  - in a well-ventilated area.
  - away from emergency food or water supplies.

DURING A TORNADO

Signs of an Approaching Storm

Some tornadoes strike rapidly, without time for a tornado warning, and sometimes without a thunderstorm in the vicinity. When you are watching for rapidly emerging tornadoes, it is important to know that you cannot depend on seeing the funnel cloud: clouds or rain may block your view. The following weather signs may mean that a tornado is approaching:

- A dark or green-colored sky
- A large, dark, low-lying cloud
- Large hail
- A loud roar that sounds like a freight train

If you notice any of these weather conditions, take cover immediately, and keep tuned to local radio and TV stations or to an NOAA weather radio.

NOAA Weather Radios

NOAA weather radios are the best way to receive warnings from the National Weather Service. By using an NOAA weather radio, you can receive continuous updates on all the weather conditions in your area. The range of these radios depends on where you live, but the average range is 40 miles. The radios are sold in many stores. The National Weather Service recommends buying a radio with a battery backup (in case the power goes off) and a tone-alert feature that automatically sounds when a weather watch or warning is issued.

Sighting a Funnel Cloud

If you see a funnel cloud nearby, take shelter immediately (see the following section for instructions on shelter). However, if you spot a tornado that is far away, help alert others to the hazard by reporting it to the newsroom of a local radio or TV station before taking shelter as described later. Use common sense and exercise caution: if you believe that you might be in danger, seek shelter immediately.

Taking Shelter

Your family could be anywhere when a tornado strikes—at home, at work, at school, or in the car. Discuss with your family where the best tornado shelters are and how family members can protect themselves from flying and falling debris.

The key to surviving a tornado and reducing the risk of injury lies in planning, preparing, and practicing what you and your family will do if a tornado strikes. Flying debris causes most deaths and injuries during a tornado. Although there is no completely safe place during a tornado, some locations are much safer than others.

At Home

Pick a place in the home where family members can gather if a tornado is headed your way. One basic rule is to *avoid windows.* An exploding window can injure or kill.

The safest place in the home is the interior part of a basement. If there is no basement, go to an inside room, without windows, on the lowest floor. This could be a center hallway, bathroom, or closet.

For added protection, get under something sturdy such as a heavy table or workbench. If possible, cover your body with a blanket, sleeping bag, or mattress, and protect your head with anything available—even your hands. Avoid taking shelter where there are heavy objects, such as pianos or refrigerators, on the area of floor that is directly above you. They could fall though the floor if the tornado strikes your house.

In a Mobile Home

Do not stay in a mobile home during a tornado. Mobile homes can turn over during strong winds. Even mobile homes with a tie-down system cannot withstand the force of tornado winds.

Plan ahead. If you live in a mobile home, go to a nearby building, preferably one with a basement. If there is no shelter nearby, lie flat in the nearest ditch, ravine, or culvert and shield your head with your hands.

If you live in a tornado-prone area, encourage your mobile home community to build a tornado shelter.

On the Road

The least desirable place to be during a tornado is in a motor vehicle. Cars, buses, and trucks are easily tossed by tornado winds.

Do not try to outrun a tornado in your car. If you see a tornado, stop your vehicle and get out. Do not get under your vehicle. Follow the directions for seeking shelter outdoors (see next section).

Outdoors

If you are caught outside during a tornado and there is no adequate shelter immediately available:

- Avoid areas with many trees.
- Avoid vehicles.
- Lie down flat in a gully, ditch, or low spot on the ground.
- Protect your head with an object or with your arms.

Long-Span Buildings

A long-span building, such as a shopping mall, theater, or gymnasium, is especially dangerous because the roof structure is usually supported solely by the outside walls. Most such buildings hit by tornados cannot withstand the enormous pressure. They simply collapse.

If you are in a long-span building during a tornado, stay away from windows. Get to the lowest level of the building—the basement if possible—and away from the windows.

If there is no time to get to a tornado shelter or to a lower level, try to get under a door frame or get up against something that will support or deflect falling debris. For instance, in a department store, get up against heavy shelving or counters. In a theater, get under the seats. Remember to protect your head.

Office Buildings, Schools, Hospitals, Churches, and Other Public Buildings

Extra care is required in offices, schools, hospitals, or any building where a large group of people is concentrated in a small area. The exterior walls of such buildings often have large windows.

If you are in any of these buildings:

- Move away from windows and glass doorways.
- Go to the innermost part of the building on the lowest possible floor.
- Do not use elevators because the power may fail, leaving you trapped.
- Protect your head and make yourself as small a target as possible by crouching down.

Shelter for People with Special Needs

Advance planning is especially important if you require assistance to reach shelter from an approaching storm.

- If you are in a wheelchair, get away from windows and go to an interior room of the house. If possible, seek shelter under a sturdy table or desk. Cover your head with anything available, even your hands.
- If you are unable to move from a bed or a chair and assistance is not available, protect yourself from falling objects by covering up with blankets and pillows.
- If you are outside and a tornado is approaching, get into a ditch or gully. If possible, lie flat and cover your head with your arms.

AFTER A TORNADO

Injury may result from the direct impact of a tornado, or it may occur afterward when people walk among debris and enter damaged buildings. A study of injuries after a tornado in Marion, Illinois, showed that 50% of the tornado-related injuries were related to rescue attempts, cleanup, and other post-tornado activities. Nearly one-third of the injuries resulted from stepping on nails. Other common causes of injury included falling objects and heavy, rolling objects. Because tornadoes often damage power lines, gas lines, or electrical systems, there is a risk of fire, electrocution, or an explosion. Protecting yourself and your family requires promptly treating any injuries received during the storm and using extreme care to avoid further hazards.

Injuries

Check for injuries. Do not try to move seriously injured people unless they are in immediate danger of further injury. Get medical assistance immediately. If someone has stopped breathing, begin CPR if you are trained to do so. Stop a bleeding injury by applying direct pressure to the wound. Have any puncture wound evaluated by a physician. If you are trapped, try to attract attention to your location.

General Safety Precautions

Here are some safety precautions that could help you to avoid injury after a tornado:

- Continue to monitor your battery-powered radio or television for emergency information.
- Be careful when entering any structure that has been damaged.
- Wear sturdy shoes or boots, long sleeves, and gloves when handling or walking on or near debris.
- Be aware of hazards from exposed nails and broken glass.
- Do not touch downed power lines or objects in contact with downed lines. Report electrical hazards to the police and the utility company.
- Use battery-powered lanterns, if possible, rather than candles to light homes without electrical power. If you use candles, make sure they are in safe holders away from curtains, paper, wood, or other flammable items. Never leave a candle burning when you are out of the room.
- Hang up displaced telephone receivers that may have been knocked off by the tornado, but stay off the telephone, except to report an emergency.
- Cooperate fully with public safety officials.
- Respond to requests for volunteer assistance by police, firefighters, emergency management, and relief organizations, but do not go into damaged areas unless assistance has been requested. Your presence could hamper relief efforts, and you could endanger yourself.

Inspecting the Damage

- After a tornado, be aware of possible structural, electrical, or gas-leak hazards in your home. Contact your local city or county building inspectors for information on structural safety codes and standards. They may also offer suggestions on finding a qualified contractor to do work for you.
- In general, if you suspect any damage to your

home, shut off electrical power, natural gas, and propane tanks to avoid fire, electrocution, or explosions.

- If it is dark when you are inspecting your home, use a flashlight rather than a candle or torch to avoid the risk of fire or explosion in a damaged home.

- If you see frayed wiring or sparks, or if there is an odor of something burning, you should immediately shut off the electrical system at the main circuit breaker if you have not done so already.

- If you smell gas or suspect a leak, turn off the main gas valve, open all windows, and leave the house immediately. Notify the gas company, the police or fire departments, or the state fire marshal's office, and do not turn on the lights, light matches, smoke, or do anything that could cause a spark. Do not return to your house until you are told it is safe to do so.

Safety During Cleanup

- Wear sturdy shoes or boots, long sleeves, and gloves.

- Learn proper safety procedures and operating instructions before operating any gas-powered or electric-powered saws or tools.

- Clean up spilled medicines, drugs, flammable liquids, and other potentially hazardous materials.

Children's Needs

After a tornado, children may be afraid the storm will come back again and they will be injured or left alone. Children may even interpret disasters as punishment for real or imagined misdeeds. Explain that a tornado is a natural event.

Children will be less likely to experience prolonged fear or anxiety if they know what to expect after a tornado. Here are some suggestions:

- Talk about your own experiences with severe storms, or read aloud a book about tornadoes.

- Encourage your child to express feelings of fear. Listen carefully and show understanding.

- Offer reassurance. Tell your child that the situation is not permanent, and provide physical reassurance through time spent together and displays of affection.

- Include your child in cleanup activities. It is comforting to children to watch the household begin to return to normal and to have a job to do.

Note: Symptoms of anxiety may not appear for weeks or even months after a tornado. They can affect people of any age. If anxiety disrupts daily activities for any member of your family, seek professional assistance through a school counselor, community religious organization, your physician, or a licensed mental health professional.

INTRODUCTION
Healthy Lifestyle Self-Assessment
1. True
2. False
3. True
4. False
5. False
6. False
7. True
8. True
9. False
10. True

CHAPTER 1
Learning Checkpoint 1
1. False. First aid usually does not replace the need for medical care (calling 9-1-1 or the victim seeing a healthcare provider). First aid is intended to help the victim until professional help can be given. With minor injuries, however, the victim sometimes does not need to see a healthcare provider.
2. True. First aid such as giving CPR or rescue breathing or stopping bleeding can make the difference between the victim living or dying. In other cases, an injury or illness could become worse if first aid is not given before the victim gets professional help.

Learning Checkpoint 2
1. d. All of the above. These are all important aspects of first aid training.
2. d. All of the above. You should have a first aid kit available wherever an injury may occur.

Learning Checkpoint 3
1. d
2. d
3. Usually first at the scene is a first responder, who may be a law enforcement officer, fire-fighter, ski patroller, or other official with more advanced training.
4. When you call 9-1-1, be ready to give the following information:
   - Your name
   - The phone number you are using
   - The location and number of victims
   - What happened to the victim(s) and any special circumstances
   - The victim's condition
   - The victim's approximate age and sex
   - What is being done for the victim(s)

Learning Checkpoint 4
1. False. Never move a victim unless faced with a life-threatening situation such as fire. Moving a victim is likely to make an injury worse.
2. d. If your job description requires you to provide first aid, then you have a duty to act.
3. a, unresponsive victim; b, child without guardian; d, a victim who nods consent; and e, a child whose parent or guardian consents. All these are expressed or implied consent.
4. b, d, e. Do *not* try techniques you have not been trained to perform, and do not move most victims by trying to transport them yourself, which may lead to more serious injury.

Review Questions
1. d
2. b
3. a
4. a
5. d
6. d
7. c
8. c
9. d
10. a

CHAPTER 2

Learning Checkpoint 1

1. False. Bloodborne diseases may be transmitted by contact with several different body fluids, or by objects contaminated with any of those body fluids.

2. True. You can almost always avoid getting an infectious disease if you use precautions such as protective equipment and follow standard precautions.

3. d. All of the above. These are basic precautions based on the assumption that any person's body fluids may carry pathogens, and any contact with these fluids may lead to infectious disease.

4. a (there may be pathogens in the blood on that bandage) and d (a cut on the finger could easily let pathogens enter your body). Shaking hands does not transmit HIV; being vaccinated for HBV prevents infection and does not cause it; coughing does not transmit hepatitis C; and urine does not normally transmit pathogens (unless it contains blood), although to be safe you should wear gloves when possibly contacting a victim's urine.

5. Signs and symptoms of latex allergy may include skin rashes, hives, itching eyes or skin, flushing, watery or swollen eyes, runny nose, or an asthmatic reaction.

Learning Checkpoint 2

1. False. The first thing to do is check the scene for safety. If you enter an unsafe scene to help a victim, you could become a second victim for EMS professionals to have to care for.

2. d. All of the above. These are all general principles for giving first aid.

3. All four of these are dangerous scenes you should not enter. Stay at a safe distance and call 9-1-1.

Review Questions

1. a
2. d
3. b
4. c
5. b
6. d
7. a
8. d

CHAPTER 3

Learning Checkpoint 1

1. heart, lungs
2. d
3. pharynx (throat)
4. a
5. These are cardiac problems that can affect tissue oxygenation: cardiac arrest, myocardial infarction, fibrillation, and dysrhythmia. Asthma is a respiratory problem, not a cardiac problem, although it too can affect tissue oxygenation.

Learning Checkpoint 2

1. All eight listed injuries and illnesses may result in altered mental status.
2. c
3. A dislocation is the movement of one or more bones out of their normal position in a joint.
4. b; a femur fracture can cause severe bleeding, which may be life threatening; the fracture may also cause soft tissue damage in the leg, but this is unlikely to be a life-threatening injury.
5. Even a small break in the skin can be very serious if a pathogen can enter the body, such as those pathogens causing serious illnesses (e.g., HIV).

Learning Checkpoint 3

1. d
2. People need a tetanus vaccine booster at least every 10 years to ensure immunity against tetanus infection, which may occur after any break in the skin.
3. a
4. c; blood in urine may result from different injuries or illnesses but should always be investigated by a healthcare professional.

Review Questions

1. d
2. a
3. b
4. c
5. b
6. a
7. a
8. d
9. c
10. c

Chapter 4
Learning Checkpoint 1

1. b (check for responsiveness), c (open airway), a (check for breathing).
2. Listen for breathing sounds, feel for breaths exhaled, and look for chest movement.
3. True. A victim who is coughing is breathing.

Learning Checkpoint 2

1. d. The secondary assessment is performed after the initial assessment and only if the victim has no life-threatening conditions requiring care.
2. S = signs and symptoms, A = allergies, M = medications, P = previous problems, L = last food or drink, and E = events leading to current situation.
3. As you examine each part of a victim's body you are looking for anything out of the ordinary, such as pain, bleeding, a swollen or deformed area, unusual skin color, temperature, or moisture, or abnormal movement or sensation in an area.

Review Questions

1. b
2. a
3. c
4. a
5. b
6. b
7. a
8. d

Chapter 5
Learning Checkpoint 1

1. breathing. Basic life support keeps victims who are not breathing (and whose heart has stopped) alive until they receive advanced medical care.
2. One to eight years: this is the definition of a child for purposes of CPR, and use of an AED.

Learning Checkpoint 2

1. a. Rescue breaths move oxygen into the victim's lungs to be transferred into the blood. (Chest compressions move that blood to vital organs.)
2. False. Blowing too hard can put air in the victim's stomach and cause vomiting. Blow only hard enough to make the chest rise.

3. c. Watch the victim's chest rise and fall. This is the best way to confirm that your breaths are going into the victim's lungs.
4. Give each breath over one second.

Review Questions

1. b
2. a
3. b
4. c
5. d

Chapter 6
Learning Checkpoint 1

1. b. Cardiopulmonary resuscitation. "Cardio" refers to the heart (chest compressions) and "pulmonary" means the lungs (rescue breathing).
2. Risk factors for cardiovascular disease include:
   • Smoking
   • High cholesterol levels
   • Inactivity
   • High blood pressure
   • Family history of heart disease
   • Growing older
3. The first crucial link in the cardiac chain of survival is early access—calling 9-1-1 to access EMS.
4. Call first for any nonbreathing, unresponsive adult victim. Give two minutes of CPR first for a nonbreathing, unresponsive infant or child.

Learning Checkpoint 2

1. c. Start CPR as soon as you determine the victim is unresponsive and not breathing (unless an AED is present and ready to be used).
2. In an adult or child, the correct position for chest compressions is on the lower half of the breastbone (sternum) midway between the nipples.
3. Chest compression depth for adults: $1\frac{1}{2}$ to 2 inches. For an infant or child: $\frac{1}{3}$ to $\frac{1}{2}$ the depth of the chest.
4. d. 30 to 2 (in all victims regardless of age).
5. a. Use the AED as soon as it is set up and ready. The AED unit will check the heart rhythm and determine whether the victim needs a shock to restore regular rhythm or needs CPR.

Review Questions

1. d
2. a
3. b
4. c
5. d
6. b
7. a
8. a
9. c
10. d

CHAPTER 7

Learning Checkpoint 1

1. Trying to swallow large pieces of food, eating too quickly, eating while engaged in other activities, eating under the influence of alcohol or drugs, eating with dentures
2. These items on the list should not be given to a child under age three:
   - Popcorn
   - Grapes
   - Marshmallows
   - Gum

Learning Checkpoint 2

1. c. Give abdominal thrusts to a choking adult *unless* he or she is coughing or able to speak.
2. True. A forcefully coughing victim is getting at least some air, and the coughing may dislodge the obstructing object.
3. True. Without air a victim will become unresponsive and the heart will stop; the victim then needs CPR.
4. d. All of the above.
5. The chest compressions of CPR may dislodge the obstructing object. Even if not, the chest compressions will circulate blood to vital organs.

Review Questions

1. d
2. a
3. b
4. a

CHAPTER 8

Learning Checkpoint 1

1. True. The shock from the AED can restore a normal heart rhythm when the heart is fibrillating.

2. False. There is almost no risk in using an AED because the unit will not indicate a shock unless it determines that the victim's heart is fibrillating; in this case the shock is appropriate and can restart a normal heartbeat.
3. About 50% of cardiac arrest victims are in fibrillation and require a shock to restore the heart to a normal rhythm.

Learning Checkpoint 2

1. a. The two pads of the AED must be correctly positioned on the victim's chest.
2. c. Give the shock when the unit indicates it, after first making sure no one is in contact with the victim.
3. CPR is given to unresponsive victims who are not breathing while the AED is being brought and set up and after the unit advises not to give a shock.

Learning Checkpoint 3

1. A situation such as drowning or poisoning may cause cardiac arrest in a child, in which case the AED may restore a normal rhythm.
2. Do not put the pad on or very near to an implanted pacemaker or defibrillator; place it several inches away.
3. Remove any medication patches before applying the AED pads.

Review Questions

1. c
2. c
3. d
4. a
5. b
6. b
7. a
8. b

CHAPTER 9

Learning Checkpoint 1

1. True. The body can quickly lose much blood from arterial bleeding.
2. False. The first thing to do always is to stop the bleeding first.
3. A victim who has been bleeding severely may show the signs of shock, including cool, clammy skin.
4. Many different materials can form a barrier between you and the victim's blood, including

bulky clothing or a plastic bag. (This topic is more fully discussed in **Chapter 2**.)

Learning Checkpoint 2

1. False. Internal bleeding can be life threatening because significant blood may be lost from internal organs or blood vessels. The blood is lost from the circulation even if it remains within a body cavity—the fact that it is still inside the body does not mean it reaches vital organs through the circulation.
2. All these are signs or symptoms of internal bleeding. Significant blood loss may cause shock, resulting in cool, clammy skin and confusion or light-headedness.
3. d

Review Questions

1. b
2. a
3. d
4. b
5. c
6. c
7. a
8. d

CHAPTER 10

Learning Checkpoint 1

1. False. Never give fluids to a shock victim. The victim is likely to vomit.
2. True. A spinal injury can cause shock if it causes nervous system damage.
3. a. Stop the bleeding. Severe bleeding is life threatening and must be managed before you do anything else.
4. b. Nausea, thirst, clammy skin. These are common signs and symptoms of shock.
5. Calling 9-1-1 is the most important action (after treating any life-threatening injuries) because the victim may need advanced medical care very soon to survive.

Learning Checkpoint 2

1. True. A victim who has experienced an allergic reaction in the past may have an emergency kit you can help them use. (Also tell the arriving EMS crew about the allergy.)
2. True. Allergic reactions to bee and wasp stings are common—and can be severe.
3. d. Breathing problems. These are caused by

swelling of the airway and are most serious because they can be life threatening.
4. Help the victim into whatever position is easiest for breathing, which is often sitting partway up.

Review Questions

1. a
2. c
3. d
4. b
5. d
6. a
7. b
8. a
9. a
10. c

CHAPTER 11

Learning Checkpoint 1

1. Include these actions in wound care:
   Irrigate minor wounds with running water.
   Use tweezers to remove large dirt particles from a minor wound.
   Cover any wounds with a sterile dressing and bandage.
   See a healthcare provider for a deep or puncture wound.
2. Soak a dressing in water if it sticks to the wound.
3. False. Puncture wounds have a greater risk of infection because germs may be trapped inside.
4. False. With *all* victims, assume there may be pathogens in the blood; follow standard precautions.
5. Use an antibiotic ointment only on abrasions.
6. Signs of wound infection include a red, swollen area, warmth in the area, fever, and pus draining from the wound.
7. These victims need to seek medical attention:
   Jose, because his wound is deep (regardless of the fact that you stopped the bleeding).
   Rebecca, because any animal bite should be seen by a healthcare provider.
   Kim, because significant face wounds should be seen by a healthcare provider.
8. False. The bandage should be tight enough to put pressure on the wound to control bleeding, but if it is too tight it may cut off circulation.

9. In this situation the bandage is too tight and is cutting off her circulation. Unwrap the bandage and reapply it less tightly.

10. c. The bandage should cover the entire dressing to secure it in place. It should be dry and should not be able to be slid to one side because a bandage that loose will not adequately protect the wound.

Learning Checkpoint 2

1. Promote some bleeding of a shallow puncture wound to "wash out" any germs that may be deep inside.

2. False. Leave an impaled object in a wound because removing it could worsen the injury.

3. True. Keep an amputated part cold to help preserve it, but do not put it in direct contact with ice (which could freeze tissue).

4. With an eye injury you should cover the uninjured eye also, because movement of the uninjured eye will also cause the injured eye to move, which could worsen the injury.

5. Three ways to remove a small particle from the eye are:
   Pull the upper eyelid out and down over the lower eyelid.
   Flush the eye with water
   Try to brush it out with a dampened cotton-tip swab or sterile dressing.

6. False. Let blood or fluid drain out.

7. 10 minutes. During this time, do not tilt the victim's head backward, do not have the victim lie down, and do not let the victim speak, swallow, cough, or sniff.

8. True. A dentist can usually reimplant a knocked-out tooth if it is kept in milk and the victim reaches the dentist soon.

9. False. Rinsing the mouth with cool water will not stop bleeding but will keep the blood from clotting in the wound.

Review Questions

1. b
2. a
3. c
4. a
5. a
6. d
7. d
8. b
9. c
10. b

CHAPTER 12
Learning Checkpoint 1

1. Following are the most common causes of fires leading to injury or death (list any three):
   - Smoking
   - Heating
   - Cooking
   - Playing with fire
   - Electrical wiring
   - Open flames
   - Appliances or other equipment

2. Specific actions to prevent fires in the kitchen:
   - Keep a fire extinguisher in the kitchen and know how to use it.
   - Tie back long hair or loose clothing when cooking or working around flames.
   - If food catches on fire in a microwave or toaster oven, leave the food there and turn the appliance off; keep other objects away until the flames go out.
   - Keep electrical cords away from counter edges where children may pull on them.

   In addition, other general measures such as these can help prevent fires in the kitchen or elsewhere in the home or workplace:
   - Make sure enough smoke detectors are installed and have good batteries (change batteries twice a year when you change clocks for daylight savings time).
   - Do not allow smoking, or ensure that it is done safely and materials safely extinguished. Never allow smoking in bed.
   - Keep curtains and other flammable objects away from fireplaces and stoves; use fireplace screens.
   - Have chimneys regularly inspected and cleaned to prevent chimney fires.
   - Never store gasoline or other highly flammable liquids indoors.
   - Prevent fires caused by electricity.
   - Keep power cords safely out of the way and away from children.
   - Check appliance cords for damaged areas or fraying.
   - Do not overload electrical outlets or use multiple extension cords.

- Unplug appliances and extension cords when not in use.
- Keep children from playing with fire.

3. False. The first thing to do is to make sure everyone is evacuated from the building.

4. Four factors that affect how serious a burn may be:
- The type of burn (first-, second-, or third-degree)
- How extensive the burn is (how much body area)
- The specific body area burned
- Special circumstances such as the victim's age and health status

Learning Checkpoint 2

1. False. Never break blisters on a burn, which could cause infection.
2. Small (less than 20% of the body).
3. First, stop the fire (have him stop, drop, and roll to put out the flames, or cover him with a coat or blanket).
Cool the area with water immediately to stop the burning (but not more than 20% of body). Remove any tight clothing or jewelry.
Call 9-1-1. Then treat for shock and cover the burned area with a dressing.

Learning Checkpoint 3

1. c. Immediately flush the eye with running water to stop the burning.
2. First, brush the chemical off the skin to stop the burning. (Wear gloves or otherwise protect yourself.)
3. False. The signs and symptoms of an injury caused by smoke inhalation may not become manifest for up to 48 hours. Any victim of smoke inhalation should receive medical attention.

Learning Checkpoint 4

1. False. The first thing to do is to unplug or turn off the electrical power.
2. Unplug the appliance or shut off the circuit breaker. Do not try to pull the victim away from the appliance or the appliance from the victim, because you too could be shocked.
3. a. Call 9-1-1 first. You cannot safely reach the victim or move the high-voltage wires yourself—you could make the situation worse.

Review Questions

1. a
2. b
3. d
4. c
5. d
6. a
7. a
8. b
9. c
10. d

CHAPTER 13

Learning Checkpoint 1

1. Signs of a possible skull fracture include a deformed area of skull, a depressed area felt in your examination, blood or fluid loss from the ears or nose, and an object impaling the skull. Do not put pressure on a bleeding wound with skull fracture.
2. False. Symptoms of brain injuries including concussion, bleeding, or swelling can be variable and may be confusing. Call 9-1-1 with any suspected brain injury.
3. Headache, memory loss, dizziness or confusion, and nausea and vomiting.
4. d. None of the above. There is no one assessment that can always determine the presence of a spinal injury. Do not assume a victim without specific symptoms does not have a possible spinal injury.
5. Signs and symptoms of a serious brain injury may occur as late as 48 hours after a blow to the head.

Learning Checkpoint 2

1. True. Suspect a spinal injury in a victim with a head injury because head trauma may also injure the spine.
2. b. Check for breathing without moving the victim, if you suspect a spinal injury. Move the victim only if necessary.
3. Always suspect a spinal injury in these situations: fall from a roof, motor vehicle crash, and a blow to the head.
4. Signs and symptoms of a spinal injury include tingling in the hands, breathing problems, and a twisted neck.
5. a. Call 9-1-1 for *all* victims who may have a spinal injury.

6. Stabilize the head of a victim with a suspected spinal injury in the position in which you find the victim, because movement could worsen the injury.

7. Vomits. The victim could choke on the vomit and therefore must be rolled onto his side, while still supported at the head. Otherwise there is no reason to move the victim and risk further injury.

8. Stabilize the victim's head by holding it still with the victim staying in the driver's seat. Call for someone to call for 9-1-1. Monitor the victim's breathing.

Review Questions

1. a
2. b
3. c
4. d
5. d
6. a
7. b
8. d
9. c

CHAPTER 14

Learning Checkpoint 1

1. False. Loosely bandage a pillow or other support over the ribs. A tight bandage could cause further injury or breathing problems.

2. d. All of the above: Preventing movement of the arm helps prevent movement of that side of the chest. Preventing movement will also ease pain. A sling and binder may be used to immobilize the arm.

3. Do not remove the impaled screwdriver, which could worsen the injury. Instead, use bulky dressings to stabilize it, and bandage around it. Then call 9-1-1.

4. Treat a sucking chest wound by covering the wound dressing with a piece of plastic taped on three sides; this prevents air from being sucked in but allows air to escape. Then keep the victim lying down and call 9-1-1.

Learning Checkpoint 2

1. The signs and symptoms of a closed abdominal injury include bruising and a swollen abdomen.

2. A victim with an open or closed abdominal wound should lie on his back with knees

slightly bent if this eases the pain.

3. True. Keep a victim in shock from becoming cold. If necessary, cover him with a coat or blanket, and place something between him and the cold ground.

4. d. Cover organs protruding from a wound with a nonadherent dressing and plastic wrap to keep the organs from drying out.

5. Call 9-1-1 for *any* victim with an open or closed abdominal wound.

Learning Checkpoint 3

1. Movement. Movement of a fractured pelvis could increase the bleeding and worsen the injury.

2. True. Pelvic bones themselves may bleed heavily, or internal organs may be damaged and bleed profusely.

3. True. Do not force the victim to bend his knees, however, if this seems to increase the pain.

Review Questions

1. a
2. b
3. d
4. a
5. c
6. b
7. b
8. d

CHAPTER 15

Learning Checkpoint 1

1. a. Most musculoskeletal injuries. You do not need to know the exact nature of the injury before using RICE.

2. False. Do not put a cold pack directly on the skin because tissue damage could occur. Place a pad or cloth between the cold pack and the skin.

3. d. All of the above.

4. Rest the ankle.
   Put an ice or cold pack on the injured area (no more than 20 minutes).
   Compress the ankle with a roller bandage (over the cold pack).
   Elevate the ankle.

Learning Checkpoint 2

1. True. Call 9-1-1 for any serious fractures or fractures of large bones.

2. c. Immobilize the joints above and below a fracture area to keep the fractured bone from moving.
3. True. Shock may result in a fracture from blood loss or pain.
4. The signs and symptoms of a bone or joint injury include a deformed area, pain, swelling, and an inability to use the part.
5. False. Moving or exerting a sprained joint will only make the injury worse.

Learning Checkpoint 3

1. False. Use an ice or cold pack, but remove it after 20 minutes, and wait at least 30 minutes before reapplying it.
2. False. Treat a muscle contusion with a cold pack, compression bandage, and elevation of the limb.
3. False. An area of skin discoloration can be caused by a fracture, dislocation, or sprain as well as by a contusion.
4. Gently stretch the muscle, and massage the muscle.

Review Questions

1. d
2. a
3. d
4. b
5. c
6. d
7. b
8. a
9. c
10. b

Chapter 16

Learning Checkpoint 1

1. You can make a rigid splint from many different materials, including a board, a piece of plastic or metal, a rolled newspaper or magazine, or thick cardboard.
2. Following are all actions to take when using a splint:
   - Pad the splint.
   - Put a cold pack around the splint.
   - Dress an open wound before splinting.
   - Splint in the position found.
3. Signs that circulation has been cut off in an extremity below the splint include swelling,

skin cold and pale or discolored, and tingling or numbness.
4. Two things you should not do when contemplating putting a victim's arm in a sling are:
   - Do not move the arm into position for a sling if this causes more pain.
   - Do not cover the fingers inside the sling, since you need to check circulation.

Learning Checkpoint 2

1. Soft
2. Elbow, hand
3. a. A binder provides additional support and helps prevent movement of the arm.

Learning Checkpoint 3

1. You do not need to know for certain if the bone is broken, since there are signs and symptoms of a fracture (pain, inability to move the leg). Take these actions:
   - Have the victim stay lying down and immobilize the leg.
   - Call 9-1-1.
   - Put an ice or cold pack on the area.
   - Splint the leg if help may be delayed, using either an anatomic splint or a rigid splint from the upper leg to the foot.
2. d. A victim with a fracture of the femur may experience severe bleeding that can cause shock. The injury may be either open or closed.
3. With any fracture of an extremity, ideally the fracture should be splinted on both sides, using two rigid splints.

Review Questions

1. d
2. d
3. a
4. c
5. c
6. a
7. d
8. d

Chapter 17

Learning Checkpoint 1

1. True. With an unknown sudden illness, the victim should not eat or drink.
2. The common signs and symptoms of a heart

attack include shortness of breath, chest pain or pressure, sweating, nausea, pale skin, and dizziness.

3. The chest pain of angina usually occurs following exertion and lasts only a few minutes. If it persists 10 minutes or more, or the victim has other signs and symptoms of a heart attack, give first aid as for a heart attack.

4. Call 9-1-1. Do not delay, because the victim needs advanced medical care immediately.

5. a. Fluids drain from the mouth. A stroke victim may vomit or drool, possibly causing choking if the fluid does not drain out.

Learning Checkpoint 2

1. False. You do not need to know the specific cause of the breathing difficulty but can care for the victim anyway: call 9-1-1, help the victim to rest in the position for easiest breathing, assist with any prescribed medications, and be prepared to give basic life support.

2. d. Let the victim find the position for easiest breathing.

3. The best thing an asthma victim can do during an attack is to use his or her prescribed inhaler; the medication should control the attack.

4. False.

5. Call 9-1-1 for a hyperventilating victim if breathing does not return to normal within a few minutes.

Learning Checkpoint 3

1. Call 9-1-1 for a victim who faints if the victim does not regain responsiveness soon or faints repeatedly.

2. False. Lay the victim down and raise his or her legs, not the head, about 12 inches.

3. c. Place something flat and soft under the victim's head. Do not try to hold the victim still, and do not put anything between the teeth.

4. Call 9-1-1 for a seizure victim:
   • if the seizure lasts more than five minutes.
   • if the victim is not known to have epilepsy.
   • if the victim recovers very slowly or has trouble breathing.
   • if the victim has another seizure.
   • if the victim is pregnant.
   • if the victim is wearing another medical ID.
   • if the victim is injured.

5. Seek urgent medical care for a young child whose abdomen is swollen and feels hard.

6. Common signs and symptoms of a low blood sugar diabetic emergency include dizziness, hunger, clumsiness, sweating, and confusion.

7. If you cannot judge whether the victim has low or high blood sugar, give sugar to the victim as for low blood sugar. Seek medical attention if the victim does not improve within 15 minutes.

Review Questions

1. d
2. a
3. c
4. a
5. b
6. d
7. c
8. a
9. d
10. b

CHAPTER 18
Learning Checkpoint 1

1. The common signs and symptoms of a swallowed poisoning include nausea, dizziness, drowsiness, vomiting, and unresponsiveness.

2. Give the victim lots of fluids to drink.

3. c. Move the victim to fresh air.

4. This is likely a poisoning situation. Call 9-1-1 and give basic life support as needed. Put the child in the recovery position. Tell the 9-1-1 dispatcher and the arriving crew about the open cleaning product.

Learning Checkpoint 2

1. False. Use soap and water to wash the area to minimize the reaction as much as possible.

2. See a healthcare provider for severe reactions or swelling of the face or genitals, or signs of infection (fever, pus).

3. a. Hydrocortisone cream. (Also colloid oatmeal, baking soda paste, or calamine lotion.)

Review Questions

1. b
2. a
3. d
4. c
5. a
6. d
7. d

8. c
9. b
10. b

CHAPTER 19

Learning Checkpoint 1

1. a. Remember: alcohol is still a drug even though legal for those of age.
2. Because alcohol and other drug abuse typically begin at young ages, prevention efforts focus on children and adolescents.
3. Following are appropriate actions to help prevent misuse of prescribed drugs:
   - Read product information that comes with prescription medications.
   - Keep medications in their original labeled containers.
   - Ensure that a person with diminished judgment cannot accidentally take too much medication.

   In addition:
   - *Always* take medications as prescribed—not only when feeling symptoms. Many medical conditions requiring drug treatment do not cause noticeable symptoms.
   - *Never* use medications prescribed for someone else—even when you are certain you have the same condition as the person with the medication. People vary in their responses to medications, and only a healthcare provider can know what medication is appropriate for you.

Learning Checkpoint 2

1. For an intoxicated person who becomes unresponsive, take these actions:
   - Check the person for injuries or illness.
   - Position the victim in the recovery position; be prepared for vomiting.
   - Monitor the victim and provide BLS if necessary.
   - Call 9-1-1 if the victim's breathing is irregular, if seizures occur, or if the victim cannot be roused (coma).
   - In a cold environment, protect the person from hypothermia.
2. b
3. Following are appropriate actions to take for a person with a drug or medication overdose:
   - Call 9-1-1 or the Poison Control Center.
   - Check for injuries that may require first aid.
   - Try to keep the person awake and talking.
   - Try to find out what the person took.

   In addition:
   - Position an unresponsive victim in the recovery position because vomiting is likely—*not* on the back.
   - Because of the risk of being injured, *never* try to restrain a potentially violent person—leave this to law enforcement personnel.
   - Do not try to induce vomiting with any victim at any time unless so instructed by the Poison Control Center.

Review Questions

1. a
2. d
3. b
4. a
5. c
6. c
7. a
8. d

CHAPTER 20

Learning Checkpoint 1

1. a. See a healthcare provider immediately. Do not wait until you develop symptoms, and do not try to capture the animal. You cannot kill the rabies germs by treating the wound site.
2. Human bites can be serious because human mouths usually contain many germs.

Learning Checkpoint 2

1. Have the victim stay calm and lie down with the bitten area below the level of the heart. Call 9-1-1.
   Wash the bite wound with soap and water.
2. Call 9-1-1 for a spider bite if the victim has trouble breathing or the bite is from a brown recluse spider.
3. Tweezers.
4. b. Bull's-eye rash is a common early sign of Lyme disease. Tick bite does not usually cause pain or burning at the site. Fever may occur with Lyme disease but usually not until much later.

Learning Checkpoint 3

1. A credit card or piece of rigid plastic.
2. Since she seems to be having an allergic reaction to the bee sting, you should first call 9-1-1, ask if she has an epinephrine kit, monitor breathing, and treat for shock.

3. c. Vinegar or baking soda applied in a compress or paste help stop the stinging and itch. Boiling water would cause a burn. Catsup and mayonnaise are not treatments.

Review Questions

1. d
2. d
3. a
4. c
5. b
6. a
7. c
8. c
9. b
10. d

CHAPTER 21

Learning Checkpoint 1

1. False. Rubbing frostbitten skin can cause damage. Instead, warm it against warm skin or in warm water.
2. Waxy white, gray, yellow, or bluish.
3. Warm his ears with your warm hands (gently). Protect the ears from being rubbed on clothing or other objects. The victim needs immediate medical care.

Learning Checkpoint 2

1. False. Hypothermia can occur any time the climate is cool enough to feel cold.
2. True. Shivering does produce body heat but is not always enough. If the victim has signs and symptoms of hypothermia, help warm his body even if he is shivering.
3. d. Remove damp clothing and warm a hypothermic person with a blanket. Do *not* let him drink alcohol, and do *not* warm him too quickly with a heat source like a fire or a hot shower.
4. Answers may vary depending on equipment the first aider is thought to have. Ideally, get the hypothermic victim out of the cold environment into a tent. Remove his cold, damp clothing and get him into dry clothing and a sleeping bag. If there is a stove, heat water to make him a warm drink.

Learning Checkpoint 3

1. False. Have the victim rest comfortably and drink a sports drink.
2. b. Give a sports drink or water to drink because the body needs fluids.

3. False. Do not give salt tablets. Give a sports drink if the victim is awake and alert.
4. Fluids.
5. Three ways to cool a heat exhaustion victim:
   - Put wet cloths on the forehead and body.
   - Sponge the skin with cool water.
   - Spray the skin with water from a spray bottle and fan the area.
6. First, get him out of the sun and into a cool place. Loosen or remove unnecessary clothing. Give a sports drink or water. Have him lie down and raise his legs 8 to 12 inches. Cool his body with one of the methods previously described.

Learning Checkpoint 4

1. False. Heatstroke is a medical emergency, and the victim may still be at risk. Call 9-1-1.
2. Call 9-1-1 for *all* instances of heatstroke.
3. A heatstroke victim may be acting very confused or disoriented, dizzy, and irrational; the victim may become unresponsive.
4. a. Have plenty of nonalcoholic fluids present. Be sure there is a shady spot for resting.

   b. Tell everyone to avoid too much exertion (especially those who are older or overweight). Make sure you keep drinking enough fluids. Stop and rest in the shade if you start feeling overheated. Tell everyone to watch for signs and symptoms of heat exhaustion in others: heavy sweating, thirst, fatigue, heat cramps, headache or dizziness, or nausea and vomiting. (Also be alert for the signs and symptoms of heatstroke—but it is better to stop and treat the person in the earlier stages of heat exhaustion.)

   c. Call 9-1-1 for a heatstroke victim.

Review Questions

1. a
2. d
3. b
4. c
5. a
6. c
7. b
8. b
9. a
10. d

CHAPTER 22

Learning Checkpoint 1

1. d
2. All of the conditions listed may cause altered mental status.
3. Following are guidelines to help calm an emotional victim:
    - Tell the victim who you are and say you are there to help. Avoid seeming judgmental.
    - Do not assume the victim is intoxicated, using drugs, or otherwise impaired.
    - Reassure the victim that help is on the way (after 9-1-1 has been called).
    - Ask the victim for his or her name, and use it when speaking to him or her.
    - If possible, try to involve any victim's friend or family member present at the scene.
    - Let the victim tell you what he or she thinks is wrong.
    - Let the victim know you understand his or her concerns.
    - Make eye contact with the victim.
    - Speak in a caring, reassuring voice, but do not give false reassurances or lie about the victim's condition.
    - Do not argue with the victim. Show that you understand the victim's concerns by repeating or rephrasing what the victim tells you.
    - If the victim seems irrational or delusional, do not make statements that support his or her false beliefs, but do not challenge them, either.
    - Stay a safe distance away from the victim until your help is accepted. If the victim does not accept your help, do not attempt to restrain him or her or force care on him or her.
    - Tell the victim what you plan to do before doing it.
    - Move calmly and slowly, touching the victim only as necessary.
4. False. It is better to encourage the victim to talk: acknowledge that the person seems sad and ask why.
5. False. This is a common myth. Talking about suicide is a warning sign that the person is contemplating suicide.
6. To ensure your own safety and get help fast, take these steps in this order:
    a. Do not enter the scene if there is a risk to your safety. Encourage others present in the scene to withdraw.
    b. Call 9-1-1.
    c. Talk to the person calmly and quietly, and try to divert the person from any violent action by keeping him or her talking.

Learning Checkpoint 2

1. c
2. Following are common characteristics of victims of domestic violence:
    - They love their partners.
    - They feel guilty and may blame themselves for the violence.
    - They often have low self-esteem.
    - They depend emotionally and/or financially on their partners.

    In addition:
    - They *are* afraid of their partners.
    - They are often *isolated from* family and friends.
3. d
4. Important first aid actions for a victim injured in a rape include:
    - Be sensitive to the victim's psychological trauma and provide emotional support.
    - Ensure that 9-1-1 has been called.
    - Ensure privacy for the victim.
    - Try to involve a friend or family member of the victim or at least a first aider of the same sex.
    - Give needed first aid and stay with the victim until help arrives.
    - Preserve evidence of the rape.

Review Questions

1. b
2. a
3. d
4. b
5. c
6. d
7. a
8. b
9. a
10. a

CHAPTER 23

Learning Checkpoint 1

1. Following are generally accepted guidelines for a healthy pregnancy:
   - Minimize caffeine and alcohol consumption.
   - Take dietary supplements as recommended.
   In addition:
   - Eat a healthy diet.
   - Accept normal weight gain.
   - Stop smoking.
   - Do not use illicit drugs.
   - Get exercise.
   - Rest sufficiently.
   - Prevent injury.
2. b
3. b

Learning Checkpoint 2

1. Call 9-1-1 for heavy vaginal bleeding. Calm the woman and help her into a comfortable position. Give the woman a towel or sanitary napkins to absorb the blood, but do not try to pack the vagina.
2. a
3. All six of the signs and symptoms listed could indicate a possible problem with the pregnancy; the woman should see her healthcare provider for any of these.

Learning Checkpoint 3

1. False. Childbirth is a natural process that seldom involves complications or requires elaborate medical care.
2. Signs and symptoms that childbirth may occur soon include:
   - Woman feels urge to push.
   - Amniotic sac has ruptured.
   - Infant's head is crowning.
   In addition:
   - Contractions are less than five minutes apart.
   - Childbirth may occur sooner in woman who has given birth before.
3. d
4. When assisting with childbirth follow these guidelines for things not to do:
   - Do not try to delay the birth by having the woman hold her legs together or any other maneuver.
   - Do not place your hands or anything else in the woman's vagina.
   - Do not interfere with the childbirth or touch the infant until the head is completely out.
   - Do not pull on the head or shoulders.
   - Do not try to wash the infant's skin, eyes, or ears.
   - Do not pull on the umbilical cord in an effort to pull out the afterbirth.
5. c
6. True. Some bleeding does normally occur with childbirth and delivery of the placenta. If bleeding does not stop soon after delivery of the placenta, massaging the abdomen may help the uterus to contract and stop bleeding.

Review Questions

1. b
2. b
3. a
4. d
5. c
6. d
7. b
8. c
9. c
10. d

CHAPTER 24

Learning Checkpoint 1

1. Rescue or medical help may be delayed in emergencies in situations such as this:
   - Rural areas
   - When hiking or camping in wilderness areas
   - When boating
   - During or after a natural disaster
2. d

Learning Checkpoint 2

1. Following are important principles for planning a trip into a wilderness location:
   - Do not go alone.
   - Tell someone where you are going and when you will return.
   - Take more food and water than you expect to need.
   In addition:
   - Take a first aid kit equipped for the location.
   - Be prepared for weather emergencies.
   - Know where you are at all times.

- Do not use alcohol or other drugs.
- Study the location in advance.

2. False. When dealing with a complex emergency in a remote location, the leader should be flexible, continually reassess the situation, and change the plan as needed.

3. A cell phone may have a dead battery, may not have a signal, or may stop working because of temperature extremes, moisture, or other problems.

4. c

Learning Checkpoint 3

1. d

2. False. If you suspect a victim in a remote location may have a spinal injury, if it is unlikely that help will arrive soon, you should assess the victim more carefully to see if a spinal injury can be ruled out so that the victim can move.

3. False. The condition of a victim with a brain injury will not improve by itself. This is a medical emergency—call for a helicopter if possible, or if you cannot communicate the need for rescue, consider evacuating the victim if it can be done safely.

4. b. (It will be difficult to warm the victim and keep him warm while walking or being carried through a cold environment for three hours; with severe hypothermia he would probably not be able to walk, and three people generally cannot effectively carry someone. It is better to build an emergency shelter and warm the victim with dry clothing, extra clothing from others, warm fluids, and even the body warmth of the other hikers.)

5. 30 minutes

Learning Checkpoint 4

1. To rescue someone in deep water, use these actions in this order (from safest to least safe):
   a. Reach to the victim with a stick or long object.
   b. Throw a rope or floating object to the victim.
   c. Go to the victim in a boat or other craft.
   d. Swim to the victim.

2. Three to five gallons

3. The typical signs and symptoms of acute mountain sickness include:
   - Headache
   - Dizziness

- Fatigue
- Nausea

Review Questions

1. d
2. b
3. b
4. d
5. a
6. c
7. a
8. b
9. d
10. c

CHAPTER 25

Learning Checkpoint 1

1. a. Get everyone out. Any delay spent calling 9-1-1, using a fire extinguisher, or taking other actions could result in someone being harmed by the fire.

2. d. All of the above. Stay low because there will be more oxygen near the floor; feel doors before opening them to avoid entering a fiery area; and use the stairs because a power outage caused by the fire could stall the elevator.

3. True. OSHA guidelines for fire prevention and safety apply in most workplaces.

4. False. Stay away from potentially hazardous materials; call 9-1-1 and let the professionals clean up the spill.

5. True. But since you cannot usually know if fumes from a spilled liquid are poisonous, act as if they are.

6. Support the victim's head and neck but do not move the victim unless there is an immediate threat. Give basic life support as needed.

7. c. The safest order in which to attempt a water rescue is reach-throw-go.

Learning Checkpoint 2

1. False. A victim with only a broken arm is considered stable and can walk and is therefore a third priority.

2. True. Victims with life-threatening injuries are the first priority.

3. Following are the ranked priorities for these four victims:
   First—b. A man on the ground with no apparent external injuries but who is unresponsive

Second—d. A man leaning against the rubble, looking very pale, who says he feels nauseous

Third—a. A woman with a bruised face and abrasions on her arms, who is walking around holding her bleeding forehead

Fourth—c. A man who is not breathing, whose chest has caved in under a steel beam, and who is surrounded by a pool of blood

Learning Checkpoint 3

1. Consider moving a victim in these situations:
   - Fire is present.
   - There is a strong smell of natural gas in the room.
   - One victim is lying on top of another.
2. d. The blanket drag is an effective way to move a victim by yourself and provide some support for the victim's head.

Review Questions

1. c
2. d
3. d
4. a

5. b
6. c
7. c
8. b
9. a
10. d

CHAPTER 26
Review Questions

1. a
2. c
3. a
4. d
5. b

CHAPTER 27
Review Questions

1. c
2. b
3. d
4. a
5. b

Glossary

Abandonment a type of negligence that occurs if someone who has begun to provide first aid then stops and the injury or illness becomes worse

ABCS acronym for airway, breathing, circulation—the three things to check in an unresponsive victim in the initial assessment to find threats to life

Abdomen the area below the ribs and above the hips

Abrasion a wound in which the top layer of skin is scraped off

Abuse an intentional inflicting of injury or suffering on someone under the abuser's power, such as a child, spouse, or elderly parent

Acquired immunodeficiency syndrome (AIDS) fatal disease caused by the human immunodeficiency virus (HIV)

Acute mountain sickness severe form of altitude sickness

Acute myocardial infarction (AMI) condition of a sudden reduced blood flow to the heart muscle; heart attack

Advanced cardiac life support (ACLS) medical procedures needed to restore a heartbeat beyond the procedures of basic life support

Airborne transmission process by which a pathogen existing in an infected person is transmitted into a different person through the air, usually via small fluid droplets the infected person coughs or sneezes out

Airway the path air takes from the nose and mouth to the lungs

Airway (adjunct) a shaped tube-like device inserted into the mouth or nose that helps keep a victim's airway open during resuscitation or until the victim receives advanced medical attention

Airway obstruction condition in which the victim's airway is partially or completely obstructed by the tongue, vomit or other body tissue or fluids, or a foreign object, preventing the flow of air to the lungs; choking

Allergen a substance that causes an allergic reaction in a person

Allergic contact dermatitis an allergic skin reaction

Aloe vera a type of plant; usually refers to a lotion or gel made with the plant's extract, which may be soothing for first-degree burns

Altered mental status a phrase used to describe a change from a person's normal responsiveness and awareness, such as confusion, disorientation, dizziness, drowsiness, or partial or complete unresponsiveness

Altitude sickness a syndrome caused by low oxygen levels at high altitudes, causing headache, dizziness, fatigue, shortness of breath, nausea, and other symptoms

Alveoli tiny air sacs in the lungs where oxygen and carbon dioxide pass into and out of small blood vessels

Amniotic fluid the fluid surrounding the embryo and fetus within the amniotic sac; often called "water"

Amniotic sac a membrane surrounding the embryo and fetus in the uterus, containing amniotic fluid

Amputation the complete cutting or tearing off of all or part of an extremity: a finger or toe, hand or foot, arm or leg

Anaphylactic shock shock resulting from an extreme allergic reaction, typically to an insect sting, a particular food, medication, or some other substance; also called anaphylaxis

Anaphylaxis another term for anaphylactic shock

Anatomic splint splinting one part of the body to another part

Angina pectoris chest pain caused by heart disease, usually occurring after intense activity or exertion; often just called angina

Ankle drag an emergency move for an unresponsive victim or one who cannot walk, but which provides no head support for a potential spinal injury

Antibiotic a medication that kills bacteria

Antivenin an antidote to the poisonous venom of a particular species, administered to counteract the effects of a bite or sting

Anxiety fear or apprehension of impending danger usually producing physical signs and symptoms

Arteries blood vessels that carry oxygenated blood from the heart to body tissues

Aspiration the movement of vomit or other fluids or solids into the lungs

Assessment process of checking a victim for conditions requiring treatment or first aid, divided into an initial assessment for life-threatening conditions and a secondary assessment for other problems

Asthma a chronic disease in which at times the airway becomes narrow and the person has difficulty breathing

Atherosclerosis a narrowing and "hardening" of the arteries caused by plaque

Aura a generalized sensation or a hallucinated sensation involving any of the senses that occurs before a seizure

Automated external defibrillator (AED) device used to shock a fibrillating heart to return it to a regular rhythm

Avulsion an open wound in which an area of skin or other soft tissue is torn partially from the body

B

Bag-valve-mask (BVM) a resuscitation mask unit connected to an airbag that is squeezed to provide air to a nonbreathing victim

Barrier device a device like a pocket mask or face shield used to provide a barrier between a victim and first aider when giving rescue breathing to reduce the risk of disease transmission

Basic life support (BLS) first aid given to a victim with a life-threatening problem of the airway or circulation; refers to rescue breathing, CPR, and use of AED

Beach drag a method for removing an unresponsive victim from shallow water that provides some head support for a potential spinal injury

Behavioral emergency situation in which the victim's behavior, whether caused by injury or illness or by personality or mental health factors, results in an emergency situation, such as potential suicide or violence

Bladder organ that stores urine until it is passed to the outside

Blanket drag an emergency move for an unresponsive victim or one who cannot walk, providing some support for the victim's head as the rescuer pulls the blanket

Blood pressure the pressure of blood on the walls of blood vessels

Bloodborne disease a disease that can be transmitted from one person to another through contact with the infected person's blood or certain other body fluids

Bloodborne transmission process by which a pathogen existing in an infected person's blood or other body fluid is transmitted into a different person through contact with that body fluid

Body mass index (BMI) a measure of weight in relation to a person's height, used to determine overweight and obesity

Body substance isolation (BSI) an infection control concept, used primarily in healthcare facilities, that assume that *any* body fluid or moist body tissue is potentially infectious

Body system a group of organs that work together to perform a major body function

Brachial pulse the pulse felt over the brachial artery in an infant's upper arm on the inside about midway between the shoulder and elbow

Breech presentation the position in which the infant's buttocks or feet move first into the birth canal rather than the head; also called breech birth

Bronchi (singular: bronchus) the passageways from the trachea to the lungs

Bronchodilator a drug that relaxes the muscles of the airway, often used in an inhaler by people with asthma

Burn damage caused to skin and other tissue by heat, chemicals, or electricity

C

Capillaries tiny blood vessels between the arteries and veins where oxygen and nutrients in the blood pass into tissues and carbon dioxide passes into the blood

Carbon monoxide an invisible, odorless, tasteless, and highly lethal gas resulting from fires, gasoline engines, furnaces, and other causes

Cardiac refers to the heart

Cardiac arrest the condition in which the heart stops beating effectively

Cardiogenic shock shock resulting when any condition, such as heart attack, causes the heart function to be reduced to the point that blood is not circulating sufficiently

Cardiopulmonary resuscitation (CPR) basic life support procedure for victim who is not breathing and has no heartbeat, consisting of rescue breathing combined with chest compressions

Cardiovascular system the body system that moves the blood, which transports both oxygen and nutrients, throughout the body to supply cells and remove wastes

Carotid pulse the pulse felt over the carotid artery in a neck of an adult or child

Central nervous system that part of the nervous system formed by the brain and spinal cord

Cervix the lower part of the uterus, opening into the vagina

Chain of survival a concept emphasizing four steps needed for cardiac arrest victims: early recognition and access, early bystander CPR, early defibrillation, and early advanced medical care

Chest compressions technique used in CPR to circulate the blood or with a choking victim to expel an object

Choking a physical obstruction of the airway, such as by food or the tongue in an unresponsive person

Cholesterol a fatty substance the body needs to carry out important functions but that in high levels is a risk factor for cardiovascular disease

Chronic refers to an illness or health condition, often incurable, that the person has had for some time; chronic conditions often make the individual more susceptible to the effects of injuries or sudden illnesses

Chronic obstructive pulmonary diseases (COPD) a group of respiratory diseases, including emphysema and chronic bronchitis, in which breathing can become difficult

Cincinnati Prehospital Stroke Scale (CPSS) a screening process for rapid identification of a stroke outside the hospital

Closed injury an injury in which the skin is not broken

Clothes drag an emergency move for an unresponsive victim or one who cannot walk, providing some support for the victim's head against the pulled clothing and rescuer's hands

Clotting process in which fibrin and platelets clump together with other blood cells to seal a leak in a blood vessel

Competence the victim is able to understand what is happening and the implications of his or her decision to receive or refuse first aid

Concussion a type of brain injury resulting from a blow to the head, involving a temporary impairment of brain function but usually not permanent damage

Confidentiality the general principle that one should not give out private information about a victim to anyone except for those caring for the victim

Consent the victim's permission for you to provide first aid

Contraction the pumping action of the heart

Contusion a bruised muscle

Coronary heart disease blockage of vessels supplying heart muscle with blood, often leading to heart attack

Cradle carry an emergency move for a light unresponsive victim or one who cannot walk, in which the rescuer carries the victim in his or her arms

Cramp a tightening of a muscle that usually results from prolonged use

Cravats strips of cloth used to tie a splint

Crepitus grating sensation felt or heard when fractured bone ends rub against each other

Cricoid pressure a technique of applying pressure to an area of cartilage in the neck to prevent the air given during rescue breathing from reaching the stomach; also called the Sellick maneuver

Crowning the stage of childbirth when the infant's head is passing into the birth canal and is visible

D

Defibrillation the process of administering an electrical shock to a fibrillating heart to restore a normal heart rhythm

Dependence a pattern of physical and behavioral changes resulting from frequent use of a substance, including tolerance to its effects and the occurrence of withdrawal symptoms after cessation

Depressant a drug that slows certain central nervous system functions and produces dulled feelings

Depression a temporary state or a chronic psychological illness involving feelings of sadness, hopelessness, and worthlessness often along with physical symptoms

Dermis the middle layer of skin, damaged in second- and third-degree burns

Diabetes a metabolic disorder in which not enough insulin is produced or the body has developed resistance in the use of insulin, resulting in blood sugar (glucose) levels not being well regulated by the body

Diaphragm a muscle between the abdomen and lungs that moves with breathing

Direct contact disease transmission that occurs when someone directly contacts an infected person, or fluids or substances from that person

Disinfectant a substance, such as a bleach solution, that kills most pathogens on contaminated surfaces

Dislocation movement of one or more bones out of their normal position in a joint, usually with ligament damage

Dispatcher EMS professional who answers 9-1-1 calls, determines the nature of the emergency, and sends the appropriate emergency personnel to the scene

Duty to act a legal obligation to provide first aid as trained, obligated by one's job requirements or role as a child's parent or guardian

Dysrhythmia an irregular heartbeat; sometimes called arrhythmia

E

Elder abuse physical, emotional, or financial abuse or neglect inflicted on someone over age 60, often by someone else in the home

Electrodes the pads of an automated external defibrillator (AED), which attach to the main unit with cables and deliver the shock to a victim's chest when indicated

Embryo a developing human from the time of implantation in the uterus through the first 8 weeks

Emergency Medical Services (EMS) a comprehensive network of professionals linked together to provide appropriate levels of medical care for victims of injury or sudden illness

Emergency medical technician (EMT) emergency personnel trained to give prehospital medical treatment to injured or ill victims and to transport victims to advanced care facilities

Emergency position indicating radio beacon (EPIRB) an emergency device for marine uses that emits a signal that is picked up by satellites and relayed to rescue personnel

Endocrine system the body system that produces hormones that help regulate many body functions

Enhanced 911 an EMS system that automatically provides the dispatcher with the caller's phone number and the location of a land telephone line being used

Entrance/exit wounds terms referring to two related wounds such as burned areas on the body where electricity entered and left the body or wounds caused by a bullet entering and exiting the body

Epidermis the outer layer of skin, the layer damaged in first-degree burns

Epiglottis a tissue flap that prevents solids and liquids from entering the trachea

Epi-Pen® a commercial emergency epinephrine kit used for anaphylactic reactions

Esophagus the tube that carries food to the stomach from the throat

Evacuation the process of removing a victim from a remote location that cannot be reached by ambulance, including carrying the victim out and helicopter rescue

Evisceration protrusion of abdominal organs through an open wound in the abdominal wall

Expressed consent consent explicitly given by the victim for first aid

External respiration the process by which oxygen enters the blood from air that is inhaled and carbon dioxide exits the blood into air that is breathed out

Extremities the arms and legs

F

Family radio service (FRS) small short-distance radios (often called walky-talkies) that do not require a special license

Febrile seizure a seizure caused by high fever

Femur the long bone of the upper leg

Fetal alcohol syndrome a pattern of growth and development problems found in infants whose mothers drank significant amounts of alcohol during pregnancy

Fetus a developing human in the uterus from the age of 8 weeks until birth

Fibrillation an abnormal heart rhythm, common after a heart attack, in which muscles of the heart are quivering instead of beating rhythmically; see *Ventricular fibrillation*

Fibrin a protein substance in blood that with platelets forms blood clots to prevent bleeding

First responder the first professionally trained person to arrive at the emergency scene, such as a police officer, fire fighter, industrial safety officer, ski patroller, or similar professional who is often close to the scene

First-degree burn a minor burn that damages only the skin's outer layer

Flail chest a fracture of two or more ribs in two or more places, allowing a segment of chest wall to move apart from rest of the chest

Flowmeter a piece of oxygen equipment that is used to adjust the rate of oxygen delivery to the victim

Food poisoning a type of poisoning that occurs after eating food that is contaminated with microorganisms, usually bacteria, or their toxins

Fracture a broken bone

Frostbite condition in which localized skin and other tissue freezes and dies, caused by exposure to freezing temperatures

Full-thickness burn another term for a third-degree burn

G

Gastrointestinal system the body system that extracts nutrients from food to meet the body's needs for energy

Genitals the male and female sex organs

Good Samaritan law a state law designed to protect people who give first aid in an emergency from lawsuits

GPS a small device, named for the global positioning system, that reads satellite signals to inform the user of location in longitude and latitude

Ground fault circuit interrupter (GFCI) a shock-preventing device that can be added to electrical circuits near water sources, such as in bathrooms and kitchens, that immediately interrupts the flow of electricity if an electrical appliance contacts water

H

Hammock carry an emergency move with which three to six rescuers carry the victim in a "hammock" made with their arms

Haz-Mat abbreviation for "hazardous materials," often used to refer to a haz-mat incident or a haz-mat team of professional rescuers

Heat cramps muscle cramps, often in the lower legs or abdominal muscles, that result from activity in a hot environment when sweating lowers the body's sodium levels

Heat exhaustion a condition of dehydration and depletion of salt and electrolytes in the body caused by heavy sweating if the person does not get enough fluids when active in a hot environment

Heatstroke a life-threatening condition in which the body's core temperature rises abnormally high when heat loss mechanisms fail to maintain a normal body temperature in a hot environment

Heimlich maneuver another term for abdominal thrusts given to a responsive choking victim to expel the obstructing object

Hemorrhage bleeding, usually significant bleeding

Hemorrhagic shock shock caused by severe external or internal bleeding

Hepatitis the various forms of liver disease caused by the bloodborne hepatitis B virus (HBV), hepatitis C virus (HCV), or other hepatitis viruses

High altitude cerebral edema (HACE) a rare but serious type of altitude sickness involving a life-threatening fluid buildup in the brain

High altitude pulmonary edema (HAPE) a rare but serious type of altitude sickness involving a life-threatening fluid buildup in the lungs

History information about what happened with an injury or illness and other relevant facts about the victim and the condition

Homeostasis a balanced state within the body necessary for effective functioning

Hormone a chemical messenger carried in the blood that affects the functioning of one or more organs

Human immunodeficiency virus (HIV) the bloodborne virus that causes acquired immunodeficiency syndrome (AIDS)

Humerus the bone of the upper arm

Hyperglycemia high blood sugar

Hypertension high blood pressure

Hyperventilation fast, deep breathing usually caused by anxiety or stress

Hypoglycemia low blood sugar

Hypothermia lowering of the body's core temperature, a life-threatening emergency caused when the body cannot produce enough heat to compensate for heat loss in a cold environment

Hypovolemic shock shock that occurs when blood volume drops

I

Immune system the body system that helps fight disease

Immunity state of being protected against an infectious disease

Implied consent consent for first aid for an unresponsive victim or a child without a parent or guardian present

Indirect contact disease transmission that occurs when someone contacts contaminated objects, food or drink, droplets in the air, or vectors such as insects

Infection an invasion of the body by a pathogen that may potentially cause disease

Initial assessment a quick first check of the victim for life-threatening problems, involving a check for responsiveness and breathing

Inline stabilization supporting the head in line with the body to prevent movement in a victim thought to have a spinal injury

Insulin a hormone secreted by the pancreas that helps regulate blood sugar levels

Integumentary system the body system that protects the body from the environment and germs and helps regulate body temperature; the skin, hair, and nails

Internal respiration the process of oxygen and carbon dioxide moving into and out of the blood within internal body tissues

Irrigation the process of washing out a wound under running water or saline solution

J

Joint the point where two bones meet; most joints are capable of movement

K

Kidneys organs that filter wastes from the blood and produce urine

L

Laceration a cut in the skin that may penetrate and also damage underlying tissue

Latex a rubber material, commonly used in medical exam gloves, to which some people are allergic

Ligament tough, fibrous band that holds bones together in a joint

Log roll a technique in which several rescuers turn a victim with a suspected spinal injury either onto the back or side while keeping the head supported in line with the body

Lyme disease a potentially serious bacterial infection that may result from the bite of a tick carrying the bacteria

M

Medical direction the process by which EMS personnel are guided in certain medical interventions in the field by a physician

Miscarriage spontaneous death of the embryo or fetus before the middle of the second trimester

Morning sickness nausea and vomiting common in early pregnancy

Musculoskeletal system the body system that gives the body shape and strength and makes movement possible

Myocardial infarction see *Acute myocardial infarction (AMI)*

Myocardium heart muscle

N

Nasal cannula oxygen delivery device usually used with a breathing victim who does not require a high concentration of oxygen; also called nasal prongs

Nasopharyngeal airway a nasal airway inserted through the nose and into the pharynx

Needlestick an accidental puncture of the skin with a used medical (syringe) needle, which may be contaminated with pathogens

Negligence a breach of duty, when one has a duty to act, that results in injury or damages to a victim

Nervous system the body system that controls all body functions and movement and allows for sensory perception and consciousness

Neurogenic shock shock that occurs when a nervous system problem allows vessels to dilate to the point that blood volume is not sufficient to fill blood vessels and be pumped to vital organs

Nitroglycerin prescription medication for angina and heart attack, increases blood flow through partially restricted coronary arteries

Nonrebreathing mask an oxygen delivery device composed of a mask and a reservoir bag, used with a breathing victim

O

Occlusive dressing an air- and water-tight dressing used to seal a wound

Open wound injury in which the skin is torn or cut open, often leading to bleeding

Organ a body part that accomplishes one or more specific functions

Oropharyngeal airway an oral airway inserted through the mouth and into the pharynx

Osteoporosis a bone condition involving a loss of calcium, common in old age

Overdose taking too much of a drug or substance, causing detrimental or life-threatening effects

P

Pacemaker a small electronic device implanted under the skin in some patients with heart disease, which helps the heart maintain a regular rhythm

Packstrap carry an emergency move for an unresponsive

victim or one who cannot walk, in which the rescuer carries the victim over the shoulders

Panic attack a sudden, overwhelming fear that is excessive for the situation

Paradoxical movement the movement of a segment of the chest in a patient with flail chest, in which the flail segment moves in the opposite direction of the rest of the chest wall

Paralysis an inability to move a body part, such as the arms or legs, caused by nerve damage

Paraphernalia things used in the preparation or taking of drugs, such as needles and syringes, eye droppers, straws used for snorting, pipes, razor blades, plastic bags, and pill bottles

Partial-thickness burn another term for a second-degree burn

Pathogen a microorganism such as bacteria and viruses that can cause infectious disease

Pelvis refers generally to the area below the abdomen and specifically to the pelvic bones between the hip and the lower spine

Personal locator beacon (PLB) a type of emergency position indicating radio beacon intended to be used by individuals in emergencies in remote land locations

Personal protective equipment (PPE) any equipment used to protect against contact with blood or other body fluids, including gloves, barrier devices, and other devices

Pharynx the throat

Physical examination process of examining an injured or ill victim head to toe to find conditions requiring first aid or medical attention

Piggyback carry an emergency move for a light responsive victim, in which the rescuer carries the victim on his or her back with arms under the victim's legs

Placenta an organ that develops in pregnancy to supply the embryo and fetus with oxygen and nutrients from the mother by means of the umbilical cord

Plaque a buildup of cholesterol and other substances inside arteries, eventually causing atherosclerosis and potentially blocked arteries

Platelet plug platelets sticking together at the site of an injury in a blood vessel, which may reduce or stop minor bleeding

Platelets structures in blood that assist in clotting at the site of an injured blood vessel to prevent bleeding

Poison Control Center (PCC) one of a national network of centers designed to provide information about specific poisons in an emergency

Poison any substance that enters or touches the body with effects that are injurious to health or life threatening

Prenatal before birth

Presentation the position of the infant in the uterus and vagina at the time of birth

Pressure bandage a bandage applied over a wound to maintain pressure to control bleeding

Pressure regulator a piece of oxygen equipment that connects to the oxygen tank to reduce the pressure of oxygen leaving the tank to a safe level

Prolapsed cord a situation in which a segment of the umbilical cord protrudes through the birth canal before childbirth

Pulse rhythmic changes in blood pressure in arteries caused by the heartbeat, which can be felt in certain body locations

Puncture a hole into the skin caused by a sharp penetrating object that may also damage deeper tissues

R

Rabies a viral disease, fatal if not treated in time, that is transmitted by the bite of an infected animal

Rape forced sexual intercourse, including vaginal, anal or oral penetration by the offender, including with a foreign object

Recovery position a position used for breathing unresponsive victims while waiting for help to arrive; the victim is positioned on the side to keep the airway open and allow fluids to drain from the mouth

Reproductive system the body system that makes human reproduction possible

Rescue breathing a BLS technique to get needed oxygen into the lungs of a nonbreathing victim

Respiratory arrest condition in which breathing has completely stopped

Respiratory distress condition in which the victim's breathing is ineffective or difficult

Respiratory system the body system that provides the oxygen needed by body cells and removes the waste product carbon dioxide

Resuscitation alternate term for basic life support skills for a victim in cardiac or respiratory arrest

RICE acronym standing for rest, ice, compression, and elevation; a procedure used with most musculoskeletal injuries

Rigid splint a splint made from something unbendable, such as a board

Risk factor anything that makes it more likely that a person will develop a particular disease

Rule of nines method calculating the percentage of body surface area of a burn

S

SAMPLE acronym referring to the SAMPLE history of an ill or injured victim, standing for Signs and symptoms, Allergies, Medications, Previous problems, Last food or drink, and Events leading up to the injury or illness

Scope of care actions one is qualified to perform, such as specific first aid techniques one learns in a first aid course

Secondary assessment an assessment performed after determining the victim does not have life-threatening problems, including obtaining a history and performing a physical examination

Second-degree burn a burn that damages the skin's deeper layers but does not penetrate to tissues beneath the skin

Sedative a drug that calms and sedates certain nervous system responses; a type of depressant

Seizure a brain disturbance caused by many different conditions, including epilepsy and high fever in infants and children; may produce convulsions

Sexual abuse any kind of sexual activity with a minor—including fondling, rape, sodomy, indecent exposure, or exploitation through prostitution or the production of pornographic materials—or with an adult without consent

Sexual assault a wide range of victimizations, generally involving unwanted sexual contact, with or without force, including grabbing or fondling as well as verbal threats

Sharps general term referring to medical needles and other sharp objects that may be contaminated with an infected person's blood and which could easily penetrate another person's skin to spread the infection, therefore requiring safe disposal

Shepherd's crook a rescue pole with a hook at the end to reach a victim from the edge of a swimming pool

Shock a life-threatening condition that occurs when vital body organs are not receiving enough oxygenated blood, usually results from bleeding

Shoulder drag an emergency move for an unresponsive victim or one who cannot walk, providing some support for the victim's head as the rescuer pulls the victim by the shoulders

Skeletal muscles muscles that attach to bones and create body movements

Sling a device used to support and immobilize the arm, made of a wide bandage or cloth tied around the neck

Soft splint a nonrigid splint made from a pillow or folded blanket

Spinal column refers generally to the vertebrae, extending from the base of the brain to the "tailbone," as well as to the nerves, or spinal cord, running through the vertebrae

Spinal cord the nerves running through the vertebrae

Splint device for immobilizing a part of the body

Sprain damage to ligaments and other structures in a joint

Standard precautions infectious disease prevention behaviors combining the major features of universal precautions and BSI precautions

Standards of care refers generally to how first aid should be performed; what others with the same training would do in a similar situation

Sternum the breastbone

Stimulant a drug that stimulates the central nervous system and produces feelings of energy and well being

Stoma a hole in the neck used for breathing that was surgically created as a result of an injury or illness

Strain a tearing of muscle or tendon tissue

Stroke a sudden impairment of blood circulation to a part of the brain; also called a cerebrovascular accident (CVA) or brain attack

Subcutaneous layer the deepest layer of skin, damaged in third-degree burns

Substance abuse the intentional and often frequent non-medical use of a substance for its effects, typically without regard for potential negative health effects

Substance misuse using a drug for an unintended purpose or using in larger amounts than prescribed, perhaps unintentionally

Sucking chest wound an open wound in the chest caused by a penetrating injury that lets air move in and out of the chest during breathing

Sudden illness any medical condition that occurs suddenly and requires first aid until the person can be seen by a medical professional

Sudden infant death syndrome (SIDS) a condition, whose exact cause is poorly understood, that results in an apparently otherwise healthy infant dying suddenly in its sleep

Sun protection factor (SPF) a numerical rating of sunblock and sunscreen products, indicating how well the skin is protected; with an SPF of 20, for example, 20 hours of sun exposure to skin covered with the sun block is the equivalent of 1 hour of exposure of unprotected skin

Superficial burn another term for a first-degree burn

Supplemental oxygen oxygen in a tank administered to ill or injured victims

T

Tendon fibrous band of tissue that attaches muscle to bone

Tetanus a serious infection caused by common bacteria, also called lockjaw

Third-degree burn a burn that damages the skin all the way through and may burn muscle or other tissues, a medical emergency

Thorax the chest area enclosed by the ribs (including the back of the body)

Tourniquet a band, such as a rope or belt, tightened around a limb above a wound to stop bleeding by cutting off circulation to the limb below the band; used only as an extreme last resort because usually the limb has to be amputated

Toxemia a hypertensive problem of pregnancy

Trachea the tube carrying air from the larynx to the bronchi

Tranquilizer a drug with calming, anxiety-reducing effects

Transient ischemic attack (TIA) a temporary interruption to blood flow in an artery in the brain; sometimes called a mini-stroke

Trauma dressings thick, bulky dressings used with large or irregular wounds, or dressings used to stabilize an impaled object

Triage a process of setting priorities for the care of multiple victims

Tripod position position often taken by a person in respiratory distress: sitting and leaning forward, with hands on knees

Two-handed seat carry an emergency move for a responsive victim, in which two rescuers carry the victim in a "seat" made with their arms

U

Umbilical cord an organ containing an artery and vein that connects the embryo and fetus to the mother

Universal precautions a set of preventive behaviors, used with all victims, all the time, always assuming that blood and other body fluids may be infected; includes handwashing, using gloves and other personal protective equipment, and other actions to prevent transmission of bloodborne diseases

Urinary system the body system that removes liquid wastes from the body and helps maintain the body's water balance

V

Vaccine a form of a dead or weakened pathogen that triggers the body's immune response, creating immunity

Vascular spasm a mechanism in which the damaged blood vessel constricts to slow the bleeding and allow clotting to occur

Vasoconstriction contraction of blood vessels

Vasodilation dilation of blood vessels

Vector transmission process by which a bloodborne pathogen is transmitted from an infected person or animal through the bite of a tick, mosquito, or other insect

Veins blood vessels that carry deoxygenated blood back to the heart from body tissues

Ventricles two of the heart's four chambers, which pump blood to the body and lungs

Ventricular fibrillation (v-fib) an abnormal heart rhythm, which commonly occurs with heart attacks, in which the ventricles of the heart are quivering instead of beating rhythmically

Vertebrae the bones the back and neck

VHF radio very-high frequency radios typically used on boats, typically for distances under 30 miles

W

Walking assist a method to help a victim walk by supporting part of the victim's weight with your arm around the victim

West Nile virus (WNV) a bloodborne disease spread mostly by the bite of infected mosquitoes

Withdrawal a physical or psychological reaction caused by abrupt cessation of a drug in someone who has become dependent on it

Index